Minimally Invasive Surgical Oncology

Ronald Matteotti • Stanley W. Ashley
(Editors)

Minimally Invasive Surgical Oncology

State-of-the-Art Cancer Management

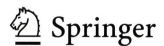

Editors
Ronald Matteotti, MD, FMH
Surgical Oncologist/Minimally
Invasive Surgeon
263 Osborn Street
Philadelphia, PA 19128
USA
ronald.matteotti@gmail.com

Stanley W. Ashley, MD, FACS
Brigham and Women's
Hospital/Harvard Med
Chief, General Surgery
Department of Surgery
Francis St. 75
Boston, MA 02115
USA
sashley@partners.org

ISBN 978-3-540-45018-4   e-ISBN 978-3-540-45021-4
DOI 10.1007/978-3-540-45021-4
Springer Heidelberg Dordrecht London New York

Library of Congress Control Number: 2011922048

© Springer-Verlag Berlin Heidelberg 2011

This work is subject to copyright. All rights are reserved, whether the whole or part of the material is concerned, specifically the rights of translation, reprinting, reuse of illustrations, recitation, broadcasting, reproduction on microfilm or in any other way, and storage in data banks. Duplication of this publication or parts thereof is permitted only under the provisions of the German Copyright Law of September 9, 1965, in its current version, and permission for use must always be obtained from Springer. Violations are liable to prosecution under the German Copyright Law.

The use of general descriptive names, registered names, trademarks, etc. in this publication does not imply, even in the absence of a specific statement, that such names are exempt from the relevant protective laws and regulations and therefore free for general use.

Product liability: The publishers cannot guarantee the accuracy of any information about dosage and application contained in this book. In every individual case the user must check such information by consulting the relevant literature.

Cover design: eStudioCalamar, Figueres/Berlin

Printed on acid-free paper

Springer is part of Springer Science+Business Media (www.springer.com)

To our patients suffering from cancer:
May new scientific discoveries, improved treatments and technologies
contribute to a better quality of life.

To my grandmother Margarethe Matteotti, my father Werner and
Mary
the greatest supporters in my life.

We would like to express a special thank you to
Stephanie Benko and Gabriele Schroeder
from Springer Verlag who greatly supported this project along the way.

Ronald Matteotti

Foreword I

The view of a pioneer in open approaches to Surgical Oncology

It must seem surprising that an 'open surgery' surgical dinosaur should be invited to write a foreword for this text on minimally invasive surgical oncology. I accepted with some trepidation, expecting to be faced with the unpleasant task of writing a critical foreword of a technical text. But the title misled me, this is not a technical treatise but a disease focused management text in which the technical issues of minimally invasive approaches are emphasized.

Above all, the text is comprehensive; from history to surgical education, research, robotics, to immunological response. Organ specific summaries are all covered in great depth. The authorship is a 'who's who's' of minimally invasive surgery and perhaps more importantly, a 'who will be a who', as the next generation develops these technical refinements. For me trying so long to focus on cancer management as a disease-based entity rather than a discipline-based entity it is most encouraging to see a text emphasizing technique but not neglecting important issues of underlying biology, evaluation and a synthesized approach to management. Having started my surgical career prior to the use of CT or MRI, I reflect how seamlessly we incorporated these techniques into patient management. I am encouraged that this will be similarly encompassed by the current generation of surgical oncologists.

The trend is clear. They are courageous enough to address natural orifice surgery in oncology. Except for the increasing use of cesarean section as opposed to transvaginal delivery surgical procedures are progressively moving from large incisions to small incisions to natural orifice surgery. While debate will no doubt continue as to the relative importance of minimally invasive approaches over the more open approaches, it is clear to me that where applicable the avoidance of a large abdominal incision with its accompanying significant risk of subsequent incisional hernia, should be replaced with a minimally invasive approach. Whether the relevant merits of minimally invasive surgery change other issues of outcome should not be a debate. Minimally invasive surgery is a technique; it does not change the disease and one would hope would not change the discipline with which surgeons approach the appropriate operation regardless of the technique employed. This then makes it an oncologic text that allows support for a minimally invasive approach where appropriate.

It is not surprising that the minimally invasive approach has not been extensively embraced in technically challenging procedures particularly those that require not only resection but subsequent reconstruction. In situations where the techniques by which tumors are removed, for example pancreaticoduodenectomy, is less of an issue than the consequences of the reconstruction; it is no surprise that minimally invasive approaches have not been embraced. Indeed, the choice of the minimally invasive approach in pancreatic surgery chooses the cases that are most amendable to success regardless of technical approach. We would all like to approach the "easy" case regardless of technique. Where minimally invasive approaches have most appeal is in the more challenging case, in the more challenging patient where the ability to perform by a minimally invasive approach has very significant benefits to the patient. An obvious example of this is in hysterectomy and bilateral salpingo oophorectomy in the morbidly obese where morbidity of the resection is often associated with the extensive abdominal incision when approached conventionally. Some MIS approaches still appear to me to be techniques looking for an indication. When asked how minimally invasive surgery has altered my approach to thyroid and parathyroid surgery, I do confess my incision is smaller and the patient goes home earlier. But I still use less pre- and intra-operative testing than most (at least when I control the plethora of tests often ordered) and my morbidity and success rate seems unchanged.

We should welcome a text, which focuses on the technical aspects of minimally invasive surgery, but remains comprehensive and inclusive of disease management approaches which ultimately are the only way to improve overall outcome.

I am cautiously optimistic that by the time I need my first procedure for malignancy minimally invasive techniques will be at such a level that I can contemplate the same outcome as I might from the open approach but with less pain, morbidity, and no need for an incisional hernia repair! I shall not need a hysterectomy; I will be pleased to have a distal pancreatectomy. But if you need to convert, convert early [1]. As for my thyroidectomy, a robot assisted thyroidectomy by the bilateral axillo-breast approach (BABA) is not for me [2]. A small neck incision cannot possibly make me look worse than I do now, and I do not want to risk lymphedema.

In the meantime, given my secondary interest in sarcoma, it is hard to envision minimally invasive surgery dealing with a 15-kg retroperitoneal soft tissue sarcoma. So my timing is right; it will take a little longer to solve that problem with a minimalist approach. I congratulate the editors and their authors.

Prof. Murray F. Brennan, M.D.
Memorial Sloan-Kettering Cancer Center,
1225 York Avenue, New York, NY 10065, USA

References

1. Jayaraman, S., Gonen, M., Brennan, M.F., D'Angelica, M.I., DeMatteo, R.P., Fong, Y., et al.: Laparoscopic distal pancreatectomy: evolution of a technique at a single institution. J. Am. Coll. Surg. **211**(4), 503–509 (2010)
2. Lee, K.E., Koo do, H., Kim, S.J., Lee, J., Park, K.S., Oh, S.K., et al.: Outcomes of 109 patients with papillary thyroid carcinoma who underwent robotic total thyroidectomy with central node dissection via the bilateral axillo-breast approach. Surgery. **148**(6), 1207–1213 (2010)

Foreword II

The view of a pioneer in Minimally Invasive Surgery

There can be little doubt that the introduction of laparoscopic surgery in the mid 1980s has had a far reaching effect on surgical practice. In many ways, this development has to be categorized as *disruptive* as defined by Christensen in his book the *Innovator's Dilemma,* because it has radically changed the way in which we, as clinical surgeons, manage and treat our patients. From the early years of cholecystectomy and appendectomy, the scope of laparoscopic surgery has expanded to the safe execution of major operations for life threatening disorders across all surgical specialties, imparting significant benefits primarily to the immediate outcome of patients and to surgical healthcare in general. The technology has continued to progress as has the surgical approaches exemplified by natural orifice and single incision laparoscopic surgery, in the quest for reduction of the traumatic insult to our patients. In some respects this progress has exceeded the expectations of the early pioneers with the advent of HDTV imaging systems and robotic surgery. To a very large extent, traditional open surgery now serves as a fall-back approach used whenever the minimally access approach proves difficult for whatever reason. This is as it should be, as surgical operations must never be considered as feats (the macho phenomenon) but simply as the appropriate means to cure or palliate patients for whom our profession exists to serve.

The concerns that the laparoscopic approach by virtue of the positive capnoperitoneum somehow compromises the clinical outcome including cure rates of patients with cancer by enhancing the risks of wound recurrence and distant spread have been disproved by seminal studies including RCTs, such that we have now level I evidence on the equivalent cure rates between the open and the laparoscopic approach for cancer surgery, certainly for colon cancer. Paradoxically, the major expansion of the laparoscopic approach witnessed in the last 10–15 years has been in surgery for solid cancers. It is timely therefore that all these significant advances are brought together for the benefit of practicing surgeons. In this respect the two Editors, Ronald Matteoti and Stanley Ashley, are to be complimented for recruiting leading contributors for *Minimally Invasive Surgical Oncology* which, in my view, achieves its objective in providing a state-of-the art account. It provides a wealth of information on all the topics which should be of considerable interest to both established surgical oncologists and residents. Appropriately in my opinion, the first 10 chapters deal with general issues and technological advances relevant to oncological practice and are followed by specific chapters on the laparoscopic treatment of the various solid cancers within the specialties of general surgery, endocrine surgery, gynecology, thoracic surgery, and urology. I know of no other reference textbook which covers the entire subject matter in such detail, and compliment the two Editors and all their Contributors for a seminal volume which has been long overdue.

Prof Sir Alfred Cuschieri, FRSE
Institute for Medical Science and Technology,
University of Dundee, Wilson House,
1 Wurzburg Loan, Dundee Medipark,
Dundee, DD2 1FD, UK

Preface

Minimally Invasive Surgical Oncology: State-of-the-Art Cancer Management offers a unique compendium of the current knowledge and applied techniques in treating cancer with a minimally invasive approach. It is a comprehensive text trying to cover all fields in oncology where minimally invasive surgery is currently used. The book is divided into two sections. Section one covers general topics ranging from historical aspects of the field to research in oncology, covering topics like residency training and includes contributions special to oncology like immunology and changes in elderly patients. Section two is subdivided into 25 chapters, organ-based, covering all aspects of minimally invasive surgery in the cancer patient in a unique way. At the end of each chapter the reader will find a section about future trends and a quick reference guide to the specific topic and procedure. More so, the accompanying DVD offers tips and tricks by experts in the field explaining their surgical approach in a step-by-step fashion.

The ever growing field of minimally invasive surgery in combination with a better understanding of the consequent immunological and pathophysiologic changes has led to applications of minimally invasive approaches to maximally invasive disease processes. Over almost 2 decades, this field has rapidly evolved and there is almost no disease process and organ which has not been addressed. Despite this, oncologic diseases have always been addressed with great reservation and, for a long time, it was thought that cure could only be safely achieved with traditional open surgery.

When we first talked about the concept of the book we quickly realized that there is no existing book focused on the topic. All that was available were surgical atlases, case reports, and some randomized studies, particularly for covering colorectal malignancies. There was no clear guide of how to apply these techniques with maximal short- and long-term benefit to cancer patients. Our goal was to give the reader a better understanding of how the proven advantages of minimally invasive surgery could factor into an individualized surgical treatment plan, understanding that management of cancer is always multidisciplinary.

Minimally Invasive Surgical Oncology: State-of-the-Art Cancer Management brings together the expertise of not only experts but true leaders and pioneers in the field. It provides clear explanations of all surgical procedures as outlined in the table of contents but is, by far, more than just another surgical atlas. Current nonsurgical therapies, future trends, and alternative procedures are discussed with a quick reference guide and a multimedia section. We hope that the unique structure of this book will particularly be helpful to those engaged in treating oncological patients, contribute to a wider acceptance of the application of minimally invasive techniques in malignancies and might open up new avenues for future research.

Philadelphia, PA, USA Ronald Matteotti
Boston, MA, USA Stanley W. Ashley

Quotes

"The smaller the incision, the bigger the surgeon's concern should be to do the right procedure for the right patient at the right time."

2010   Ronald Matteotti

"The cleaner and gentler, the act of operation, the less pain the patient suffers, the smoother and quicker the convalescence, the more exquisite his healed wound, the happier his memory of the whole incident."

1920   Lord Moynihan

Editor's Biographies

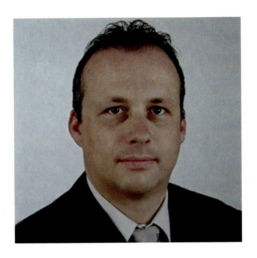

Ronald S. Matteotti, MD, FMH
Editor in Chief
Surgical Oncologist/Minimally
Invasive Surgeon
263 Osborn Street
Philadelphia, PA 19128, USA

Ronald Matteotti, MD is a graduate of Gymnasium Vaduz, Principality of Liechtenstein and Medical College University of Basel, Switzerland. He completed a residency in general surgery and thereafter joined the faculty of Kreisspital Männedorf, Faculty of Surgery, University of Zurich, Switzerland. In Zurich, he was responsible for building up a minimally invasive surgical unit. In 2003 he joined the research staff of Prof. Gagner at his Minimally Invasive Surgical Unit at Mount Sinai Hospital, New York, NY and Weill-Cornell College of Medicine. After 2 years in research with Prof. Gagner he completed an advanced laparoscopy fellowship at Boston University in Boston, Massachusetts as the first Karl Storz "Surgical Innovation and Advanced Laparoscopy fellow." Realizing the tremendous opportunities in the USA he completed a second residency at University Hospital of Cleveland, Case Western Reserve, Cleveland, OH. He moved on to Fox Chase Cancer Center in Philadelphia, where he served as a fellow in surgical oncology. Dr Matteotti holds specialty certificates in general, gastrointestinal, and trauma surgery. His primary interest is hepatobiliary disease and gastrointestinal cancer, especially minimally invasive approaches to gastric and colo-rectal malignancies. His research founded at Mount Sinai Hospital and further at Fox Chase Cancer Center includes pathophysiological changes during laparoscopy in a sepsis model and currently novel targets to treat hepato-cellular cancer. He has multiple publications in the field of minimally invasive surgery and was the founding editor of the open access journal "Annals of Surgical Innovation and Research" where he currently is the editor in chief. He is a member of multiple professional societies especially SAGES – Society of Gastrointestinal end Endoscopic Surgeons.

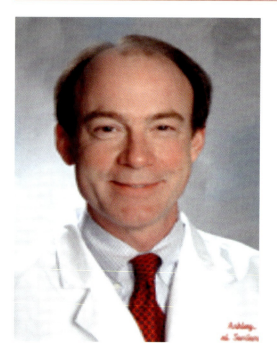

Stanley W. Ashley, MD, FACS
Coeditor-in-Chief
Frank Sawyer Professor
and Vice Chairman
Department of Surgery
Brigham and Women's Hospital/
Harvard Medical School
Boston, MA 02115, USA

Stanley W. Ashley, MD is a graduate of Oberlin College and Cornell University Medical College. He completed a residency in general surgery at Washington University in St. Louis and subsequently joined the faculty. He spent 7 years at UCLA before assuming his current position at Brigham and Women's Hospital/ Harvard Medical School in 1997. He is currently the Frank Sawyer Professor and Vice Chairman of the Department of Surgery. He is also Program Director of the General Surgery Residency and Chief of General Surgery for Harvard Vanguard Medical Associates. Dr. Ashley is a gastrointestinal surgeon whose primary interests are diseases of the pancreas and inflammatory bowel disease. His research, which has been funded by both the VA the NIH, has examined the pathophysiology of the small bowel and pancreas. He has more than 250 publications. He serves on numerous editorial boards, including the Journal of Gastrointestinal Surgery, the Journal of the American College of Surgeons, Current Problems in Surgery, and ACS Surgery. He is currently a director of the American Board of Surgery and will serve as Vice Chair and then Chair from 2010 to 2012. He is a member of the Board of Trustees of the Society for Surgery of the Alimentary Tract.

Acknowledgements

For Sandra who stood at my side all this time.

Ronald Matteotti

To
Stanley W. Ashley
Who always supported this project as coeditor without any reservations, adding his invaluable input and experience.

Ronald Matteotti

To
Michel Gagner and Jeffrey Ponsky
Two pioneers, creative minds, thought leaders, and real friends.
Without you two as mentors I would not be where I am right now and this book would never have been possible without your continued inspiration.

Ronald Matteotti

To
Ronald Matteotti
Without whose vision and effort this project would not have been possible.

Stanley W. Ashley

Contents

Part I   General Topics

1. **Minimally Invasive Surgery – The Pioneers** 3
   George Berci and Masanobu Hagiike

2. **Evolution of Minimally Invasive Surgery and Its Impact on Surgical Residency Training** 11
   Adrian E. Park and Tommy H. Lee

3. **Laparoscopy and Research in Surgical Oncology: Current State of the Art and Future Trends** 23
   Dominic King, Henry Lee, and Lord Ara Darzi

4. **Moral and Ethical Issues in Laparoscopy and Advanced Surgical Technologies** 39
   Richard M. Satava

5. **Robotic Applications in Surgical Oncology** 47
   Scott J. Belsley

6. **Laparoscopy and Malignancy – General Aspects** 59
   Shigeru Tsunoda and Glyn G. Jamieson

7. **Laparoscopy and Immunology** 69
   Michael J. Grieco and Richard Larry Whelan

8. **Pneumoperitoneum and Its Effects on Malignancy** 83
   Alan T. Lefor and Atsushi Shimizu

9. **Laparoscopy in the Elderly** 97
   Michael Ujiki and Nathaniel Soper

10. **Transluminal Surgery: Is There a Place for Oncological Procedures?** 107
    Patricia Sylla and David W. Rattner

Part II Special Topics: Cancer of the Esophagus and the Gastro-Esophageal Junction

11 **Cancer of the Esophagus and the Gastroesophageal Junction: Two-Cavity Approach**.............................. 125
Christopher R. Morse, Omar Awais, and James D. Luketich

12 **Cancer of the Esophagus and the Gastroesophageal Junction: Transhiatal Approach**... 137
Lee Swanstrom and Michael Ujiki

Part III Special Topics: Cancer of the Stomach

13 **Laparoscopic Distal Gastrectomy – *LADG***...................... 149
Mutter Didier, O.A. Burckhardt, and Perretta Silvana

14 **Laparoscopic Total Gastrectomy – *LATG***...................... 159
Seigo Kitano, Norio Shiraishi, Koji Kawaguchi, and Kazuhiro Yasuda

15 **Endoluminal Procedures for Early Gastric Cancer**............... 167
Brian J. Dunkin and Rohan Joseph

Part IV Special Topics: Small Bowel

16 **Laparoscopic Management of Small Bowel Tumors**............. 183
Miguel Burch, Brian Carmine, Daniel Mishkin, and Ronald Matteotti

Part V Special Topics: Cancer of the Colon and Rectum

17 **Right Hemicolectomy and Appendix**......................... 199
Antonio M. Lacy

18 **Left Hemicolectomy and Sigmoid Colon**...................... 219
Joel Leroy, Ronan Cahill, and Jacques Marescaux

19 **Laparoscopic Rectal Procedures**............................ 235
Rolv-Ole Lindsetmo and Conor P. Delaney

Part VI Special Topics: Cancer of the Hepato-Biliary System

20 **General Considerations**................................... 253
Jonathan P. Pearl and Jeffrey L. Ponsky

21 **Liver: Nonanatomical Resection**............................ 263
Fumihiko Fujita, Susumu Eguchi, Yoshitsugu Tajima, and Takashi Kanematsu

22	**Liver – Anatomical Liver Resections**...........................	273
	Bruto Randone, Ronald Matteotti, and Brice Gayet	
23	**Cancer of the Gallbladder and Extrahepatic Bile Ducts**...........	297
	Andrew A. Gumbs, Angel M. Rodriguez-Rivera, and John P. Hoffman	

Part VII   Special Topics: Spleen

24	**Spleen: Hematological Disorders**............................	311
	Eduardo M. Targarona, Carmen Balague, and Manuel Trias	

Part VIII   Special Topics: Endocrinology

25	**Cancer of the Thyroid**.....................................	331
	Prashant Sinha and William B. Inabnet	
26	**Cancer of the Parathyroid**..................................	355
	Paolo Miccoli, Gabriele Materazzi, and Piero Berti	
27	**Cancer of the Pancreas: Distal Resections and Staging of Pancreatic Cancer**...................................	363
	Vivian E. Strong, Joshua Carson, and Peter J. Allen	
28	**Cancer of the Pancreas: The Whipple Procedure**................	379
	Michael L. Kendrick	
29	**Cancer of the Adrenal Gland**................................	389
	Ronald Matteotti, Luca Milone, Daniel Canter, and Michel Gagner	

Part IX   Special Topics: Gynecology

30	**Minimally Invasive Management of Gynecologic Malignancies**.....	407
	Farr Reza Nezhat, Jennifer Eun Sun Cho, Connie Liu, and Gabrielle Gossner	

Part X   Special Topics: Urology

31	**Cancer of the Kidney**......................................	447
	Daniel J. Canter and Robert G. Uzzo	
32	**Cancer of the Prostate**.....................................	465
	Gino J. Vricella and Lee E. Ponsky	
33	**Cancer of the Urinary Bladder**...............................	487
	Kevin P. Asher and David S. Wang	

Part XI Special Topics: Pediatrics

34 Minimally Invasive Management of Pediatric Malignancies 501
Arjun Khosla, Todd A. Ponsky, and Steven S. Rothenberg

Part XII Special Topics: Lung and Mediastinum

35 Minimally Invasive Management of Intra-Thoracic Malignancies 515
Philip A. Linden

Index 533

Abbreviations

5-FU	5-Fluorouracil
ABC	Argon Beam Coagulation
ABMS	American Board of Medical Specialties
ABVD	Adriamycin, Bleomycin, Vinblastine, Dacarbazine
AC	Anesthesia Control
ACC	Adrenocortical Carcinomas
ACGME	Accreditation Council for Graduate Medical Education
ACS	American College of Surgeons
ACTH	Adreno Cortico Tropes Hormon
ADEPT	Advanced Dundee Endoscopic Psychomotor Tester
AESOP	Animated Endoscopic System for Optimal Positioning
AGES	Age, Tumor Grade, Extent, Size
AHPBA	The American Hepato-Pancreato-Biliary Association
AJCC TNM	American Joint Committee on Cancer Tumor Node Metastasis
AJCC/UICC	American Joint Committee on Cancer/International Union Against Cancer
AMES	Age, Metastasis, Extent, Size
ANED	Alive with No Evidence of Disease
AP	Anterior-Posterior
APDS	Association of Program Directors in Surgery
APR	Abdominoperineal Resection
APUD	Amine Precursor Uptake and Decarboxylation
ARR	Aldosterone to Renin Ratio
ASCRS	American Society of Colon and Rectal Surgeons
ASGE	American Society of Gastrointestinal Endoscopy
ASIS	Anterior Superior Iliac Spine
ASMBS	American Society for Metabolic and Bariatric Surgery
ASTRO	American Society of Therapeutic Radiology and Oncology
ATA	Anterior Transabdominal
AWD	Alive With Disease
BABA	Bilateral Axillary-Breast Approach
BCR-ABL	Breakpoint Cluster Region-Abelson Murine Leukemia
bDFS	biochemical Disease-Free Survival
BEACOPP	Bleomycin, Etoposide, Adriamycin, Cyclophosphamide, Vincristin = Oncovine, Procarbazine, Prednisone
BED	Biologic Effective Dose
BMI	Body Mass Index

BNS	Bilateral Nerve Sparing
CA	Carbohydrate Antigen
CAR	Compression Anastomosis System
CBC	Complete Blood Count
CBD	Common Bile Duct
CCD	Charged Coupled Device
CCG	Children's Cancer Group
CDR	Complimentary Determining Region
CEA	Carcino-embryonic Antigen
CEM	Confocal Endomicroscopy
CHF	Chronic Heart Failure
CHOP	Cytoxan, Hydroxyrubicin (Adriamycin), Oncovin (Vincristine), Prednisone
CIS	Carcinoma In Situ
CLASICC	Conventional versus Laparoscopic-assisted Surgery in Colorectal Cancer
CLASSIC	Conventional versus Laparoscopic-assisted Surgery in Colorectal Cancer
CLL	Chronic Lymphocytic Leukemia
CML	Chronic Myeloid Leukemia
CO	Converted to Open
COG	Children's Oncology Group
COLOR	COlon Cancer Laparoscopic or Open Resection
COST	Clinical Outcomes of Surgical Therapy
CP	Pancreatic Cyst
CRC	Colorectal Cancer
CRM	Circumferential Resection Margin
CRP	C-Reactive Protein
CSF	Cerebrospinal Fluid
CT	Computerized Tomography
CVA	Cerebrovascular Accident
CVP	Central Venous Pressure
CVP	Cyclophosphamide, Vincristine, and Prednisone
CXR	Chest X-ray
DC	Descending Colon
DCUE	Dual-Channel Endoscope
DOF	Degrees of Freedom
DP	Distal Pancreas
DPAM	Disseminated Peritoneal Adenomucinosis
DRE	Digital Rectal Examination
DTC	Differentiated Thyroid Cancer
DTH	Delayed-Type Hypersensitivity
DVD	Digital Versatile Disc
DVT	Deep Venous Thrombosis
EBL	Estimated Blood Loss
EBRT	External Beam Radiotherapy
ECOG	Eastern Cooperative Oncology Group
EEG	Electroencephalogram
EGC	Early Gastric Cancer

EGD	Esophagogastroduodenoscopy
EKG	Electrocardiography
EMR	Endoscopic Mucosal Resection
EN	Enucleation
ENT	Ear, Nose & Throat
EORTC	European Organization for Research and Treatment of Cancer
EPO	Erythropoietin
ERCP	Endoscopic Retrograde Cholangio Pancretography
ESD	Endoscopic Submucosal Dissection
ESR	Erythrocyte Sedimentation Rate
EUS	Endoscopic Ultrasound
FACT-G	Functional Assessment of Cancer Therapy-General
FAP	Familial Adenomatous Polyposis
FC	Fellowship Council
FDA	Food and Drug Administration
FDG	Fluorodeoxyglucose
FDG-PET	Fluorodeoxyglucose Positron Emission Tomography
FDG-PET	^{18}F-fluorodeoxy Glucose Positron Emission Tomography
FIGO	International Federation of Obstetrics and Gynecology
FLS	Fundamentals of Laparoscopic Surgery
FNA	Fine-Needle Aspiration
FTC	Follicular Thyroid Cancer
FU	Fluorouracil
FVC	Forced Vital Capacity
FvPTC	Follicular Variant of Papillary Thyroid Cancer
GB	Gallbladder
GI	Gastrointestinal
GIA	Gastro Intestinal Anastomosis
GIST	Gastrointestinal Stromal Tumor
GMCSF	Granulocyte-Macrophage-Colony-Stimulating-Factor
GOALS	Global Operative Assessment of Laparoscopic Skills
GOG	Gynecologic Oncology Group
GOO	Gastric Outlet Obstruction
GU	Genitourinary
HAIC	Hepatic Arterial Infusion Chemotherapy
HALS	Hand-assisted Laparoscopic Surgery
HBV	Hepatitis B Virus
HCC	Hepatocellular Carcinoma
hCG	Human Chorionic Gonadotropin
HCV	Hepatitis C Virus
HD	High Definition
HDTV	High-Definition TV
HGD	High-Grade Dysplasia
HIFU	High-Intensity Focused Ultrasound
HIFU	High Intensity Focused Ultrasound
HL	Hodgkin's Lymphoma
HLA-DR	Human Leukocyte Antigen DR
HMD	Head-Mounted Display
HPT	Hyperparathyroidism

HPT-JT	Hyperparathyroidism-Jaw Tumor Syndrome
HPTN	Hyperparathyroidism
HRPT2	Hyperparathyroidism 2
HU	Hounsfield Unit
IC	Integrated Circuit
ICAM-1	Inter-Cellular Adhesion Molecule 1
ICG R15	Indocyanine Green Retention Rate at 15 min
ICSAD	Imperial College Surgical Assessment Device
ICU	Intensive Care Unit
IFN	Interferon
IGS	Image-Guided Surgery
IL	Interleukin
IMA	Inferior Mesenteric Artery
IMRT	Intensity-Modulated Radiation Therapy
IMV	Inferior Mesenteric Vein
INSS	International Neuroblastoma Staging System
IPC	Intraperitoneal Chemotherapy
IPMN	Intraductal Papillary Mucinous Neoplasm
IPSID	Immunoproliferative Small Intestinal Disease
iPTH	Intact PTH
IPTMT	Intrapapillary Tumor/Mucinous Tumor
IRB	Institutional Review Board
IT	Insulation Tipped
ITP	Idiopathic Thrombocytopenic Purpura
IVC	Inferior Vena Cava
JCOG	Japan Clinical Oncology Group
JGCA	Japanese Gastric Cancer Association
JP	Jackson–Pratt
JSES	The Japanese Society of Endoscopic Surgery
LAC	Laparoscopic-Assisted Colectomy
LACR	Laparoscopic Colon Resection
LADG	Laparoscopic-Assisted Distal Gastrectomy
LAK	Lymphokine-Activated Killer
LAPG	Laparoscopic-Assisted Proximal Gastrectomy
LAR	Low Anterior Resection
LATG	Laparoscopic Total Gastrectomy
LAVH	Laparoscopic Assisted Vaginal Hysterectomy
LC	Laparoscopic Cholecystectomy
LCS	Laparoscopic Ultrasonic Coagulation Shears
LDH	Lactate Dehydrogenase
LDP	Laparoscopic Distal Pancreatectomy
LDS	Laparoscopic Dissection Shears
LED	Light-Emitting Eiode
LEn	Laparoscopic Enucleation
LESS	Laparo-Endoscopic Single-Site Surgery
LESS	Laparo Endoscopic Single Port Surgery
LG	Laparoscopic Gastrectomy
LK	Left Kidney
LLL	Left Lower Lobectomy

LN	Lymph Node
LOS	Length of Stay
LPD	Laparoscopic Pancreaticoduodenectomy
LPNs	Laparoscopic Partial Nephrectomies
LPS	Lipo-Polysaccharide
LRN	Laparoscopic Radical Nephrectomy
LRP	Laparoscopic Radical Prostatectomy
LS	Laparoscopic Splenectomy
LTA	Lateral Transabdominal
LTE	Laparoscopic Transhiatal Esophagectomy
LUL	Left Upper Lobectomy
MAC-1	Membrane-Activated Complex 1
MACC	Methotrexate, Adriamycin, Cyclophosphamide, CCNU
MACIS	Metastases, Age, Completeness of Surgical Resection, Invasion, Size of the Primary Tumor
MALT	Mucosa-Associated Lymphoid Tumor
MC	Mammary Cancer Cells
MCT	Microwave Coagulation Therapy
MEMS	Micro Electro Mechanical Systems
MEN	Multiple Endocrine Neoplasm
MEN 1	Multiple Endocrine Neoplasia 1
MEN 2	Multiple Endocrine Neoplasia type 2
MHC-II	Major HistocompatibilityComplex-II
MI	Myocardial Infarction
MIBG	Metha-Ido-Benzo-Guanidine
MIE	Minimally Invasive Esophagectomy
MIRS	Minimally Invasive Robotic Surgery
MIS	Minimally Invasive Surgery
MISTELS	McGill Inanimate System for Training and Evaluation of Laparoscopic Skills
MIST-VR	Minimally Invasive Surgical Trainer-virtual Reality
MIT	Minimally Invasive Open Technique
MIT	Minimally Invasive Open Thyroidectomy
MIVAT	Minimally Invasive Video Assisted Thyroidectomy
MMPs	Matrix Metalloproteins
MN	Minnesota
MR	Magner Resonance
MRC CLASIC	Multicenter Randomized Comtrolled Trial of Conventional versus Laparoscopic-Assisted
MRI	Magnetic Resonance Imaging
MSI-H	High Microsatellite Instability
MTC	Medullary Thyroid Cancer
mTOR	Surgery in Colorectal Cancer
MVP	Maryland Virtual Patient
NCCN	National Comprehensive Cancer Network
NCI	National Cancer Institute
NE	Neuroendocrine
NED	No Evidence of Disease
NET	Neuroendocrine Tumor

NG	Naso-Gastric
NHANES	National Health and Nutrition Examination Survey
NHL	Non-Hodgkin's Lymphoma
NIS	Sodium Iodide Symporter
NK	Natural Killer
NK-LGL	NK-Large Granular Lymphocyte
NOSCAR	Natural Orifice Surgery Consortium for Assessment and Research
NOTES	Natural Orifice Transluminal Endoscopic Surgery
NOTUS	Natural Orifice Trans Umbilical Surgery
NPO	Nil Per Os
NS	Not Significant
NSADS	Non-Steroidal Antiinflammatory Drugs
NSQUIP	National Surgical Quality Improvement Program
NSS	Nephron-Sparing Surgery
OC	Open Colectomy
ODG	Open Equivalent Gastrectomy
OGT	Oral Gastric Tube
OPUS	One Port Umbilical Surgery
OR	Operating Room
OR	Open Reconstruction
OR time	Mean Operating Room Time
OSATS	Objective Structured Assessment of Technical Skill
OST	Overnight Low-Dose Dexamethasone Suppression Test
PACE	Preoperative Assessment of Cancer in the Elderly
PALND	Para Aortic Lymph Node Dissection
PBMC	Peripheral Blood Mononuclear Cells
PDS	Polydioxanone Suture
PDT	Photodynamic Therapy
PE	Pulmonary Embolism
PECAM1	Platelet Endothelial Cell Adhesion Molecule 1
PEG	Percutaneous Endoscopic Gastrostomy
PET	Positron Emission Tomography
PF	Pancreatic Fistula
PFT	Pulmonary Function Test
PGE2	Prostaglandin E2
PHP	Primary Hyperparathyroidism
PIP	Picture-In-Picture
PL	Pure Laparoscopic
PlGF	Placental Growth Factor
PLN	Pelvic Lymph Node
PLND	Pelvic Lymph Node Dissection
PMCA	Peritoneal Mucinous Carcinomatosis
PME	Partial Mesorectal Resection
PMN	Polymorphonuclear Leukocyte
PMP	Pseudomyxoma Peritonei
PN	Partial Nephrectomy
POD	Postoperative Day
POG	Pediatric Oncology Group
PRAD1	Parathyroid Adenomatosis 1

PSA	Prostate-specific Antigen
PTC	Papillary Thyroid Cancer
PTH	Parathyroid Hormone
PV	Portal Vein
QOL	Quality of Life
R/O	Ruled/Out
RA	Renal Artery
RAI	Radioactive Iodine
RALPN	Robot-Assisted Laparoscopic Partial Nephrectomy
RAS	Rat Sarcoma
RB	Retinoblastoma
RCC	Renal Cell Carcinomas
RCT	Randomized Controlled Trial
REA	Retroperitoneal Adrenalectomy
RFA	Radiofrequency Ablation
RLL	Right Lower Lobectomy
RLN	Recurrent Laryngeal Nerve
RML	Right Middle Lobectomy
RMS	Rhabdomyosarcoma
RN	Radical Nephrectomy
RPP	Radical Perineal Prostatectomy
RRP	Radical Retropubic Prostatectomy
RTOG	Radiation Therapy Oncology Group
RT-PCR	Reverse Transcription Polymerase Chain Reaction
RUL	Right Upper Lobectomy
RUQ	Right Upper Quadrant
SAE	Splenic Artery Embolization
SAGES	The Society of American Gastrointestinal and Endoscopic Surgeons
SARA	Single Access Retroperitoneoscopic Adrenalectomy
SCD	Sequential Compression Device
SCM	Sternocleidomastoid Muscle
SCT	Sacro Coccygeal Teratoma
SCUE	Single-Channel Endoscope
SD	Standard Definition
SEER	Surveillance Epidemiology and End Results
SEMS	Self-Expandable Metal Stents
SILS	Single-Incision Laparoscopic Surgery
SILS	Single Port Laparoscopic Surgery
SIOP	International Society for Pediatric Oncology
SMA	Superior Mesenteric Artery
SMV	Superior Mesenteric Vein
SPA	Single Port Access
SRMs	Small Renal Masses
SSAT	The Society for Surgery of the Alimentary Tract
TACE	Transarterial Chemoembolization
TAE	Transarterial Embolization
TAH	Total Abdominal Hysterectomy
TCC	Transitional Cell Carcinoma
TA™	Triangular Anastomosis

TEM	Trans-Anal Endoscopic Microsurgery
TEMS	Trans-Anal Endoscopic Microsurgery
TG	Transgastric
THOR	Conventional Thoracotomy
TID	Ter in Die (Thrice Daily Dosage)
TLH	Total Laparoscopic Hysterectomy
TLRP	Transperitoneal Laparoscopic Radical Prostatectomy
TME	Total Mesorectal Excision
TNsyF	Tumor Necrosis Factor
TNF-a	Tumor Necrosis Factor Alpha
TNM	Tumor, Node, Metastases
TRH	Thyrotropin-Releasing Hormone
TRUS	Transrectal Ultrasound
TSH	Thyroid-Stimulating Hormone
TUES	Trans Umbilical Endoscopic Surgery
TULA	Trans Umbilical Laparoscopic Assisted
TUR-B	Transurethral Resection of the Bladder
TUR-P	Transurethral Resection of the Prostate
TV	Television
UFC	Urinary-Free Cortisol Evaluation
UGI	Upper Gastro-Intestinal Imaging
UNS	Unilateral Nerve Sparing
US	Ultrasound
UTI	Urinary Tract Infection
UVF	Uretero-Vaginal Fistula
VATS	Video-Assisted Thoracic Surgery
VC	Vena Cava
VCAM	Vascular Cell Adhesion Molecule
VEGF	Vascular Endothelial Growth Factor
VHS	Video Home System
VR	Virtual Reality
VVF	Vesico Vaginal Fistula
WIT	Warm Ischemia Time
YAG	Yttrium Aluminum Garnet

List of Videos

Chapter 11 Cancer of the Esophagus and the Gastroesophageal Junction: Two-Cavity Approach
Christopher R. Morse, Omar Awais, and James D. Luketich

The two cavity approach to esophageal cancer

Chapter 12 Cancer of the Esophagus and the Gastroesophageal Junction: Transhiatal Approach
Lee Swanstrom and Michael Ujiki

Chapter 13 Laparoscopic Distal Gastrectomy – *LADG*
Mutter Didier, O.A. Burckhardt, and Perretta Silvana

Laparoscopic distal gastrectomy – *LADG*

- Clip 1   Division of the gastro-colic ligament (case 1)
- Clip 2   Division of the gastro-colic ligament (case 2)
- Clip 3   Dissection of the right gastro-omental vessels and of the inferior side of the proximal duodenum (case 1)
- Clip 4   Dissection of the right gastro-omental vessels (case 2)
- Clip 5   Vascular lesions on the right gastro-omental vessels
- Clip 6   Dissection of the gastro-hepatic ligament up to the hepatic common artery (case 2)
- Clip 7   Dissection of the gastro-hepatic ligament up to the hepatic common artery (case 1)
- Clip 8   Division of the right gastric artery
- Clip 9   Posterior dissection and division of the duodenum (case 2)
- Clip 10 Posterior dissection and division of the duodenum (case 1)
- Clip 11 Dissection of the common hepatic artery
- Clip 12 Lymphadenectomy of nodal stations 7, 8 and 9
- Clip 13 Division of the stomach
- Clip 14 Exposure of the stomach by trans-abdominal suspension
- Clip 15 Trans-mesocolic route and approximation of the stomach to the mesocolon
- Clip 16 Gastro-jejunal anastomosis, closure of the mesocolic window and extraction of the specimen (case 1)
- Clip 17 Gastrojejunal anastomosis (case 2)

Chapter 14 Laparoscopic Total Gastrectomy – *LATG*
Seigo Kitano, Norio Shiraishi, Koji Kawaguchi, and Kazuhiro Yasuda

Laparoscopic total gastrectomy with Roux-En-Y reconstruction

Chapter 15 Endoluminal Procedures for Early Gastric Cancer
Brian J. Dunkin and Rohan Joseph

Endoluminal procedures for early gastric cancer

Chapter 16 Laparoscopic Management of Small Bowel Tumors
Miguel Burch, Brian Carmine, Daniel Mishkin, and Ronald Matteotti

Laparoscopic management of small bowel tumors

Chapter 17 Right Hemicolectomy and Appendix
Antonio M. Lacy

Right hemicolectomy and appendectomy for cancer

Chapter 18 Left Hemicolectomy and Sigmoid Colon
Joel Leroy, Ronan Cahill, and Jacques Marescaux

Laparoscopic Sigmoidectomy for cancer

Chapter 19 Laparoscopic Rectal Procedures
Rolv-Ole Lindsetmo and Conor P. Delaney

Laparoscopic procedures of the rectum

Clip 1   Transanal endoscopic microsurgery
Clip 2   Laparoscopic Low anterior resection with colo-anal anastomosis
Clip 3   Laparoscopic Abdominoperineal resection - colonic division
Clip 4   Laparoscopic Abdominoperineal resection - perineal portion

Chapter 21 Liver: Nonanatomical Resection
Fumihiko Fujita, Susumu Eguchi, Yoshitsugu Tajima,
and Takashi Kanematsu

Laparoscopic Hepatectomy: Non-Anatomical resection

Chapter 23 Cancer of the Gallbladder and Extrahepatic Bile Ducts
Andrew A. Gumbs, Angel M. Rodriguez-Rivera, and John P. Hoffman

Laparoscopic approaches to gallbladder cancer

Chapter 24 Spleen: Hematological Disorders
Eduardo M. Targarona, Carmen Balague, and Manuel Trias

1   Hand-assisted laparoscopic splenectomy in cases of massive splenomegaly
2   Laparoscopic splenectomy and splenomegaly: Anterior-Posterior approach and 'hanged' technique

Chapter 26 Cancer of the Parathyroid
Paolo Miccoli, Gabriele Materazzi, and Piero Berti

Minimally invasive video-assisted parathyroidectomy

Chapter 27 Cancer of the Pancreas: Distal Resections and Staging of Pancreatic Cancer
Vivian E. Strong, Joshua Carson, and Peter J. Allen

Laparoscopic distal pancreatectomy

Chapter 29 Cancer of the Adrenal Gland
Ronald Matteotti, Luca Milone, Daniel Canter, and Michel Gagner

Laparoscopic left adrenalectomy-Lateral Transabdominal Approach-*LTA*

Chapter 30 Minimally Invasive Management of Gynecologic Malignancies
Farr Reza Nezhat, Jennifer Eun Sun Cho, Connie Liu, and Gabrielle Gossner

1 **Robotic assisted ovarian transposition and pretreatment surgical staging in ovarian cancer**
2 **Robotic radical hysterectomy**

Chapter 31 Cancer of the Kidney
Daniel J. Canter and Robert G. Uzzo

Minimally Invasive Renal Surgery

Chapter 35 Minimally Invasive Management of Intra-Thoracic Malignancies
Philip A. Linden

Left VATS lingular resection

Part I

General Topics

Minimally Invasive Surgery – The Pioneers

George Berci and Masanobu Hagiike

1.1 Introduction

It is always interesting to learn how pioneers conceived an idea, the motives behind it, and the circumstances under which a theoretical concept was transformed to a functioning unit. Sometimes, we wonder at the simplicity of a particular solution and we wonder why no one else thought about this obvious answer. Alternatively, we wonder at the ingenuity of the inventor to be able to complete this sophisticated design in a perfect operating condition without the support of an armada of consulting specialists from various disciplines or access to data-compiling libraries linked with computers, microfilm fiches, Internet, etc. The discoveries at the turn of the century, or even earlier, needed much more individual depths, because in the majority the originators were left on their own. Perhaps, one great asset of those times was the availability of time for thinking. No deadlines for submission had to be met, or preprogrammed phases completed. If the mood or spirit was not present, the sketch or draft was put aside to be taken into consideration again when the inventor felt he could accomplish his task.

"Inter arma Silent Musae" is valid for the creative act, not only during wartime, but whenever pressure or tension is high or constant. The creative solution is difficult today because there is support only for the "earth-shaking" invention or preprogrammed revolutionary ideas.

G. Berci (✉) and M. Hagiike
Department of Surgery, Cedars-Sinai Medical Center,
8700 Beverly Boulevard, Los Angeles, CA 90048, USA
e-mail: bercig@cshs.org

1.2 Definition and Evolution of Endoscopy

The word Endoscopy was inherited from the Greek, meaning to "examine within." The meaning was later interpreted as the examination of the interior of a deep, hollow viscus that communicates with the outside through an orifice of the body by means of a channel through which an instrument can be introduced. The speculum was already mentioned in the time of Hippocrates where the exploration of an orifice and the illumination of deeply located organs was the first issue to be solved.

If we divide the evolution of Endoscopy in certain stages, then definitely the first dominant ones were:

- How to get light in the depth.
- How can we keep the orifice and the deeply located organ explored?
- What type of instrument should we design that would be able to transmit the image of a deeply located organ to the eye (telescope)?
- At a later stage, can we perform tissue sampling or other more complex manipulations under visual control?
- If we are recognizing certain changes, how to document our findings?

1.3 Light Source – *Bozzini and Desormeaux*

Bozzini (1806) recognized the need for direct light to facilitate the examination of a more deeply seated organ. He employed a candle enclosed in a tubular-shaped holder with a mirror reflector. The attachable and detachable empty tubes were attached according to the shape, size, and depths of the organ, which was kept explored. The light was reflected into the tube [1]. In the early stages before Bozzini, reflected sunlight with a mirror was used for illumination. Desormeaux, a French surgeon (1867), described an open tube for the examination of the genitourinary passages, and used, as an improved light source, a mixture of alcohol and turpentine. A condenser lens with a reflector was employed to deviate the increased illumination into a tube attached to this light source. No doubt, there was more light at the end of the tube, but the burning flame created heat and the unit was very cumbersome [2].

1.4 Open Tube – *Kussmaul*

Kussmaul, a surgeon in 1870, was very fortunate that in his time malpractice insurance did not exist. He was able to insert a rigid tube through the mouth and pharynx into the esophagus. Allegedly, the first patient was a professional sword swallower [3].

Kussmaul was interested in removing foreign bodies from the esophagus and came later to the idea to explore some pathological entities in this tubular-shaped organ. The open tube system, with its inherited problem of difficulties in the introduction because of the size, pain, complication, and poor illumination, did not find too many followers.

1.5 Telescope

1.5.1 Galileo Galilei

Galileo Galilei, an Italian astronomer and physicist, described the telescope. It is true that he had great difficulties in constructing the first unit, which magnified the remote object only three times. He was able to improve it later to the power of 32 times. He was able to observe the moons of Jupiter, the phases of Venus, and sunspots, but was unfortunately placed on trial in 1633 and was forced to recall his views; he died under house arrest [4].

1.5.2 Maximilian Frederick Nitze

The inventor of the medical telescope was Maximilian Frederick Nitze, a German general practitioner, who was very interested in the pathology of the bladder. He devoted his time to urology. He designed a tube in which he placed small optics to transmit the image of an organ, located, in this case, the bladder, to the external surface. He created a chapter in endoscopy and urology by the invention of his cystoscope. Viewing the anatomy of the male urethra, he made an instrument to introduce it more easily, and therefore designed the angulated tip. At that time, he used a platinum filament, which was heated by a battery, to glow to create illumination. Due to the heat production, this "globe" had to be water-cooled (Fig. 1.1). A telescope was made with a prism at the end, creating a right-angle direction of the view. We are talking about 1879 [5]. It is amazing that a few years later, after the discovery of Edison's electric globe, a miniature filament lamp was made and the clumsy and large water-cooled platinum wire illuminator was replaced by the smallest electric globe. It made it also possible to decrease the tip of the instrument, and at a later stage to insert a small channel where a catheter could be advanced into the ureter. A part of prostatomegaly, bladder stones were extremely common. The other entity was from the field of oncology, bladder tumors. It was also his amazing ingenuity that a few years later, at the turn of the century, he designed and made with his instrument maker a photo cystoscope. There was a rotating disc at the proximal end where he inserted many miniature film plates. Despite the slight overburning of the globe (exposure time 3–5 s), he was able to obtain photos in an apnoic condition. At the turn

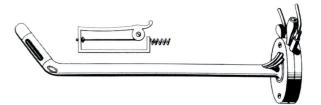

Fig. 1.1 Nitze's first cystoscope with a platinum wire *"globe"*: heated by a battery to create light, it needed water cooling. The tip was angulated with the globe. Below the opening window of the 90° direction of view telescope. The platinum wire illumination was changed few years later with a miniaturized Edison filament globe

of the century, he published an atlas of pathologies of the urinary bladder. Perhaps, this was the first documented endoscopic finding of oncology diseases.

Nitze had an excellent optician (Beneche from Berlin) and outstanding instrument maker, (Leiter from Vienna), who designed the first cystoscope without computers or other advanced technical tools.

1.5.3 Johann Mikulicz

Mikulicz, a surgeon, in 1881, introduced a gastroscope, which was based on the principles of the cystoscope but in an elongated version. It was put together with an articulated joint. At that time, it was 13 mm in diameter and 650 mm in length attached to a straight rigid part in a 150° angulation at the distal tip. He even used a cover plate, which was protecting the objective during the introduction and was withdrawn after the scope was in position. Mikulicz recommended that patients should fast the evening before the examination and the stomach was washed out with water before the procedure. Air insufflation was used to distend the stomach and the patient was put in a lateral position. Morphine was injected to premedicate the patient. He described three physiological phenomena of the stomach: peristalsis, respiration, and transmission of aorta pulsation [6].

1.5.4 Theodor Rosenheim and Rudolf Schindler

Rosenheim, in 1896, reported 20 successful gastroscopies, and mentioned the existence of "blind spots." One case was described as suspicious for a malignant lesion [7].

Schindler introduced a gastroscope, which was semiflexible, 77 cm long and 12 mm in diameter at the flexible portion but only of 8.5 mm diameter in the rigid part. An electric globe was used for illumination. A lateral view was provided. The system contained more than 48 lenses. He reported in several chapters of gastric carcinoma of the cardia, prepyloric lesions, and elaborated on the gastroscopic diagnosis of linitis plastica. He also described metastatic lesions and created the first endoscopic atlas, a textbook of oncological pathology.

In the later models, there was a channel inserted for a biopsy to also provide tissue samples [8].

1.5.5 Fritz Lange and C.A. Meltzing

Two surgeons, Drs. Lange and Meltzing, became interested in the endoscopic diagnostic modalities of the stomach. In 1898, after years of hard work, they had the idea to design a flexible rubber tube called a "photo gastroscope" with an outside diameter of 11 mm. There was no viewing component, but the rigid head was 20 mm long and contained an electric filament globe and a 5-mm wide film strip, which could be pulled into the rubber tube of this flexible "photo gastroscope." There was also a small channel for air insufflation of the stomach. It was inserted after the patient was fasted and the stomach was rinsed with saline. The globe was discharged, and after each exposure the exposed film was pulled into a tubular-shaped magazine. They were able to perform 50 exposures per patient. It took approximately 10–15 min. It is interesting to note that at the turn of the century, a photocystoscope was already developed with specific oncologic diagnostic aims and was revived or reinvented 70 years later [9].

1.6 The Endoscopic Exploration of the Abdominal Cavity: *Coelioskopie, Peritoneoscopy, or Laparoscopy*

1.6.1 Christian Jacobeus – 1910

A very interesting report came from a Swedish surgeon Christian Jacobeus in 1910, who explored the oncology aspect of the abdominal cavity. He selected, cleverly, in the first small series, patients with ascitic fluid where he did not need to perform a pneumoperitoneum employing Nitze's cystoscope. He described the appearance of tuberculosis and liver metastases. At a later stage, he also performed a pneumoperitoneum with room air and inspected the abdominal cavity, particularly the liver. He also became interested in thoracoscopy [10].

1.6.2 George Kelling – 1923

After the discovery of the telescope by Nitze, which mainly explored the urinary bladder, a surgeon, George Kelling, in 1923, reported the creation of a pneumoperitoneum by insufflation of air, and the introduction of a trocar and a telescope with a cystoscope optic. The procedure was carried out with sedation and local anesthesia. Kelling was mainly interested to obtain compression of the abdominal organs, especially the stomach and duodenum, thinking on arresting bleeders from these organs. He did not publish a larger series [11].

1.6.3 Heinz Kalk – 1929

A gastroenterologist, Kalk, improved the laparoscopic technique by introducing a telescope instead of the cystoscope from Nitze by changing the direction of view from 90° to 135°, calling it forward oblique [12]. He also introduced a double trocar technique for tissue sampling. In 1951, he published a monograph based on 2,000 patients without mortality. He became very interested in liver disease and performing biopsies but providing hemostasis with a very primitive coagulation technique. He also mentioned primary and secondary liver tumors and claimed this minimal procedure as a very accurate diagnostic and staging technique [13].

1.6.4 John Ruddock – 1934

John Ruddock, an American cardiologist, became interested in peritoneoscopy and in 1934 he reported at the Pacific Coast Surgical Association on his first 200 cases. In 1957, he published over 5,000 laparoscopies with eight bowel perforations and one mortality due to bleeding after liver biopsy. He diagnosed several metastatic carcinoma cases [14].

1.6.5 Swierenga J., Michael J. Mack, Mark J. Krasna – 1974–1994

Swierenga (1974) developed thoracoscopic diagnosis of mediastinal tumors, and performed 200 thoracoscopies based on this indication. A positive diagnosis was made in a high percentage of cases [15]. Mack and Krasna published an atlas of thorascopic surgery with special reference to oncology [16].

There were many attempts made to diagnose pathological entities in the abdominal and thorax cavities, but the limitation of the Nitze optical system was problematic and therefore did not gain wide acceptance.

1.7 Illumination – *Heinrich Lamm*

Light was a great problem with those small miniature filament globes, which worked through a rheostat. If we did not have enough light, we would ask the nurse to "crank it up." The globes burn out, the instrument had to be withdrawn, and the globe exchanged and reintroduced, which was not easy for the patient in case of a cystoscopy or a bronchoscopy. A great breakthrough was made by a gynecologist, Lamm, in 1930, who put fiber threads in a bundle (10–20 μm in size) and bent it and was able to transmit, even in this position, light. In other words, he was able to use a larger external light source and transmit light to a remote point, even if the line was not straight (Fig. 1.2). This phenomenon was not recognized for endoscopy until 1950 [17]. Today, the overwhelming majority of rigid or flexible endoscopes have a light guide fiber bundle, which creates a much more convenient illumination. It is true that light loss through the light guide and endoscope fiber light guides is significant, but it is still more practical to work with an external light source.

The other breakthrough in lighting systems was the light source itself. A variety of filament globes with

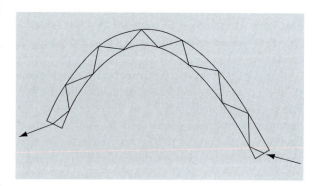

Fig. 1.2 Principles of light transmission through a bent fiber bundle: published by Heinrich Lamm in 1930. This idea replaced 30 years later the distal globes with an external light source and a flexible fiber light transmitter

condenser lenses and mirrors were built creating enormous heat. This was followed by the quartz glass arc globe, which gave a significant amount of light with proper color temperature, but the heat reduction here, too, was significant.

The size was large and had to be placed in a stainless steel cover in case of an explosion. Finally, a 1-in. miniature Xenon arc globe light source in a ceramic explosion proof housing was found, which was tested and released in 1975 [18]. Today, every endoscopic manufacturer is still using the same light source. The advantages are good color, temperature, high intensity, small size, safety, and ease of use. Light is crucial for any endoscopic procedure.

1.8 Image Transmission – *Harold Hopkins, Basil Isaac Hirschowitz, Shigeto Ikeda, Wolff WI, Shinya H*

The real breakthrough was, of course, the improvements in image transmission. In the rigid section (telescopes) we had Nitze system for decades which somehow was improved but still the absorption of the light was significant (over 90%). There were problems with the image quality at the edges, difficulties in recording and manufacturing. Harold Hopkins, a physicist in London (later Professor of Physics at University of Redding, UK) invented two major contributions.

- A flexible image-transmitting system based on fiber microthreads properly arranged, which was published in 1955 (Fig. 1.3). This system created the area of modern gastroscopy, colonoscopy, bronchoscopy, ERCP, and other flexible instruments. Without this invention, we would have been greatly set back in the diagnosis of malignancies of the upper and lower GI tracts and the extra hepatic biliary system and pancreatic organs [19].
- A similar breakthrough was achieved with the Hopkins (rigid) rod lens system, which opened new vistas in diagnostic and therapeutic diagnostic procedures [20] (Fig. 1.4).

In reality, Hopkins' two inventions, the flexible image and the new rigid image guiding system, created new chapters of endoscopic diagnosis and treatment of oncologic entities.

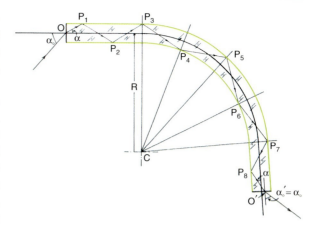

Fig. 1.3 The basic principle of the Hopkins flexible fiber image transmission through a fiber thread: If the 6–10 μm fiber threads are in a bundle but assorted (coherent), an image can be transmitted. The next generations of flexible fiberscopes were based on this innovation

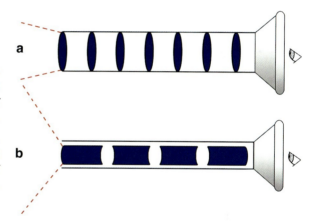

Fig. 1.4 Schematic diagram of telescopes: (**a**) The classic (slightly improved) Nitze's idea. Small little lenses are placed in certain air intervals, resulting in a dim image because of the significant (light) absorption. The scope has a narrow viewing angle and was difficult to manufacture. (**b**) The air interspace is replaced by glass rods. Results: Brighter image with more resolution, wider viewing angle, larger image, easier orientation, and smaller diameter

Hirschowitz published his first results of the endoscopic exploration of the esophagus, stomach, and duodenum, including the possibility of taking tissue samples in 1958 and 1963. Today, this examination plays a leading role in early diagnosis as well as in staging of upper GI malignancies [21, 22].

In 1962, Ikeda et al. introduced the flexible bronchoscope. This new instrument made it possible to visualize the bronchial tree and to perform aimed biopsies under visual control. It was a great help to thoracic oncologists in diagnosing and staging certain lung disorders [23].

This was followed by the flexible colonoscopic examination of the colon by Wolff and Shinya in 1973, who taught us to remove a colonic polyp without exploration. A huge number of patients escaped unnecessary open colectomies. It became an important tool of diagnosing, assessing, and staging colonic malignancies [24].

A few years later after the introduction of UGI, flexible instruments with a lateral view were designed to explore the extrahepatic biliary system and the pancreatic ducts [25, 26]. Further refinement of instruments took the flexible endoscopic examination with improved image quality and instrumentation to new treatment modalities.

Hopkins invented the rod lens system, which replaced the almost century old Nitze telescope. He replaced the air interval with glass rods, which resulted in a brighter and detailed image (resolution), which is crucial in endoscopic observation, and increased contrast, which improves the assessment of inflammatory components and smaller lesions (Figs. 1.5 and 1.6).

Nitze would have been happy and proud to see or to read the results of the Hopkins cyst scope and the recto scope in 1969 [27]. It was a particular help in transitional cell carcinomas of the bladder, where previously with the old system and poor vision it was difficult to take accurate biopsies or remove smaller lesions without the hazard of perforating the bladder.

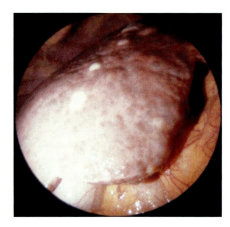

Fig. 1.6 Hopkins rod lens telescope: Laparoscopic photograph from a left lobe of the liver with metastases

This was followed by the opening of a larger number of laparoscopic explorations of the abdominal cavity. It is true that it started 37 years ago already indicating the importance of diagnosing and staging oncology cases. The gynecologists were the first discipline who at an early stage of laparoscopy praised the value of this procedure [28]. It is surprising that it took the general surgeons decades to get the message that a large number of diagnostic open surgeries could have been avoided [29, 30]. Finally, it took a well-deserved place in the armamentarium of the surgical oncologists. Needless to say, the brilliant image, fine details, and additional bonus of recording possibilities contributed to wider acceptance. Thoracoscopy followed oncology in endoscopically exploring lung cancer cases, combined with mediastinoscopy for staging or to determine whether the disease entity allowed thoracoscopic removal of lobes or lungs [15, 16].

In general, endoscopic exploration added a significant advantage to patient care because of the shorter hospitalization, less postoperative discomfort, and faster returns to activities. It became a patient's demanded operation.

1.9 From Vision to Television – *Soulas A., Dubois De Montreynaud*

Five decades ago, a French Endoscopy group discovered that improved recording is of crucial importance. Using a Nitze-type optical system, more light was

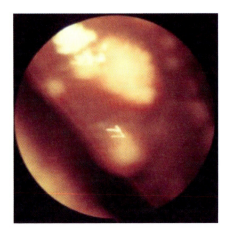

Fig. 1.5 Old telescope by the author (GB) in 1959: Laparoscopic photograph of a right liver lobe metastases

required to obtain a photo or a television image. Therefore, they introduced a 2-mm rigid quartz rod, which has superb light-carrying parameters (more light than we are producing today). A small little 15-W projector globe in an air-cooled housing projected through a prism and a condenser lens the light into the quartz rod and body cavity. Outstanding 16-mm movie film strips of high quality were produced. Unfortunately, this light transmission system could be attached only to a rigid endoscope. It has to be handled very carefully, because it breaks easily. It drew a lot of attention to see superb films from the pathology [31]. Television at the time was at a very early stage. Soulas, in 1956 [32], reported the first televised bronchoscopy showing the inside of the lung using a 150-lb Orthicon camera (Fig. 1.7). It was a real performance but it clearly predicted the vision that looking through a monocular eyepiece, holding the scope with one hand, having only the other hand "free" does not work. Having no coordinating assistant was another disadvantage. It was clear that if they can produce a smaller and better television camera, the method of choice would be to observe the procedure from a large screen, at a convenient distance with both eyes. Montreynaud used a 20-lb Vidicon camera for the same reason [31]. My research team at the University Department of Surgery Melbourne (Australia) designed and produced the first miniature endoscopic television camera: diameter 45 mm, length 120 mm, weight 350 g (12 oz) (Fig. 1.8). Fortunately, it was only a monochrome or black and white display and did not generate many followers [33]. It was clear to us that television is one of the major issues of the future success of endoscopic procedures. With the Hopkins rod lens system, we had an optical transmitter, which permitted more light and better image to be obtained and gave us hope for future developments. We changed from the Vidicon cameras to the Charged Coupled Devices (CCDs), which became smaller and smaller and more sensitive. During the years, television technique became a central part of endoscopic procedures. There is no question that we would have been unable to extend the activities to more complex procedures, and to perform laparoscopies, hysterectomies, colectomies, prostatectomies, lobectomies, or liver resections, just to mention a few, without TV. The ability to have a coordinated four-hand approach observing an enlarged excellent image and ability to teach are dominant advantages. It is also important that the OR team, including the scrub nurse, sees what is going on and what is needed. The value of recording cannot be underestimated starting a couple of decades ago with the 16-mm movie film,

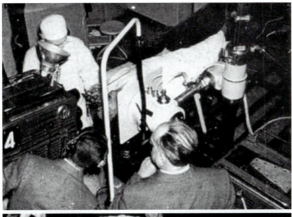
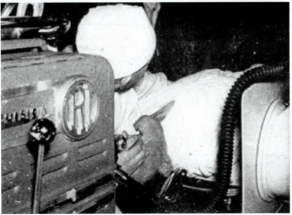

Fig. 1.7 The first published Television bronchoscopy by Soulas in 1956 TV camera: Orthicon tube, black and white display, and 150 lb in weight.

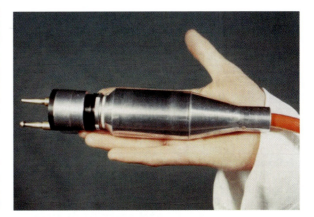

Fig. 1.8 The first miniature endoscopic TV Vidicon tube camera (1962) Diameter 45 mm, length 120 mm, weight 350 g, monochrome display

continuing with the VHS and ending up today with the DVD, particularly in documenting the findings of malignant lesions as well as the teaching value [34]. The recent advantages of using the distal (video) chip technique instead of a fiber image bundle improved the image quality. The future probably lies in the evolution of the distal chip CCD technology and particularly the new C-Mos technique to place a chip at the distal end of the scope.

High definition (HDTV) is in its infancy, but with further developments in display, recording, and electronic refinements, higher resolution, magnification, and excellent color reproduction can play a role in observing a better image with easier perception, which could be a great contribution to the endoscopic diagnosis in treatment modalities of oncology cases.

With this large number of invention coordination developments, we were able to report a more important role of endoscopy in cancer patients. The superfast speed of technology dictates that there will come a time in the near future when we can have a super-endo-confocal-microscope, which will perhaps provide histological tissue diagnosis on the spot, or perhaps can even deliver a therapeutic modality to the individual malignant cell.

We came a long way since Nitze and his followers joined the historical and early period of endoscopy.

References

1. Bozzini, P.H.: Lichtleiter, eine Erfindung zur Anschauung innerer Teile und Krankheiten. J. Prak. Heilk. **24**, 107 (1806)
2. Desormeaux, A.J.: Endoscope and its application to the diagnosis and treatment of the genitor-urinary passages. Chicago. Med. J. **24**, 177–194 (1867)
3. Kussmaul, J.: Uber Magenspiegelung. Verh Naturforschenden Ges. Freiburg. **5**, 112 (1870)
4. Morgenstern, L.: A tale of two telescopes: far in and far out. Surg. Innov. **14**(1), 7–8 (2007)
5. Nitze, M.: Beobachtungs and Untersuchungsmethode fur Harnrohre Harnblase und Rectum. Wien. Med. Wochenschr. **24**, 651 (1879)
6. McCallum, R.W., Berci, G.: Laparoscopy in hepatic disease. Gastroint. Endosc. **23**, 20–24 (1976)
7. Rosenheim, T.: Uber gastroskopie. Klin. Wochenschr. **13**, 275 (1896)
8. Schindler, R.: Gastroscopy with a flexible gastroscope. Am. J. Digest. Dis. Nutr. **2**, 656 (1936)
9. Lange, F.: Meltzing: Die Photography des Mageninnern. Münch. Med. Wochenschr. **50**, 1585 (1898)
10. Jacobaeus, H.C.: Ueber die Moglichkeit die Zystoskopie bei Untersuchung seroser Hohlungen anzuwenden. Münch. Med. Wochenschr. **57**, 2090–2092 (1910)
11. Kelling, G.: Zur Colioskopie. Arch. Klin. Chir. **126**, 226–229 (1923)
12. Kalk, H.: Erfahrungen mit der Laparoskopie. Z. Klin. Med. **111**, 303–348 (1929)
13. Kalk, H., Bruhl, W.: Leitfaden der Laparoskopie und Gastroskopie. Stuttgart, Thieme (1951)
14. Ruddock, J.C.: Peritoneoscopy: a critical clinical review. Surg. Clin. North Am. **37**, 1249 (1957)
15. Swierenga, J.: Thoracoscopy, Chap. 52. In: Berci, G. (ed.) Endoscopy. Appleton-Century-Crofts, New York (1976)
16. Mack, M.J., Krasna, M.J.: Thorascopic Surgery. Quality Medical Publishing, St. Louis (1994)
17. Lamm, H.: Biegsame optische Geraete. Z. Instr. **50**, 579 (1930)
18. Olson, V.: Light sources, Chap. 3. In: Berci, G. (ed.) Endoscopy, pp. 64–69. Appleton-Century-Crofts, New York (1976)
19. Hopkins, H.H., Kapany, N.S.: A flexible fiberscope, using static scanning. Nature **173**, 39–41 (1954)
20. Hopkins, H.H.: Optical principles of the endoscope, Chap. 1. In: Berci, G. (ed.) Endoscopy, pp. 3–27. Appleton-Century-Crofts, New York (1976)
21. Hirschowitz, B.I.: A fibre optic flexible oesophago-gastroscope. Lancet **2**, 338 (1963)
22. Hirschowitz, B.I., Curtis, L.E., Peters, C.W., Pollard, H.M.: Demonstration of a new gastroscope: "the fiberscope" Gastroenterology **35**, 50 (1958)
23. Ikeda, S., Yanai, N., Ishikawa, S.: Flexible bronchofiberscope. Keio J. Med. **17**, 1 (1968)
24. Wolff, W.I., Shinya, H.: A new approach to colonic polyps. Ann. Surg. **178**, 367 (1973)
25. Oi, I., Kobayashi, S., Kondo, T.: Endoscopic pancreatocholangiography. Endoscopy **2**, 103 (1970)
26. Oi, I., Takemoto, T., Nakayama, K.: "Fiberduodenoscopy" – early diagnosis of cancer of the papilla of Vater. Surgery **67**, 561 (1970)
27. Berci, G., Kont, L.A: A new optical endoscope with special reference to cystoscopy. Br. J. Urol. **41**, 564–571 (1969)
28. Reich, H., McGlynn, F., Wilkie, W.: Laparoscopic management of stage I ovarian cancer. J. Reprod. Med. **35**, 601–605 (1990)
29. Berci, G.: Laparoscopy in oncology, Chap. 4. In: Surgical oncology Arnold, New York (2002)
30. Mikulicz, J.: Uber Gastroskopie und Osophagoskopie. Wien. Med. Presse. **45**, 1405 (1881)
31. Montreynaud, J.M., Bruneau, Y., Jomain, J.: Traite Pratique de Photography et de Cinematography Medicales. Montel, Paris (1960)
32. Soulas, A.: Televised bronchoscopy. Presse Méd. **64**, 97 (1956)
33. Berci, G., Davids, J.: Endoscopy and television. Br. Med. J. **1**, 1610 (1962)
34. Berci, G., Schwaitzberg, D.: The importance of understanding the basics of imaging in the era of high tech endoscopy. Logic, reality and utopia Part II. Surg. Endosc. **16**, 1518–1523 (2002)

2 Evolution of Minimally Invasive Surgery and Its Impact on Surgical Residency Training

Adrian E. Park and Tommy H. Lee

2.1 Introduction

Upon reflection, it is remarkable how little has been written on the subject of the evolution of minimally invasive surgery (MIS). It is likely that history will judge the impact of MIS on patient-care practices and healthcare economics on par with the introduction of antibiotics for surgical patients.

As we are frequently reminded in the American popular press, the first wave of the approximately 79 million "Baby Boomers" turns 65 in 2011, thus becoming eligible for healthcare benefits under Medicare [1]. Imagine for a moment a scenario in which there had occurred no MIS revolution and, therefore, no MIS approaches to common surgical disorders existed. In this day of healthcare funding crises and limited hospital bed access, if cholecystectomy potentially still required a 4- to 6-day hospital stay and 4- to 6-week postoperative recuperation and paraesophageal hiatal hernia repairs occasioned a 7- to 10-day hospital stay and 6- to 8-week recovery period, our current volumes of patients – let alone the anticipated infusion of senior citizens – could not possibly be accommodated within such a strained system. The advent of MIS has been most fortuitous on many levels.

In its most recent incarnation, MIS is only about 20 years old. Despite laparoscopy having been described more than a century ago [2] and practiced to some degree over the intervening years, the introduction of laparoscopic cholecystectomy (LC) by Phillip Mouret in 1987 is largely credited with launching the revolution in MIS with which most readers will be familiar [3]. The purist will insist that Muhe, in fact, performed the first truly minimally invasive cholecystectomy in 1985 [4].

These remarkable procedures were first reported on North American shores by 1988. Although many surgeons' imaginations were captured by the possibilities that the new techniques promised, the response of the surgical "establishment" and "academic surgery" was largely that of viewing MIS as surgical heresy, to be spurned! Thus, LC was first learned and practiced and promulgated in the US by community or private practice surgeons. Patients soon took notice of LC and voted with their feet en masse to have the procedure done.

Such a manner of introduction of a new technique or technology into the surgical mainstream was a marked departure from historical practice. Whether or not advances in surgical care and practice can or should only originate in academic centers is not this chapter's argument; however, the lack of effective, deliberate, coordinated oversight that accompanied the introduction of LC to North American practice brought with it many foreseeable problems.

More than a decade earlier, Fineberg had stated, "It is crucial that a process is identified by which the rate of diffusion of technologies is controlled by evidence related to their costs and benefits" [5]. It is certainly fair to say that no such evidence existed at the time that LC was being widely adopted in the United States (US). Historically, new techniques or technologies that had been developed in academic surgical centers emerged having been built on a foundation of basic research-derived knowledge and early clinical work that had occurred under the strict aegis of an

---

A.E. Park (✉) and T.H. Lee
Department of Surgery, University of Maryland Medical Center, 22 South Greene Street – Room S4B14, Baltimore, MD 21201-1595, USA
e-mail: apark@smail.umaryland.edu

institutional review board with its requisite accountabilities. Furthermore, these new techniques were taught or trained in the context of a surgical residency or fellowship where oversight through apprenticeship was the model.

Such a model of development and training through the failing of no particular party did not greet the dissemination of LC in the US. Private practice surgeons, referred to as the "early adopters" [6], had neither the resources nor the time to set up comprehensive training programs. The academic surgical establishment, for the most part, perceived both LC and MIS as "passing fads" over which they had little control and with which they had not been adequately engaged early enough to contribute significantly either in terms of training or dissemination of the techniques [6].

2.2 Recognizing the Need for Training, Proctoring, and Preceptoring

As a result, there arose in short order a great unmet need for training in LC and other MIS techniques. It is estimated that between 1990 and 1992, approximately 15,000 general surgeons in the US were trained in LC [2]. Most of the training was accomplished without any form of recognized oversight or accreditation by means of "short courses" involving animal labs. Predictably, there followed a spike of surgical misadventures and an increased rate of common bile duct injury [7]. It was soon apparent that the "weekend" or short course without ongoing proctoring was not the optimal training format for the adoption of these new techniques. The inadequacies of such a surgical educational model were well described by Rogers et al. [8]. There is, however, evidence that by adding a disciplined regimen of proctoring and preceptoring of cases to the successful completion of a short course, a surgeon could safely assimilate a new laparoscopic technique into his or her practice [9]. Even so, there remained further training challenges to address, such as who would fund such a labor-intensive process? Could proctors or preceptors perform their role via telesurgery? If so, how were issues of liability and licensing requirements to be addressed? Many of these questions remain unanswered.

2.3 Competency in Laparoscopic Training During Surgical Residency in the US

In time, academic surgical centers recognized that this new field of surgery was here to stay and began a process of "catch up" that is still underway. Clearly, the most ideal framework within which to teach and train MIS techniques was the surgical residency program. This, obviously, would not meet the needs of that large cohort of surgeons who were out in practice without the benefit of learning MIS during their residency training. More than a decade following the introduction of MIS techniques to North America, Park et al. conducted a national survey of MIS and surgical education leaders to determine how much progress had been made in residency training of MIS techniques [10]. It was determined that (over a range of 13 laparoscopic procedures) American surgical residency programs did not meet the MIS case volumes required for competency as determined by experts. Five years later in 2007, residents were still performing far fewer cases on average [11] than what was felt necessary for competence in a poll of 2006 MIS fellows [12]. In fact, with the exception of LC, in which residents had more than adequate case volumes (average 103.1 cases for a graduating chief in 2007, compared with the 35.6 thought needed for competency by 2006 MIS fellows), for no other procedures was the average resident exposure/case volume close to the required numbers set by the fellows themselves to attain competence. This was the case even for operations such as fundoplication for which a laparoscopic approach is undisputedly the standard of care – graduating chiefs in 2007 performed 4.6 on average, while the competence standard was estimated at 22.0 by fellows in 2006. Among the conclusions of these studies were proposals for the development of a national MIS skills curriculum and the development and recruitment of MIS expert faculty to train residents and identification of the need to move training out of the operating room (OR) through new methodologies and technologies such as simulation to address the ongoing deficit in resident training in MIS.

2.4 Fellowship Council and Advanced MIS Postgraduate Training

Fortunately, a great deal of intentional progress in the provision of minimally invasive training, as this chapter will specify, has been made over the subsequent years. While much in terms of laparoscopic education has been instituted within residency programs, a telling and important development has been the emergence of the Fellowship Council (FC), dedicated to bring order to the chaos of postgraduate advanced gastrointestinal (GI) surgery and MIS training. As larger numbers of graduating general surgical residents began to pursue fellowship training to gain adequate exposure to and experience with MIS, there arose tandem efforts to bring standards, accreditation, and a "match" to that process [13]. These efforts came to maturity in the form of the FC, a coalescence to work toward the ends of the stake-holding surgical societies: The Society of American Gastrointestinal and Endoscopic Surgeons (SAGES), The Society for Surgery of the Alimentary Tract (SSAT), The American Hepato-Pancreato-Biliary Association (AHPBA), and the American Society for Metabolic and Bariatric Surgery (ASMBS). Currently, the estimate is that one quarter of all graduating general surgery residents engage in the application process for an FC-sanctioned GI/MIS fellowship [11, 14]. This suggests that American surgical residency programs have still not consistently bridged the deficit in MIS training; otherwise, surgical residents would not still be "voting with their feet" in such large numbers.

2.5 Development of Resident Education Guidelines for Basic and Advanced Laparoscopy

On a more positive note, it should be emphasized that a movement is afoot nationally to bring coherence and focus to the challenge of surgical training in the era of rapid technology development and technique progression. The benefits promised by this movement will accrue not just to surgical residents but also to practicing surgeons. The ultimate benefits, of course, will be to enhance patient safety and outcomes. Within this movement, the resources and efforts being directed toward a few initiatives in particular are worth examination: standardized curricular development, objective metrics establishment for surgical performance/competence assessment, transfer of training, and simulation's role in surgical training. These will be the foci of the remainder of this chapter.

In 1998 (with a 2009 revision), the Resident Education Committee of SAGES published resident education guidelines for basic and advanced laparoscopy. Intended to aid program directors in planning an educational curriculum, these guidelines recommended starting with the acquisition of a core group of technical skills. The safe learning and refinement of these skills prior to OR deployment would be accomplished through use of surgical trainers, animal models, virtual reality (VR) trainers, or other simulated operating conditions housed within skills laboratories, the recommended learning environment [15]. Simulation came to the fore, showing promise as a gateway technology in terms of providing both objective metrics and training transfer, characteristics that among others continue to secure its role as a primary tool in the armamentarium of minimally invasive surgical training [16].

2.6 Simulation Training

2.6.1 General Remarks

In laparoscopic skill acquisition, many of the initial challenges are related to a loss of depth perception, the fulcrum effect, and the use of new, unfamiliar instruments. Certainly, the first time one is faced with these challenges should not be when working on a living patient, and it seems reasonable that as much skill acquisition as possible should be moved out of the OR and into arenas where mistakes do not compromise patient safety.

At the mid-point of the 1990s, the view that simulation was a technology promising both as a tool for laparoscopic training and as a cornerstone of the OR of the future began to take hold [17–19]. Although objective evidence is relatively sparse, there is no question that simulation must be an important part of education for the future. What remains in question, however, is what type of simulator and what will simulation's part in training be.

Simulators and training models, for the most part, fall into three broad categories:

- Virtual reality (VR) trainers
- Box or mechanical trainers
- Biological models

Use of animal models for skill acquisition allows the trainee to work with tissue prior to doing so surgically in a human. Few places, however, have either ready lab access or the monetary resources necessary to make animal models a regular part of a training curriculum. Additionally, there are ethical considerations in regard to acquiring technical skills by regularly using live animals. For over 100 years, for instance, since the 1876 enactment of the Cruelty to Animals Act, the performance of surgical procedures on live animals has been prohibited in Great Britain.

2.6.2 Reliability and Validation

Although mechanical and VR trainers are increasingly relied on in surgical teaching programs, validation studies have been limited. Proving the value of a trainer means demonstrating the reliability of its associated tests and metrics. Reliability is the degree to which consistent results are obtained each time the test is used. Validation is the next step and it is here that surgical literature is most lacking. In its simplest form, validity refers to whether a test actually measures what it purports to do. The depths and breadths to which such assessments are proven subdivide validity into dozens of subcategories.

2.6.2.1 Face Validity

Face validity assesses only whether a test "looks" as if it will measure what it claims to – a basic and subjective measure at best.

2.6.2.2 Content Validity

Content validity ascertains if test content truly is representative of what a test claims to measure. A test capable of maintaining its results across varied settings, procedures, and participants is said to have external validity. Three validities – concurrent, construct, predictive – address actual participant skills in meaningful ways.

2.6.2.3 Concurrent and Construct Validity

Concurrent validity establishes that a test is able to measure accurately the skill level of a test-taker at the time of the test, and construct validity presents proof that a test is able to differentiate subjects by their skill levels. Demonstrating correlation with performance in the real world – predictive validity – is in terms of training usefulness, the most important while also the most difficult to determine and least reported.

2.6.3 Mechanical or Box Trainers

For basic and demanding skills associated with MIS, a variety of simple to complex physical objects, referred to as mechanical trainers, can be used for the purpose of simulated learning (Fig. 2.1). Another common method for introducing such skills to trainees is that of using a simple box-trainer comprising essentially the same equipment as would be found in the OR. These trainers come in various forms, but the basic components are the same – an enclosure with integrated skill

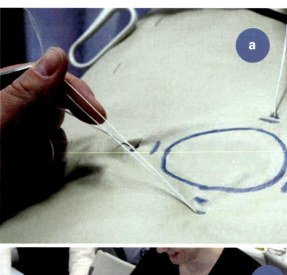

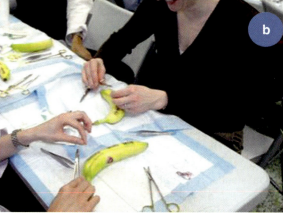

Fig. 2.1 Two instances of mechanical model use: (**a**) Physical abdominal model used for training the technique of placing transfascial sutures. (**b**) Students trained in open suturing using bananas

or task components, a camera system, and a light source. The cheapest and simplest of these training options are constructed from a simple plastic or cardboard box, a webcam, and a computer display [20–22]. On the high end, some mechanical trainers consisting of an actual laparoscope with accompanying fiberoptic light source and display are available (Fig. 2.2). Tasks to be practiced and perfected with the use of simulators can be as simple as moving laparoscopic instruments along a piece of rope in a fashion similar to that practiced with bowel or as sophisticated as actual procedural mock-ups.

2.6.3.1 Reliability and Validation

Demonstrations of the validities and reliability of box trainers are commonplace in clinical literature. One of the earliest examples demonstrating validity in surgical education is the Objective Structured Assessment of Technical Skill (OSATS). OSATS, developed initially for use in the open surgical environment, utilizes bench tasks, the performance of which surgeon-observers using task-specific checklists rate and also assign a global rating to. Its reliability and construct validity were initially established in 1996 [23]. OSATS and other variants that rely on procedure-related checklists have become common teaching tools in the assessment of surgical trainees [24, 25].

2.6.3.2 McGill Inanimate System for Training and Evaluation of Laparoscopic Skills (MISTELS)

The best studied of the mechanical box trainers designed specifically for laparoscopic surgery, the McGill Inanimate System for Training and Evaluation of Laparoscopic Skills (MISTELS) now also forms the basis of the Fundamentals of Laparoscopic Surgery (FLS) training and assessment system (Fig. 2.3). In a trainer-box environment, MISTELS allows performance practice and acquisition of five basic laparoscopic exercises, scored for both efficiency (time) and precision. The validity of MISTELS has been demonstrated on multiple levels. Two 1998 reports introducing MISTELS provided evidence of the simulator's construct validity [26] and substantiated it with additional research [27]. Studies confirming MISTELS' construct and establishing its concurrent validities have also appeared [28–32] as has evidence of its predictive and face validity [33]. Additionally, the reliability of MISTELS has been described [34].

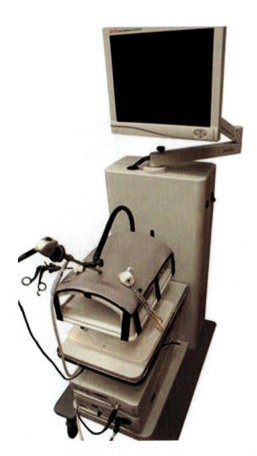

Fig. 2.2 The ergonomically designed Park training stand and box (San Jose, USA)

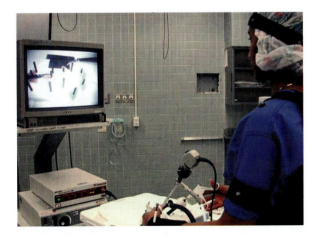

Fig. 2.3 Performance of FLS in a traditional laparoscopic box skills trainer

2.6.3.3 Limitations of Box Trainers

Box trainers in comparison to VR trainers are relatively cheap with both providing similar access to basic skills practice (Fig. 2.4). Box trainers do necessitate some ongoing costs as they use consumable materials and require maintenance. The complexity of tasks performable in a box trainer is limited since tasks requiring cutting, clipping, or suturing generally damage these models irreversibly, making them mostly single-use only. The limitations in regard to single usage and inability to accommodate practice of complex tasks dictate the impracticality of high-cost box trainers. When box trainers are low-cost overall, use very inexpensive consumables, are reusable, and are primarily for practice of simple tasks, they make satisfactory single-use models.

2.6.4 Virtual Reality

VR simulation has been made possible by ongoing advances in computer power and technology. In comparison to even the simplest biologic system, man-made machines such as automobiles and airplanes have proven easy to model accurately. Vehicle VR simulators are increasingly realistic, while VR simulators in surgery still provide very crude approximations of life in most cases. The first VR surgical simulators had limited or absent tactile (haptic) feedback, and this type of simulator continues to have a strong presence today. MIST-VR (Mentice, Göteborg, Sweden), built on the Virtual Laparoscopic Interface hardware platform from Immersion Medical Inc (Gaithersburg, USA), is one of the first and probably the most widely known of these simulators. The Virtual Laparoscopic Interface continues to be the platform for several simulators currently in use today, such as LapSim (Surgical Science, Göteborg, Sweden) – which was recently investigated by Aggarwal et al. [35] in a study that demonstrated that its proficiency-based curriculum of basic tasks at varying difficulties shortened the learning curve of a laparoscopic procedure, specifically a porcine cholecystectomy.

2.6.4.1 Limitations and Challenges of Virtual Reality Simulation

While VR simulations are visually becoming increasingly life-like, with image-quality approaching photo-realism (Fig. 2.5), the development of interface

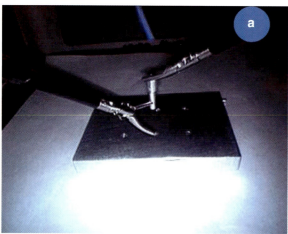
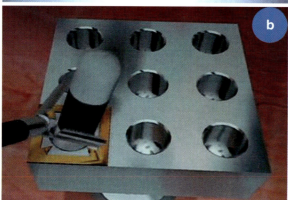

Fig. 2.4 The same basic laparoscopic skill performed in (**a**) Basic trainer box and (**b**) VR simulator

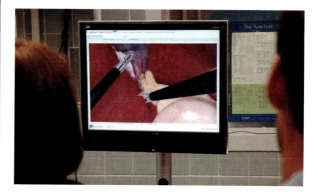

Fig. 2.5 Screen shot of students performing a cholecystectomy in a VR trainer

technology that provides users with haptic feedback lags. Haptics do not yet convey well the real anatomic situation [36]. Challenges to creating a realistic virtual environment include the modeling of tissue properties, rendering of the flow dynamics of hemorrhage and smoke, and simulating the operating environment on a larger scale including components such as patient physiology, personnel, and equipment. [37] Additionally, although the technological developments being made are exciting, true scientific evidence in support of VR simulators is still lacking overall. For this reason, VR simulation, though it holds great promise for the future, is not yet ready for wholesale incorporation into mainstream surgical curricula.

2.6.4.2 Comparison Between Virtual Reality, Box Trainer, and Their Impact in Clinical Practice

Whatever claims – positive or not – are bandied about in terms of types or models of simulators, the ultimate considerations must be how effectively and successfully they contribute to the acquisition of laparoscopic or other surgical skills. To date, no single type of trainer has been demonstrated to be superior to the other. In fact, one recent systematic review of the spectrum of surgical simulators, covering VR, video simulation (defined as box trainers with simple tasks), and model simulation (defined as box trainers with anatomic models) by Sutherland et al. [38] ultimately concluded that no single training method was consistently superior to the others. Their review, however, was limited by the tremendous heterogeneity of the current published literature. Nonetheless, a few trends emerged. VR training was found to be superior to no training and to standard training, although the benefits over the latter were less pronounced. Compared to training on a video simulator (box trainer with simple tasks), VR was neither consistently better nor worse. Surprisingly, video simulation did not show a consistent advantage over either no training or standard training. Again however, this heterogeneity is likely due to the broad range of simulators and training standards currently in use. Similarly, model simulation also had mixed results. No "gold standard" has been established in laparoscopic training; therefore, the methodologies compared in studies tend to be chosen arbitrarily. No research has yet established a relationship between simulation training and improved patient outcomes. For the time being, their educational contributions must be measured in terms of their capabilities to provide objective performance metrics and to assure that simulated training once acquired is transferable to the OR.

2.7 Objective Metrics

Objective metrics, when obtainable, provide certainty toward assessment of progress of trainee proficiency and competency in addition to the continuance of acquired skills. In little more than a decade, interest and research have considerably expanded and improved reliable, objective metrics. A measure of success has been enjoyed by two similarly computer-controlled objective evaluation tools.

2.7.1 ICSAD and ADEPT

- Imperial College Surgical Assessment Device (ICSAD)
- Advanced Dundee Endoscopic Psychomotor Tester (ADEPT) [39–42]

The evaluative data accumulated by ICSAD, for example, are focused on the time taken and the distance covered by a surgeon's hands as they are engaged in the performance of basic surgical tasks or an actual procedure. Additionally, ICSAD has claimed the number of hand movements in surgical performance as a qualitative objective performance measurement although that has been challenged [43]. Other systems of metric acquisition include the Blue Dragon and its successor the Red Dragon, which in addition to instrument movement measure the torque and force applied by a surgeon during laparoscopic tasks [44, 45].

2.7.2 Measuring Performance in the Operating Room – GOALS

Measuring performance in the OR in a reliable, unobtrusive fashion can be done using assessment instruments such as the Global Operative Assessment of

Laparoscopic Skills (GOALS) rating scale described by Vassiliou et al. [46]. Developed for the assessment of cholecystectomy performance, GOALS utilizes a combination of a five-item global rating scale, a ten-item task checklist, and two visual analogue scales (one for competence and the other for difficulty). GOALS has been successfully used to differentiate novices from more experienced surgeons [47] and is potentially adaptable to other laparoscopic procedures.

2.8 Transfer of Training

Transfer of training refers to whether acquiring proficiency in one task is of benefit in developing proficiency in another related, possibly more complex task. Issues of transfer of training are particularly germane in two aspects of teaching MIS. The first relates to whether open surgical skills carry over to laparoscopic skills. Figert et al. [48] found no correlation between the amount of open surgical experience and laparoscopic suturing performance in residents. This highlights the important of training specifically targeting laparoscopic skills.

Transfer of training is again an important consideration when examining the benefit of various simulators currently in use. Studies tying simulator practice to skills transferable to the OR have steadily proliferated though the need for such proof is far from satisfied. Transfer of training has been seen in regard to both box trainers (Fig. 2.6) and VR simulators [37, 49–52]. The endpoints for these studies are heterogeneous, ranging from tasks in a live animal model to performance in a real human OR. This highlights the lack of a consensus metric or technique of assessing "real" operative performance – a significant challenge yet to be overcome.

2.9 Work-hour Restrictions

Medical work-hour restrictions are becoming increasingly enforced around the world. Surgical trainees in the US are now limited to working 80 h per week. Although the literature on this topic continues to grow, thus far the 80-h work week has been found to have no measurable impact on the quality of patient care [53]. Concerns persist, however, that trainee education will be hampered by the 80-h regulation. Diminishment of exposure to real clinical scenarios increases the importance of considering and proving simulation training as a viable alternative. Still, residents must be motivated to use their own time in simulator practice as it may fall outside of the 80-h work week. In a survey of resident perception of simulator training, Boyd et al. [54] found that a majority of residents felt that such training should be mandatory (though it should be considered that this was the answer given by 75% of the junior residents and only 27% of the senior residents). Furthermore, junior residents ranked simulation training as the best way to learn new skills, whereas seniors preferred proctorship.

2.10 Cost Considerations

Surgical training costs money, space, and time. Money must be available to purchase simulators, there must be space to train and practice, and surgical instructors must make time for their trainees. Mounting evidence supporting the efficacy of laparoscopic skills training outside of the OR should encourage improved support resulting in increased amounts of educational resources. Ideally, the specific advantages and disadvantages of each type of simulator suggest that some exposure to each would likely be of benefit to the trainee. When working with limited resources, however, simulator training of basic laparoscopic skills can be provided cost-effectively through creative and frugal use of materials. In fact, low-tech (and relatively inexpensive)

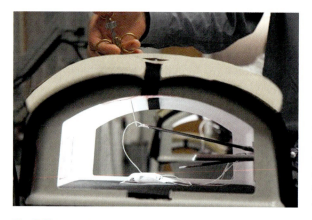

Fig. 2.6 Example of simulation aimed to improve transfer of suture passing technique to OR

simulators are at this date the best studied. Low costs make these simulators accessible and easily incorporated into most training programs. Berg et al. [55] described a yearly laparoscopic training cost of $982 per resident that included the price of constructing simulators by using combined materials of the type that could be found in research labs and retail stores or donated by industry. Similarly, Adrales et al. [56] described anatomic models constructed from inexpensive materials such as elastics for vessels and crinoline fabric for hernia mesh. Mirrors have also been described as low-cost alternatives to both cameras and monitors [57].

2.11 Value and Relevance of Simulator Training

The success of simulation training hinges on residents, in particular whether they trust its educational value and future relevance and believe that they will have opportunities to use the skills thus acquired in the OR during residency and practice. Trusting and believing thus are crucial attitudes in terms of determining whether residents will be motivated, as many believe they must use their own time for simulator practice. Few residents will see the benefit of mastering laparoscopic suturing in a training box, if they are never given the chance to suture in the OR. With limited time available, most residents will need to be able to reap the rewards of practice and training in the OR to realize the worth of their time spent in the simulation environment.

2.12 Cognitive Skills

In MIS, the process of decision-making occurs from the moment a patient is encountered, and continues as a diagnosis is made and surgical or other treatment is selected and performed. In the OR, as a surgeon proceeds through a case, many moment-to-moment decisions, including whether to convert to laparotomy, must be made. Tissues and planes must be identified, respected, and manipulated in an appropriate fashion. While there is a growing complement of educational tools for teaching the purely technical aspects of surgery (simulation exercises have in the majority been based on tasks most notable for their potential development of the basic hand–eye coordination necessary for performing laparoscopic procedures), surgery is more than simple technical skills. Indeed, it has been argued that learning is best facilitated when training in technical skills takes place in tandem with development of cognitive skills [42]. The cognitive aspects of decision-making, however, have largely been unaddressed in surgical training; when they have been, they are learned almost solely through patient care. In this instance, it is fortunate that risks to patients may be minimized by the careful supervision of an expert, who can correct unsound or poor decisions before the possibility of any adverse patient effects. Clinic discussions of a patient or active feedback presented in the OR are two of many ways that corrections can be offered. Learning as much as possible prior to or outside of direct clinical contact, one must remember, is of benefit to trainees as it allows them to optimize their time spent with patients.

In terms of teaching decision-making, simulators currently are hindered by their design, which specifically focuses on "how" rather than "why." We have a limited example of "why" decision-making incorporated into the mock-ups of real operative procedures described by Adrales et al. [56] where items such as appropriate respect for tissues is part of the trainee's evaluation. There is the promise that VR simulators will one day better incorporate the unpredictability that typifies the decision-making necessary in real surgical scenarios and will contain also the capacity to model larger portions of procedures. At this point, however, the fidelity of VR simulators is not adequate to capture the often very fine and subtle cues that generate inputs leading to surgical decision-making.

2.12.1 Maryland Virtual Patient (MVP)

There has been the development of a novel high-level simulation approach to teaching clinical decision-making – cognitive modeling. This type of simulation models the clinical pathways that are involved in disease presentation and management. An example of this type of simulation, which based on input from expert sources fosters trainee decision-making, is the Maryland Virtual Patient (MVP). The MVP simulates disease states in a patient and allows the user to perform diagnostic tests as well as interventions [58]. At the core of the MVP is an engine built around a unique ontology that organizes medical knowledge into a form that can be processed by a computer. A natural-language, artificial-intelligence-driven user interface creates an intuitive, realistic experience – albeit through a computer monitor and keyboard. This simulator has the potential to be combined with other simulators to create a larger, even more complete simulation. For example, combination with a VR trainer would allow trainees to not only medically diagnose and treat a patient but also simulate the appropriate surgery.

2.13 Laparoscopic Training: Current Status and Future Direction

Within residency training programs, there is a significant variability in available equipment and training practices, a disparity perhaps reflective of time and money limitations. Recent surveys by Kapadia et al. [59] and Gould [60] found that 80–90% of programs possessed skills labs. These numbers likely represent a very broad spectrum of what the training programs across the country possess. However, interpretation of their findings should be tempered by the fact that these were self-reporting, voluntary surveys and that their definitions of what constituted a "skills lab" were not necessarily consistent. Still, these studies hopefully reflect increasing awareness of and resource allocation to training labs.

Another promising undertaking is the accelerated effort to bring some standardization to both the teaching and simulation processes. A combined American College of Surgeons (ACS) and Association of Program Directors in Surgery (APDS) task force is currently in the midst of rolling out a standard national curriculum for residents in surgery. Scott and Dunnington recently published a description of this program [61]. This curriculum is conceptualized in three phases.

- *Phase I*: Focuses on basic skills ranging from asepsis and instrument handling to fashioning an anastomosis
- *Phase II*: Focuses on procedures (and is still under development)
- *Phase III*: Focuses on team-based training (and is still under development)

This curriculum is promising as a comprehensive whole as its incorporation of concepts in regard to teaching and assessing judgment augments technical skill acquisition.

Throughout this chapter, it has hopefully been apparent that the advent of MIS has not only revolutionized surgical patient care but has also ushered in a new era and focus on surgical training and residency training in particular. Considerations that include surgical simulation, the development of objective measures of surgical performance, and the way in which both will come together in a standard surgical curriculum should leave little doubt of the significant impact MIS has had on surgical residency training. The actual business of training surgeons and the related surgical research that will accompany these efforts promise to be compelling endeavors for the foreseeable future.

References

1. Cauchon, D.: Senior benefit costs up 24%: 'health care crisis' leads to 8-year rise. USA Today, pp. 1A–2A (February 14, 2008)
2. Soper, N.J., Brunt, L.M., Kerbl, K.: Laparoscopic general surgery. N. Engl. J. Med. **330**, 409–419 (1994)
3. Cuschieri, A., Dubois, F., Mouiel, J., et al.: The European experience with laparoscopic cholecystectomy. Am. J. Surg. **161**, 385–387 (1991)
4. Harrell, A.G., Heniford, B.T.: Minimally invasive abdominal surgery: lux et veritas past, present, future. Am. J. Surg. **190**, 239–243 (2005)
5. Cuschieri, A.: Whither minimal access surgery: tribulations and expectations. Am. J. Surg. **169**, 9–19 (1995)
6. Rogers, E.M.: Diffusions of Innovations, 5th edn. Free Press, New York (2003)
7. The Southern Surgeons Club: A prospective analysis of 1518 laparoscopic cholecystectomies. N. Engl. J. Med. **324**, 1073–1078 (1991)
8. Rogers, D.A., Elstein, A.S., Bordage, G.: Improving continuing medical education for surgical techniques: applying the lessons learned in the first decade of minimal access surgery. Ann. Surg. **233**, 159–166 (2001)
9. Heniford, B.T., Backus, C.L., Matthews, B.D., et al.: Optimal teaching environment for laparoscopic splenectomy. Am. J. Surg. **181**, 226–230 (2001)
10. Park, A., Witzke, D., Donnelly, M.: Ongoing deficits in resident training for minimally invasive surgery. J. Gastrointest. Surg. **6**, 501–509 (2002)
11. Department of Applications and Data Analysis: General surgery case logs: national data report. Accreditation Council

for Graduate Medical Education. http://www.acgme.org/acWebsite/RRC_440/reports/GSNatData0607.pdf (2007). Accessed 05 Nov 2010
12. Park, A., Kavic, S.M., Lee, T.H., et al.: Minimally invasive surgery: the evolution of fellowship. Surgery **142**, 505–513 (2007)
13. Swanstrom, L.L., Park, A., Arregui, M., et al.: Bringing order to the chaos: developing a matching process for minimally invasive and gastrointestinal postgraduate fellowships. Ann. Surg. **243**, 431–435 (2006)
14. The Fellowship Council Newsletter: Latest accreditation & match statistics. Fellowship Council. https://fellowship-council.org/documents/FC_news_fall07_web.pdf (2007). Accessed 05 Nov 2010
15. Resident Education Committee: SAGES curriculum outline for resident education. Society of American Gastrointestinal and Endoscopic Surgeons. www.sages.org/publications/publication-pdf.php?id=28 (2009). Accessed 05 Nov 2010
16. Segan, R.D., Park, A.E.: Training competent minimal access surgeons: review of tools, metrics, and techniques across the spectrum of technology. In: Szabo, Z., Coburg, A.J., Savalgi, R.S., et al. (eds.) Surgical Technology International XIII, pp. 25–32. Universal Medical Press, San Francisco (2004)
17. Ota, D., Loftin, B., Saito, T., et al.: Virtual reality in surgical education. Comput. Biol. Med. **25**, 127–137 (1995)
18. Satava, R.M.: Medical applications of virtual reality. J. Med. Syst. **19**, 275–280 (1995)
19. Satava, R.M.: Virtual reality, telesurgery, and the new world order of medicine. J. Image Guid. Surg. **1**, 12–16 (1995)
20. Beatty, J.D.: How to build an inexpensive laparoscopic webcam-based trainer. BJU Int. **96**, 679–682 (2005)
21. Chung, S.Y., Landsittel, D., Chon, C.H., et al.: Laparoscopic skills training using a webcam trainer. J. Urol. **173**, 180–183 (2005)
22. Pokorny, M.R., McLaren, S.L.: Inexpensive home-made laparoscopic trainer and camera. ANZ J. Surg. **74**, 691–693 (2004)
23. Reznick, R.R., Regehr, G., MacRae, H., et al.: Testing technical skill via an innovative "bench station" examination. Am. J. Surg. **172**, 226–230 (1996)
24. Martin, J.A., Regehr, G., Macrae, H., et al.: Objective Structured Assessment of Technical Skill (OSATS) for surgical residents. Br. J. Surg. **84**, 273–278 (1997)
25. Szalay, D., MacRae, H., Regehr, G., et al.: Using operative outcome to assess technical skill. Am. J. Surg. **180**, 234–237 (2000)
26. Derossis, A.M., Fried, G.M., Abrahamowicz, M., et al.: Development of a model for evaluation and training of laparoscopic skills. Am. J. Surg. **175**, 482–487 (1998)
27. Derossis, A.M., Bothwell, J., Sigman, H.H., et al.: The effect of practice on performance in a laparoscopic simulator. Surg. Endosc. **12**, 1117–1120 (1998)
28. Derossis, A.M., Antoniuk, M., Fried, G.M.: Evaluation of laparoscopic skills: a 2-year follow-up during residency training. Can. J. Surg. **42**, 293–296 (1999)
29. Feldman, L.S., Hagarty, S.E., Ghitulescu, G., et al.: Relationship between objective assessment of technical skills and subjective in-training evaluations in surgical residents. J. Am. Coll. Surg. **198**, 105–110 (2004)
30. Fried, G.M., Derossis, A.M., Bothwell, J., et al.: Comparison of laparoscopic performance in vivo with performance measured in a laparoscopic simulator. Surg. Endosc. **13**, 1077–1081 (1999)
31. Ghitulescu, G.A., Derossis, A.M., Feldman, L.S., et al.: A model for evaluation of laparoscopic skills: is there correlation to level of training? Surg. Endosc. **15**(Supp 1), S127 (2001)
32. Ghitulescu, G.A., Derossis, A.M., Stanbridge, D., et al.: A model for evaluation of laparoscopic skills: is there external validity? Surg. Endosc. **15**(Supp 1), S128 (2001)
33. Fried, G.M., Feldman, L.S., Vassiliou, M.C., et al.: Proving the value of simulation in laparoscopic surgery. Ann. Surg. **240**, 518–528 (2004)
34. Vassiliou, M.C., Ghitulescu, G.A., Feldman, L.S., et al.: The MISTELS program to measure technical skill in laparoscopic surgery. Evidence for reliability. Surg. Endosc. **20**, 744–747 (2006)
35. Aggarwal, R., Ward, J., Balasundaram, I., et al.: Proving the effectiveness of virtual reality simulation for training in laparoscopic surgery. Ann. Surg. **246**, 771–779 (2007)
36. Picod, G., Jambon, A.C., Vinatier, D., et al.: What can the operator actually feel when performing a laparoscopy? Surg. Endosc. **19**, 95–100 (2005)
37. Seymour, N.E., Rotnes, J.S.: Challenges to the development of complex virtual reality surgical simulations. Surg. Endosc. **20**, 1774–1777 (2006)
38. Sutherland, L.M., Middleton, P.F., Anthony, A., et al.: Surgical simulation – a systematic review. Ann. Surg. **243**, 291–300 (2006)
39. Hanna, G.B., Cuschieri, A.: Influence of the optical axis-to target view angle on endoscopic task performance. Surg. Endosc. **13**, 371–375 (1999)
40. Hanna, G.B., Drew, T., Clinch, P., et al.: A microprocessor controlled psychomotor tester for minimal access surgery. Surg. Endosc. **10**, 965–969 (1996)
41. Hanna, G.B., Drew, T., Clinch, P., et al.: Computer-controlled endoscopic performance assessment system. Surg. Endosc. **12**, 997–1000 (1998)
42. Poulin, E.C., Gagne, J.P., Boushey, R.P.: Advanced laparoscopic skills acquisition: the case of laparoscopic colorectal surgery. Surg. Clin. N. Am. **86**, 987–1004 (2006)
43. Lee, G., Lee, T., Dexter, D., et al.: Methodological infrastructure in surgical ergonomics: a review of tasks, models, and measurement systems. Surg. Innov. **14**, 153–167 (2007)
44. Brown, J.D., Rosen, J., Chang, L., et al.: Quantifying surgeon grasping mechanics in laparoscopy using the Blue DRAGON system. Stud. Health Technol. Inform. **98**, 34–36 (2004)
45. Gunther, S., Rosen, J., Hannaford, B., et al.: The red DRAGON: a multi-modality system for simulation and training in minimally invasive surgery. Stud. Health Technol. Inform. **125**, 149–54 (2007)
46. Vassiliou, M.C., Feldman, L.S., Andrew, C.G., et al.: A global assessment tool for evaluation of intraoperative laparoscopic skills. Am. J. Surg. **190**, 107–113 (2005)
47. Vassiliou, M.C., Feldman, L.S., Fraser, S.A., et al.: Evaluating intraoperative laparoscopic skill: direct observation versus blinded videotaped performances. Surg. Innov. **14**, 211–216 (2007)

48. Figert, P.L., Park, A.E., Witzke, D.B., et al.: Transfer of training in acquiring laparoscopic skills. J. Am. Coll. Surg. **193**, 533–537 (2001)
49. Hyltander, A., Liljegren, E., Rhodin, P.H., et al.: The transfer of basic skills learned in a laparoscopic simulator to the operating room. Surg. Endosc. **16**, 1324–1328 (2002)
50. Korndorffer, J.R., Dunne, J.B., Sierra, R., et al.: Simulator training for laparoscopic suturing using performance goals translates to the operating room. J. Am. Coll. Surg. **201**, 23–29 (2005)
51. Stefanidis, D., Korndorffer, J.R., Markley, S., et al.: Closing the gap in operative performance between novices and experts: does harder mean better for laparoscopic simulator training? J. Am. Coll. Surg. **205**, 307–313 (2007)
52. Youngblood, P.L., Srivastava, S., Curet, M., et al.: Comparison of training on two laparoscopic simulators and assessment of skills transfer to surgical performance. J. Am. Coll. Surg. **200**, 547–551 (2005)
53. Haluck, R.S., Marshall, R.L., Krummel, T.M., et al.: Are surgery training programs ready for virtual reality? a survey of program directors in general surgery. J. Am. Coll. Surg. **193**, 660–665 (2001)
54. Boyd, B.K., Olivier, J., Salameh, J.R.: Surgical residents' perception of simulation training. Am. Surg. **72**, 521–524 (2006)
55. Berg, D.A., Milner, R.E., Fisher, C.A., et al.: A cost-effective approach to establishing a surgical skills laboratory. Surgery **142**, 712–721 (2007)
56. Adrales, G.L., Chu, U.B., Witzke, D.B., et al.: Evaluating minimally invasive surgery training using low-cost mechanical simulations. Surg. Endosc. **17**, 580–585 (2003)
57. Bruynzeel, H., de Bruin, A.F.J., Bonjer, H.J.: Desktop simulator: key to universal training? Surg. Endosc. **21**, 1637–1640 (2007)
58. Jarrell, B., Nirenburg, S., McShane, M., et al.: An interactive, cognitive simulation of gastroesophageal reflux disease. Stud. Health Technol. Inform. **125**, 194–199 (2007)
59. Kapadia, M.R., DaRosa, D.A., MacRae, H.M., et al.: Current assessment and future directions of surgical skills laboratories. J. Surg. Educ. **64**, 260–265 (2007)
60. Gould, J.C.: Building a laparoscopic surgical skills training laboratory: resources and support. JSLS **10**, 293–296 (2006)
61. Scott, D.J., Dunnington, G.L.: The new ACS/APDS skills curriculum: moving the learning curve out of the operating room. J. Gastrointest. Surg. **12**, 213–221 (2008)

Laparoscopy and Research in Surgical Oncology: Current State of the Art and Future Trends

Dominic King, Henry Lee, and Lord Ara Darzi

3.1 Introduction

Minimally Invasive Surgery (MIS) is the most important revolution in surgical technique since the early 1900s [1]. It is generally agreed that MIS emerged when it did because the enabling technology permitting this approach had matured [2]. The technologies that facilitated this shift were the development of

- The charge coupling device (CCD) chip that allowed for high-resolution video images
- High-intensity xenon and halogen light sources that improved visualization of the surgical field
- Improved hand instrumentation designed for endoscopic approaches [3]

MIS is now established in all areas of surgery and has developed through the marriage of surgical expertise with technological advances [4]. Cholecystectomy was the first laparoscopic procedure to be widely accepted by the surgical community, and pioneers of laparoscopic surgery have subsequently carried out ever more ambitious procedures, with major developments in the field of surgical oncology.

Excellence in MIS requires skilled surgeons and the right equipment and facilities. The development of laparoscopic surgery has been limited by a number of technical factors including: restricted freedom of movement within the body cavity, two-dimensional vision and the lack of tactile feedback from instruments. Surgeons have largely accommodated these deficiencies through development of their own expertise; however, the last few years have brought continued advances in the technology behind MIS. The sizes of the laparoscopic ports we use have decreased in size as the usability of instruments has improved and we are able to see clearer images of the structures we are operating on. MIS represents a new era of technology-dependent surgical intervention, and its future progress depends on the growth of interventional technologies and devices [2].

In Cuschieri's view, advances in MIS fall into three categories:

- Facilitative
- Enabling
- Additive technologies

Facilitative technologies improve the efficiency of performance of the procedure and reduce the level of its difficulty. Examples of such technologies include ultrasonic dissection systems and impedance-controlled bipolar coagulation. Enabling technologies allow procedures to be carried out, which would be near impossible without the instrument or device. Examples include endostaplers for colonic surgery and inflatable bands for obesity surgery. Additive technologies whilst not essential enhance the effectiveness of the procedure. Examples of additive technologies include the DaVinci system (Intuitive Surgical, California, USA), which can aid the precision of surgery.

While we have seen remarkable changes in surgery in the last two decades, commentators such as Satava would say that this is just a preview of what is to come as we enter the "Bio intelligence Age" [5]. The future of MIS will build on the work that has already been done and pursue additional technological innovations to improve surgical outcomes, advance surgical technique and decrease peri-operative morbidity.

D. King, H. Lee, and L.A. Darzi (✉)
Department of Surgery and Cancer, Imperial College London, Praed Street, London, W2 1NY, UK
e-mail: a.darzi@imperial.ac.uk

3.2 Instrument Technology and Research

MIS requires instruments "on the end of the stick" that allow the surgeon to carry out a safe and effective operation. Traditionally instruments for MIS were simply narrower and thinner than the equivalents used in open surgery. Shaft instruments for MIS should provide ergonomic handling, high functionality and additional degrees of freedom at the instrument's tip [6]. The development of laparoscopic instruments has occurred in response to the demands of undertaking more complicated procedures. Traditional equipment is now being replaced by purpose-designed instruments, which provide for better and safer access, more effective tissue retraction and more versatile dissection. Examples of progress in this area include internal stapling devices that enable internal anastomosis and harmonic scalpels that facilitate haemostasis without ligatures.

New instruments for MIS must fulfil essential criteria such as being inherent stable, safe and being able to be sterilized if necessary. Commonly, MIS instruments consist of three functional units: the handle, the force transmission unit inside the shaft and the effector manipulating the tissue. Research has looked at both complex mechanical constructions and miniature hydraulic actuators to improve on current instruments [7].

3.2.1 Problems with Current Instruments for MIS

The majority of current laparoscopic instruments are rigid and do not provide the degrees of freedom needed by a surgeon in certain situations. Laparoscopic instruments are usually limited to four (five with instrument actuation) degrees of freedom (DOF) including pitch, jaw, rotation, extraction/insertion plus the actuation of the instrument. They lack the extension/flexion and tilt function of the wrist [8]. The position of the trocars acts as a pivot point restricting translational movement and resulting in a fulcrum effect. Therefore, every motion is mirrored to the opposite site so that moving the instrument up results in intra-abdominal downward movement. The leverage effect caused by most of the laparoscopic instrument being outside the body also leads to considerable scaling effects. 2D systems, lack of haptic feedback and poor ergonomic design also make complex tasks such as suturing difficult for surgeons [9].

3.2.2 Instrument Development in MIS

Progress in the development of tools for MIS has led to thinner and smaller instruments being produced. Instruments in MIS must be capable of performing several functions, and modular instruments have been introduced to avoid the need for frequent changes of instruments. Minimally invasive surgery (MIS) often requires the complete removal of one tool and reinsertion of another. Modular or multifunctional tools can be used to avoid this step. A device that has six interchangeable tips which can be changed through the tools shaft has shown decreased operating times [10].

MEMS (Micro Electro Mechanical Systems) technology is a micro-fabrication technique that deals with the fabrication of mechanical structures on silicon wafers using integrated circuit (IC) processing techniques such as photolithography and silicon etching. MEMS devices can incorporate several functions such as sensor, actuator and microelectronics. These functions can then be incorporated into instruments for the realization of high performance and multifunctional minimally invasive medical tools [11].

A new generation of laparoscopic instruments are available that offer the ability to articulate their end-effectors. This gives the surgeon the flexibility needed to perform complex tasks in a constricted surgical site. There is evidence from non-clinical studies that experienced surgeons are readily able to transfer their skills from conventional to articulating laparoscopic instruments [12].

To overcome the limitations and drawbacks of assisted manipulation, other instruments have been produced that can transfer the actions of the surgeon into the target without the restriction of laparoscopic ports fixed on the abdominal wall. A magnet-retracting forceps has been used in an animal model, which takes advantage of the attractive force between two magnets, one inserted into the peritoneal cavity and the other located outside the abdominal wall. This device was found to offer the surgeon excellent endoscopic views, as retraction forces could be applied without any shaft device in the abdomen. In addition, this reduced the number of laparoscopic ports required [13].

3.2.3 Instruments to Enable Tissue Approximation and Anastomosis

In surgical oncology, most of the advanced resections and procedures require suturing skills to perform tissue approximation and anastomosis. Restricted ergonomics, limited degrees of freedom and the two-dimensional (2D) image associated with MIS make suturing a demanding operative technique for the surgeon [14]. Mechanical stapling devices were introduced into open practice in the 1970s and have since become part of routine practice in many surgical operations. The role of MIS in advanced oncological surgery is in a large part due to advances in suturing and stapling technologies [15].

Suturing still has to be used in certain circumstances in advanced MIS. It is considered to be one of the most complex tasks within the discipline and requires specialist training. Improvements in needles, sutures and needle holders have overcome some of these difficulties. Specifically designed MIS instruments for suturing include the Endo-Stitch (Tyco, Massachusetts, USA) [16]. Robotic systems have also facilitated the performance of a complex sutured anastomosis enormously [17].

Stapling techniques used in MIS are based on developments in open surgery and modifications allow for both circular end-to-end stapling as well as the use of endoscopic linear cutting staplers. There has been recent interest in compression anastomosis in gastrointestinal anastomosis. This involves compressing two bowel walls together with the aim of joining the two lumens together. Compression devices have been used in the past and although high efficacy and safety rates were seen in many experimental and clinical trials, they were substituted largely for staplers due to their cost and awkwardness of use [18]. Nitinol (Nickel Titanium Naval Ordnance Laboratory) contains almost equal amounts of nickel and titanium and was invented in the 1960s and has been used in various stents and grafts subsequently. It has characteristic features of shape memory and super-elasticity. Nitinol is manufactured in a certain form and will stay in this form as long as it

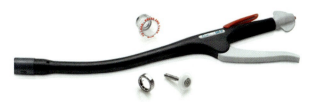

Fig. 3.1 CAR 27 compression anastomosis system: ring, anvil, applier and ring loader (With permission by NiTi™ Surgical Solutions)

is kept at or above a core temperature. When cooled below this temperature, it can be easily deformed into other temperatures. Once warmed back to the stable temperature, it regains its original form exactly. The properties of Nitinol make it a good candidate as a new compression anastomosis device and this concept was revitalized by NiTi Medical Technologies, Ltd (Netanya, Israel) with the design of a new instrument specifically for end-to-end anastomosis, the *CAR 27* (Endoluminal Compression Anastomosis Ring). This leads to a sutureless anastomosis. Compression devices have been FDA approved for open and laparoscopic procedures [19] with good results in clinical studies [20,21]. Further studies may prove the efficacy of this device as an additional tool or even as a replacement for currently available suturing and stapling technologies (Fig. 3.1).

3.2.4 Instruments to Enable Haemostasis

The ability to carry out increasingly sophisticated procedures using MIS has depended on the development of techniques to achieve haemostasis [22]. Laparoscopic surgery brings particular demands for strict haemostasis compared to open surgery. In MIS, high-quality images are essential to safe and effective operating and even small bleeds can significantly impair surgical vision and impact on quality and safety. As in open surgery, patient selection and preparation is essential to reduce the risk of peri-operative bleeding. Simple measures to control bleeding should be remembered and include compression with the tip of a suction probe or using a laparoscopic sponge stick. Further methods for haemostasis include physical modalities, thermal modalities and tissue sealants.

3.2.4.1 Mechanical Methods of Hemostasis

Sutures remain an effective tool for haemostasis in MIS. Loss of tactile feedback and loss of degrees of freedom with laparoscopic instruments can make suturing challenging and time-consuming, especially for less-experienced surgeons. Instruments simplifying intra-corporeal knot tying include the Endo-stitch device (US Surgical, Connecticut, USA) and Endoloops (Ethicon, New Jersey, USA). Other mechanical methods of haemostasis include titanium clips, which are practical and easy to use and circumvent the need for intra-corporeal suturing. Polymer clips are also available and have an advantage over titanium clips as they have a self-locking feature designed to prevent slippage. Vascular endo-staplers are used for control of major vessels or tissue stumps and have dual stapling and cutting functions. Robotic systems may facilitate advanced laparoscopic suturing through additional capabilities including enhanced DOF and 3D visualization. Experimental work shows that robotic suturing tends to be superior to traditional laparoscopic suturing in terms of time, safety and patency when seven DOF systems are used although this needs to be proven in further clinical series [14]. High costs and set-up times will continue to be limiting steps in the widespread uptake of robotic surgery at this time [23].

3.2.4.2 Thermal Methods of Hemostasis

Thermal methods can provide a fast and effective mode of hemostasis. Monopolar cauterization can be applied to various instruments such as hooks and scissors but is disadvantaged by the heat scatter, which can damage adjacent tissue. The argon beam coagulator, which uses an argon jet for control of minor capillary bleeding, is a monopolar electrocautery instrument. The Tissuelink Floating Ball (Tissuelink, Hew Hampshire, USA) device uses monopolar radiofrequency energy with low-volume saline irrigation for simultaneous blunt dissection, haemostatic sealing and coagulation.

Bipolar cautery can be a safer alternative to its monopolar counterpart and acts through current that flows between the forceps jaws. This minimizes the risk of damage to adjacent tissue. Ligasure (Valleylab, Colorado, USA) uses bipolar cauterization to produce a permanent haemostatic seal by applying a high current and low voltage to the vessel and can be used on vessels up to 7 mm [24]. The Harmonic scalpel (Ethicon Endo-Surgery, Cincinnati, USA) is an instrument that simultaneously excises and coagulates tissue with high-frequency ultrasound causing coagulation within vessels through protein denaturation. Ligasure can seal vessels and its strength has been found by certain authors to be superior to that of the harmonic scalpel and equivalent to mechanical clips [25]. Other studies have demonstrated that the harmonic scalpel has been found to be quicker, causes less thermal injury and performs better as a grasper than the Ligasure [26]. Both devices have advocates and detractors, and as with many areas of surgery there remains a strong element of surgeon preference in this field.

3.2.4.3 Tissue Sealants

Tissue sealants are substances that are often derived from human or animal blood or tissue components and include gelatin matrix (FloSeal, Baxter), fibrin glues (Crosseel, Johnson & Johnson) and fibrin and thrombin materials (Tachosil, Baxter). These products can be applied laparoscopically and have proven effectiveness in a number of clinical areas including laparoscopic prostatectomy [27] and vascular surgery [28].

3.2.4.4 Laser

Experimental work on the use of lasers in haemostasis has been undertaken [29]. Lasers have also been used for haemostasis in MIS. Carbon dioxide and neodymium: yttrium aluminum garnet (Nd: YAG) lasers have been evaluated with varying degrees of success. The Holmium:YAG laser has been shown to be an effective tool for the bloodless division of renal parenchyma [30].

3.2.5 NOTES and Instrument Development

The surgical community has developed new techniques and technologies to make MIS even more "minimal." Work has been carried out to reduce the size and number of trocars and in the case of Natural Orifice Transluminal Endoscopic Surgery (NOTES) transcutaneous trocars are eliminated completely. The motivation for making MIS even less invasive has been to reduce the cosmetic impact of surgery as well as the morbidity. Laparo-endoscopic Single-Site Surgery (LESS) also known as Single Incision Laparoscopic Surgery (SILS) and One Port Umbilical Surgery (OPUS) involves single port access to the body cavity being operated in. This has been made possible by advances in instrument design and technology including the use of articulating or bent instruments through a single large caliber trocar or multiple small, adjacent trocars [31]. New laparoscopic access ports have been developed (Quadport, Advanced Surgical Concepts, Wicklow, Ireland). Instruments that still permit triangulation despite the close proximity of instruments via a single port have been designed including laparoscopic needle drivers (Cambridge Endo) and endoshears (Cambridge Endo). Instrument design for NOTES and LESS is likely to lead to advancements in instrument design that can be equally applied to conventional laparoscopic surgery (Fig. 3.2). The development of endoscopic instruments may allow the further use of endoscopy for definitive treatment in surgical oncology. Endoscopic submucosal dissection (ESD) permits the resection of gastrointestinal epithelial neoplasms in an en bloc manner. A novel endosurgical knife called the "splash-needle" is a thin, short needle with a water-irrigation function that has shown promising results in a case series with few associated complications [32].

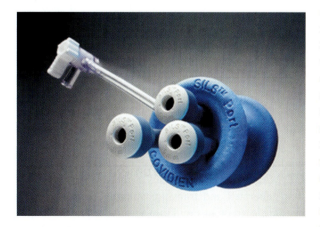

Fig. 3.2 SILS Port (Covidien, Massachusetts, USA) is a multi-instrument access port for laparoscopic surgery (With permission by Covidien©, Mansfield, MA, USA)

3.3 Device Technology and Research

New techniques and devices have been used to improve outcomes in MIS. No chapter or textbook can fully do justice to the efforts of researchers who push the frontiers of MIS as new innovations and developments are continually being realized. Recent examples that have had an impact in MIS include the development of hand-assisted laparoscopic surgery and the application of ablative techniques in surgical oncology.

3.3.1 Hand-assisted Laparoscopic Surgery (HALS)

Hand-assisted laparoscopic surgery involves the intra-abdominal placement of a hand or forearm through a mini-laparotomy incision while pneumoperitoneum is maintained. In this way, the hand can be used as in an open procedure to palpate organs or tumors, reflect organs atraumatically, retract structures, identify vessels, dissect bluntly along a tissue plain, and provide finger pressure to bleeding points while proximal control is achieved. Some advocates of this technique claim that it is easier to learn and perform than totally laparoscopic approaches and that it may be more economical as there are reduced laparoscopic ports and instruments required [33].

Early handports used in HALS were not sufficiently successful as they impaired movement of the hand and were associated with a loss of pneumoperitoneum. The technology of these devices has improved considerably over the years and they now allow the surgeon to insert their hand into the abdominal cavity through a relatively small incision whilst preserving the ability to work with an adequate pneumoperitoneum. This has allowed better exposure, retraction and facilitation of specimen removal [34]. The advantages of HALS seem to eliminate a substantial part of the technical challenges of conventional MIS as well as providing a more acceptable learning curve. Recent systematic reviews have looked at the role of HALS in surgery for colorectal cancer comparing it to both open and minimally invasive procedures. HALS proved to be a valid alternative to conventional laparoscopic procedures reducing operative times and conversion rates although morbidity and length of stay did not differ [35]. In a systematic review comparing HALS to open surgery, it was clearly seen that HALS has the advantages of laparoscopic surgery over open surgery while reducing some of the disadvantages of laparoscopic surgery (shorter operative time, lower conversion rate and flatter learning curves) [36].

3.3.2 Tissue Ablation

Tumor ablation is a treatment modality based on in situ destruction of tumor tissue. Thermal ablation therapies have been used to treat benign and malignant tumors for many years. Thermal ablation can destroy tumor cells that are not otherwise surgically resectable. Thermal ablation can be carried out either by heating the tissue above 60°C, which leads to protein denaturation or cooling the tissue to below −40°C where intracellular crystallization occurs. Methods of heat generation include high-frequency focused ultrasound [37], radiofrequency [38], microwave [39] and laser-induced thermal therapy [40]. The key for a thermal ablation technique is to generate a clear boundary in a desired time, and to prevent surrounding tissue from being burned.

3.3.2.1 Radiofrequency Ablation (RFA)

Radiofrequency ablation (RFA) is probably the most commonly used method of ablation by heat. It induces temperature change by using high-frequency alternating current applied via electrodes placed within the tissue to generate areas of coagulative necrosis and tissue desiccation. Radiofrequency ablation can be applied percutaneously, laparoscopically or at open surgery. One of the problems with all ablative techniques has been how to hit the target as exactly as required. Despite improvements in imaging, treatment of certain lesions is still difficult to perform percutaneously. Laparoscopic RF ablation can offer better access to difficult lesions than via the percutaneous route and is less invasive than open surgery and has been proven to be a viable option [41]. However, laparoscopic RF has been hampered by the limited maneuvering space and the lack of specialized instruments to complete procedures effectively. A dedicated set of instruments is required to improve the effectiveness of this procedure and initial work in this area has shown promising results [42]. Continued improvement in the technology associated with this procedure and increased clinical experience is likely to lead to improved patient outcomes.

3.3.2.2 High-intensity Focused Ultrasound (HIFU)

Focused ultrasound is a promising treatment of malignant tumors and no skin incision is necessary. Dramatic developments in imaging technology have driven the resurgence in interest in this technology. Both ultrasound and MRI can be incorporated into high-intensity focused ultrasound (HIFU) devices to guide each stage of the treatment. HIFU raises the temperature in the focal area by using ultrasonic energy of sufficient strength. This leads to tissue ablation and should not lead to damage of the surrounding tissue. The purpose of HIFU treatment is to either achieve a cure or palliate. Types of HIFU devices being used clinically include extracorporeal and transrectal devices, with transrectal devices being used to manage prostate cancer [43]. Extracorporeal devices include the ExAblate 2000 (InSightec-TxSonics Ltd, Haifa, Israel), which uses MRI-guidance and the Mode-JC HIFU system (Haifu Technology Co. Ltd, Chongqing, China), which uses ultrasound guidance. The MRI-guided HIFU device has been used to treat breast neoplasms and uterine fibroids and the ultrasound-guided device has been used for various solid malignancies [44]. Like many surgeries, HIFU is a locally ablative technology and it is essential to combine HIFU with other therapies including chemotherapy and radiotherapy when necessary. Large prospective, randomized clinical trials are necessary before HIFU becomes a widespread conventional treatment.

3.3.2.3 Microwave Ablation

Microwave ablation is an emerging treatment option for patients with unresectable hepatic cancers and is guided by imaging modalities such as ultrasound and CT. Microwave ablation uses a microwave coagulator that generates and transmits microwave energy to a needle electrode inserted into a tumor to induce coagulative necrosis. Initial microwave ablation had limited applications due to the small area of necrosis. Larger diameters of necrosis were not possible due to the high temperatures necessary causing associated soft tissue damage. A new novel cooled-tip electrode may expand the use of this technology in MIS [45].

Compared with conventional thermal ablation, an injectable NaK alloy-induced exothermic reaction has been shown to achieve localized, irreversible thermochemical ablation of tissue both in vitro and in vivo, although at an early stage, initial results demonstrate that this technique has a potential role in the treatment of malignant tumors [46].

3.3.2.4 Cryoablation

Cryoablation or thermal ablation by freezing is an old principle that was amongst the first of the thermal ablative techniques widely used as a treatment of liver tumors. The mechanism of action of cryoablation is of direct cellular injury and microvascular injury. Cryoablation of liver tumors commonly use liquid nitrogen and argon gas and are applied with cryoprobes whose number, size and position vary according to the tumor size and location. Traditionally, cryosurgery has been performed by open surgery but cryoprobe can be placed percutaneously or laparoscopically [47]. At present, long-term outcome data are not properly documented and cryoablation has not been adequately evaluated against the other ablative [47].

At present, firm evidence for the type of ablation that should be used in oncology is not conclusive [48]. Further work in this area combined with improvements in imaging technologies has the potential to offer real improvements in patient care.

3.4 Imaging Technology and Research

Advances in imaging technology have changed the way surgeons operate. Visualization of the operative field in MIS requires optimal image capture, processing and display. The introduction of technological advances such as three-dimensional (3D) laparoscopy, miniaturization of high-resolution digital video cameras and high-definition image display has led to significantly enhanced opportunities in MIS.

3.4.1 Light Sources

In the 1950s, there were two milestone inventions in the evolution of endoscopy: the rod lens system and the fiber-optic light transmitting system [49,50]. The light source and the structure of rigid endoscopes have remained pretty much unchanged since this work. Current endoscopic illumination systems have several limitations and the coupling mismatches at the fiber-optic interfaces results in light loss and heat production. In addition, the illuminated field from an arc lamp endoscope is not uniform and the intensity of the directed light beam decreases radially, which results in darker peripheries and an overexposed centre. Light-emitting diodes (LEDs) are solid-state semiconductor devices, which convert electrical potential energy to electromagnetic energy in the form of light. High-power white LEDs are readily available at a cost of less than US $10 and have a long life span of over 10,000 h. LEDs already have a role in capsule endoscopy [51] and in overhead operating lights in the operating room. A newly developed LED endo-illuminator using a white LED mounted at the tip of a steel rod gave more uniform illumination, less flickering and better illumination for visual perception compared to the arc-lamp-based system currently used [52].

3.4.2 Image Transmission

Imaging transmission is being revolutionized most importantly by replacing optical with digital transmission. Analog imaging was the first type of imaging technology used in MIS and the technique required separate units to convert information about an object into an image on the video monitor. Digital imaging allows for direct transfer of images to the display unit without the need for further processing. The latest high-definition monitors have the potential to improve detail recognition and visualization to bring the operative field closer to the surgeon than is possible with open procedures. The miniaturization of chip cameras also means that they can be mounted at the tip of the endoscope, rendering traditional rod lenses or fiber-optical systems unnecessary.

There have been relatively few studies looking at the objective imaging characteristics of high-definition (HD) laparoscopes against standard-definition (SD) laparoscopes. In a comparative study, an Olympus SD 10 mm, zero degree laparoscope (Olympus Surgical & Industrial America Inc, Pennsylvania, USA) was compared with the Olympus HD 10 mm, zero degree laparoscope. The Olympus HD laparoscope has the charge-coupled device in the tip of the laparoscope rather than the camera head attached to it. It was found that the image resolution with the HD laparoscope was greater than the SD laparoscope and that there was less distortion and greater depth of field. There were no significant differences between the HD and SD laparoscope with reference to color reproduction and grayscale discernment [53]. HD imaging has also been seen to contribute to improved surgical task performance [54].

HD laparoscopy has superior objective performance characteristics compared with standard laparoscopes and may lead to easier identification of anatomical structures, finer dissection and enhanced 3D spatial positioning during HD laparoscopic procedures. Better display monitors with higher resolution, better light sources and 3D vision systems promise to bring vision to a level unsurpassed by direct vision.

3.4.3 Image-guided Surgery

Image-guided surgery is set to revolutionize how we operate and will have particular application in minimally invasive cancer surgery. Images from ultrasound (US), computerized tomography (CT) and magnetic resonance imaging (MRI) can be used in combination with imaging technology to plan a procedure, define the surgical target or resection margin and to guide laparoscopic instruments. In advanced systems, currently available surgeons are provided with a three-dimensional (3D) "road map," which incorporates imaging of the patient's anatomy with real-time visualization of tracked surgical instruments.

Image-guided surgery (IGS) involves a number of steps including preoperative image acquisition, intraoperative visualization which can make use of updated data and postoperative imaging for adequate evaluation of the treatment. Much of the work in this field has been carried out in neurosurgery [55], but other clinical applications are being developed in many surgical disciplines.

Preoperative patient data registration can be characterized as point-based, surface-based or volume-based [56]. Tracking technologies for medical instruments determine the position through instruments and there are mechanical, electromagnetic, optical and acoustic mechanisms of achieving this. Currently intraoperative visualization in minimally invasive surgery is limited by the view from the laparoscope or endoscope. Techniques such as US, CT and MRI can be used but the challenge is how to update preoperative registered data with new information.

Using ultrasound has the potential to compensate for some of the intraoperative limitations such as the lack of tactile feedback and restricted view associated with MIS. Fukuda first introduced laparoscopic ultrasound with screening of the liver during diagnostic laparoscopy [57], Computerized Tomography (CT) and Magnetic Resonance Imaging (MRI) have also been used in MIS, but advancements in ultrasound technologies and its portability and low relative cost have led to increasing attention on its applications. The use of ultrasound in MIS has included support in visualizing relevant surgical anatomy and the detection of hepatic metastasis [58,59]. It has been demonstrated that 2D and 3D ultrasound can be integrated with navigation technologies to improve laparoscopic surgery by improving orientation and image display user-friendliness. Navigation technology has been shown to solve the orientation problems and makes it possible to show real-time 2D ultrasound images in their correct orientation relative to the patient and the surgeon's view [60,61]. Using fast-rendering algorithms and morphing technologies will allow synthesis of updated information from real-time intraoperative ultrasound with preoperative CT or MRI imaging.

As with all surgery, safety is paramount in IGS. IGS cannot operate under the assumption that the tissue being operated on is within a rigid body whose appearance has not changed since the preoperative imaging was carried out. It must take account of any changes since the registered image were taken and any dynamic movements that occur during surgical manipulation. At present, the most important approaches are based on ultrasound imaging [62].

Future areas of development in this field will include markerless registration for the patient, as registration can be inconvenient, inefficient and time-consuming.

Developments in multimodality visualization will require image fusion techniques to be further developed. This will allow the surgeon to better target pathological structures but also aid them to avoid important structures such as blood vessels especially with the shifting anatomy that is inherent during surgical manipulation [63].

3.4.4 Magnifying Endoscopy

Magnifying endoscopy has been used to visualize the microstructure of mucosa and mucosal vascularity, particularly in the gastrointestinal tract and may avoid the multiple or blind biopsies required in conventional MIS. Magnifying endoscopy enhances mucosal detail by enlarging the image. Chromo endoscopy was introduced as the mucosal pattern can be enhanced by the addition of contrast agents [64]. Chromo endoscopic agents are characterized by their working principle. Methylene blue is absorbed into cells whilst indigo carmine accumulate in the pits and valleys between cells [65].

Confocal endomicroscopy (CEM) is a recent advancement in imaging technology that incorporates a confocal laser microscope into the tip of a flexible endoscope. CEM allows 1,000-fold magnification with high resolution allowing for real-time in vivo histology or "virtual biopsies" [66]. Endomicroscopy opens a new door for immediate tissue and vessel analysis. Other techniques have been used to improve visualization and detection of mucosal lesions such as auto-fluorescence imaging [67], but biopsy is still required to look for and confirm atypia.

CEM has been used to visualize the mucosa of the bowel for the early detection of dysplasia and cancer and allows high-resolution, cross-sectional imaging of mucosa at different depths [68]. Confocal miniprobes were initially inserted through the endoscope working channel to obtain dynamic imaging of the mucosa; however, initial images produced were unsatisfactory. The main CEM system in use in clinical gastroenterology at present is a joint collaboration between Pentax (Tokyo, Japan) and Optiscan (Victora, Australia), which provides a superior resolution with reduced image noise with confocal images generated simultaneously with the endoscopic images. This model integrates a confocal fluorescence microscope into the distal tip of a conventional flexible endoscope. CEM requires contrast agents to achieve the high-contrast images necessary for adequate examination (Fig. 3.3).

CEM is carried out much as a conventional endoscopy to visualize the gastrointestinal tract. Expertise requires the endoscopist to have adequate skills and

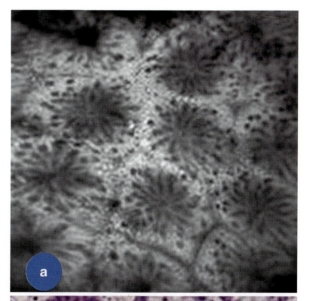
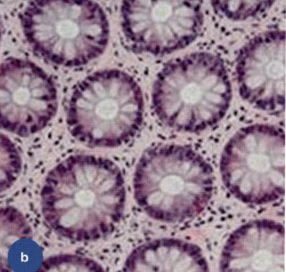

Fig. 3.3 (**a**) Optiscan confocal endomicroscopy image showing welldefined and ordered crypts projecting onto the surface of colonic mucosa. (**b**) Corresponding histology image from a biopsy (With permission by Optiscan™, Victoria, Australia)

knowledge of pathological and histological images to make the correct diagnosis, and this may require significant training. CEM has been shown to be effective in surveillance of Barrett's esophagus [69] and early gastric neoplasia [70].

CEM is a promising optical technology that may play a critical role in one stop endoscopic surgery for gastrointestinal tract neoplasms. CEM may have applications in other types of MIS including laparoscopic procedures such as tumor staging. It may become common that people will undergo histological examination of areas of interest by CEM followed immediately by endoscopic submucosal dissection of the lesion or other minimally invasive procedure. For the use of CEM technology to become more widespread, further advancement in its technology will be necessary. Equally important is the adequate training of individuals using the system.

3.4.5 Head-mounted Display in Laparoscopic Surgery

Image displays in endoscopic surgery have not changed much in the last two decades and the default set-up consists of a monitor atop of a tower structure. Laparoscopic surgery is limited by the difficulties of two-dimensional (2D) projection and the loss of depth perception and spatial orientation. Laparoscopic surgery is also limited by the reliance of a single image capture displayed on one or two overhead monitors, which is not ergonomic and can lead to hand–eye dissociation, loss of image detail and neck strain [71]. Current technology does not allow adequate image projection in daylight necessitating the theatre in MIS usually being in the dark, which can cause additional problems to circulating staff.

Head-mounted display (HMD) goggles offer freedom from staring at a stationery monitor and may improve ergonomics [71] and display the image in lighted surroundings [72]. Previous HMD systems have been troubled by being bulky, uncomfortable and offering a poor image. More recently, the image quality has greatly improved and the systems are much more comfortable and portable. HMDs offer a solution to many of the shortcomings of traditional monitored displays of the surgical field. A study has found that high-quality HMDs improve endoscopic performance over the traditional overhead display [73]. Advances in the merging of videoscopic and archival images [74] and enhanced reality imaging [75] may also lead to improvements in HMD units.

3.5 Robotics, Haptics and Telesurgery Technology

3.5.1 Robots

Robotics was first introduced into the surgical world in 1996 when AESOP was produced by Computer Motion Inc. (California, USA). This device controlled the position of a laparoscopic camera during MIS and stimulated a flurry of activity and development in this area. The role of robotic-assisted surgery is continuing to expand in the field of MIS, which is evidenced by the exponential growth of the DaVinci robotic surgical system worldwide, with more than 867 systems sold up to May 2008 [76].

The challenges of using laparoscopic instruments in MIS include a loss in the degrees of freedom that are usually produced by the human wrist. Laparoscopic instruments are unable to articulate up and down and from left to right as the wrist can do in open surgery. Manipulators were introduced to address the handling problems instruments in MIS. Although sometimes termed robots, these manipulators are under the direct control of a human being and not a computer program. The surgeon (master) initiates the movements; the manipulator (slave) carries them out. It is essential that despite the technology, the manipulator functions in a safe and effective environment and the set-up time and effort are not too burdensome.

Robotic assistants or scope positioning systems have been shown to be of value in the operating room. Surgical assistants sometimes have to stand at the operating table in a way that constrains the surgeon, and the position for the assistant may also be uncomfortable and unergonomic and this may result in tremor and uncoordinated movements [77]. Robotic assistants offer many of the advantages of a traditional human assistant with additional benefits of freeing up working space and allowing surgeons to operate on their own in a controlled manner. To be successful, these systems need to be OR and procedure ready and this set-up should be fast and easy. AESOP (Animated Endoscopic System for Optimal Positioning; Computer Motion, California, USA) was the first clinically available scope positioning system and the device is attached directly on the OR table and can be controlled by a button control or by voice activation. The ENDOASSIST system (Prosurgics, Bracknell, UK) is a robotic arm placed next to the OR table and the position is controlled by a footswitch and the surgeons head movements, which are tracked by a headband sensor.

The DaVinci Robotic system (Intuitive Surgical, California, USA) is a telemanipulator using robotic technology. As a manipulator, the DaVinci system can be better considered as a sophisticated remote control of the laparoscopic instruments. The DaVinci system has three major components. The first component is the console, in which the surgeon sits ergonomically behind to control the robotic system remotely. The console can be placed anywhere in or even outside the operating theatre. The second component is the Insite Vision System through which a 3D view is created with the use of two camera control units and two light sources, built into the unit. The viewer can get a 6–10 times magnification of the operation field. The 3D view as well as high-definition resolution can provide excellent visual feedback. The patient side cart with the robotic arms forms the third component. EndoWrist instruments are attached to the arms that provide DOF similar to the human hand. The system provides enhanced dexterity, articulation, motion scaling, tremor filtration and the potential for telesurgery. Robotic surgical systems have the theoretical ability to compensate the most important drawbacks of laparoscopy and have been used in a wide variety of procedures and have the potential to allow more complex procedures in the future (Fig. 3.4).

Radical prostatectomy has been the fastest growing application of robotic surgery in urology and is the standard procedure for this condition in many North American Centers [8]. Robotic surgery has also been used in a number of procedures for oncology including radical nephrectomy [78] and colectomies [79].

As with every innovation that introduces new technology, robotic surgery has met skepticism with regard to necessity, applicability and affordability. It is likely that in the near future robotic systems will become

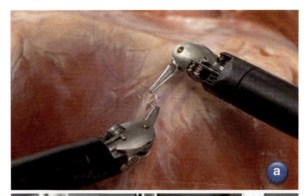
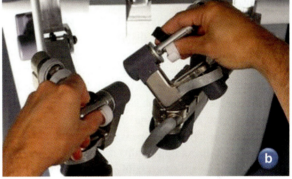

Fig. 3.4 The Da Vinci System: (**a**) Operator's view. (**b**) Hand controls (With permission by Intuitive Surgical, Inc. Sunnyvale, CA, USA)

smaller and more user friendly and be more integrated into modern operating theatres. The first MRI-compatible robot was introduced in neurosurgery in 2007 [80] and we are likely to see further fusion of imaging techniques with robotic systems.

3.5.2 Development of Haptics in Minimally Invasive Surgery

MIS brings difficulty to the operating surgeon through a loss of perception, which can lead to a higher number of errors and complications [81]. Indirect visualization of tissue through a laparoscope or endoscope and manipulation of tissue with long instruments leads to disturbed hand–eye coordination, reduced depth perception and reduced haptic feedback [34]. In open surgery, the sense of touch (though reduced by a glove) is maintained and the surgeon can adjust the forces applied to tissue to reduce damage. MIS instruments do provide some degree of haptic feedback and can perceive the texture, shape and consistency of objects, but the feedback is reduced by indirect tissue contact, trocar friction and scaling [34]. In conventional laparoscopy, surgeons are provided with some haptic feedback, and with experience they learn to better understand the haptic feedback they do receive [82]. Haptic information feedback in MIS can help the surgeon to apply and control forces and this can be done through improving mechanical construction or adding extra information feedback (sensory substitution). Sensory substitution uses sensors to measure forces applied to the tissue and then reflect them electronically to the surgeon using a haptic, auditory or visual display [83]. Experimental research in this field has shown promise with instruments providing audio feedback [84], tactile feedback [85] and visual feedback [86]. In MIRS, the potential for offering feedback is made easier as an electromechanical device connects the surgeon (master) to the slave (instrument) and compensation mechanisms can be introduced. Providing feedback is complicated and expensive and is still not readily available [87]; however, it has been found experimentally at least to lead to more precise dissection and fewer errors [88].

3.5.3 Telemedicine

Telemedicine permits the viewing, monitoring, collaborating and performance of medical procedures from a distance. Telemedicine has the potential to improve the performance of surgery and provide expertise to underserved and remote areas. There have been vivid demonstrations showing how a surgeon can carry out procedures when they are not physically located by the patient, but telemedicine can be expanded to include telementoring, teleproctoring and teleconsulting.

Using current robotic systems, the usual displacement between the Surgeon and the patient is approximately 5–10 m. Extending master–slave control may introduce powerful, new capabilities [89]. Telesurgery is defined as the performance of robotic surgery over long distances with a communication link. One of the earliest cases of telesurgery was a cholecystectomy performed in September 2001 by Surgeons in New York on a patient in France [90]. Subsequently, the world's first telerobotic surgical service was set up in Canada [91]. Telesurgery was believed to have the potential to extend surgical expertise, provide care for remote communities and reduce the costs of providing specialist care; however, uptake has been relatively slow compared to the great strides seen in other areas of MIS. The data transferred for telesurgery include the video and audio signals in addition to the digital signals representing the surgeon's movements and this can take up significant bandwidth. Latency or time lag is the time difference that occurs from when an action occurs till the surgeon perceives and can be another significant limitation with this technology. Reliability and security are further technical barriers that must be overcome before both the surgeon and patient will be comfortable with telesurgery.

3.6 Ergonomic and Operating Theatres Technology

Most minimally invasive surgical procedures are performed in operating rooms that were originally designed for traditional open surgery. New equipment is often placed inconveniently around the operating room and can create potential mechanical, electrical, and biological hazards to the patient and operating staff.

Hippocrates wrote that the surgeons should be seated comfortably and work in good light [92]. Many operating rooms (ORs) function poorly through under-funding or poor design. Progress in medicine and the development of a multitude of new technologies has made the task to be performed in operating theatres increasingly complex. In a place where people work under extreme physical and mental stress, it is important that the OR is not just cost-effective but also ergonomically correct. Design and configuration of operating theatres is unsuitable for MIS and purpose-designed theatres are required. Specialist publications on operating room design and function exist [93].

Operating room design needs to be looked at from the standpoints of the various disciplines, which include surgery, anesthetics, hygiene, engineering and architecture. Integrated systems are required to meet the challenges of MIS and increase benefits to our patients. When we actually ask surgeons how we can improve the OR, we get a wide variety of responses [94]. The main concerns focused on poor equipment, lack of training of staff in using new technologies and poor interaction between the designers of OR's and the end users. In designing new ORs, essential features may be overlooked and it is suggested that a checklist is put in place to ensure the key characteristics of a successful OR are in place [95].

The operating room of the future needs to accommodate procedural and technological developments. Increasingly, surgery and interventional procedures require image guidance or real-time imaging to localize pathology and guide treatments. Operating rooms may therefore need to accommodate imaging systems including CT and MRI.

3.6.1 Surgeon Comfort in MIS

More thought must be given to optimizing operator comfort through intelligent design and ergonomics. In most operating rooms, the surgeon has to use instruments that place their hands in an awkward position and also have to use foot pedals that do not allow safe standing on both feet. Recommendations for working posture, lighting levels, information design and management structures are widely available in standard ergonomic textbooks [96].

Technological solutions can also be found to improve operator comfort. For example, surgeons have been reported to experience heat-related discomfort during long surgical procedures due to increased physical and mental effort and poor ergonomic working conditions. An efficient and comfortable cooling vest to relieve thermal stress for surgeons has been developed. Preliminary results have shown physiological benefits of reduced seat rate and lower mean skin temperature and increased personal comfort of the surgeon [97].

3.6.2 Operator Panels

The actual operating team is blocked at the sterile field in the OR. The devices necessary for MIS including camera and lighting equipment and the operating table usually have different user panels, which are sometimes difficult to reach and are also often in the dark. In order to overcome these challenges, integrated OR systems have been developed that connect all electronic equipment in the OR to a single central controller unit.

The settings on these central systems may be adjusted by a member of the operating team or from somebody outside of the sterile field. Examples of commercially available systems include HERMES (Computer Motion, CA, USA) and EndoALPHA (Olympus, Tokyo, Japan). A number of these systems have additional capabilities including being able to import imaging from the hospital network and use teleconferencing systems to enable telementoring. Voice activation and control of the OR environment are future directions.

3.7 Surgery Without External Scars and Technology Development

There is an increasing interest in treating a number of pathological conditions through operative flexible endoscopic procedures. In common, these procedures attempt to leave no external scars. Examples include endoscopic stenting for malignant strictures, endoscopic treatment of gastrointestinal lesions such as polyps, trans-anal endoscopic microsurgery (TEMS) for removal of lower gastrointestinal tract lesions and natural orifice transluminal endoscopic surgery (NOTES) [98]. Trans-gastric cholecystectomies and appendectomies have been performed successfully applying this technique. The literature is replete with the pros and cons of treating abdominal pathologies by opening a healthy viscus to complete a procedure. Earlier recovery and improved cosmoses have to be balanced against the risks of contamination and the lack of capability to manage intraoperative complications. In terms of further research in the field of MIS, it is often the case that new areas of interest stimulate research. NOTES is one area that is pushing the multidisciplinary team into developing new technologies. Even if NOTES and related procedures do not take hold in the wider surgical community, developments in technology will translate into tools that will improve more mainstream practice.

Quick Reference Guide

1. MIS has established itself in all areas of surgical oncology as a result of advancements in surgical expertise and the enabling technologies.
2. Facilitative technologies improve the efficiency of performance and reduce the level of difficulty of MIS.
3. A new generation of laparoscopic instruments are available that provide greater flexibility that allow the surgeon to work in more complex areas.
4. Further research and development is required to facilitate operations using Natural Orifice Transluminal Endoscopic Surgery (NOTES) and Single Incision Laparoscopic Surgery (SILS).
5. Visualization of the operative field is improving and there are promising developments in three-dimensional (3D) laparoscopy and the miniaturization of high-definition (HD) digital video cameras.
6. Robotic technology is becoming smaller and more user friendly and will be increasingly integrated into modern operating rooms.

References

1. Darzi, A., Mackay, S.: Recent advances in minimal access surgery. BMJ **324**, 31–34 (2002)
2. Cuschieri, A.: Laparoscopic surgery: current status, issues and future developments. Surgeon **3**, 125–130, 132–133, 135–138 (2005)
3. Mack, M.J.: Minimally invasive and robotic surgery. JAMA **285**, 568–572 (2001)
4. Jones, S.B., Jones, D.B.: Surgical aspects and future developments of laparoscopy. Anesthesiol. Clin. N. Am. **19**, 107–124 (2001)
5. Satava, R.M.: Information age technologies for surgeons: overview. World J. Surg. **25**, 1408–1411 (2001)
6. Disch, A., Lutze, T., Schauer, D., et al.: Innovative polymer-based shaft instruments for minimally invasive surgery. Minim. Invasive Ther. Allied Technol. **17**, 275–284 (2008)
7. de Volder, M., Piers, J., Reynaerts, A., et al.: A novel hydraulic microactuator sealed by surface tension. Senors Actuat. A **123**, 547–554 (2005)
8. Rassweiler, J., Hruza, M., Teber, D., et al.: Laparoscopic and robotic assisted radical prostatectomy–critical analysis of the results. Eur. Urol. **49**, 612–624 (2006)
9. Rassweiler, J., Safi, K.C., Subotic, S., et al.: Robotics and telesurgery–an update on their position in laparoscopic radical prostatectomy. Minim. Invasive Ther. Allied Technol. **14**, 109–122 (2005)
10. Miller, D.J., Nelson, C.A., Oleynikov, D.: Shortened OR time and decreased patient risk through use of a modular surgical instrument with artificial intelligence. Surg. Endosc. **23**(5), 1099–105 (2009)
11. Haga, Y., Matsunaga, T., Makishi, W., et al.: Minimally invasive diagnostics and treatment using micro/nano machining. Minim. Invasive Ther. Allied Technol. **15**, 218–225 (2006)
12. Martinec, D.V., Gatta, P., Zheng, B., et al.: The trade-off between flexibility and maneuverability: task performance with articulating laparoscopic instruments. Surg. Endosc. **21**, 1223–1232 (2009)
13. Kume, M., Miyazawa, H., Abe, F., et al.: A newly designed magnet-retracting forceps for laparoscopic cholecystectomy in a swine model. Minim. Invasive Ther. Allied Technol. **17**, 251–254 (2008)
14. Kenngott, H.G., Muller-Stich, B.P., Reiter, M.A., et al.: Robotic suturing: technique and benefit in advanced laparoscopic surgery. Minim. Invasive Ther. Allied Technol. **17**, 160–167 (2008)
15. Lirici, M.M.: How advances in tissue approximation technology and technique influence progress in minimally invasive therapy. Minim. Invasive Ther. Allied Technol. **17**, 149–150 (2008)
16. Dorsey, J.H., Rese, T.C., Zucker, K.A.: Laparoscopic suturing and knot tying. In: Zucker, K. (ed.) Surgical laparoscopy. Lippincott Williams & Williams, Philadelphia (2001)
17. Arvidsson: Anastomotic devices for minimally invasive surgery. Minim. Invasive Ther. Allied Technol. **13**, 32–35 (2004)
18. Ravitch, M.M., Rivarola, A.: Enteroanastomosis with an automatic instrument. Surgery **59**, 270–277 (1966)
19. Szold, A.: New concepts for a compression anastomosis: superelastic clips and rings. Minim. Invasive Ther. Allied Technol. **17**, 168–171 (2008)
20. Nudelman, I., Fuko, V., Waserberg, N., et al.: Colonic anastomosis performed with a memory-shaped device. Am. J. Surg. **190**, 434–438 (2005)
21. Kopelman, D., Lelcuk, S., Sayfan, J., et al.: End-to-end compression anastomosis of the rectum: a pig model. World J. Surg. **31**, 532–537 (2007)
22. Lattouf, J.B., Beri, A., Klinger, C.H., et al.: Practical hints for hemostasis in laparoscopic surgery. Minim. Invasive Ther. Allied Technol. **16**, 45–51 (2007)
23. Hanly, E.J., Talamini, M.A.: Robotic abdominal surgery. Am. J. Surg. **188**, 19S–26S (2004)
24. Constant, D.L., Florman, S.S., Mendez, F., et al.: Use of the LigaSure vessel sealing device in laparoscopic living-donor nephrectomy. Transplantation **78**, 1661–1664 (2004)
25. Kennedy, J.S., Buysse, S.P., Lawes, K.R.: Recent innovations in bipolar electrosurgery. Minim. Invasive Ther. Allied Technol. **8**, 95–99 (1999)
26. Landman, J., Kerbl, K., Rehman, J., et al.: Evaluation of a vessel sealing system, bipolar electrosurgery, harmonic scalpel, titanium clips, endoscopic gastrointestinal anastomosis vascular staples and sutures for arterial and venous ligation in a porcine model. J. Urol. **169**, 697–700 (2003)
27. Ahlering, T.E., Eichel, L., Chou, D., et al.: Feasibility study for robotic radical prostatectomy cautery-free neurovascular bundle preservation. Urology **65**, 994–997 (2005)
28. Pupka, A., Rucinski, A., Pawlowski, S., et al.: Use of mesh fibrous dressing covered with fibrin glue (TachoComb) in hemostasis after vascular anastomoses in the groin. Polim. Med. **34**, 47–51 (2004)

29. Lotan, Y., Gettman, M.T., Ogan, K., et al.: Clinical use of the holmium: YAG laser in laparoscopic partial nephrectomy. J. Endourol. **16**, 289–292 (2002)
30. Lotan, Y., Gettman, M.T., Lindberg, G., et al.: Laparoscopic partial nephrectomy using holmium laser in a porcine model. JSLS **8**, 51–55 (2004)
31. Kommu, S.S., Rane, A.: Devices for laparoendoscopic single-site surgery in urology. Expert Rev. Med. Devices **6**, 95–103 (2009)
32. Fujishiro, M., Kodashima, S., Goto, O., et al.: Technical feasibility of endoscopic submucosal dissection of gastrointestinal epithelial neoplasms with a splash-needle. Surg. Laparosc. Endosc. Percutan. Tech. **18**, 592–597 (2008)
33. Darzi, A.: Hand-assisted laparoscopic colorectal surgery. Semin. Laparosc. Surg. **8**, 153–160 (2001)
34. van der Westebring, P.E.P., Goossens, R.H., Jakimowicz, J.J., et al.: Haptics in minimally invasive surgery – a review. Minim. Invasive Ther. Allied Technol. **17**, 3–16 (2008)
35. Aalbers, A.G., Biere, S.S., van Berge Henegouwen, M.I., et al.: Hand-assisted or laparoscopic-assisted approach in colorectal surgery: a systematic review and meta-analysis. Surg. Endosc. **22**, 1769–1780 (2008)
36. Aalbers, A.G., Doeksen, A., Van Berge Henegouwen, M.I., et al.: Hand-assisted laparoscopic versus open approach in colorectal surgery: a systematic review. Colorectal Dis. **12**(4), 287–295 (2009)
37. Curiel, L., Chavrier, F., Souchon, R., et al.: 1.5-D high intensity focused ultrasound array for non-invasive prostate cancer surgery. IEEE Trans. Ultrason. Ferroelectr. Freq. Control **49**, 231–242 (2002)
38. McGhana, J.P., Dodd 3rd, G.D.: Radiofrequency ablation of the liver: current status. AJR Am. J. Roentgenol. **176**, 3–16 (2001)
39. Sterzer, F.: Microwave medical device. IEEE Microwave Mag. **3**, 65–70 (2002)
40. Orth, K., Russ, D., Durr, J., et al.: Thermo-controlled device for inducing deep coagulation in the liver with the Nd:YAG laser. Lasers Surg. Med. **20**, 149–156 (1997)
41. Tait, I.S., Yong, S.M., Cuschieri, S.A.: Laparoscopic in situ ablation of liver cancer with cryotherapy and radiofrequency ablation. Br. J. Surg. **89**, 1613–1619 (2002)
42. Raggi, M.C., Schneider, A., Hartl, F., et al.: A family of new instruments for laparoscopic radiofrequency ablation of malignant liver lesions. Minim. Invasive Ther. Allied Technol. **15**, 42–47 (2006)
43. Chaussy, C., Thuroff, S., Rebillard, X., et al.: Technology insight: high-intensity focused ultrasound for urologic cancers. Nat. Clin. Pract. Urol. **2**, 191–198 (2005)
44. Wu, F.: Extracorporeal high intensity focused ultrasound in the treatment of patients with solid malignancy. Minim. Invasive Ther. Allied Technol. **15**, 26–35 (2006)
45. Zhang, X., Zhou, L., Chen, B., et al.: Microwave ablation with cooled-tip electrode for liver cancer: an analysis of 160 cases. Minim. Invasive Ther. Allied Technol. **17**, 303–307 (2008)
46. Rao, W., Liu, J.: Injectable liquid alkali alloy based-tumor thermal ablation therapy. Minim. Invasive Ther. Allied Technol. **18**, 30–35 (2009)
47. Mala, T.: Cryoablation of liver tumors – a review of mechanisms, techniques and clinical outcome. Minim. Invasive Ther. Allied Technol. **15**, 9–17 (2006)
48. Fosse, E.: Thermal ablation of benign and malignant tumors. Minim. Invasive Ther. Allied Technol. **15**, 2–3 (2006)
49. Hopkins, H.H., Kapany, N.S.: A flexible fibrescope, using static scanning. Nature **173**, 39–41 (1954)
50. Hopkins, H.H., Berci, G.: Optical principle of the endoscope. In: Hopkins, H.H. (ed.) Endoscopy. Appleton-Century-Crofts, New York (1976)
51. Iddan, G., Meron, G., Glukhovsky, A., et al.: Wireless capsule endoscopy. Nature **405**, 417 (2000)
52. Lee, A.C., Elson, D.S., Neil, M.A., et al.: Solid-state semiconductors are better alternatives to arc-lamps for efficient and uniform illumination in minimal access surgery. Surg. Endosc. **23**, 518–526 (2009)
53. Pierre, S.A., Ferrandino, M.N., Simmons, W.N., et al.: High definition laparoscopy: objective assessment of performance characteristics and comparison with standard laparoscopy. J. Endourol. **23**, 523–528 (2009)
54. Hagiike, M., Phillips, E.H., Berci, G.: Performance differences in laparoscopic surgical skills between true high-definition and three-chip CCD video systems. Surg. Endosc. **21**, 1849–1854 (2007)
55. Gronningsaeter, A., Kleven, A., Ommedal, S., et al.: SonoWand, an ultrasound-based neuronavigation system. Neurosurgery **47**, 1373–1379 (2000). discussion 1379-80
56. Maintz, J.B., Viergever, M.A.: A survey of medical image registration. Med. Image Anal. **2**, 1–36 (1998)
57. Fukuda, M., Mima, F., Nakano, Y.: Studies in echolaparoscopy. Scan. J. Gastroenterol. **17**(Supplement 78), 186 (1982)
58. Jakimowicz, J.J.: Intraoperative ultrasonography in open and laparoscopic abdominal surgery: an overview. Surg. Endosc. **20**(Suppl 2), S425–S435 (2006)
59. Patel, A.C., Arregui, M.E.: Current status of laparoscopic ultrasound. Surg. Technol. Int. **15**, 23–31 (2006)
60. Unsgaard, G., Gronningsaeter, A., Ommedal, S., et al.: Brain operations guided by real-time two-dimensional ultrasound: new possibilities as a result of improved image quality. Neurosurgery **51**, 402–411 (2002). discussion 411-2
61. Ellsmere, J., Stoll, J., Rattner, D., et al.: A navigation system for augmenting laparoscopic ultrasound. Lect. Notes Comput. Sci. **2879**, 184–191 (2003)
62. Lange, N., Becker, C.D., Montet, X.: Molecular imaging in a (pre-) clinical context. Acta Gastroenterol. Belg. **71**, 308–317 (2008)
63. Solberg, O.V., Lango, T., Tangen, G.A., et al.: Navigated ultrasound in laparoscopic surgery. Minim. Invasive Ther. Allied Technol. **18**, 36–53 (2009)
64. Wong Kee Song, L.M., Adler, D.G., Chand, B., et al.: Chromoendoscopy. Gastrointest. Endosc. **66**, 639–649 (2007)
65. Boeriu, A.M., Dobru, D.E., Mocan, S.: Magnifying endoscopy and chromoendoscopy of the upper gastrointestinal tract. J. Gastrointestin. Liver Dis. **18**, 109–113 (2009)
66. Nguyen, N.Q., Leong, R.W.: Current application of confocal endomicroscopy in gastrointestinal disorders. J. Gastroenterol. Hepatol. **23**, 1483–1491 (2008)
67. Mayinger, B.: Endoscopic fluorescence spectroscopic imaging in the gastrointestinal tract. Gastrointest. Endosc. Clin. N. Am. **14**, 487–505 (2004). viii-ix
68. Hoffman, A., Goetz, M., Vieth, M., et al.: Confocal laser endomicroscopy: technical status and current indications. Endoscopy **38**, 1275–1283 (2006)
69. Kiesslich, R., Gossner, L., Goetz, M., et al.: In vivo histology of Barrett's esophagus and associated neoplasia by con-

69. focal laser endomicroscopy. Clin. Gastroenterol. Hepatol. **4**, 979–987 (2006)
70. Kitabatake, S., Niwa, Y., Miyahara, R., et al.: Confocal endomicroscopy for the diagnosis of gastric cancer in vivo. Endoscopy **38**, 1110–1114 (2006)
71. Hanna, G., Cuschieri, A.: Image display technology and image processing. World J. Surg. **25**, 1419–1427 (2001)
72. Hua, H., Gao, C.: Design of a bright polarized head-mounted projection display. Appl. Opt. **46**, 2600–2610 (2007)
73. Prendergast CJ, Ryder BA, Abodeely A, et al (2008) Surgical performance with head-mounted displays in laparoscopic surgery. J. Laparoendosc. Adv. Surg. Tech. A **19**(Suppl 1), S237–S240 (2009)
74. Caversaccio, F.: Computer assistance for intraoperative navigation in ENT surgery. Minim. Invasive Ther. Allied Technol. **12**, 36–51 (2003)
75. Marescaux, J., Rubino, F., Arenas, M., et al.: Augmented-reality-assisted laparoscopic adrenalectomy. JAMA **292**, 2214–2215 (2004)
76. Schreuder, H.W., Verheijen, R.H.: Robotic surgery. BJOG **116**, 198–213 (2009)
77. Deinhardt: Manipulators and integrated OR systems - requirements and solutions. Minim. Invasive Ther. Allied Technol. **12**, 284–292 (2003)
78. Klingler, D.W., Hemstreet, G.P., Balaji, K.C.: Feasibility of robotic radical nephrectomy – initial results of single-institution pilot study. Urology **65**, 1086–1089 (2005)
79. Rawlings, A.L., Woodland, J.H., Vegunta, R.K., et al.: Robotic versus laparoscopic colectomy. Surg. Endosc. **21**, 1701–1708 (2007)
80. Sutherland, G.R., Latour, I., Greer, A.D., et al.: An image-guided magnetic resonance-compatible surgical robot. Neurosurgery **62**, 286–292 (2008). discussion 292-3
81. Wentink, Dankelman, Stassen: Human reliability and training in minimally invasive surgery. Minim. Invasive Ther. Allied Technol. **12**, 129–135 (2003)
82. Bholat, O.S., Haluck, R.S., Murray, W.B., et al.: Tactile feedback is present during minimally invasive surgery. J. Am. Coll. Surg. **189**, 349–355 (1999)
83. Wall, S.A., Brewster, S.: Sensory substitution using tactile pin arrays: human factors, technology and applications. Signal Process. **86**, 3674–3695 (2006)
84. Prasad, S.K., Kitagawa, M., Fischer, G.S., et al.: A modular 2-Dof force-sensing instrument for laparoscopic surgery. In: Ellis, R.E., Peters, T.M. (eds.) Lecture notes in computer science. Springer Berlin, Heidelberg (2003)
85. Schostek, S., Ho, C.N., Kalanovic, D., et al.: Artificial tactile sensing in minimally invasive surgery – a new technical approach. Minim. Invasive Ther. Allied Technol. **15**, 296–304 (2006)
86. Ottermo, M.V., Ovstedal, M., Lango, T., et al.: The role of tactile feedback in laparoscopic surgery. Surg. Laparosc. Endosc. Percutan. Tech. **16**, 390–400 (2006)
87. Sim, H.G., Yip, S.K., Cheng, C.W.: Equipment and technology in surgical robotics. World J. Urol. **24**, 128–135 (2006)
88. Wagner, C.R., Stylopoulos, N., Howe, R.D.: The role of force feedback in surgery: analysis of blunt dissection. Proceedings – 10th symposium on haptic interfaces for virtual environment and teleoperator systems. HAPTICS **2002**, 68–74 (2002)
89. Rayman, R., Croome, K., Galbraith, N., et al.: Robotic telesurgery: a real-world comparison of ground- and satellite-based internet performance. Int. J. Med. Robot. **3**, 111–116 (2007)
90. Marescaux, J., Leroy, J., Gagner, M., et al.: Transatlantic robot-assisted telesurgery. Nature **413**, 379–380 (2001)
91. Anvari, M., McKinley, C., Stein, H.: Establishment of the world's first telerobotic remote surgical service: for provision of advanced laparoscopic surgery in a rural community. Ann. Surg. **241**, 460–464 (2005)
92. Hippocrates.:The genuine works of Hippocrates; tr. from the Greek, with a preliminary discourse and annotations, 1st edn. W Wood, New York (1886)
93. Johnson, I.D.A., Hunter, A.R.: The design and utilization of operating theatres, 1st edn. Edward Arnold, London (1984)
94. Patkin: What surgeons want in operating rooms. Minim. Invasive Ther. Allied Technol. **12**, 256–262 (2003)
95. Patkin: A checklist for components of operating room suites. Minim. Invasive Ther. Allied Technol. **12**, 263–267 (2003)
96. Salvendy, G. (ed.): Handbook of human factors, 1st edn. New York, Wiley (1987)
97. Lango, T., Nesbakken, R., Faerevik, H., et al.: Cooling vest for improving surgeons' thermal comfort: a multidisciplinary design project. Minim. Invasive Ther. Allied Technol. **18**, 1–10 (2009)
98. Lirici, M.M., Arezzo, A.: Surgery without scars: the new frontier of minimally invasive surgery? Controversies, concerns and expectations in advanced operative endoscopy. Minim. Invasive Ther. Allied Technol. **15**, 323–324 (2006)

Moral and Ethical Issues in Laparoscopy and Advanced Surgical Technologies

Richard M. Satava

4.1 Introduction

The Golden Age of Surgery toward the end of the nineteenth century represents the origins of modern surgery – with its roots in the Industrial Age and the simultaneous rise of the scientific method and the disciplines of chemistry, biology, pharmacology, and engineering, both mechanical and shortly thereafter electrical. The resulting combination of the analogous medical applications – asepsis, anesthesia, antibiotics, histology, physiology, instrumentation – was integrated in a multidisciplinary effort that resulted in making surgery not only safe, but also superior to many of the nonsurgical options of the past. Pain and patient struggling were overcome with anesthesia, overwhelming sepsis yielded to antiseptics and antibiotics, accurate diagnosis was made with histological examination, and postoperative care became routine with physiologic monitoring – all of which dramatically improved patient safety. The moral and ethical question of whether it was within Man's province to cut open what God had created yielded to pragmatic triumphs of science. Over the 100 years of the Industrial Age, there had been small but impressive incremental changes that continued to improve the art and science of surgery, but there had not been revolutionary changes that shook the very foundations of surgery or raised major ethical questions – until the Information Age.

R.M. Satava
Department of Surgery, University of Washington Medical Center, 1959 N.E. Pacific St., BB430, Box 356410, Seattle, WA 98195-6410, USA
e-mail: rsatava@u.washington.edu

4.2 Dissociation of Surgeon and Patient

Using video technologies coupled with older laparoscopic technologies, the first steps into minimally invasive surgery (MIS) began at the end of the twentieth century. This was a true revolution, because for the first time surgeons were operating upon patients through tiny incisions without looking at the patient – they were looking at the video monitor (an information representation of what the camera was seeing, and not looking directly at the organs themselves). Then immediately came the next part of the revolution – not touching the patient – with robotic surgery: Not only does the surgeon not look at the patient, but the hand motions are transmitted electronically to remote instruments (end effectors) that perform the cutting, suturing, and other such actions. The surgeon has, in effect, become an "information manager." Other variations are rapidly emerging, such as natural orifice transluminal endoscopic surgery (NOTES) and single incision laparoscopic surgery (SILS) for the near term, and speculative new technologies such as intracellular surgery (genetic surgery), regenerative (and artificial organ) surgery, noninvasive directed-energy surgery (such as radio-surgery and other image-guided surgical options), and additionally suspended animation (instead of anesthesia) and spectrographic analysis (instead of histology).

Each of these foundational advances over the preceding accomplishments introduces an entire new set of profound moral and ethical questions in addition to the pragmatic economic and patient safety issues. Until present times, most of the philosophical and theological conundrums addressed individual patient issues, such as "do not resuscitate," who receives a transplant, etc.; however, the emerging technologies go beyond individual concerns and affect national priorities, entire populations, and even the human species as a whole.

4.3 Laparoscopic Surgery – The Start of a New Era

In the late 1980s, laparoscopic surgery arrived at the shores of the United States as it was beginning to spread over the European continent. However, it came not to the academic community, which opposed it violently (with only a few exceptions), but to the private sector. The benefits of laparoscopic cholecystectomy for the patient were self-evident: less pain, shorter hospital stay, and quicker return to work or activities. For the first time ever, patients began to *demand* the surgery. Opportunistic surgeons began "marketing" the new surgery, and were using terminology such as "laser surgery," though the expensive laser did not provided significant benefit over standard electrocoagulation. Because of patient pressure, insurance companies began reimbursement, which was well above the cost of conventional cholecystectomy.

> *Did the patient have the right to demand a surgical procedure that had a priori huge benefits even though science had not validated the efficacy or safety?*
>
> –
>
> *What is the surgeon's responsibility toward the patient's demands – to refuse the surgery, or to explain the risks, and then proceed with the surgery even though there is increased risk?*

The academic community responded responsibly, with numerous retrospective studies which precipitated a windfall of prospective studies. The initial findings [1] confirmed not only the efficacy (equivalent to or better than open cholecystectomy) but also revealed the increased complications, morbidity, and mortality. Analysis demonstrated that the primary factor in compromising patient safety was due mainly to lack of standardized curriculum and supervised training. Interestingly, a new technology (for healthcare and surgery) arose to meet the need: surgical skills simulation.

4.3.1 Objective Structured Assessment of Technical Skills (OSATS)

With objective structured assessment of technical skills (OSATS) by Reznick et al. [2], a clear standardized methodology for certification of surgical skills was established. Then validation of not only simple and cost-effective training of the fundamentals of laparoscopic surgery (FLS) by Fried et al. [3], but even more sophisticated virtual reality (VR) "surgical simulators" by Seymour et al. [4] resulted in a clear lowering of the procedure complications to the same level of patient safety for both the open and laparoscopic procedures. Fortunately, at the same time, advances in new technologies and instruments in addition to intense competition within the marketplace led to a significant decrease in the cost of laparoscopic procedures. Combined with the dramatic decrease in hospital stay (including the rise of same-day surgery), the laparoscopic approach became even more cost-effective than the open approach. However, initial success with cholecystectomy prompted surgeons to extend the MIS approach to literally every other surgical procedure, once again with the same results of decreased patient safety during the "learning curve" phase of the new procedure. Fortunately, prior experience led to pioneers in new procedures rapidly developing stringent training and assessment programs, so the compromise to patient safety was minimized. It is interesting that the demand and response for patient safety led to another barrier to achieving patient safety – the protest of animal use for training. The objection to using animal training to insure patient safety significantly decreased the opportunity to train new surgeons – however, this had the unintended good consequence of spurring on the development of alternate forms of surgical simulation.

4.3.2 Gartner's Hype Cycle of Innovation

Thus we have seen the typical "Gartner's hype cycle of innovation" [5] response of a new technology – the initial trigger with the inflated expectations, followed by a rapid disillusionment as the expectations are not met (and unintended consequences occur) and the final rigid scientific validation (slope of enlightenment) that results in generalized acceptance and safe application (Fig. 4.1 and Tables 4.1 and 4.2).

Once laparoscopic surgery matured, new nuances emerged. With the demonstrated safety and dramatic decrease in pain and discomfort of the procedure, the indications for the procedure became more relaxed to a point where nearly anyone with right upper quadrant

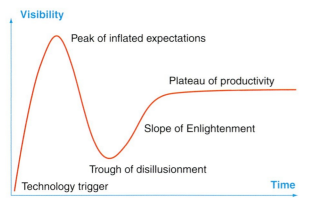

Fig. 4.1 Gartner's hype cycle of innovation

Table 4.1 The six competencies

2001 Consensus by the ACGME and ABMS	
I	Knowledge
II	Patient care
III	Interpersonal and communication skills
IV	Professionalism
V	Practice-based learning and improvement
VI	Systems-based practice

Table 4.2 Standardized curriculum – suggested template

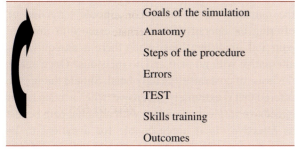

	Goals of the simulation
	Anatomy
	Steps of the procedure
	Errors
	TEST
	Skills training
	Outcomes

4.4 Robotic Surgery – The Second Step Forward in Clinical Practice

Close on the heels of laparoscopic surgery came robotic MIS. Because of the experience with the introduction of laparoscopic surgery, robotic surgery underwent a much more deliberate and stringent validation phase. Yet once again, the benefits for certain procedures was obvious and in a short time clear improvements in quality were demonstrated – though in some cases that improvement in quality did not necessarily result in a significant improvement in overall outcome. However, a new factor was introduced – cost. While laparoscopic surgery systems cost approximately $100,000 with per case costs of a few hundred dollars, the robotic surgery system cost over $1,500,000 with an annual service cost in hundreds of thousands of dollars, and a per case cost of disposable instruments in the thousands – orders of magnitude more expensive than laparoscopic surgery.

> *Was the slight improvement in quality, with questionable improvement in long-term results, worth the significant increase in cost?*

From another perspective there was a great "marketing value" of having "the latest in technology," which results in substantial financial gain. And, while most surgeons carefully analyzed not only the quality of the surgery, but also the importance in advancement in surgical science and teaching to residents (in academic centers), there were clearly some "entrepreneurs" who exploited the technology. Therein is a huge conundrum – how to determine when there is true scientific merit in advancing a new technology to benefit patients, especially when the improvement is initially small, as opposed to when the underlying motive is for profit or self-aggrandizement? And, like in the case of laparoscopic surgery, patients are actually coming to a specific surgeon or hospital because of the perceived benefits of robotic surgery – in this competitive world of healthcare, should not a hospital strive to provide the very best of care, even if the quality improvement is marginal?

Next-generation robots are certain to reduce the price while improving performance. There is always the concern raised that the "robot will take over the surgery" or "what happens if the robot goes 'berserk'." While this is a reasonable question, the likelihood is extremely small, and over 100,000 robotic surgical procedures have been performed to date, with not a single episode of the robot

pain ended up undergoing laparoscopic cholecystectomy, following a diagnosis of acalculus cholecystitis. This relaxing of indications has had a pervasive and subtle influence. Once again, because of the minimal discomfort to the patient, there is a rise in live donors of kidneys – and perhaps other organs. While justified usually within the family, there is a growing opportunity to exploit underprivileged persons in this new "marketplace." While some might extol the humanitarian aspect of living organ donation, there is greater concern for the financial gain and exploitation.

being the problem. The Food and Drug Administration (FDA) has done an excellent job of insuring safety, as have the manufacturers. These robotic systems are built with redundancy, fault tolerance, graceful degradation, and other safety features that insure that no mechanical misadventure can occur. Yet, in spite of all of these safeguards, inevitably something might go wrong.

> *Should science deprive healthcare of a significant advance because of the possibility of a one in a million chance of something going wrong?*

No other systems (for example laparoscopic surgery, where there were a number of mechanical problems that resulted in significant complications, such as stripping of insulation from the instruments with arching, inadvertent unrecognized bowel injury, and death) are foolproof and yet we continue to use them. Should we hold robotic surgery systems to an unreasonable level of accountability beyond where we hold other systems? Should patients be deprived of a new technology because of the "potential" to cause harm, even long after the new technology has a proven safety record which is better than the previous gold standard? There are a number of generally accepted steps in research, development, and validation (including FDA approval) that maximize patient safety – some of these issues will be raised with the following technologies that are not FDA-approved and still in the laboratory development or early clinical trial phase.

4.5 NOTES, SPA, and Cyberknife – Out of the Lab and onto the Bedside

The above technologies of laparoscopic and robotic surgery have been tried, tested, and FDA-approved to a high level of safety. There are other developing technologies that have not met FDA approval – as a matter of fact they require clinical trials to insure their safety and efficacy. NOTES and single port access (SPA) are two new categories of procedures, each with a different set of dilemmas. With NOTES, the question is mainly one of safety – is it prudent and justifiable to create a hole in the gastrointestinal tract (GI) (or other natural orifice) with a greater risk of complication and with a longer operating time simply to avoid an abdominal scar? Can the "discomfort" and/or length of stay be reduced to less than what it is today for standard laparoscopic surgery – and, if so, is the minimal improvement worth the significant increased risk of surgery? Clinical trials are under way to determine safety and efficacy – this is all very carefully controlled and monitored and a necessary step forward in the process of advancing the science; however, is it justified to move forward when there is no reasonable expectation that there would be a significant improvement over the current approach? This is a specious argument, for it presumes two things: (1) that we cannot do better than what we currently have and (2) that during the investigation, we won't learn something not anticipated that will provide a major advance forward and benefit the patient. Should a new technology not be explored because we are not sure what the result would be and because there might (though not certain) be more harm than good?

Another technology undergoing clinical trials is the CyberKnife – a form of x-ray (proton beam) therapy for cancer. The recent advances are in controlling the proton beam with much greater precision, such that only the tumor mass receives the maximal lethal dose, and the intervening tissue receives minimal dosage – and there are no incisions, and virtually no pain. At this time, the technology is extraordinarily expensive – and appropriate for those cancers that are not amenable to surgical resection. However, the difficult decision comes when comparing CyberKnife to alternative proven effective surgical therapies – especially when the outcomes are comparable. Should surgeons be offering an operative procedure, even with minimal pain and small incisions, when there is an equivalent alternative with no pain and no incisions? Once again, the issue of cost raises its ugly head. Should therapy be offered that is extremely expensive, when a much lesser expensive surgical procedure with minimal pain be just as effective? Is it unreasonable for a patient to be expected to suffer a minor amount of pain in order to have their disease treated or cured? Such questions (as with robotic surgery) have become even more germane in the light of the recent crisis in healthcare costs.

4.6 Micro-robots, Genetic Surgery, Tissue Engineering, and Beyond

Thus far, technologies that have been proven or which are carefully being investigated in clinical trials have been reviewed for their moral and ethical issues. There are more momentous issues that will be raised with the "promising" technologies that are in the laboratory, and their impact will revolutionize civilization and the adverse consequences will likewise be more profound.

4.6.1 Micro-robots

The next generation of robots are getting smaller – micro-robots, tiny robots that can be inserted into the body and controlled from the outside [6]. The current prototype that has recently become an approved device is the Given Endoscopic Capsule – a tiny camera inside a pill that is swallowed and passively goes through the GI tract, transmitting images of the mucosal surface, very similar to endoscopy. Already, new versions are being designed which can be controlled, and with micromanipulators attached for biopsy or therapy. Eventually the question will arise – should we insert these into the body for prophylactic purposes, leaving "dormant" medical "probes" in place in case we need them in the future? When they are miniaturized to be small enough to be injected into the blood stream, will they be able to be controlled at that microscopic level, and if so, should there be millions of "tiny robots" circulating in our blood stream? It is one thing to have a pacemaker, hip prosthesis, or other macroscopic artificial object placed in the body which can be easily be removed; it is yet another issue to have millions of microscopic objects which may not be able to be completely removed – would this be an unacceptable safety risk?

4.6.2 Intracellular Surgery

As these micro-robots are perfected and the safety issues resolved, the next level of miniaturization will follow – intracellular surgery. Using femtosecond (ultrafast, pulsed) lasers, it is possible to make an incision in the cell membrane and "operate" upon individual cell components with optical tweezers, magnetic nano-probes to manipulate the mitochondria, Golgi apparatus, and even inside the nucleus. Recent research at Dundee Scotland [7] has demonstrated the ability to "operate" on individual chromosomes. This is but the first step to surgeons performing genetic engineering, removing certain genes and directly inserting desired genes, without the use of viral transfection. While it is likely that it is morally acceptable to change genetic material that causes severe physical disease, would it be acceptable for changing "emotional disorders"? Currently there is the practice of "savior babies" – if a child is born with a known correctable genetic disorder (such as vonWillebrands Disease or phenylketonuria or more severe impairments), it is possible to procreate another child who is genetically engineered to insure that it will be normal, and then harvest some of the cells of the normal child to correct the disease of the "defective" child. Should the parents have the right to not conceive a second child, and be allowed to nurture the disabled child but not allow the child to reach their full potential? Should the government have the right to step in, and demand another child because of the first "child's rights," as well as the significant financial burden to the healthcare system? Even more controversial, if genetic manipulation is acceptable for clear therapeutic benefit, would it also be acceptable to enhance a person beyond current human limitations? Transgenic (genes from one species to another) manipulation is commonplace in genetic engineering research. It is known that the pit viper snake finds it prey using infrared vision, and the humming bird finds flowers in the ultraviolet light portion of the spectrum, and that humans have the same genetic sequences for vision as these species, but these have not been completely activated. Would it be ethical to genetically engineer a young child with either of the above genetic sequences, allowing them to see in the dark or beyond – they clearly would be enhanced beyond what humans could normally do. Who would decide exactly what enhancements were allowable, and who would be able to acquire such enhancements (only the privileged who can pay for them)? What about the initial investigational trials, should unintended consequences occur – is it ethical to offer an enhancement to a perfectly normal healthy person, with the chance of some horrible unforeseen consequence, perhaps as bad as or worse than the stunted arms and legs in the Thalidomide babies?

4.6.3 Tissue Engineering and Regeneration

Somewhat less controversial, and on the macro scale, is tissue engineering, including growing artificial organs or regenerating lost or injured "parts." In tissue engineering, clinical trials on synthetically grown urinary bladders have been successful: using the patient's own stem cells and bio-resorbable scaffolding, synthetically grown bladders were implanted, without the need for immunosuppression, with excellent 5-year follow-up of normally functioning bladders [8]. In the laboratory, every organ and tissue has been grown (except the brain) and animal trials are in progress. Thus, in the future, there is the possibility that any organ will be replaceable, and without rejection because the body does not reject its own stem cells. While replacing normal artificial organs has little moral implications, what happens if nearly all of a person's organs and tissues are replaced with prostheses and/synthetic organs – if 95% of them are artificial, are they still "human"?

What determines whether a person is "human"?

4.6.4 Suspended Animation

Recent advances in research in hibernation and suspended animation have revealed that the Arctic ground squirrel does not hibernate because it is cold; it hibernates because it turns itself off [9]. It is not clear what the stimulus is (light, decreased food, etc.); however, signaling molecules from the hypothalamus are dispersed to all cells of the body, at the mitochondrial membrane, blocking the uptake of oxygen and essentially "turning off" all metabolic processes. Similar results have been induced in mice using hydrogen sulfide [10]. Following induction with hydrogen sulfide, the metabolism is reduced to non-detectable levels – no heart rate, electrocardiography (EKG) is flat, no respiration, body temperature is ambient, and no detectable brain activity by electroencephalogram (EEG) – meeting all the physiologic criteria of death. However, after 6 h of hydrogen sulfide, the oxygen is returned and the mice awaken and run through a maze to feed themselves, inferring that their brains are intact. Currently, similar experiments are being performed in larger animals. Should this be successful, this could be the ideal anesthetic agent – the patient would not die on the operating table, not move, not bleed when cut, and not feel any pain. When the procedures were finished, it would be similar to "rebooting" the system, by reactivating all the metabolic pathways. While the application to surgery is not that controversial, major ethical issues arise if suspended animation is accomplished for significantly longer time frames – in terms of years. Then the frequently cited moral and ethical questions would include: Should a patient with a terminal disease be placed in suspended animation until a cure is possible? Is it even possible to afford to support thousands or millions of people waiting for a cure? What would happen (psychologically, behaviorally) when they were awakened years in the future?

Should we try to keep people alive beyond their "natural" life span, if we already have too many people on the planet to support and feed?

4.7 Summary – And the Ultimate Moral and Ethical Question

It is clear that the rapidly accelerating pace of technological advancement is outstripping the ability to respond to the moral and ethical implications. This must instill in the medical community a responsibility to participate in the debate, regulation, and legislation (if needed) of measures to insure a responsible solution for these changes – it is unconscionable to totally abdicate such responsibilities to non-healthcare professionals such as lawyers and politicians – and we must be at the table providing advice and counsel. The ultimate moral and ethical question lies immediately before us, as first proposed by Francis Fukuyama, the Chairman of the President's Commission on Biomedical Ethics, and later included in his book, *Our Post Human Future*. To paraphrase this challenge:

*For the first time in the history of our planet, there walks upon this planet a **species** so powerful that it can control its own evolution to its own time and its own choosing – **homo sapiens**.*
What shall we choose to make as the species which follows humans?

References

1. The Southern Surgeons Club: A prospective analysis of 1518 laparoscopic cholecystectomies. N. Engl. J. Med. **324**, 1073–1078 (1991)
2. Resnick, R., Regehr, G., MacRae, H., Martin, J., McCulloch, W.: Testing technical skill via an innovative bench station examination. Am. J. Surg. **173**, 226–230 (1997)

3. Derossis, A.M., Fried, G.M., Abrahamowicz, M., Sigman, H.H., Barkun, J.S., Meakins, J.L.: Development of a model of evaluation and training of laparoscopic skills. Am. J. Surg. **175**, 482–487 (1998)
4. Seymour, N.E., Gallagher, A.G., Roman, S.A., O'Brien, M.K., Bansal, V.K., Andersen, D., Satava, R.M.: Virtual reality training improves operating room performance: results of a randomized, double-blinded study. Ann. Surg. **236**, 458–464 (2002)
5. Feen, J.: Understanding Gartner's Hype Cycles, 2007, Gartner Research, ID Number: G00144727 (2007)
6. Shah, B.C., Buettner, S.L., Lehman, A.C., Farritor, S.M., Oleynikov, D.: Miniature in vivo robotics and novel robotic surgical platforms. Urol. Clin. North Am. **36**(2), 251–263 (2009 May)
7. Konig, K., Riemann, I., Fischer, P., Halbhuber, K.G.: Intracellular nanosurgery with near infrared femtosecond laser pulses. Cell Mol Biol (Noisy-le-grand) **45**(2), 195–201 (1999 Mar)
8. Atala, A.: Advances in tissue and organ replacement. Curr. Stem Cell Res. Ther. **3**, 21–31 (2008)
9. Blackstone, E., Morrison, M., Roth, M.B.: H2S induces a suspended animation-like state in mice. Science **308**(5721), 518 (2005 Apr 22)
10. Fukuyama, F.: Our Posthuman Future. Picador, New York (2003)

Robotic Applications in Surgical Oncology

Scott J. Belsley

5.1 Introduction

Robotic applications in surgical oncology range from systems biology and the categorization of the genomic variations responsible for increased susceptibility to cancer as well as an elaboration of the causative mutations. Robots are involved in sequencing the genome, aiding diagnoses and developing new chemotherapeutic agents, as well as testing these agents in virtual environments. Parallels in the development of robotics in genomic analysis and systems biology extend from protein chemistry to proteomics with the latter further extending to the three-dimensional structure analysis of proteins, structural genomics and manipulation of the genome.

Robotics is also prevalent in the diagnostic phases of surgical oncology in the more traditional sense. Computer-controlled end-effectors of varying degrees of automation exist across the spectrum of treatment modalities which range from the development of chemotherapeutic agents, robotic brachytherapy, automated stereotactic radiation with beam intensity modulation, as well as the more traditional and increasingly relevant da Vinci robot. Patterns of the da Vinci's oncological application throughout the specialties are briefly discussed.

The da Vinci robot is a master-slave device that was introduced to the market without an obvious application. The success of the device with increased dexterity of the endowrists and improved visualization remains somewhat enigmatic.

S.J. Belsley
Department of Robotic Surgery, St. Luke's – Roosevelt Hospital Center, Columbia College of Physicians and Surgeons, 425 West 59th Street, Suite 7B, New York, NY 10014, USA
e-mail: sjb47@columbia.edu

5.2 Oncologic Predictive Algorithms

There are a plethora of definitions describing what exactly composes a robot. The evolution that the Intuitive device brought to oncological surgery is the introduction of a computerized surgical console with the ability to assemble visual and tactile information in a manner that adds increased precision and accuracy to the end-effectors. The end-effectors in the case of the Intuitive machine are metal laparoscopic instruments controlled by piano wire. As wristed technology exists in simplistic laparoscopic instrumentation, the significance of robotic-wristed instrumentation lies not in its increased flexibility but rather the computer algorithms that can filter tremor and interact in the same multidimensional environment that is transmitted in the console eyepieces.

For purposes of this chapter, the Intuitive robot will be considered relevant not as a device that popularized wristed instrumentation nor as a device that provides three-dimensional vision but rather as the computer platform that allows a creation of three-dimensional space and the ability of the surgeon to interact in that three-dimensional space. Vision stereopsis is the most rudimentary of these initial calculations but represents a foundation for more complicated coalescing including visual overlay, use of immunofluorescence and advanced haptics. Tremor-cancelling algorithms and the filters involved represent a second level of potential that suggest a more advanced programming path for future automatizaton.

This computerized brain of the da Vinci allows the creation and recognition of multidimensional space by combining images and creating stereopsis; an operating language allows interaction inside a three-dimensional visual space with the potential to overlay other sources of information. Allowing this abstraction, a discussion of the oncological implications of robotics must also include the computer algorithms that encompass the forerunners of artificial intelligence including the mathematical disciplines of dynamic programming, hidden Markov models and advanced algorithms with predictive capabilities that function to elucidate probabilities in the expansive genome.

5.3 Relational Databases and Search Algorithms for Genetic Abnormalities

On one level, the idea of proteomics and structural genomics might seem an abstraction from traditional robotic applications in surgical oncology. To begin with, robotics and computer automation are intimately involved in the construction of genomic databases. Robotic algorithms and automatization allow the identification of oncological targets and the advance from gene transcription to the level of protein biochemistry including injection of novel agents into living cells and advances in clinical development.

Hagler was one of the first to describe the formation of protein tertiary structure on a computer [1] and this finding represents a forerunner of the dynamic interplay between protein chemistry to structural genomics and ultimately to the manipulation of the genome.

Computational power allowing large-scale sequencing projects facilitate an evolution from one-way data analysis into a system of networked dynamic computer systems that allow further investigation such as the development of translational matrices. Protein chemistry has evolved into proteomics [2]. Computational approaches allow better understanding of three-dimensional structures with modeling that incorporates data from different sources. Bioinformatics analysis includes functions such as structure alignment, homology structure modeling and protein functional analysis.

The relevance of machine learning is demonstrated by the multitude of Internet-based search engines as well as stand-alone analytical mining tools [3]. Interlinked systems allow integration of database entries with related resources [4]. Software packages allow varying options on candidate gene screening and annotation of microarray results [5]. Flexible frameworks for detecting and interpreting gene–gene interactions utilize advances in information theory to elucidate single-nucleotide polymorphisms. Constructive induction used for analysis of epistasis is one such example of machine learning to provide classification [6].

5.4 Artificial Intelligence

Although in the past proteomics has been primarily used for discovery, significant efforts are being made to develop proteomic technologies into clinical tools. Reverse-phase protein arrays offer a robust new method of quantitatively assessing expression levels and the activation status of protein panels [7].

Computational servers use mathematical algorithms to form predictions [8]. Network-distributed autonomous agents allow genome alignments and protein homology inference with efficiency and high throughput [9]. Advances in information theory allow interpretations of gene–gene interactions [6].

Genetic regulators including small regulatory RNAs, known as microRNAs, are identified using context-sensitive Hidden Markov Models [10]. Machine learning applied to databases of reference metabolic pathways can predict hypothetical pathways and the possible function of newly sequenced proteins [11]. Variable penetrance and the influence of environmental risk factors are related using computer simulations that apply multi-logistic modeling to escape the limitations of logistic regression and multifactor dimensionality reduction [12].

5.5 Automated Identification of Cancer Cells

Robotic automation is also used to standardize DNA bench work by providing the highly repetitive precise movements required at an exponential frequency as our understanding of the intricacies of the genome evolves. Robotic-automated microscopy allows the ability to capture and analyze images in multiple focal planes of fluorescence with in situ hybridization. This sensitivity allows the ability to identify DNA sequences in less than one epithelial cell per millimeter of blood [13].

High-density DNA arrays automated with robotic deposition of 1 ng of material placed at intervals of 100–300 μm are devices used to measure levels of gene expression and allow complex mixtures of RNA and DNA to be interrogated in a parallel and quantitative fashion simultaneously [14].

5.6 Transitions from Protein Chemistry into Proteomics and Structural Genomics

Databases allow indexing and searching. Machine-learning algorithms facilitate genomic analysis and are used to identify polymorphisms and statistical areas of epistasis. These algorithms will eventually allow proteomic technologies to evolve into clinical tools. Computational approaches are the most powerful way to infer the biological function including structure analysis, prediction and functional annotation.

DNA hybridization used to be manually labor-intensive; now the level of automation has progressed beyond robotics so much so that it is better described as computerization. DNA microarrays make use of high-density cDNA libraries printed on microchips and allow genetic tests in parallel [15]. Slightly larger in scale, motorized autonomous micromanipulators with three degrees of freedom demonstrate the feasibility of large-scale screening of biomolecules when used for the microinjection of zebrafish embryos [16].

The widespread use of robotics in protein crystallography has had a huge impact at every stage of the pipeline from protein cloning, over-expression, purification, crystallization, data collection, structure solution, refinement, validation and data management. All of these processes have become more or less automated requiring minimal human intervention [17].

Outside the scope of this chapter is the next stage of nanorobots, which currently are better described as biodegradable polycationic polymers for the delivery of RNAi therapeutics. Other esoteric delivery systems such as carbon nanotubes, gold nanorads and nanoparticles will likely once again redefine the role of what can be categorized as a robotic oncologic application [18].

5.7 Augmented Reality for Tumor Localization

The introduction of robotic assistance hypothetically enhances applied manual dexterity as well as the precision and accuracy of instrument manipulation. A hybrid evolution from master-slave robotics includes a category of stereotactic biopsy robotic technologies designed to facilitate

- Needle biopsy
- Guidance of radiofrequency ablation
- Insertion of brachytherapy

The need to reconstruct a three dimensional radio-opaque target from two-dimensional data sources from different axes holds obvious potential for improvement with robotic automation.

The da Vinci canvas was developed to solve the inconsistencies arising from varying position and probe pressure during laparoscopic ultrasonography. A dexterous robotic arm integrated with the da Vinci robot incorporates a rigid laparoscopic ultrasound probe into the da Vinci operating system. The device does not just serve as a stable platform but also allows video tracking of the probe motions, calibration, registration and the display of both two-dimensional and three-dimensional images [19].

Another system aligns needles for image-guided needle biopsy to planned entry paths using three-dimensional ultrasound reconstructed from freehand two-dimensional scans. At this stage in the development, this ultrasound-guided robotic system is significantly more accurate than single manual insertions when only one opportunity to hit the target is allowed. When multiple reinsertions are allowed, differences in improved accuracy drop. This drop is also seen in in vivo experiments that require compensation for heartbeat and respiratory effects [20]. An augmented reality visualization and haptic feedback system uses cooperative control to allow

- Accurate planning of needle trajectory
- Adjustments in planned trajectory
- Compensation for target motion
- Overcoming needle deflection

The robotic arm with a six-degree-of-freedom force sensor has demonstrated utility with an ultrasound phantom [21].

A promising fusion of unique data sources is exemplified in an image-guided robotic system used to measure oxygen tension in rodent tumor xenografts. Fiducial markers in the rodent bed visible on positron emission tomography (PET) images were registered to interstitial probes guided by tumor hypoxia. The robotic fusion suggests a point-by-point comparison of physiological probe measurements and image volumetric pixel values as a means of validating molecularly targeted radiotracers [22].

Early technologies allow visual overlay; however, registration of the images is computer-intensive and problematic. Further challenges arise with real-time tissue deformation and the need to constantly re-register visual information with the radiographic results. This phenomenon of accurate but limited fusion imaging potential is demonstrated in a system that combines ultrasound and computed tomography (CT) in the targeting and subsequent radiofrequency ablation of radio-opaque targets in bovine livers. Registration and the simulated ablations were accurate when conducted optimally in an ideal experimental setting without patient movements and breathing [23].

5.8 Dynamic Active Constraints and Haptics

Fusion of visual data from radiologic sources is only one example of augmented reality. Tremor filtration as well as the ability to scale motions on the da Vinci system (i.e. the fine setting on the machine) is an example of the potential of advanced haptic interfaces. Future tissue navigation will use tissue deformation tracking in a manner that combines preoperative data and image guidance into the surgical navigation framework in order to minimize collateral damage during dissection [24].

A single-degree-of-freedom magnetic resonance imaging (MRI)-compatible needle driver system was combined with a haptic feedback device for radiofrequency ablation of breast tumors. This was tele-operated under continuous MRI from outside the scanning room and allowed experimenters to detect healthy versus cancerous tissue in a phantom model when provided with the data from both visual feedback and haptic feedback [25].

A new, intuitive augmented reality system for presentation of force information through sensory substitution has been developed and evaluated. The augmented reality system consists of force-sensing robotic instruments, a kinematic tool tracker, and a graphic display that overlays a visual representation of force levels on top of the moving instrument tips [26]. The intentional transformation of haptic information from touch into a visual representation on top of the moving instrument highlights an additional difficulty with haptics – that of returning the haptic information to the operator in a manner that is easily understood.

5.9 Registration Difficulties

Techniques of augmented reality can hypothetically be used in preoperative planning of laparoscopic and robotic procedures as well as to guide surgical dissection and enhance its accuracy. The organ anatomy that lends itself easiest to registration is one that is relatively static with definite, high-contrast borders. Marker registration systems typically have two stages, hypothesis generation from unique image features and then a combination of both identification and verification. The hypothesis stage is most accurate with an edge-based method that can efficiently detect subtle changes in lighting and partial occlusion [27].

Augmented reality overlay is possible using iterative closest point and image-based surface-tracking technology in organs with definite borders such as renal anatomy [28]. Physiologic markers on the body surface for noninvasive markerless registration have also been described for hypothetical use in gastrointestinal, hepatobiliary and pancreatic surgery [29].

Real-time tracking of surgical tools during robotic surgery can be used to demonstrate the ability to automatically position and control surgical robotic arms in three dimensions [30]. Frame rate and alignment precision with potential clinical utility is demonstrated in a machine vision method which augments stereoscopic images by mixing volumetric CT or MRI radiological images with live patient camera images [31]. An intraoperative cone-beam CT on a mobile arm demonstrates real-time utility for guidance during head and neck surgery in cadavers [32].

5.10 Arterial Targets Used for Overlay

Although not yet applicable in an oncologic setting, vasculature overlay has great potential for tumor dissection. Benefits were found in a model that allows a surgeon to see a patient's anatomy in transparency using an environmental infrared localizer and a stereoscopic helmet. Optimal positioning of trocars and focus of dissection on top of a splenic aneurysm left the blood supply from the short gastric vessels and other collaterals intact [33]. Optimal arterial target selection was also demonstrated in a coronary artery bypass grafting model. Augmented reality and applied alignment algorithms were designed to register with any bifurcations seen in the endoscopic image. The program used these registrations to compare landmark information and look for compatibility within the segmented coronary tree [34].

Augmented reality and tumor tracking is challenging. Although radiologic fixed points can be selected in various systems instead of externally placed fiducial markers, the true challenge of image overlay remains in the ability to track tissue deformation throughout the course of the operation. While early success has been demonstrated in the overlay of relatively fixed vascular structures, the ability to register more ambiguous organs, such as the movement of the small bowel throughout an operation, is still far into the future.

5.11 Tumor Tracking and Motion Compensation

More refined concepts and clinical applications of optical tracking systems are currently in use for stereotactic radiation therapy [35]. Respiratory gating with fiducially based respiratory motion tracking on a robotic radio-surgery system exemplifies a forerunner of more advanced fiducially based tracking systems [36].

Algorithms needed to achieve a geometrically ideal dose delivery to moving tumors can be categorized into those necessary to track the tumor and those needed for real-time beam adaptation [37]. Adaptive tumor-tracking systems allow real-time tumor tracking for compensated lung trajectory prediction [38]. Intensity-modulated radiation therapy with variable beam fluence is capable of generating extremely conformal dose distributions. Accurate isodose volumes provide conformal target volume coverage and avoidance of normal structures [39].

5.12 Robotic Stereotactic Radio-surgery

Stereotactic radio-surgery is a relatively novel treatment modality which allows high radiation dose delivery with sub-millimeter precision utilizing a linear accelerator mounted on a robotic arm. The field is non-invasive compared to the minimally invasive categorization of robotics and laparoscopy and currently falls under the realm of radiation oncologists. Since the introduction of the harmonic scalpel in 1995, surgeons have respected the increasing relevance of energy delivery devices. Unlike single-incision laparoscopic surgery (SILS) and natural orifice translumenal endoscopic surgery (NOTES), the modality truly represents scarless surgery. The Cyberknife represents an evolution from Gamma Knife target radiation therapy, which moved the patient in sub-millimeter increments during the treatment but was only applicable for lesions of the brain.

Although this technology represents an evolution from traditional medical linear accelerators, its application is still limited to the early stages of development. Very high-risk patients with difficult treatment options are selected in order to balance the level of risk with yet unproven benefit.

Robotic stereotactic radio-surgery is used on relapse of gynecological malignancies and other cancers where options are limited by prior surgical, chemotherapeutic or radiation treatments [40]. The Cyberknife has treated locally recurrent nasopharyngeal carcinoma with fractionated stereotactic radiotherapy [41]. Image-guided robotic radio-surgery is suggested as a feasible, safe and comfortable treatment option for patients with uveal melanoma [42].

Proprietary motion compensation software packages are becoming more common. There are compensation systems that employ different methods of fiducially based respiratory gating. Using external markers in conjunction with diagnostic x-ray images allows the robotic arm to move in real time such that the beam always remains aligned with the target [43].

The ability to use split-volume treatment planning in clinical situations where stringent dose limits are required is another benefit [44].

Although long-term data are lacking, computerized precision applied to energy therapies represents an area of great clinical potential. In the short term, clinical outcomes of robotic radio-surgery with its typical hypo-fractionation characteristics will be based on assumptions of equivalence [45].

5.13 Robotic Brachytherapy

Robotic brachytherapy employs robotic technology to deploy indwelling energy therapy and therefore represents a hybrid between master-slave surgical robots and stereotactic radio-surgery. The placement of seeds based on radiographic imaging is an area with potential for automation.

A robotically assisted prostate brachytherapy system co-registers data from transrectal ultrasound and integrates information with a Food and Drug Administration (FDA)-approved commercial treatment-planning system. The device shows improvement in tip-positioning errors when compared to manual template guidance [46]. Another device uses MRI guidance calibrated with fiducially based image coordinates and allows for interactive target planning and generates rapidly updated registered two-dimensional images [47].

A fourth-generation thoracic brachytherapy robot incorporates modified electromagnetic navigation and ultrasound image guidance with robotic assistance and a seed injector [48]. The advantages of the da Vinci robot's articulating instrumentation to reduce damage to diseased lung parenchyma makes robotic surgical brachytherapy seed placement after sub-lobar resection in medically compromised patients a potential option [49].

5.14 Da Vinci™ Oncological Trends

The introduction of the robotic technology throughout each of the specialties waxes and wanes. While the increased precision of the device suggests that ideal applications would lie in technically challenging, complicated procedures, the driving market force of the technology comprises in the procedures that can be performed in bulk in high numbers and with low complications.

Robotics allows a stable platform for the surgical procedure. The importance of a stable platform should not be underestimated. On a purely technical level, it allows increased independence of the primary surgeon away from a secondary surgeon. The stable platform also serves to help surgeon orientation and will ultimately facilitate image registration with other technologies.

5.14.1 Applications in Urology

5.14.1.1 Robotic Prostatectomy

Prostatectomy represents an ideal platform to evaluate different modalities for cancer treatment. Prostate cancer has both a high prevalence and a multitude of treatment options extending from surgery, radiation, cryotherapy and expectant management [50,51]. Robotic prostatectomy is currently limited to localized disease (stage cT2 or less) without evidence of clinical or radiographic metastatic disease. The contraindications to robotic prostatectomy are relatively few and include severe bleeding diatheses and cardiopulmonary compromise contradicting general anesthesia [52].

Although robotic and laparoscopic prostatectomy is associated with a shorter hospital stay and a lower bladder neck/urethral obstruction rate, when an analysis is broadened to a multitude of outcomes, laparoscopic prostatectomy and open radical prostatectomy share similar rates of postoperative morbidity and need for additional treatment [53]. There is no considerable improvement in postoperative pain with robotic and laparoscopic prostatectomy versus the open operation [54,55].

Assessment of the comparative effectiveness and harms of localized prostate cancer treatments is, however, difficult because of limitations in the feasibility of prospective study design. Despite the enthusiasm with which robotic prostatectomy continues to be embraced, no large randomized trial evaluates brachytherapy, cryotherapy, robotic radical prostatectomy, or photon-beam or intensity-modulated radiation [56].

The technical abilities of the robot may allow an improvement on the design of the surgical technique to improve functional outcomes. There is potential demonstrated by the robotic technique of preserving the peri-prostatic fascia. This layer on histological analysis demonstrates neuro-vascular bundles assumed best to preserve and is not appreciated during the laparoscopic and open techniques. Results with the robotic approach suggest an increase in potency [57]. Other investigators report small improvements in potency after robotic bilateral-nerve sparing procedures [58]. Although there is an increasing need to standardize assessment techniques, complications and learning curves for robotic procedures, [59] there is a trend toward consistently better outcomes following robotic versus laparoscopic prostatectomy and it seems that the technology can successfully diminish the learning curve for the minimally invasive approach [60].

Within the narrow bony pelvis, the da Vinci robot seems ideally situated vis-à-vis the prostate. The use of the da Vinci robot to assist laparoscopic urologic surgery is embraced as a platform to enhance the surgeon's technical skills with the ultimate goal of a merge of technology to improve surgical outcomes [61]. Lack of significant advantages of the minimally invasive approaches may be due to sacrificed visual and tactile assessment of tumor stage afforded by the open approach and may represent an area of potential improvement with future technology [62].

5.14.1.2 Robotic Resection of Renal Cancer

Although long-term outcome data are presently lacking, early experience with robotic partial nephrectomy shows promise. The technique should continue to evolve as it gains acceptance as an alternative to the traditional laparoscopic approach [63]. There have been few recently published papers regarding the robotic approach to the management of renal cancer with few clear benefits [64]. Until some technological advantage, most likely some visual overlay of tumor or vasculature, is added to the robotic procedure, robotic minimally invasive nephron-sparing nephrectomy will have difficulty showing benefit over the laparoscopic approach.

5.14.2 Robotic Gynecological Surgery

Robotic gynecological oncologic surgery is gaining acceptance and is rapidly growing as evidenced by an increased number of publications on the topic; these publications demonstrate the safety, efficacy, and improved outcomes compared to open surgery and conventional laparoscopy [65]. Institutions are discovering that the introduction of a robotic system can actually change referral patterns and outcomes [66] and that these changes occur over a relatively short time in a manner that has been both feasible and safe [67].

The introduction of laparoscopic cholecystectomy led to an increased frequency of the procedure [68] largely because of a sustained lowering in the threshold of patients and physicians. Despite the improvement afforded by technology, this caused an increase in the consumption of health-care resources [69] ultimately not leading to cost savings. Although a portion of the increased trends of robotic gynecological approaches are due to this same phenomenon, with robotic gynecological surgery there is an expansion of the perceived indications for minimally invasive surgery as endometrial cancer staging has become an accepted indication for laparoscopy, with many surgeons planning on increasing their use of robotic-assisted surgery in the next year [70].

Robotic gynecological surgery is similar to other specialties in that current advantages are due to its abilities to allow a more rapid transition to minimally invasive surgery and that in the hands of experienced minimally invasive surgeons, final outcomes are likely similar with or without the use of the robot [71].

5.14.3 Robotic Applications in Skull Base Surgery and ENT

Robotic equipment for laryngeal surgery has hypothetical potential to overcome many of the limitations of endo-laryngeal procedures [72]. Transoral robotic surgery has technical limitations due to instrumentation and challenges with regard to the bony skull base and intracranial work. Transoral formal neck dissection for cervical metastases is not currently feasible [73]. Early applications will likely require a combined approach to enhance access to the midline and anterior skull base [74]. Another problem to overcome will be the risk of cerebrospinal fluid (CSF) leak after endoscopic approaches, which has been reported to be as much as tenfold higher than after the open approach [75].

Robotic endoscopic thyroidectomy using a gasless, trans-axillary approach for bilateral total thyroidectomy with ipsilateral central compartment node dissection is feasible and safe in selected patients with a benign or malignant thyroid tumor [76,77]. Similar results were found using a bilateral axillary breast approach (BABA), where similar cosmetic results and minimal postoperative pain were suggested to be improved [78]. Conventional open thyroidectomy requires a shorter operative time but the robotic cases may also reduce postoperative neck discomfort with fewer adverse swallowing symptoms [79]. Robotic thyroid surgery currently has a longer length of stay than its open counterpart; with increases in surgeon experience, this improves [80].

Technical challenges with adequate protection of the contralateral recurrent largyngeal nerve as well as limited benefit have slowed the robotic procedure's widespread adoption other than in parts of Asia. There is a chance, however, that with increasing patient awareness, popularity may be gained among consumers [81].

5.14.4 Applications in Thoracic Surgery

5.14.4.1 Robotic Thymectomy and Resection of Mediastinal Tumors

The upper mediastinum is an anatomic area with large vulnerable vessels and nerves that is difficult to reach when approached by conventional thoracoscopy. The improved maneuverability of robotics might be suggested as the optimal approach for select mediastinal dissection including extended thymectomy [82]. The robot is thought to facilitate complete resection of the thymus and perithymic fat with benefit over thoracoscopic approaches and may have potential for early, low-grade thymoma resection [83]. Technical expertise with thoracoscopy allows similar outcomes as robotics [84]. Posterior mediastinal tumors are neurogenic tumors and commonly adherent to the posterior mediastinal skeleton. Although robotic resection has been reported [85,86], a widespread adoption seems unlikely.

5.14.4.2 Robotic Resection of Lung Cancer

Technological improvements are required to popularize applications for lung cancer. Robotic I[125] brachytherapy seed placement tailored by a radiation oncologist working with the surgeon in the operating room facilitates an exact dosing regimen. Although a feasible adjuvant procedure to reduce the incidence of recurrence after sub-lobar resection in medically compromised patients, this procedure can be improved with better technology [49]. Robotic lung lobectomy for lung cancer with mediastinal lymph node dissection has similar complications and median number of lymph nodes harvested as in other approaches. Median postoperative hospitalization improves with increasing experience [87].

5.14.4.3 Robotic Esophageal Resection

The phenomenon of a less invasive access approach not corresponding to improved outcomes is seen in transhiatal esophagectomy. This approach does not seem to have the assumed potential benefits in terms of recovery when compared to three-hole esophagectomy and also requires endoscopic dilatation at increased incidence [88]. Minimally invasive robotic esophagectomy represents a challenging application because of the already high morbidities associated with the operations, partially due to the associated comorbidities of the patient population.

Early data suggest that the robotic approach facilitates an extended three-field esophago-lymphadenectomy even after induction therapy and abdominal surgery. Complications are similar to other approaches but with the potential for a decreased need for an intensive care unit (ICU) stay [89]. The technique of robotic esophagectomy is oncologically acceptable [90]; however, the identifiable benefit of robotics relative to other approaches still needs to be demonstrated [91].

5.14.5 Applications in General Surgery

5.14.5.1 Robotic Gastric Surgery

Robot-assisted gastrectomy with lymphadenectomy can be applied safely and effectively for patients with gastric cancer [92]. The extent of lymphadenectomy and postoperative morbidity is similar. Estimated blood loss and length of stay are significantly less in patients who undergo robotic gastrectomy compared to patients operated with laparoscopic or open approaches [93].

The robotic approach may enable the surgeon to perform atypical gastrectomies for oncologically safe resections in challenging locations with respect to the gastro-esophageal junction or pylorus and allow their preservation [94].

The use of endoscopic mucosal resection pioneered in Japan for the treatment of early gastric cancer has expanded to include therapy for other early gastrointestinal malignancies including pre-cancerous lesions such as adenomas in the colorectal tract [95,96]. This area may represent potential for further mechanization of the instruments and the application of robotics.

5.14.5.2 Robotic Large Bowel Procedures

Robotic colon and rectal resections are safe and feasible options but without proven utility and efficacy [97]. The conversion rate is significantly lower for robotic anterior rectal resection when compared to traditional laparoscopic approaches for anterior rectal resection [98].

An operation that makes use of the da Vinci's advantages with increased visualization and dexterity in the bony pelvis is robotic-assisted total mesorectal excision. When performed for primary rectal cancer, the operation in experienced hands is safe with equivalent recurrence and survival rates as other approaches [99,100].

One-stage resection of primary colon cancer and synchronous liver metastases is considered an effective strategy of cure. A pilot study suggests that robot assistance may facilitate liver resection and increase the number of patients who may benefit from a minimally invasive operation [101].

5.14.5.3 Robotic Resection of Solid Organ Lesions

Robotic pancreatico-duodenectomy can be accomplished using robotic instrumentation [102]. Robot-assisted laparoscopic middle pancreatectomy with pancreatico-gastrostomy presents an interesting, less invasive option for resection of benign tumors of the neck and proximal body of the pancreas [103]. Complication and mortality rates are comparable to those of open surgery but with some of the advantages typically associated with minimally invasive surgery [104].

From a purely technical level, robotic adrenalectomy is an acceptable option in high-volume robotic centers from the standpoints of outcomes, feasibility, and cost [105].

5.15 Conclusion

Robotics plays a role in the oncologic classification of genomic targets with applications that include the use of DNA impregnated on microchips, automated robotic microscopes and machine-learning methods for classification and identification of polymorphisms. Future devices will allow direct manipulation of embryonic cells and later provide more esoteric delivery systems for RNAi.

The Intuitive robot has proven oncologic outcomes throughout all of the surgical specialties. The improvements provided by the technology make certain procedures more amenable to surgeons with less minimally invasive surgery training. The robot may serve as a bridge device for those not completely comfortable with laparoscopic approaches. The use of the robot in the pelvis for urologic and gynecologic procedures as well as total mesorectal excisions maximizes the current benefits of the da Vinci with its increased visualization and articulating instruments. Procedures where a large intra-corporeal working area is needed such as thoracoscopy and general surgery are less applicable to the current advantages of the da Vinci system. Oncological procedures in these areas are limited by exposure, retraction, tactile sense and not necessarily by an instrument's ability to articulate with increased dexterity. The delay in availability of robotic sealing devices including energy devices and staplers has also resulted in decreased application of robotics in these areas.

Oncological operations occur only after the patient has undergone multiple radiological studies and an exhaustive medical work-up. Currently the surgeon is required to merge these multiple sources of information into an operative plan. Intra-operative decisions are based on the recollection of these sources. The da Vinci device has obvious potential as a computer platform to merge patient data from multiple sources in real time.

Energy devices will be of increasing importance in an oncologic surgeon's armamentarium. In the near future there will be a further bifurcation between the categories of robotic surgical devices based on the types of end-effector. One fork will be represented by automated stereotactic radiation devices such as the Cyberknife and the other represented by more traditional surgical operations performed by machines similar to the da Vinci surgical robot. A parallel evolution with redundant technologies that include a more robust visual processor and those that allow overlay of information will solve the surgical tenants of increased precision and accuracy while at the same time limiting damage to contiguous structures.

As technology develops exponentially, the categorization of robotic applications in oncologic surgery becomes merely semantic. Robotic oncologic surgery is the undeniable future when classified as broadly as any technology that requires a microchip as an intermediary for control. The short-term utility of the current clinical devices will depend on their ability to coalesce multiple sources of information and provide augmented reality to the operator.

References

1. Hagler, A.T., Honig, B.: On the formation of protein tertiary structure on a computer. Proc. Natl. Acad. Sci. USA **75**(2), 554–558 (1978)
2. Patterson, S.D., Aebersold, R.H.: Proteomics: the first decade and beyond. Nat. Genet. **33**(Suppl), 311–323 (2003)
3. Wilkins, M.R., et al.: Protein identification and analysis tools in the ExPASy server. Methods Mol. Biol. **112**, 531–552 (1999)
4. Gasteiger, E., et al.: ExPASy: The proteomics server for in-depth protein knowledge and analysis. Nucleic Acids Res. **31**(13), 3784–3788 (2003)
5. Smedley, D., et al.: BioMart–biological queries made easy. BMC Genomics **10**, 22 (2009)
6. Moore, J.H., et al.: A flexible computational framework for detecting, characterizing, and interpreting statistical patterns of epistasis in genetic studies of human disease susceptibility. J. Theor. Biol. **241**(2), 252–261 (2006)
7. Ornstein, D.K., Petricoin III, E.F.: Proteomics to diagnose human tumors and provide prognostic information. Oncology (Williston Park) **18**(4), 521–529 (2004). discussion 529-32
8. Pal, D., Eisenberg, D.: Inference of protein function from protein structure. Structure **13**(1), 121–130 (2005)
9. Severin, J., et al.: eHive: an artificial intelligence workflow system for genomic analysis. BMC Bioinform. **11**(1), 240 (2010)
10. Agarwal, S., et al.: Prediction of novel precursor miRNAs using a context-sensitive hidden Markov model (CSHMM). BMC Bioinform. **11**(Suppl 1), S29 (2010)
11. Dale, J.M., Popescu, L., Karp, P.D.: Machine learning methods for metabolic pathway prediction. BMC Bioinform. **11**, 15 (2010)
12. Amato, R., et al.: A novel approach to simulate gene-environment interactions in complex diseases. BMC Bioinform. **11**, 8 (2010)
13. Ntouroupi, T.G., et al.: Detection of circulating tumour cells in peripheral blood with an automated scanning fluorescence microscope. Br. J. Cancer **99**(5), 789–795 (2008)
14. Lockhart, D.J., Winzeler, E.A.: Genomics, gene expression and DNA arrays. Nature **405**(6788), 827–836 (2000)
15. Schena, M., et al.: Quantitative monitoring of gene expression patterns with a complementary DNA microarray. Science **270**(5235), 467–470 (1995)
16. Wang, W., et al.: A fully automated robotic system for microinjection of zebrafish embryos. PLoS ONE **2**(9), e862 (2007)
17. Manjasetty, B.A., et al.: Automated technologies and novel techniques to accelerate protein crystallography for structural genomics. Proteomics **8**(4), 612–625 (2008)
18. Higuchi, Y., Kawakami, S., Hashida, M.: Strategies for in vivo delivery of siRNAs: recent progress. BioDrugs **24**(3), 195–205 (2010)
19. Leven, J., et al.: DaVinci canvas: a telerobotic surgical system with integrated, robot-assisted, laparoscopic ultrasound capability. Med. Image Comput. Comput. Assist. Interv. **8**(Pt 1), 811–818 (2005)
20. Boctor, E.M., et al.: Three-dimensional ultrasound-guided robotic needle placement: an experimental evaluation. Int. J. Med. Robot. **4**(2), 180–191 (2008)
21. Freschi, C., et al.: Ultrasound guided robotic biopsy using augmented reality and human-robot cooperative control. Conf. Proc. IEEE. Eng. Med. Biol. Soc. **2009**, 5110–5113 (2009)
22. Chang, J., et al.: A robotic system for 18 F-FMISO PET-guided intratumoral pO2 measurements. Med. Phys. **36**(11), 5301–5309 (2009)
23. Crocetti, L., et al.: Targeting liver lesions for radiofrequency ablation: an experimental feasibility study using a CT-US fusion imaging system. Invest. Radiol. **43**(1), 33–39 (2008)
24. Lee, S.L., et al.: From medical images to minimally invasive intervention: computer assistance for robotic surgery. Comput. Med. Imaging Graph. **34**(1), 33–45 (2010)
25. Kokes, R., et al.: Towards a teleoperated needle driver robot with haptic feedback for RFA of breast tumors under continuous MRI. Med. Image Anal. **13**(3), 445–455 (2009)
26. Akinbiyi, T., et al.: Dynamic augmented reality for sensory substitution in robot-assisted surgical systems. Conf. Proc. IEEE Eng. Med. Biol. Soc. **1**, 567–570 (2006)
27. Fiala, M.: Designing highly reliable fiducial markers. IEEE Trans. Pattern Anal. Mach. Intell. **32**(7), 1317–1324 (2010)
28. Su, L.M., et al.: Augmented reality during robot-assisted laparoscopic partial nephrectomy: toward real-time 3D-CT to stereoscopic video registration. Urology **73**(4), 896–900 (2009)
29. Sugimoto, M., et al.: Image overlay navigation by markerless surface registration in gastrointestinal, hepatobiliary and pancreatic surgery. J. Hepatobiliary Pancreat. Surg. (2009)

30. Marescaux, J., Solerc, L.: Image-guided robotic surgery. Semin. Laparosc. Surg. **11**(2), 113–122 (2004)
31. Ferrari, V., et al.: A 3-D mixed-reality system for stereoscopic visualization of medical dataset. IEEE Trans. Biomed. Eng. **56**(11), 2627–2633 (2009)
32. Daly, M.J., et al.: Intraoperative cone-beam CT for guidance of head and neck surgery: Assessment of dose and image quality using a C-arm prototype. Med. Phys. **33**(10), 3767–3780 (2006)
33. Pietrabissa, A., et al.: Mixed reality for robotic treatment of a splenic artery aneurysm. Surg. Endosc. **24**(5), 1204 (2010)
34. Falk, V., et al.: Cardio navigation: planning, simulation, and augmented reality in robotic assisted endoscopic bypass grafting. Ann. Thorac. Surg. **79**(6), 2040–2047 (2005)
35. Wagner, T.H., et al.: Optical tracking technology in stereotactic radiation therapy. Med. Dosim. **32**(2), 111–120 (2007)
36. Afthinos, J.N., et al.: What technical barriers exist for real-time fluoroscopic and video image overlay in robotic surgery? Int. J. Med. Robot. **4**(4), 368–372 (2008)
37. Sawant, A., et al.: Toward submillimeter accuracy in the management of intrafraction motion: the integration of real-time internal position monitoring and multileaf collimator target tracking. Int. J. Radiat. Oncol. Biol. Phys. **74**(2), 575–582 (2009)
38. Wilbert, J., et al.: Tumor tracking and motion compensation with an adaptive tumor tracking system (ATTS): system description and prototype testing. Med. Phys. **35**(9), 3911–3921 (2008)
39. Purdy, J.A.: From new frontiers to new standards of practice: advances in radiotherapy planning and delivery. Front. Radiat. Ther. Oncol. **40**, 18–39 (2007)
40. Kunos, C., et al.: Stereotactic body radiosurgery for pelvic relapse of gynecologic malignancies. Technol. Cancer Res. Treat. **8**(5), 393–400 (2009)
41. Seo, Y., et al.: Robotic system-based fractionated stereotactic radiotherapy in locally recurrent nasopharyngeal carcinoma. Radiother. Oncol. **93**(3), 570–574 (2009)
42. Muacevic, A., et al.: Development of a streamlined, non-invasive robotic radiosurgery method for treatment of uveal melanoma. Technol. Cancer Res. Treat. **7**(5), 369–374 (2008)
43. Ozhasoglu, C., et al.: Synchrony–cyberknife respiratory compensation technology. Med. Dosim. **33**(2), 117–123 (2008)
44. Sahgal, A., et al.: Split-volume treatment planning of multiple consecutive vertebral body metastases for cyberknife image-guided robotic radiosurgery. Med. Dosim. **33**(3), 175–179 (2008)
45. Nijdam, W., et al.: Robotic radiosurgery vs. brachytherapy as a boost to intensity modulated radiotherapy for tonsillar fossa and soft palate tumors: the clinical and economic impact of an emerging technology. Technol. Cancer Res. Treat. **6**(6), 611–620 (2007)
46. Fichtinger, G., et al.: Robotic assistance for ultrasound-guided prostate brachytherapy. Med. Image Anal. **12**(5), 535–545 (2008)
47. Tokuda, J., et al.: Integrated navigation and control software system for MRI-guided robotic prostate interventions. Comput. Med. Imaging Graph. **34**(1), 3–8 (2010)
48. Lin, A.W., et al.: Electromagnetic navigation improves minimally invasive robot-assisted lung brachytherapy. Comput. Aided Surg. **13**(2), 114–123 (2008)
49. Blasberg, J.D., et al.: Robotic brachytherapy and sublobar resection for T1 non-small cell lung cancer in high-risk patients. Ann. Thorac. Surg. **89**(2), 360–367 (2010)
50. Barry, M.J.: The prostate cancer treatment bazaar: comment on "Physician visits prior to treatment for clinically localized prostate cancer". Arch. Intern. Med. **170**(5), 450–452 (2010)
51. Jang, T.L., et al.: Physician visits prior to treatment for clinically localized prostate cancer. Arch. Intern. Med. **170**(5), 440–450 (2010)
52. Bivalacqua, T.J., Pierorazio, P.M., Su, L.M.: Open, laparoscopic and robotic radical prostatectomy: optimizing the surgical approach. Surg. Oncol. **18**(3), 233–241 (2009)
53. Lowrance, W.T., et al.: Comparative effectiveness of prostate cancer surgical treatments: a population based analysis of postoperative outcomes. J. Urol. **183**(4), 1366–1372 (2010)
54. Webster, T.M., et al.: Robotic assisted laparoscopic radical prostatectomy versus retropubic radical prostatectomy: a prospective assessment of postoperative pain. J. Urol. **174**(3), 912–914 (2005). discussion 914
55. Smith Jr., J.A., et al.: A comparison of the incidence and location of positive surgical margins in robotic assisted laparoscopic radical prostatectomy and open retropubic radical prostatectomy. J. Urol. **178**(6), 2385–2389 (2007). discussion 2389-90
56. Wilt, T.J., et al.: Systematic review: comparative effectiveness and harms of treatments for clinically localized prostate cancer. Ann. Intern. Med. **148**(6), 435–448 (2008)
57. Menon, M., et al.: Vattikuti Institute prostatectomy: contemporary technique and analysis of results. Eur. Urol. **51**(3), 648–657 (2007). discussion 657-8
58. Hakimi, A.A., et al.: Direct comparison of surgical and functional outcomes of robotic-assisted versus pure laparoscopic radical prostatectomy: single-surgeon experience. Urology **73**(1), 119–123 (2009)
59. Murphy, D.G., et al.: Downsides of robot-assisted laparoscopic radical prostatectomy: limitations and complications. Eur. Urol. (2009)
60. Finkelstein, J., et al.: Open versus laparoscopic versus robot-assisted laparoscopic prostatectomy: the European and US experience. Rev. Urol. **12**(1), 35–43 (2010)
61. Pow-Sang, J.: Pure and robotic-assisted laparoscopic radical prostatectomy: technology and techniques merge to improve outcomes. Expert Rev. Anticancer Ther. **8**(1), 15–19 (2008)
62. Nelson, J.B.: Debate: open radical prostatectomy vs. laparoscopic vs. robotic. Urol. Oncol. **25**(6), 490–493 (2007)
63. Shapiro, E., et al.: The role of nephron-sparing robotic surgery in the management of renal malignancy. Curr. Opin. Urol. **19**(1), 76–80 (2009)
64. Murphy, D., Dasgupta, P.: Robotic approaches to renal cancer. Curr. Opin. Urol. **17**(5), 327–330 (2007)
65. Mendivil, A., Holloway, R.W., Boggess, J.F.: Emergence of robotic assisted surgery in gynecologic oncology: American perspective. Gynecol. Oncol. **114**(2 Suppl), S24–S31 (2009)
66. Hoekstra, A.V., et al.: The impact of robotics on practice management of endometrial cancer: transitioning from traditional surgery. Int. J. Med. Robot. **5**(4), 392–397 (2009)

67. Peiretti, M., et al.: Robotic surgery: changing the surgical approach for endometrial cancer in a referral cancer center. J. Minim. Invasive Gynecol. **16**(4), 427–431 (2009)
68. Orlando III, R., et al.: Laparoscopic cholecystectomy. A statewide experience. The Connecticut Laparoscopic Cholecystectomy Registry. Arch. Surg. **128**(5), 494–498 (1993)
69. Legorreta, A.P., et al.: Increased cholecystectomy rate after the introduction of laparoscopic cholecystectomy. JAMA **270**(12), 1429–1432 (1993)
70. Mabrouk, M., et al.: Trends in laparoscopic and robotic surgery among gynecologic oncologists: a survey update. Gynecol. Oncol. **112**(3), 501–505 (2009)
71. Cho, J.E., Nezhat, F.R.: Robotics and gynecologic oncology: review of the literature. J. Minim. Invasive Gynecol. **16**(6), 669–681 (2009)
72. Hillel, A.T., et al.: Applications of robotics for laryngeal surgery. Otolaryngol. Clin. North Am. **41**(4), 781–791 (2008). vii
73. O'Malley Jr., B.W., Weinstein, G.S.: Robotic skull base surgery: preclinical investigations to human clinical application. Arch. Otolaryngol. Head Neck Surg. **133**(12), 1215–1219 (2007)
74. O'Malley Jr., B.W., Weinstein, G.S.: Robotic anterior and midline skull base surgery: preclinical investigations. Int. J. Radiat. Oncol. Biol. Phys. **69**(2 Suppl), S125–S128 (2007)
75. Snyderman, C.H., et al.: Endoscopic skull base surgery: principles of endonasal oncological surgery. J. Surg. Oncol. **97**(8), 658–664 (2008)
76. Kang, S.W., et al.: Robotic thyroid surgery using a gasless, transaxillary approach and the da Vinci S system: the operative outcomes of 338 consecutive patients. Surgery **146**(6), 1048–1055 (2009)
77. Kang, S.W., et al.: Robot-assisted endoscopic surgery for thyroid cancer: experience with the first 100 patients. Surg. Endosc. **23**(11), 2399–2406 (2009)
78. Lee, K.E., Rao, J., Youn, Y.K.: Endoscopic thyroidectomy with the da Vinci robot system using the bilateral axillary breast approach (BABA) technique: our initial experience. Surg. Laparosc. Endosc. Percutan. Tech. **19**(3), e71–e75 (2009)
79. Lee, J., et al.: Differences in postoperative outcomes, function, and cosmesis: open versus robotic thyroidectomy. Surg. Endosc. (2010)
80. Miccoli, P., et al.: Minimally invasive video-assisted thyroidectomy: five years of experience. J. Am. Coll. Surg. **199**(2), 243–248 (2004)
81. Goh, H.K., Ng, Y.H., Teo, D.T.: Minimally invasive surgery for head and neck cancer. Lancet Oncol. **11**(3), 281–286 (2010)
82. Savitt, M.A., et al.: Application of robotic-assisted techniques to the surgical evaluation and treatment of the anterior mediastinum. Ann. Thorac. Surg. **79**(2), 450–455 (2005). discussion 455
83. Al-Mufarrej, F., et al.: From Jacobaeus to the da Vinci: thoracoscopic applications of the robot. Surg. Laparosc. Endosc. Percutan. Tech. **20**(1), 1–9 (2010)
84. Augustin, F., et al.: Video-assisted thoracoscopic surgery versus robotic-assisted thoracoscopic surgery thymectomy. Ann. Thorac. Surg. **85**(2), S768–S771 (2008)
85. Meehan, J.J., Sandler, A.D.: Robotic resection of mediastinal masses in children. J. Laparoendosc. Adv. Surg. Tech. A **18**(1), 114–119 (2008)
86. Bodner, J., et al.: Early experience with robot-assisted surgery for mediastinal masses. Ann. Thorac. Surg. **78**(1), 259–265 (2004). discussion 265-6
87. Veronesi, G., et al.: Four-arm robotic lobectomy for the treatment of early-stage lung cancer. J. Thorac. Cardiovasc. Surg. **140**(1), 19–25 (2009)
88. Chang, A.C., et al.: Outcomes after transhiatal and transthoracic esophagectomy for cancer. Ann. Thorac. Surg. **85**(2), 424–429 (2008)
89. Kernstine, K.H., et al.: The first series of completely robotic esophagectomies with three-field lymphadenectomy: initial experience. Surg. Endosc. **21**(12), 2285–2292 (2007)
90. Boone, J., et al.: Robot-assisted thoracoscopic oesophagectomy for cancer. Br. J. Surg. **96**(8), 878–886 (2009)
91. Watson, T.J.: Robotic esophagectomy: is it an advance and what is the future? Ann. Thorac. Surg. **85**(2), S757–S759 (2008)
92. Song, J., et al.: Robot-assisted gastrectomy with lymph node dissection for gastric cancer: lessons learned from an initial 100 consecutive procedures. Ann. Surg. **249**(6), 927–932 (2009)
93. Kim, M.C., Heo, G.U., Jung, G.J.: Robotic gastrectomy for gastric cancer: surgical techniques and clinical merits. Surg. Endosc. **24**(3), 610–615 (2010)
94. Buchs, N.C., et al.: Robot-assisted oncologic resection for large gastric gastrointestinal stromal tumor: a preliminary case series. J. Laparoendosc. Adv. Surg. Tech. A **20**(5), 411–415 (2010)
95. Puli, S.R., et al.: Meta-analysis and systematic review of colorectal endoscopic mucosal resection. World J. Gastroenterol. **15**(34), 4273–4277 (2009)
96. Jameel, J.K., et al.: Endoscopic mucosal resection (EMR) in the management of large colo-rectal polyps. Colorectal Dis. **8**(6), 497–500 (2006)
97. Zimmern, A., et al.: Robotic colon and rectal surgery: a series of 131 cases. World J Surg. **34**(8), 1954–1958 (2010)
98. Patriti, A., et al.: Short- and medium-term outcome of robot-assisted and traditional laparoscopic rectal resection. JSLS **13**(2), 176–183 (2009)
99. Baek, J.H., et al.: Oncologic outcomes of robotic-assisted total mesorectal excision for the treatment of rectal cancer. Ann. Surg. **251**(5), 882–886 (2010)
100. Pigazzi, A., et al.: Multicentric study on robotic tumor-specific mesorectal excision for the treatment of rectal cancer. Ann. Surg. Oncol. **17**(6), 1614–1620 (2010)
101. Patriti, A., et al.: Laparoscopic and robot-assisted one-stage resection of colorectal cancer with synchronous liver metastases: a pilot study. J. Hepatobiliary Pancreat. Surg. **16**(4), 450–457 (2009)
102. Narula, V.K., Mikami, D.J., Melvin, W.S.: Robotic and laparoscopic pancreaticoduodenectomy: a hybrid approach. Pancreas **39**(2), 160–164 (2010)
103. Giulianotti, P.C., et al.: Robot-assisted laparoscopic middle pancreatectomy. J. Laparoendosc. Adv. Surg. Tech. A **20**(2), 135–139 (2010)
104. Giulianotti, P.C., et al.: Robot-assisted laparoscopic pancreatic surgery: single-surgeon experience. Surg. Endosc. **24**(7), 1646–1657 (2010)
105. Hyams, E.S., Stifelman, M.D.: The role of robotics for adrenal pathology. Curr. Opin. Urol. **19**(1), 89–96 (2009)

Laparoscopy and Malignancy – General Aspects

Shigeru Tsunoda and Glyn G. Jamieson

6.1 Introduction

When compared to open surgery, the laparoscopic approach has been associated with less postoperative pain, an earlier return of bowel function, a shorter period of hospitalization and disability, and better cosmetic results. Therefore, laparoscopy has become important not only in the treatment but also in the investigation of abdominal malignancy. However, as a diagnostic tool it is still invasive and its value over and above existing noninvasive imaging techniques must be clear to outweigh its potentially detrimental effects. As a therapeutic tool, laparoscopy offers the benefits of minimalization of surgical trauma, but this needs to be balanced against any compromise of oncological principles and it needs also to be compared critically with the results of conventional surgery.

The role of laparoscopy in malignant disease can be interpreted differently by enthusiasts and nonenthusiasts.

Its use should be driven by clinical need and determined by actual rather than potential benefits and certainly not by enthusiasm for new technology. Conversely, progress should not be inhibited by leaders of opinion in surgery who remain more comfortable with conventional operative approaches and are reluctant to embrace new technology.

S. Tsunoda and G.G. Jamieson (✉)
Department of Surgery, The University of Adelaide,
Royal Adelaide Hospital, Adelaide, SA 5000, Australia
e-mail: Chris.batesbrownsword@adelaide.edu.au

6.2 General Applications of Laparoscopy for Cancer

6.2.1 Laparoscopy for Cancer – Curative Intent

The strategy of the treatment for abdominal malignancies depends on the organ, the stage of the disease, the histological type, and patient factors such as age and comorbidity. Superficial cancers of the gastrointestinal tract, except for the small intestine, are good candidates for endoscopic mucosal resection (EMR) [1, 2] or polypectomy. Total surgical removal of all or part of the involved organ is standard therapy for the vast majority of abdominal solid malignancies unless there is evidence of distant metastasis or an unresectable lesion due to the invasion of adjacent structures. Therefore, a laparoscopic approach, potentially, can be considered for any surgical patient. In addition, laparoscopic techniques usually provide excellent visualization and may, in skilled hands, minimize tumor manipulation [3]. Indeed, laparoscopic surgery has become the first choice for nonbulky colorectal cancers in a large number of hospitals and there are increasing numbers of reports of laparoscopic gastrectomy [4–6] and laparoscopic (+thoracoscopic) esophagectomy [7]. These approaches might become the standard in the next decade. There are also many anecdotal reports of laparoscopic hepatectomy for hepatocellular carcinoma [8], laparoscopic pancreatectomy for pancreatic cancer [9–11], and laparoscopic resection of small bowel tumors [12]. In the reports of laparoscopic pancreaticoduodenectomy for ductal carcinoma of the head of the pancreas and bile duct cancer, the merit of the laparoscopic approach has not been established [9, 10]. Although laparoscopic cholecystectomy has been the gold standard for benign gallbladder diseases, laparoscopic cholecystectomy is not the first option for gallbladder carcinoma due to the high rate of port-site metastasis [13]. Laparoscopic ablation therapy for hepatic tumors is also commonly performed [14].

6.2.2 Laparoscopy for Cancer – Palliation

In a palliative setting, laparoscopic gastro-jejunostomy for obstructing distal gastric cancer or duodenal obstruction due to pancreatic head cancer reportedly can be performed with less immune suppression, lower morbidity, and earlier recovery of gastro-intestinal function when compared with open surgery [15]. Laparoscopic biliary bypass is also a good option for an unresectable pancreatic cancer [16, 17]. These procedures may be particularly appropriate in the setting of preoperative staging, which demonstrates unresectable disease [18]. There seems little argument against a laparoscopic approach for palliative procedures other than the availability of the necessary laparoscopic expertise.

6.2.3 Laparoscopy for Cancer – Carcinomatosis

As far as disseminated cancer is concerned, laparoscopic intraperitoneal chemotherapy or chemohyperthermia have been reported for peritoneal carcinomatosis resulting from gastric cancer [19, 20], colon cancer [19], and ovarian cancer [19]. Although effective in terms of the control of debilitating malignant ascites [19], the survival benefit from these procedures remains unclear [20]. Currently, standard treatment for unresectable or recurrent disease is still systemic chemotherapy, radiotherapy, or their combination, and/or supportive care. With regard to immunotherapy, there is not yet enough evidence to support its use as standard practice, but active specific immunotherapy (vaccination) of the patients with colorectal cancer in an adjuvant setting has shown promise in several randomized controlled trials [21]. However, only one report is available regarding local immunotherapy via laparoscopy [22] so that at present this approach has to be regarded as experimental.

6.3 Laparoscopy and Malignancy – Special Considerations

6.3.1 Pneumoperitoneum

Most laparoscopic surgery is performed using a pneumoperitoneum with CO_2 gas at a pressure of 10–12 mmHg in order to create a large space between the anterior abdominal wall and the intraperitoneal viscera. In obese patients, higher pressure may be needed to lift the thick abdominal wall. There is good evidence that an intraabdominal pressure of 14 mmHg or lower is safe in a healthy patient [23].

During pneumoperitoneum, venous return to the heart from the infradiaphragmatic region may be compromised, and relative compression of pulmonary excursion by the elevated diaphragm may occur. Therefore, patients with severe cardiac or pulmonary disorders may be unable to tolerate the hemodynamic changes caused by the pneumoperitoneum. For these reasons, a laparoscopic approach with a pneumoperitoneum is contraindicated for patients who are in a shock state. Gasless laparoscopic surgery is an alternative procedure in such situations. However, a randomized controlled study of laparoscopic cholecystectomy reported that the gasless procedure required a longer operation time due to the limited working space and impaired videoscopic view of the underlying viscera, and so its benefit may be confined to high-risk patients with cardio-respiratory diseases [24]. An evidence-based clinical algorithm for the use of pneumoperitoneum in laparoscopic surgery was recommended by the European Association for Endoscopic Surgery [23].

6.3.2 Influence on the Immune System

In terms of the influence on the immune system, there is evidence that attenuation of the immune response occurs following laparoscopic procedures [25]. Animal studies provide ample evidence that pneumoperitoneum impairs cellular [26] and humoral [27] immune responses. The effect of laparoscopy on the human immune system has been compared with that of open surgery in several randomized trials, which documented profound effects of laparoscopy on both the systemic, cellular [28], and the humoral [29] immune response with suppression of intraperitoneal cell-mediated immunity [30]. Systemic immunity appears to be better preserved after laparoscopic surgery than after open surgery, but some studies found that the effects of laparoscopy were no different from those of laparotomy [29, 31, 32]. Thus, there is good evidence that laparoscopy influences patients' immune responses, but on the other hand there is no evidence to support the notion that this has any clinical importance in terms of patient outcome [33].

6.3.3 Port Site Metastasis

The laparoscopic era blossomed in the early 1990s, and the laparoscopic approach has been broadly accepted in various abdominal operations including malignant tumor resection. However, a disturbing report of the development of 3 (21%) wound recurrences following 14 laparoscopic colectomy cases [34] led many to voice concern regarding laparoscopic approaches for solid tumor resection. In fact, there are many reports of tumor seeding during laparoscopy as demonstrated by port-site metastases or recurrence and development of peritoneal dissemination [35]. There is anecdotal evidence of rapid peritoneal tumor spread following laparoscopy [36]. The insufflations associated with laparoscopy may have a significant effect on the invasive capacity of tumor cells and promote tumor growth. It has been suggested as a factor in the incidence of port-site metastases seen in patients following laparoscopic resection for malignancy [37–41]. There is experimental evidence, which appears to support this. Exposure of a colonic adenocarcinoma cell line to either a CO_2 or helium pneumoperitoneum causes an increase in tumor cell invasiveness, which is abolished by the presence of an inhibitor of matrix metalloproteases [42]. The invasive capacity of a pancreatic adenocarcinoma cell line is augmented by helium and CO_2 in vitro pneumoperitoneum, associated with increased gelatinase activity [43]. In a rat model, port-site metastases were significantly increased using air, CO_2, and N_2O insufflations compared with helium [44]. Tumor implantation also appears to be promoted by the presence of intraperitoneal blood during rodent laparoscopy [45].

There is conflicting evidence as to whether escape of aerosolized tumor cells around the trocar or through the port site (the so-called chimney effect) results in implantation. Experimental evidence suggests that port-site metastases are more common where gas could escape around the trocar [46, 47]. Other in vitro and in vivo studies including studies in patients with pancreatic cancer have failed to confirm such findings [48, 49]. There are a number of mechanisms listed in the literature whereby laparoscopy may contribute to cancer progression [50] (Table 6.1).

Table 6.1 Theories on how laparoscopy may contribute to cancer progression [50]

Theory	Presumed mechanism	Proposed protective measure
Pneumoperitoneum	May aerosolize shed tumor cells	"Gasless" laparoscopy
Loss of tactile feedback	Missed metastases	Hand-assisted approach
Excessive tumor	• Surgical inexperience	• Specialized training
Manipulation	• Poor patient selection	• Use of hand-assisted approach
Immune response	• Direct drying effects of prolonged insufflations	Use of humidifiers and alternative insufflation agents such as helium
	• CO_2 toxicity to peritoneal macrophages	
"Chimney effect"	Tumor-bearing gas escaping around ports permitting wound seeding	• Muscle-separating trocars
		• Perpendicular trocar placement
		• Trocar fixation with suture
"Sloshing" effect	Tumor irrigant escaping around ports permitting wound seeding	• Aspiration of peritoneal fluid prior to desufflation
		• Closure of port sites
Inadequate lymphadenectomy	Difficulty of laparoscopic node dissection	Existing data do not support this concern

Table 6.2 Laparoscopic surgery for colorectal cancer: Incidence of port-site recurrence

	Year	Tumor location	n	Port-site recurrence (%)
Lacy et al. [93]	2002	Colon	111	0.9
The COST study group [94]	2004	Colon	435	0.5
Leung et al. [68]	2004	Recto-sigmoid	203	0
Kaiser et al. [70]	2004	Colon	29	0

Table 6.3 Gallbladder cancer: Port-site recurrence after laparoscopic cholecystectomy

	Year	Study design	n	Port-site recurrence (%)
Schaeff et al. [95]	1998	Retrospective, nationwide	409	17.1
Lundberg et al. [96]	1999	Retrospective, nationwide	55	16
Paolucci et al. [97]	2001	Retrospective, nationwide	174	14
Wakai et al. [98]	2002	Retrospective	28	10.1

Although one international survey suggests that incisional metastases occur more commonly than would have been expected following open surgery [51], large controlled single-center studies suggest that the incidence is no different [52, 53]. Peritoneal implantation undoubtedly can occur if there is disruption of tumor and this may especially happen with inexperience, excessive laparoscopic manipulation, and nonprotected specimen extraction [54]. When compared with conventional surgery, expert laparoscopic colorectal surgery for colonic cancer has not been associated with an increased incidence of intraperitoneal cancer cell spillage [55] (Table 6.2). On the contrary, gallbladder cancer is known to have a high incidence of port-site recurrence after laparoscopic cholecystectomy [56] (Table 6.3). Because of this high incidence of port-site recurrence, laparoscopic cholecystectomy probably should not be undertaken for preoperatively diagnosed or suspected gallbladder cancer [13]. However, in a retrospective study from Sweden [57] involving 270 patients with documented gallbladder cancer, 210 had open surgery and 60 underwent a laparoscopic cholecystectomy. Twelve patients (12.5%) who underwent open surgery and nine patients (15%) who had laparoscopic surgery developed incisional or port-site recurrence, suggesting that the underlying cause may be the disease itself, rather than the approach used.

Ultimately, wound recurrence seems to be more related to tumor biology, tumor stage, and the degree of tumor manipulation during surgery [58, 59]. Criticism that laparoscopy itself leads to an unacceptable incidence of port-site metastases is, on the balance of evidence, unfounded.

6.4 Oncological Outcome of Different Applications

6.4.1 Laparoscopy in Gastric Cancer

Case series suggest that the results of laparoscopically assisted distal gastrectomy are broadly similar to open surgery although complications have been high with a reported anastomotic leak rate of up to 14% [60, 61]. With the laparoscopic approach, there is significantly less postoperative pain, less respiratory compromise, more rapid recovery of gastrointestinal function, earlier mobilization, and shorter postoperative stay [62–64]. However, there is some evidence that these benefits are at the expense of longer operating times and a smaller lymph node yield [65]. A prospective randomized trial [66] reported that laparoscopic radical subtotal gastrectomy for distal gastric cancer is a feasible and safe oncologic procedure with short- and long-term results similar to those obtained with an open approach along with the additional benefits of reduced blood loss, shorter time to resumption of oral intake, and earlier discharge from hospital. As far as early gastric cancer is concerned, a Japanese multicenter retrospective study recently reported 1,294 early gastric cancer patients who underwent a laparoscopic gastrectomy without any operative deaths and with only 6 patients developing recurrent disease [67].

6.4.2 Laparoscopy in Colorectal Cancer

For colorectal cancer, a laparoscopic approach has been used more commonly; so there is a lot of evidence which shows the equivalence or superiority of laparoscopic surgery to open surgery. Laparoscopic resection of recto-sigmoid cancer has been reported to be equivalent to conventional open surgery looking at 5-year survival [68], recurrence rate, pattern of recurrence [69], as well as short-term results [70–72]. A meta-analysis of three randomized controlled trials recently demonstrated the equivalence of laparoscopically assisted colectomy in terms of oncological safety [73]. Regarding the oncological clearance in rectal cancer, a meta-analysis showed equivalent results for open surgery and laparoscopic surgery [74].

6.4.3 Laparoscopy and Liver Tumors

As far as liver tumors are concerned, a meta-analysis of eight nonrandomized studies looking at 165 laparoscopic hepatic resections for benign and malignant neoplasms showed that laparoscopic resection resulted in reduced operative blood loss and earlier recovery with oncological results, especially resection margins, comparable to open surgery [75]. Therefore, it appears to be a safe and feasible alternative to open surgery as long as it is performed by specialized surgeons in selected patients [75].

Currently, there are no reports of randomized controlled trials in cancers of the esophagus or pancreas investigating the advantages or disadvantages of a laparoscopic approach.

6.5 Staging Laparoscopy

The laparoscope is a useful diagnostic tool to determine local involvement and/or dissemination of tumor in the abdominal cavity. However, the advantage of laparoscopy should be balanced carefully against potential risks. If therapeutic strategy was always surgical exploration, then preoperative staging would be unnecessary. However, with increasing nonoperative treatment strategies available, staging procedures must be sufficiently accurate to allow correct assignment of cases to specific treatment protocols.

Historically, it has not been uncommon for "open and close" laparotomies to be performed when diseases have been understaged by conventional imaging. With refinement of technique and technology, with computed tomography (CT), magnetic resonance imaging (MRI), ultrasound, and ^{18}F-fluorodeoxy glucose positron emission tomography (FDG-PET), this has become much less common. Nevertheless, cases with undetected small hepatic metastasis or peritoneal deposits are still sometimes encountered at a preliminary laparotomy. Staging or planning laparoscopy has proved useful in planning treatment and has been a proven benefit in identifying radiologically undetected hepatic and peritoneal metastasis.

Even though laparoscopic surgery has been proven to be a less invasive procedure than open surgery, its liberal use should be avoided until any adverse effects from the pneumoperitoneum on port-site recurrence and oncological outcome are better known. Diagnostic laparoscopy replaces the preliminary assessment at the commencement of a laparotomy for resection of an organ. If a laparoscopy causes a significant change from an operative to a nonoperative treatment, then such an approach allows better allocation of resources and better preparation of patients and spares patients the morbidity of a more major surgical trauma. However, such accuracy of preoperative staging is not necessary in situations where resection will remain the management plan anyway, despite the presence of small hepatic, peritoneal, or nodal deposits. Even in centers that practice staging laparoscopy, open and close laparotomies can still occur [76]. Laparoscopy may miss deep liver lesions, which are usually detected by palpation. The addition of laparoscopic ultrasound may substitute for the lack of tactile sensitivity in laparoscopy, enabling detection of deeply placed lesions [77]. In certain centers, the use of laparoscopic ultrasound has improved the assessment of nodal involvement and local invasion and has proved useful in planning treatment particularly for patients with pancreatic and peri-ampullary tumors [78, 79]. In some centers, the routine use of laparoscopic ultrasound has enhanced the role of staging laparoscopy leading to a reduction yet further in nontherapeutic laparotomies, improved respectability rate, and optimization of palliation [80, 81]. Yet, in other centers, 96% accuracy of staging is achieved by CT and external ultrasound alone, perhaps obviating the need for more invasive procedures [82, 83].

With advances in conventional imaging, the pursuit of occult intraabdominal dissemination by laparoscopy may become less necessary. For example, with modern conventional imaging, the presence of local invasion by pancreatic cancer is the most influential in deciding operability and often it is the most difficult parameter to determine preoperatively by laparoscopy [78, 83]. Other, less invasive diagnostic modalities such as color Doppler ultrasound are more effective than laparoscopy in the assessment of local invasion by pancreatic and biliary malignancy and may be a more useful and relevant tool for planning treatment [84].

The use of peritoneal cytology at the time of staging laparoscopy has been advocated to add to the technique and provide a further marker of prognosis [85]. Even molecular diagnosis can be made of laparoscopic peritoneal washings [86, 87], which may reveal more information on prognosis [86]. Some practice "extended diagnostic laparoscopy" [88], which involves not merely inspection but dissection, laparoscopic ultrasound, peritoneal lavage, and biopsy. This has been reported to result in a modification of therapeutic strategy in up to 40% of patients [88–90]. However, as yet there does not appear to be strong evidence to support such individualized treatment strategies. In gastric cancer, for example, peritoneal washings may be performed but the technology risks exceeding our ability to correctly interpret the information provided. Although positive peritoneal cytology identifies a poor prognosis group [91], it is not established whether these patients should be excluded from surgery. In certain situations, this information may aid the decision-making process, but its overall impact has not been established.

Competition between adjuncts to laparoscopy and improvements in conventional imaging means we need to constantly rebalance the role of these diagnostic tools. More so than any other investigation, because of its relatively invasive nature, laparoscopy should be planned to answer specific questions in a particular case. While laparoscopy can detect subtle macroscopic malignant disease missed on other investigations, as the precision of other investigations improve along with the expertise of their interpretation, individual centers will need to decide for themselves how much additional value is gained from staging laparoscopy. Our own view is that a selective approach to staging laparoscopy should be undertaken in patients in whom there is a suspicion of intraabdominal dissemination in situations where a palliative open procedure would be inappropriate. The evolution of the role of laparoscopy as a therapeutic tool in abdominal malignancy may yet lead to further adjustment of its preoperative role.

6.6 Future Trends

Laparoscopy has unleashed a new wave of surgical inventiveness. It seems highly likely that in the future, new developments and modifications of technique will expand the role of laparoscopic surgery in abdominal malignancy. Indeed, the telerobotic Zeus and da Vinci surgical systems have emerged to replace the surgeon's hands with robotic instruments and serve as a master–slave relationship for surgeons. "Computer-assisted" laparoscopic gastrointestinal surgery such as bowel resection and distal pancreatectomy has been reported to be feasible and safe with regard to operating time and patient recovery [92]. This technology is expensive and the setup time-consuming. Therefore, its use in routine procedures at present is hard to justify. It remains to be seen if it will provide easier and safer anastomoses and superior lymphadenectomies in malignant diseases.

However, it is important to realize that it is just a technique we are talking about. The fact that such things as the role of lymphadenectomy in open surgery remain unresolved only makes it harder to assess laparoscopic techniques in abdominal malignancy, which is why randomized controlled trials are important in this field.

Quick Reference Guide

1. Define a clear indication addressing the specific oncological problem.
2. Select only appropriate patients for laparoscopy.
3. Keep abdominal pressure as low as possible and certainly lower than 14 mmHg.

4. Have trocars fixed to the abdominal wall to prevent air escape.
5. "No-touch-technique" is key! Manipulate a tumor as little as possible.
6. Avoid all forceps movement unless it is visually monitored.
7. Always maintain oncological accuracy. Don't compromise surgical margin.
8. If a port-site metastasis occurs, excise it.
9. Use staging laparoscopy liberally if noninvasive imaging does not answer your questions.
10. Involve patients in randomized trials if possible.

References

1. Inoue, H.: Treatment of esophageal and gastric tumors. Endoscopy **33**, 119–125 (2001)
2. Williams, C.B., Saunders, B.P., Talbot, I.C.: Endoscopic management of polypoid early colon cancer. World J. Surg. **24**, 1047–1051 (2000)
3. Yahchouchy-Chouillard, E., Etienne, J.C., Fagniez, P.L., Adam, R., Fingerhut, A.: A new "No-touch" technique for the laparoscopic treatment of gastric stromal tumors. Surg. Endosc. **16**, 962–964 (2002)
4. Chau, C.H., Siu, W.T., Li, M.K.: Hand-assisted d2 subtotal gastrectomy for carcinoma of stomach. Surg. Laparosc. Endosc. Percutan. Tech. **12**, 268–272 (2002)
5. Reyes, C.D., Weber, K.J., Gagner, M., Divino, C.M.: Laparoscopic vs open gastrectomy. A retrospective review. Surg. Endosc. **15**, 928–931 (2001)
6. Tanimura, S., Higashino, M., Fukunaga, Y., Osugi, H.: Laparoscopic gastrectomy with regional lymph node dissection for upper gastric cancer. Gastric Cancer **6**, 64–68 (2003)
7. Okushiba, S., Ohno, K., Itoh, K., Ohkashiwa, H., Omi, M., Satou, K., Kawarada, Y., Morikawa, T., Kondo, S., Katoh, H.: Hand-assisted endoscopic esophagectomy for esophageal cancer. Surg. Today **33**, 158–161 (2003)
8. Descottes, B., Lachachi, F., Sodji, M., Valleix, D., Durand-Fontanier, S., Pech de Laclause, B., Grousseau, D.: Early experience with laparoscopic approach for solid liver tumors: initial 16 cases. Ann. Surg. **232**, 641–645 (2000)
9. Gagner, M., Pomp, A.: Laparoscopic pancreatic resection: is it worthwhile? J. Gastrointest. Surg. **1**, 20–25 (1997). discussion 25-26
10. Cuschieri, A.: Laparoscopic pancreatic resections. Semin. Laparosc. Surg. **3**, 15–20 (1996)
11. Cuschieri, A.: Laparoscopic surgery of the pancreas. J. R. Coll. Surg. Edinb. **39**, 178–184 (1994)
12. Ehrmantraut, W., Sardi, A.: Laparoscopy-assisted small bowel resection. Am. Surg. **63**, 996–1001 (1997)
13. Sikora, S.S., Singh, R.K.: Surgical strategies in patients with gallbladder cancer: nihilism to optimism. J. Surg. Oncol. **93**, 670–681 (2006)
14. Santambrogio, R., Podda, M., Zuin, M., Bertolini, E., Bruno, S., Cornalba, G.P., Costa, M., Montorsi, M.: Safety and efficacy of laparoscopic radiofrequency ablation of hepatocellular carcinoma in patients with liver cirrhosis. Surg. Endosc. **17**, 1826–1832 (2003)
15. Choi, Y.B.: Laparoscopic gatrojejunostomy for palliation of gastric outlet obstruction in unresectable gastric cancer. Surg. Endosc. **16**, 1620–1626 (2002)
16. Scott-Conner, C.E.: Laparoscopic biliary bypass for inoperable pancreatic cancer. Semin. Laparosc. Surg. **5**, 185–188 (1998)
17. Charukhchyan, S.A., Lucas, G.W.: Lesser sac endoscopy and laparoscopy in pancreatic carcinoma definitive diagnosis, staging and palliation. Am. Surg. **64**, 809–814 (1998). discussion 814-806
18. Croce, E., Olmi, S., Azzola, M., Russo, R., Golia, M.: Surgical palliation in pancreatic head carcinoma and gastric cancer: the role of laparoscopy. Hepatol. Gastroenterol. **46**, 2606–2611 (1999)
19. Garofalo, A., Valle, M., Garcia, J., Sugarbaker, P.H.: Laparoscopic intraperitoneal hyperthermic chemotherapy for palliation of debilitating malignant ascites. Eur. J. Surg. Oncol. **32**, 682–685 (2006)
20. Ikeguchi, M., Matsumoto, S., Yoshioka, S., Murakami, D., Kanaji, S., Ohro, S., Yamaguchi, K., Saito, H., Tatebe, S., Kondo, A., Tsujitani, S., Kaibara, N.: Laparoscopic-assisted intraperitoneal chemotherapy for patients with scirrhous gastric cancer. Chemotherapy **51**, 15–20 (2005)
21. Mosolits, S., Ullenhag, G., Mellstedt, H.: Therapeutic vaccination in patients with gastrointestinal malignancies. A review of immunological and clinical results. Ann. Oncol. **16**, 847–862 (2005)
22. Maraveyas, A., Snook, D., Hird, V., Kosmas, C., Meares, C.F., Lambert, H.E., Epenetos, A.A.: Pharmacokinetics and toxicity of an yttrium-90-citc-dtpa-hmfg1 radioimmunoconjugate for intraperitoneal radioimmunotherapy of ovarian cancer. Cancer **73**, 1067–1075 (1994)
23. Neudecker, J., Sauerland, S., Neugebauer, E., Bergamaschi, R., Bonjer, H.J., Cuschieri, A., Fuchs, K.H., Jacobi, C., Jansen, F.W., Koivusalo, A.M., Lacy, A., McMahon, M.J., Millat, B., Schwenk, W.: The European association for endoscopic surgery clinical practice guideline on the pneumoperitoneum for laparoscopic surgery. Surg. Endosc. **16**, 1121–1143 (2002)
24. Uen, Y.H., Liang, A.I., Lee, H.H.: Randomized comparison of conventional carbon dioxide insufflation and abdominal wall lifting for laparoscopic cholecystectomy. J. Laparoendosc. Adv. Surg. Tech. **12**, 7–14 (2002)
25. Hartley, J.E., Mehigan, B.J., Monson, J.R.: Alterations in the immune system and tumor growth in laparoscopy. Surg. Endosc. **15**, 305–313 (2001)
26. Gitzelmann, C.A., Mendoza-Sagaon, M., Talamini, M.A., Ahmad, S.A., Pegoli Jr., W., Paidas, C.N.: Cell-mediated immune response is better preserved by laparoscopy than laparotomy. Surgery **127**, 65–71 (2000)
27. Iwanaka, T., Arkovitz, M.S., Arya, G., Ziegler, M.M.: Evaluation of operative stress and peritoneal macrophage function in minimally invasive operations. J. Am. Coll. Surg. **184**, 357–363 (1997)
28. Leung, K.L., Lai, P.B., Ho, R.L., Meng, W.C., Yiu, R.Y., Lee, J.F., Lau, W.Y.: Systemic cytokine response after

laparoscopic-assisted resection of rectosigmoid carcinoma: A prospective randomized trial. Ann. Surg. **231**, 506–511 (2000)
29. Perttila, J., Salo, M., Ovaska, J., Gronroos, J., Lavonius, M., Katila, a., Lahteenmaki, M., Pulkki, K.: Immune response after laparoscopic and conventional nissen fundoplication. Eur. J. Surg. Acta Chirurgica **165**, 21–28 (1999)
30. Gupta, A., Watson, D.I.: Effect of laparoscopy on immune function. Br. J. Surg. **88**, 1296–1306 (2001)
31. Hewitt, P.M., Ip, S.M., Kwok, S.P., Somers, S.S., Li, K., Leung, K.L., Lau, W.Y., Li, A.K.: Laparoscopic-assisted vs. Open surgery for colorectal cancer: comparative study of immune effects. Dis. Colon Rectum **41**, 901–909 (1998)
32. Squirrell, D.M., Majeed, A.W., Troy, G., Peacock, J.E., Nicholl, J.P., Johnson, A.G.: A randomized, prospective, blinded comparison of postoperative pain, metabolic response, and perceived health after laparoscopic and small incision cholecystectomy. Surgery **123**, 485–495 (1998)
33. Urbach, D.R., Swanstrom, L.L., Hansen, P.D.: The effect of laparoscopy on survival in pancreatic cancer. Arch. Surg. **137**, 191–199 (2002)
34. Berends, F.J., Kazemier, G., Bonjer, H.J., Lange, J.F.: Subcutaneous metastases after laparoscopic colectomy. Lancet **344**, 58 (1994)
35. Bouvy, N.D., Marquet, R.L., Jeekel, H., Bonjer, H.J.: Impact of gas(less) laparoscopy and laparotomy on peritoneal tumor growth and abdominal wall metastases. Ann. Surg. **224**, 694–700 (1996). discussion 700-691
36. Gave, A.A., Hopkins, M.A.: Laparoscopy and unsuspected intra-abdominal malignancy with rapid peritoneal spread. Surg. Endosc. **15**, 518 (2001)
37. Bouvy, N.D., Marquet, R.L., Jeekel, J., Bonjer, H.J.: Laparoscopic surgery is associated with less tumour growth stimulation than conventional surgery: an experimental study. Br. J. Surg. **84**, 358–361 (1997)
38. Ishida, H., Murata, N., Yamada, H., Nomura, T., Shimomura, K., Fujioka, M., Idezuki, Y.: Influence of trocar placement and co(2) pneumoperitoneum on port site metastasis following laparoscopic tumor surgery. Surg. Endosc. **14**, 193–197 (2000)
39. Wu, J.S., Jones, D.B., Guo, L.W., Brasfield, E.B., Ruiz, M.B., Connett, J.M., Fleshman, J.W.: Effects of pneumoperitoneum on tumor implantation with decreasing tumor inoculum. Dis. Colon Rectum **41**, 141–146 (1998)
40. Le Moine, M.C., Navarro, F., Burgel, J.S., Pellegrin, A., Khiari, A.R., Pourquier, D., Fabre, J.M., Domergue, J.: Experimental assessment of the risk of tumor recurrence after laparoscopic surgery. Surgery **123**, 427–431 (1998)
41. Volz, J., Volz-Koster, S., Kanis, S., Klee, D., Ahlert, C., Melchert, F.: Modulation of tumor-induced lethality after pneumoperitoneum in a mouse model. Cancer **89**, 262–266 (2000)
42. Ridgway, P.F., Smith, A., Ziprin, P., Jones, T.L., Paraskeva, P.A., Peck, D.H., Darzi, A.W.: Pneumoperitoneum augmented tumor invasiveness is abolished by matrix metalloproteinase blockade. Surg. Endosc. **16**, 533–536 (2002)
43. Ridgway, P.F., Ziprin, P., Jones, T.L., Paraskeva, P.A., Peck, D.H., Darzl, A.W.: Laparoscopic staging of pancreatic tumors induces increased invasive capacity in vitro. Surg. Endosc. **17**, 306–310 (2003)
44. Neuhaus, S.J., Watson, D.I., Ellis, T., Rowland, R., Rofe, A.M., Pike, G.K., Mathew, G., Jamieson, G.G.: Wound metastasis after laparoscopy with different insufflation gases. Surgery **123**, 579–583 (1998)
45. Neuhaus, S.J., Ellis, T., Jamieson, G.G., Watson, D.I.: Experimental study of the effect of intraperitoneal heparin on tumour implantation following laparoscopy. Br. J. Surg. **86**, 400–404 (1999)
46. Reilly, W.T., Nelson, H., Schroeder, G., Wieand, H.S., Bolton, J., O'Connell, M.J.: Wound recurrence following conventional treatment of colorectal cancer. A rare but perhaps underestimated problem. Dis. Colon Rectum **39**, 200–207 (1996)
47. Tseng, L.N., Berends, F.J., Wittich, P., Bouvy, N.D., Marquet, R.L., Kazemier, G., Bonjer, H.J.: Port-site metastases. Impact of local tissue trauma and gas leakage. Surg. Endosc. **12**, 1377–1380 (1998)
48. Whelan, R.L., Sellers, G.J., Allendorf, J.D., Laird, D., Bessler, M.D., Nowygrod, R., Treat, M.R.: Trocar site recurrence is unlikely to result from aerosolization of tumor cells. Dis. Colon Rectum **39**, S7–S13 (1996)
49. Reymond, M.A., Wittekind, C., Jung, A., Hohenberger, W., Kirchner, T., Kockerling, F.: The incidence of port-site metastases might be reduced. Surg. Endosc. **11**, 902–906 (1997)
50. Kooby, D.A.: Laparoscopic surgery for cancer: historical, theoretical, and technical considerations. Oncology (Williston Park, NY) 20:917–927 (2006) discussion 927-918, 931-912
51. Paolucci, V., Schaeff, B., Schneider, M., Gutt, C.: Tumor seeding following laparoscopy: international survey. World J. Surg. **23**, 989–995 (1999). discussion 996-987
52. Shoup, M., Brennan, M.F., Karpeh, M.S., Gillern, S.M., McMahon, R.L., Conlon, K.C.: Port site metastasis after diagnostic laparoscopy for upper gastrointestinal tract malignancies: an uncommon entity. Ann. Surg. Oncol. **9**, 632–636 (2002)
53. Pearlstone, D.B., Feig, B.W., Mansfield, P.F.: Port site recurrences after laparoscopy for malignant disease. Semin. Surg. Oncol. **16**, 307–312 (1999)
54. Mayer, C., Miller, D.M., Ehlen, T.G.: Peritoneal implantation of squamous cell carcinoma following rupture of a dermoid cyst during laparoscopic removal. Gynecol. Oncol. **84**, 180–183 (2002)
55. Kim, S.H., Milsom, J.W., Gramlich, T.L., Toddy, S.M., Shore, G.I., Okuda, J., Fazio, V.W.: Does laparoscopic vs. Conventional surgery increase exfoliated cancer cells in the peritoneal cavity during resection of colorectal cancer? Dis. Colon Rectum **41**, 971–978 (1998)
56. Steinert, R., Nestler, G., Sagynaliev, E., Muller, J., Lippert, H., Reymond, M.A.: Laparoscopic cholecystectomy and gallbladder cancer. J. Surg. Oncol. **93**, 682–689 (2006)
57. Lundberg, O., Kristoffersson, A.: Open versus laparoscopic cholecystectomy for gallbladder carcinoma. J. Patobiliary-pancreatic Surg. **8**, 525–529 (2001)
58. Pearlstone, D.B., Mansfield, P.F., Curley, S.A., Kumparatana, M., Cook, P., Feig, B.W.: Laparoscopy in 533 patients with abdominal malignancy. Surgery **125**, 67–72 (1999)
59. Wang, P.H., Yuan, C.C., Lin, G., Ng, H.T., Chao, H.T.: Risk factors contributing to early occurrence of port site metastases

of laparoscopic surgery for malignancy. Gynecol. Oncol. **72**, 38–44 (1999)
60. Fujiwara, M., Kodera, Y., Kasai, Y., Kanyama, Y., Hibi, K., Ito, K., Akiyama, S., Nakao, a.: Laparoscopy-assisted distal gastrectomy with systemic lymph node dissection for early gastric carcinoma: a review of 43 cases. J. Am. Coll. Surg. **196**, 75–81 (2003)
61. Ballesta Lopez, C., Ruggiero, R., Poves, I., Bettonica, C., Procaccini, E.: The contribution of laparoscopy to the treatment of gastric cancer. Surg. Endosc. **16**, 616–619 (2002)
62. Shimizu, S., Uchiyama, A., Mizumoto, K., Morisaki, T., Nakamura, K., Shimura, H., Tanaka, M.: Laparoscopically assisted distal gastrectomy for early gastric cancer: is it superior to open surgery? Surg. Endosc. **14**, 27–31 (2000)
63. Kitano, S., Shiraishi, N., Fujii, K., Yasuda, K., Inomata, M., Adachi, Y.: A randomized controlled trial comparing open vs laparoscopy-assisted distal gastrectomy for the treatment of early gastric cancer: an interim report. Surgery **131**, S306–S311 (2002)
64. Adachi, Y., Shiraishi, N., Shiromizu, A., Bandoh, T., Aramaki, M., Kitano, S.: Laparoscopy-assisted billroth i gastrectomy compared with conventional open gastrectomy. Arch. Surg. **135**, 806–810 (2000)
65. Mochiki, E., Nakabayashi, T., Kamimura, H., Haga, N., Asao, T., Kuwano, H.: Gastrointestinal recovery and outcome after laparoscopy-assisted versus conventional open distal gastrectomy for early gastric cancer. World J. Surg. **26**, 1145–1149 (2002)
66. Huscher, C.G., Mingoli, A., Sgarzini, G., Sansonetti, A., Di Paola, M., Recher, A., Ponzano, C.: Laparoscopic versus open subtotal gastrectomy for distal gastric cancer: Five-year results of a randomized prospective trial. Ann. Surg. **241**, 232–237 (2005)
67. Kitano, S., Shiraishi, N., Uyama, I., Sugihara, K., Tanigawa, N.: A multicenter study on oncologic outcome of laparoscopic gastrectomy for early cancer in Japan. Ann. Surg. **245**, 68–72 (2007)
68. Leung, K.L., Kwok, S.P., Lam, S.C., Lee, J.F., Yiu, R.Y., Ng, S.S., Lai, P.B., Lau, W.Y.: Laparoscopic resection of rectosigmoid carcinoma: prospective randomised trial. Lancet **363**, 1187–1192 (2004)
69. Liang, J.T., Huang, K.C., Lai, H.S., Lee, P.H., Jeng, Y.M.: Oncologic results of laparoscopic versus conventional open surgery for stage ii or iii left-sided colon cancers: a randomized controlled trial. Ann. Surg. Oncol. **14**, 109–117 (2007)
70. Kaiser, A.M., Kang, J.C., Chan, L.S., Vukasin, P., Beart Jr., R.W.: Laparoscopic-assisted vs. open colectomy for colon cancer: a prospective randomized trial. J. Laparoendosc. Adv. Surg. Tech. **14**, 329–334 (2004)
71. Wu, F.P., Sietses, C., von Blomberg, B.M., van Leeuwen, P.A., Meijer, S., Cuesta, M.A.: Systemic and peritoneal inflammatory response after laparoscopic or conventional colon resection in cancer patients: a prospective, randomized trial. Dis. Colon Rectum **46**, 147–155 (2003)
72. Veldkamp, R., Kuhry, E., Hop, W.C., Jeekel, J., Kazemier, G., Bonjer, H.J., Haglind, E., Pahlman, L., Cuesta, M.A., Msika, S., Morino, M., Lacy, A.M.: Laparoscopic surgery versus open surgery for colon cancer: short-term outcomes of a randomised trial. Lancet Oncol. **6**, 477–484 (2005)
73. Bonjer, H.J., Hop, W.C., Nelson, H., Sargent, D.J., Lacy, A.M., Castells, A., Guillou, P.J., Thorpe, H., Brown, J., Delgado, S., Kuhrij, E., Haglind, E., Pahlman, L.: Laparoscopically assisted vs open colectomy for colon cancer: a meta-analysis. Arch. Surg. **142**, 298–303 (2007)
74. Aziz, O., Constantinides, V., Tekkis, P.P., Athanasiou, T., Purkayastha, S., Paraskeva, P., Darzi, A.W., Heriot, A.G.: Laparoscopic versus open surgery for rectal cancer: a meta-analysis. Ann. Surg. Oncol. **13**, 413–424 (2006)
75. Simillis, C., Constantinides, V.A., Tekkis, P.P., Darzi, A., Lovegrove, R., Jiao, L., Antoniou, A.: Laparoscopic versus open hepatic resections for benign and malignant neoplasms – a meta-analysis. Surgery **141**, 203–211 (2007)
76. Bhalla, R., Formella, L., Kerrigan, D.D.: Need for staging laparoscopy in patients with gastric cancer. Br. J. Surg. **87**, 362–373 (2000)
77. Hunerbein, M., Rau, B., Schlag, P.M.: Laparoscopy and laparoscopic ultrasound for staging of upper gastrointestinal tumours. Eur. J. Surg. Oncol. **21**, 50–55 (1995)
78. John, T.G., Wright, A., Allan, P.L., Redhead, D.N., Paterson-Brown, S., Carter, D.C., Garden, O.J.: Laparoscopy with laparoscopic ultrasonography in the TNM staging of pancreatic carcinoma. World J. Surg. **23**, 870–881 (1999)
79. Murugiah, M., Paterson-Brown, S., Windsor, J.A., Miles, W.F., Garden, O.J.: Early experience of laparoscopic ultrasonography in the management of pancreatic carcinoma. Surg. Endosc. **7**, 177–181 (1993)
80. Goudas, L.A., Brams, D.M., Birkett, D.H.: The use of laparoscopic ultrasonography in staging abdominal malignancy. Semin. Laparosc. Surg. **7**, 78–86 (2000)
81. Goletti, O., Buccianti, P., Chiarugi, M., Pieri, L., Sbragia, P., Cavina, E.: Laparoscopic sonography in screening metastases from gastrointestinal cancer: comparative accuracy with traditional procedures. Surg. Laparosc. Endosc. **5**, 176–182 (1995)
82. Bottger, T., Engelman, R., Seifert, J.K., Low, R., Junginger, T.: Preoperative diagnostics in pancreatic carcinoma: would less be better? Langenbecks Arch. Surg. **383**, 243–248 (1998)
83. Bottger, T.C., Boddin, J., Duber, C., Heintz, A., Kuchle, R., Junginger, T.: Diagnosing and staging of pancreatic carcinoma – what is necessary? Oncology **55**, 122–129 (1998)
84. Smits, N.J., Reeders, J.W.: Imaging and staging of biliopancreatic malignancy: role of ultrasound. Ann. Oncol. **10**(Suppl 4), 20–24 (1999)
85. Hayes, N., Wayman, J., Wadehra, V., Scott, D.J., Raimes, S.A., Griffin, S.M.: Peritoneal cytology in the surgical evaluation of gastric carcinoma. Br. J. Cancer **79**, 520–524 (1999)
86. Fujiwara, Y., Takiguchi, S., Mori, T., Yasuda, T., Yano, M., Monden, M.: The introduction of preoperative staging laparoscopy and molecular diagnosis of peritoneal lavages for the treatment of advanced gastric cancer. Gan to kagaku ryoho **29**, 2279–2281 (2002)
87. Iwasaki, Y., Arai, K., Kimura, Y., Takahashi, K., Ohue, M., Yamaguchi, T.: Preoperative diagnostic laparoscopy with local anesthesia and lavage telomerase activity for advanced gastric cancer. Gan to kagaku ryoho **29**, 2275–2278 (2002)
88. Feussner, H., Omote, K., Fink, U., Walker, S.J., Siewert, J.R.: Pretherapeutic laparoscopic staging in advanced gastric carcinoma. Endoscopy **31**, 342–347 (1999)

89. Hunerbein, M., Rau, B., Hohenberger, P., Schlag, P.M.: The role of staging laparoscopy for multimodal therapy of gastrointestinal cancer. Surg. Endosc. **12**, 921–925 (1998)
90. Asencio, F., Aguilo, J., Salvador, J.L., Villar, A., De la Morena, E., Ahamad, M., Escrig, J., Puche, J., Viciano, V., Sanmiguel, G., Ruiz, J.: Video-laparoscopic staging of gastric cancer. A prospective multicenter comparison with non-invasive techniques. Surg. Endosc. **11**, 1153–1158 (1997)
91. Ribeiro Jr., U., Safatle-Ribeiro, A.V., Zilberstein, B., Mucerino, D., Yagi, O.K., Bresciani, C.C., Jacob, C.E., Iryia, K., Gama-Rodrigues, J.: Does the intraoperative peritoneal lavage cytology add prognostic information in patients with potentially curative gastric resection? J. Gastrointest. Surg. **10**, 170–176 (2006). discussion 176-177
92. Talamini, M.A., Chapman, S., Horgan, S., Melvin, W.S.: A prospective analysis of 211 robotic-assisted surgical procedures. Surg. Endosc. **17**, 1521–1524 (2003)
93. Lacy, A.M., Garcia-Valdecasas, J.C., Delgado, S., Castells, A., Taura, P., Pique, J.M., Visa, J.: Laparoscopy-assisted colectomy versus open colectomy for treatment of non-metastatic colon cancer: a randomised trial. Lancet **359**, 2224–2229 (2002)
94. The clinical outcomes of surgical therapy study group: a comparison of laparoscopically assisted and open colectomy for colon cancer. N Engl J. Med. **350**, 2050–2059 (2004)
95. Schaeff, B., Paolucci, V., Thomopoulos, J.: Port site recurrences after laparoscopic surgery. A review. Dig. Surg. **15**, 124–134 (1998)
96. Lundberg, O., Kristoffersson, A.: Port site metastases from gallbladder cancer after laparoscopic cholecystectomy. Results of a swedish survey and review of published reports. Eur. J. Surg. Acta Chirurgica **165**, 215–222 (1999)
97. Paolucci, V.: Port site recurrences after laparoscopic cholecystectomy. J. Patobiliary Pancreatic Surg. **8**, 535–543 (2001)
98. Wakai, T., Shirai, Y., Hatakeyama, K.: Radical second resection provides survival benefit for patients with t2 gallbladder carcinoma first discovered after laparoscopic cholecystectomy. World J. Surg. **26**, 867–871 (2002)

Laparoscopy and Immunology

Michael J. Grieco and Richard Larry Whelan

7.1 Introduction

Surgery has long been suspected to affect the immune system. Long before the advent of laparoscopic surgery, open surgery was known to cause transient suppression of the innate and adaptive immune system. The advent of minimally invasive surgery led to numerous studies carried out to gain an understanding of the physiologic and immunologic impact of laparoscopic methods. This necessitated a fresh look at open surgical methods and comparisons of the two access methods. Also, for the first time it was possible to gauge the relative contributions of the abdominal wall and intra-abdominal trauma to the transient immunosuppression that accompanies open surgical procedures. These studies have led to a better understanding of perioperative immune function after open surgery in addition to providing data regarding minimally invasive procedures done under a CO_2 pneumoperitoneum. There is reasonable evidence, in regard to a fair number of immune parameters and functions, that laparoscopic operation methods are associated with significantly less postoperative immune suppression than the equivalent open abdominal operation. It is important to note that, for a fair number of parameters where differences have been noted between open and closed operations, the duration of the surgery-induced changes is brief. Also, it must be stated that the clinical importance of the immune function changes, individually and collectively, is unclear.

Although it is clear that anergic patients who cannot mount a delayed-type hypersensitivity (DTH) reaction have higher rates of infection and complications, not much data are available regarding the importance of the period of relative immunosuppression associated with surgery in immunocompetent patients. Finally, although there is controversy regarding the role of the immune system in the cancer setting, some believe that minimizing the immunosuppression associated with surgery may be oncologically advantageous.

A variety of both small animal and human studies have been carried out. Murine and rat studies have mostly assessed the impact of CO_2 pneumoperitoneum alone although some have included cecal resection, gastrotomy, splenectomy, or other relatively minor intra-abdominal procedures. It is important to note that, in addition to the trauma induced by placing ports through the abdominal wall, the CO_2 pneumoperitoneum has important local and systemic physiologic effects that must be considered when assessing laparoscopic procedures. Studies range from simple measurements of blood cytokine levels to ex vivo studies of immune cells harvested from the blood. Cytokines are elaborated by a variety of immune cells and can impact immune function and also provide information regarding the functional status of the various immune cells. The status and function of circulating T-cells, monocytes, natural killer cells, and neutrophils can be directly studied via in vitro cultures after isolation from the blood. Monocytes can also be isolated from the peritoneal cavity. It is important to note that, in addition to blood cytokine changes related to immune function, the levels of many circulating proteins are altered as a result of surgery. Recently, it has become clear that perhaps some of the most important surgery-related changes involve proteins involved with angiogenesis. Studies assessing tumor growth and

---

M.J. Grieco and R.L. Whelan (✉)
Department of Surgery, St. Luke's Roosevelt Hospital,
425 West 59th Street, St. Luke's Roosevelt Hospital Suite 7B,
New York, NY 10019, USA
e-mail: dr.michael.grieco@gmail.com; rwhelan@chpnet.org

establishment as well as apoptosis and proliferation after both CO_2 pneumoperitoneum and laparotomy have also been carried out. It is difficult to determine which of the surgery-related changes (immune related or other) are responsible for the increased tumor growth noted in the majority of studies early after surgery.

In regard to the minimally invasive literature, the most common type of immune or physiologic study conducted are the ones that compare equivalent open and laparoscopic procedures in relation to blood levels of one or several proteins. Cholecystectomy is the best studied procedure, colon resection the next most common followed by Nissen fundoplication and gastric bypass. Studies have also been done on nephrectomy and hernia repair.

7.2 Humoral Immunity – *Cytokines*

7.2.1 *The Inflammatory Cascade*

Trauma of all sorts as well as burns, infections, and malignancies induce inflammatory responses which include the production of proinflammatory mediators and, in some situations, cellular and humoral immune responses. In the case of surgery, the inflammatory response is most notable in the surgical wound, but may spillover into the blood stream and, thus, result in downstream systemic changes. The blood concentrations of a variety of cytokines, acute phase reactants, and proteins are transiently altered after surgery. In general, the more extensive the procedure, the more tissue injury occurs and the greater the response will be. In addition to mediating local and systemic inflammatory responses, these cytokines recruit phagocytes and promote wound repair. In the setting of blunt trauma and burns serum elevations of IL-6, CRP, and TNF have been noted and are associated with a high rate of infections. Largely because of this association, some believe that in situations where blood levels of these proteins are increased, after surgery for example, that immune system function is diminished or impaired. Thus, increased levels of cytokines and acute phase proteins are a general indicator of, but do not directly correlate with, the immune response. Various studies have analyzed these plasma cytokines and acute phase proteins both in isolation and in concert with one another.

It is important to note that the duration of the elevation in blood levels of the acute phase proteins after open surgery is between 1 and 5 days. Further, where significant differences in blood protein levels between open and closed procedures have been found, the duration of the difference is often short-lived. Differences are most pronounced 1–6 h after surgery and, in many cases, are no longer detectable by postoperative day (POD) 2 [1–3].

7.2.2 *C-reactive Protein (CRP)*

C-reactive protein (CRP), which is produced by the liver following burns, infections, trauma, and surgery, is the most frequently studied acute phase response protein. CRP stimulates phagocytosis of neutrophils and macrophages. Most cholecystectomy studies have found significantly higher postoperative levels of CRP in open patients when compared to the laparoscopic group [4–11]. Interestingly, a study which compared cholecystectomy carried out via mini-laparotomy with a 5- to 7-cm incision to traditional laparoscopy demonstrated equivalent postoperative CRP levels in the blood. These studies suggest that the CRP elevation is directly proportional to the extent of the abdominal wall trauma. Higher CRP levels have also been noted in laparoscopic colorectal resection patients when compare to an open cohort in some but not all studies [12–15]. In one study, CRP was elevated after both open and laparoscopic colectomy; however, levels returned to normal more rapidly after the laparoscopic procedure [16]. Higher early postoperative CRP levels have also been noted after laparoscopic Nissen fundoplication [17] and gastric bypass [18]. Interestingly, no differences in CRP levels were noted between laparoscopic and open hernia repair patients [19].

7.2.3 *Interleukin-6 (IL-6)*

Interleukin-6 (IL-6) is a multifunctional cytokine involved in inflammation. It is secreted by many cells, including T-cells and macrophages, in response to trauma. IL-6 effects the production of other acute phase proteins including CRP. Blood levels of IL-6 are increased following major open surgery and IL-6 is thought, by many, to be a measure of operative stress [20, 21]. The majority of studies comparing laparoscopy versus open cholecystectomy (8/11) have noted significant lower IL-6 levels in the laparoscopic surgery groups [7–9, 11, 22–29]. Most colectomy studies have found significantly lower IL-6 elevations after laparoscopic-assisted resection than after open colectomy; however, the differences are short lived and were usually noted during the first 24–36 h [1, 13, 30–35]. In a few studies, comparing laparoscopic colectomy to an open approach, no differences in IL-6 levels have been found. As a shortcoming of these studies it has to be noted, that only late postoperative sampling points were assessed [36–38]. In regard to gastric bypass, a randomized study noted significantly smaller increases in IL-6 levels 1, 2, and 3 days after surgery in the laparoscopic surgery group [18].

7.2.4 Tumor Necrosis Factor α (TNF-α)/Interleukin-1 (IL-1)

Tumor necrosis factor alpha (TNF-α) and Interleukin-1 (IL-1) are inflammatory mediators produced by monocytes and macrophages that act both independently and synergistically. They are capable of inducing fever and also contribute to the inflammatory response. In addition, they can induce apoptosis and inhibit tumor growth. Plasma levels of TNF-α are very low preoperatively which makes it more difficult to study. Unfortunately, there is a paucity of data concerning both parameters in the literature. A small randomized study that compared laparoscopic to open cholecystectomy done via a mini-laparotomy noted no differences in TNF-α levels at the single postoperative time point that was assessed, 12-h post surgery [7]. In the randomized gastric bypass study mentioned above nonsignificant similar TNF-α increases were noted on POD 1–3 in both groups. A porcine study of Nissen fundoplication demonstrated that the open group had a significantly greater mean level of serum TNF-α than the closed group [39]. Of uncertain significance, in a rodent model in which fecal pellets were injected intraperitoneally to induce peritonitis, much higher levels of TNF-α were noted in the laparotomy than in the CO_2 pneumoperitoneum group [40]. In a prospective human study, IL-1 levels were significantly higher in patients undergoing open cholecystectomy when compared to the laparoscopic group [41]. This limited literature does not allow any firm conclusions to be drawn regarding these parameters.

7.3 Cellular Immunity

7.3.1 T-cell Function

7.3.1.1 Delayed Type Hypersensitivity (DTH)

The Three Phases of DTH

Delayed type hypersensitivity (DTH) is a type IV hypersensitivity reaction and its testing provides an indirect assessment of multiple elements of the immune system. This type of immune response is a direct measurement of T-cell function. DTH response can be broken down into three main phases:

- Cognitive phase
- Activation phase
- Effector phase

The cognitive phase requires that the foreign antigen be processed and then presented by an antigen-presenting cell (monocyte or dendritic cell) to the appropriate CD4+ memory T cell. During the activation phase the stimulated CD4+ cell proliferates and also elaborates cytokines. The effector phase involves the accumulation of macrophages and other effector cells at the injection site followed by fibrin deposition, edema, and induration. In order to develop a response which presents as an indurated wheal at the injection site, all three main phases must be functioning. The tuberculin skin test is the most commonly performed DTH test. Mumps and Candida DTH tests are commonly used in an effort to detect anergic patients who are not able to mount a DTH response to antigens that they have been exposed to in their lives. Serial DTH testing, wherein identical antigen challenges are given before and after surgery, has been used for decades to assess postoperative immune function. The size and area of the preoperative response is compared to the postoperative result. It has been noted, after major open surgery in immunocompetent patients, that the DTH response is notably smaller or absent for the first 6–9 days [42, 43].

7.3.1.2 DTH in Animal Research

Not surprisingly, serial DTH testing has been used in both animal studies and patient related research, to compare immune function after open and laparoscopic procedures. In small animal models it has been shown that a sham laparotomy or open cecal resection results in less significant postoperative DTH responses than those noted in mice that underwent CO_2 pneumoperitoneum or laparoscopic cecectomy [44, 45]. In another murine study the length of the abdominal incision was correlated to the size of the postoperative DTH response [46]. One interesting murine study demonstrated that CO_2 pneumoperitoneum was associated with better preserved DTH responses and a greater ability to prevent the establishment of an immunogenic tumor postoperatively when compared to results after sham laparotomy [47].

7.3.1.3 DTH in Clinical Research

In the clinical setting, when serial DTH tests were carried out before and on POD 1 and POD 6 after open and laparoscopic cholecystectomy, a significantly smaller mean response was noted on POD 1 in the open group. There were no significant changes noted in the responses in the laparoscopic group [24]. Minimally invasive and open colorectal resection methods were compared in a prospective study that assessed DTH responses to a panel of antigens preoperatively, immediately after the operation, and on POD 3. Significantly smaller DTH responses were noted after open colectomy for both postoperative challenges whereas no significant change was seen in the laparoscopic colectomy patients [48]. Serial DTH testing, following a similar schedule, was carried out in a small randomized drug study that assessed the impact of perioperative granulocyte-macrophage-colony-stimulating-factor (GMCSF) in 59 patients. No significant changes in the size of the DTH responses were noted on POD 1 or POD 3 in either the GMCSF or the control group [49].

7.3.1.4 Significance of DTH in the Clinical Setting

The results of these animal and human DTH studies suggest that minimally invasive approaches are associated with notably less cell-mediated immunosuppression than the equivalent open procedures. The clinical significance of better preserved cell-mediated immune function in immunocompetent patients in the setting of laparoscopic surgery has not been clearly demonstrated, thus far. However, it is possible that the significantly lower rate of wound infections and overall decreased morbidity after laparoscopy, especially seen in the colectomy literature, may be a manifestation of this preservation of immune function after minimally invasive surgery [25, 50]. Of note, the clinical importance of the preoperative finding of anergy has been well established; anergic cancer patients undergoing resection have increased rates of sepsis, tumor recurrence, and higher perioperative mortality [51–54]. Therefore it seems to be logic to apply less invasive techniques whenever possible and not further depress the immune system.

7.3.2 Systemic Monocyte Function

7.3.2.1 Mechanism of Action and HLA-DR

Mononuclear phagocytes are formed in the bone marrow as monocytes, are disseminated via the blood stream, and differentiate into tissue macrophages upon leaving the circulation. After monocytes or macrophages phagocytize pathogens the foreign antigens they contain are broken down and peptide segments of the antigens are "presented" on their surface in conjunction with human leukocyte antigen DR (HLA-DR) to lymphocytes for recognition. Expression of HLA-DR, a class II major histocompatibility (MHC-II) molecule, on the surface of the monocyte or macrophage is required for successful antigen presentation to T-lymphocytes which results in activation of the T-cell.

Via antigen processing and presentation monocytes play a vital role in cellular immunity. Thus, it is no surprise that monocytes and macrophages evaluations have been included in studies comparing conventional and laparoscopic surgery.

7.3.2.2 Monocyte Function in Clinical Research

Improved short term outcome after major elective surgery and trauma has been shown to directly correlate with the percentage of circulating monocytes expressing surface HLA-DR [55–57]. Decreased monocyte human HLA-DR expression has been associated with a decreased ability to destroy pathogens and with a higher rate of clinical infections [58]. In one study, circulating monocyte HLA-DR expression was found to be significantly decreased in open cholecystectomy patients on POD 1 but not POD 6 when compared to preoperative expression levels; no significant differences from baseline were noted in the laparoscopic patients [24]. A second cholecystectomy study found significantly decreased monocyte HLA-DR expression in both the open and laparoscopic groups on POD 1. The extent of the decrease was noted to be greater in the open group; however, the p value for the open vs. closed comparison is not provided [59]. A randomized study that compared open and laparoscopic colorectal resection in a cancer population demonstrated significantly lower blood monocyte HLA-DR expression in the open patients at a single time point (POD 4); this was not the case for the laparoscopic patients [1]. Another study comparing open and laparoscopic surgical treatments for hepatobiliary and colorectal diseases demonstrated a significant decrease in blood monocyte HLA-DR expression after open but not after laparoscopic surgery from POD 2 to POD 8 [60]. Thus, short duration differences in monocyte HLA-DR expression between open and laparoscopic groups, of uncertain clinical importance, have been demonstrated mainly after cholecystectomy and colorectal resection.

7.3.2.3 Monocyte Function in Animal Research

Monocyte function was analyzed in a murine study by Watson et al. in which mice were randomized into four groups; controls, laparoscopy with CO_2 inflation, laparoscopy with air inflation and laparotomy [61]. Monocytes were isolated from each of the four groups and 24 h postoperatively their ability to ingest Candida albicans was compared. This study showed that the ability of the monocytes from the laparotomy and air laparoscopy groups to ingest Candida albicans was significantly decreased compared to the control or carbon dioxide inflation group. This study also investigated circulating monocyte and peritoneal expression of the molecule membrane-activated complex 1 (MAC-1) (CD11b/CD18) which is an important leukocyte β-2 integrin adhesion molecule. It has various functions including leukocyte adhesion and emigration from the bloodstream. In their study, Watson et al. found significantly decreased expression in the laparotomy group compared to the control or CO_2 insufflation group.

7.3.3 Natural Killer Cell Activity

7.3.3.1 Mechanism of Action

A major component of the innate immune system is the Natural Killer (NK) cell as well known as NK-Large granular lymphocyte (NK-LGL). The term NK cells denote a large group of granular lymphocytes without B-cell or T-cell markers that are able to kill both human cells infected by viruses as well as some tumor cells. NK cells are capable of killing cells that lack MHC class I molecules, which identify cells as being "self." The NK cell kills via its cytoplasmic perforin granules, which create pores in the target cell, as well as by granzymes, which are serine proteases that induce apoptosis in the target cell. Activated NK cells produce interferon (IFN)-γ which attracts leukocytes (chemotaxis) and also stimulates the growth, maturation, and differentiation of many cell types, including monocytes. NK cells are believed to be an important line of defense against intravascular dissemination of tumor cells which has been shown to occur during cancer resection.

7.3.3.2 Natural Killer Cell and Animal Research

A rodent study compared the activity of NK cells 24 h postoperatively in animals subjected to:

1. Pneumoperitoneum alone
2. Laparoscopic dissection of the retroperitoneum to expose the aorta and vena cava
3. The same retroperitoneal exposure carried out via laparotomy
4. Control group with no surgical intervention

No change in NK cell activity was demonstrated between the pneumoperitoneum group and the control group. However, significantly decreased NK cell cytotoxicity was noted in both the open and laparoscopic retroperitoneal dissection groups when compared to the control group. Of note, no difference was noted between the open and laparoscopic groups [62]. A murine study comparing the rate of pulmonary metastases formation following open and laparoscopic tumor resection noted an increased number of metastases in both groups postoperatively; however, the open group had significantly more lung metastases than the laparoscopic group. NK cells were harvested from blood samples at various postoperative time points and their function analyzed ex vivo. NK activity in the open mice group was significantly suppressed on POD 1, POD 7, and POD 14, whereas the laparoscopic group's NK cell function was decreased only on POD 1 and POD 14 [63].

A second murine study assessed NK and lymphokine-activated killer (LAK) cell function after laparoscopy and laparotomy using a hepatic and lung metastases model. Lymphokine-activated killer (LAK) cells are cytotoxic effector cells activated by Interleukin-2 that are capable of killing tumor cells. Laparotomy, and to a lesser extent laparoscopy, was associated with greater tumor growth and tumor establishment as well as suppressed NK and LAK cell activity. Of note, the open group's NK and LAK cell function was more significantly decreased than in the laparoscopy group animals [64].

7.3.3.3 Natural Killer Cell and Clinical Research

A nonrandomized study of 21 laparoscopic and 13 open cholecystectomy patients compared blood samples drawn preoperatively and on POD 1. Both groups were found to have a small but statistically significant decrease in NK cytotoxicity [65]. Another nonrandomized study including 70 patients compared laparoscopy to open colorectal resection. The overall count of NK cells postoperatively was similarly decreased in both laparoscopic and open surgery patients [35]. Similarly, a randomized study of 40 colon cancer patients showed no difference in postoperative NK cytotoxicity between the two groups [66]. A study of open patients reported NK cell impairment postoperatively and noted that NK cell function, as opposed to a decrease in the absolute number of NK cells, was responsible for the changes [67].

7.3.4 Lymphocytes

The term "lymphocyte" encompasses a broad category of immune cells and includes NK cells, T-cells, and B-cells. In vitro proliferation assays carried out on lymphocytes harvested from blood samples taken before and after surgery have been used to assess the proliferative function of lymphocytes postoperatively. Simple lymphocyte counts before and after surgeries have also been compared. A murine study compared anesthesia alone, pneumoperitoneum, or sham laparotomy and found that lymphocyte proliferation was significantly decreased 24 h after surgery only in the laparotomy group [65]. Similarly a nonrandomized study, including 34 patients, comparing laparoscopic and open cholecystectomy, reported a significantly decreased lymphocyte proliferation rate on POD 1 in the open patients only [65]. Conversely, a more definitive randomized colectomy study ($n=79$) that assessed total lymphocyte count noted reduced counts postoperatively in both the open and closed groups [16].

7.3.4.1 Clusters of Differentiation or CD Markers

T-helper (CD4) and cytotoxic T-cells (CD8) as well as other T-cell subpopulations can be identified by the surface molecules they express (referred to as "Clusters of differentiation or CD markers"). The numbers of each T-cell subset can be determined before and after surgery and then compared. There is a broad consensus that when compared to anesthesia alone, surgical stress in general causes a decrease in the ratio of CD4 to CD8 cells [68]. In a randomized study that compared cholecystectomy carried out via laparoscopy and mini-laparotomy a less pronounced decrease in the CD4/CD8 ratio was noted in the closed patients [69]. In the above-mentioned randomized colectomy study, the laparoscopy group had a significantly higher CD4/CD8 ratio on POD 1 than the open group ($p=0.01$) [16]. Similarly, in a prospective study of open and laparoscopic-assisted colectomy patients, although decreased from the preoperative result, the laparoscopics group's CD4/CD8 ratio, after surgery, was significantly higher than the open group's result [70]. Of note, four other colectomy studies found no difference between the open and laparoscopic groups in regards to this parameter [1, 36–38]. A prospective study of 20 patients randomized to laparoscopic or open Nissen fundoplication also demonstrated no difference in the mean CD4/CD8 ratio [71].

7.3.4.2 T-Helper 1 (Th1) and T-Helper 2 (Th2)

Some investigators have indirectly determined the ratio of two subsets of T-helper cells, namely T-helper 1 (Th1) and T-helper 2 (Th2) cells, by measuring and comparing levels of the principal cytokines that each cell type produces. Th1 cells produce IL-2 and IFN-γ, which activate macrophages, as well as TNFα and are the critical effectors of cell-mediated immunity against intracellular microbes. Th1 cells also play a key role in DTH reactions. Th2 cells promote humoral immune function and produce IL-4, IL-5, IL-10, and IL-13 which stimulate antibody production by B cells. Trauma, burns, and hemorrhagic shock have been associated with decreased production of Th1 type cytokines and increased production of Th2 type cytokines.

Surgical stress is associated with a decrease in the Th1/Th2 ratio which suggests that cell-mediated immunity is down regulated and antibody mediated immunity is up regulated [59]. A greater decrease in the Th1/Th2 ratio has been demonstrated after open surgery and less so following laparoscopic surgery. This is mainly due to a decrease in Th1 function; however, the difference between groups persists for less than 24 h [30]. In a clinical study comparing laparoscopic-assisted distal gastrectomy (LADG) and the open equivalent (ODG), Th-1 function was better preserved after LADG [72]. A human study of 43 patients reported that open cholecystectomy was associated with decreased Th1 function as determined by measuring phytohemagglutinin-induced IFN-γ secretion in cultures of peripheral blood mononuclear cells (PBMCs) and by measuring HLA-DR expression on monocytes [59]. In a second cholecystectomy study decreased levels of the following proinflammatory and Th-1 type cytokines were noted in the open patients during the first 24 h after surgery; IFN-γ (48.3% reduction), TNF-α (36.6% reduction), and IL-2 (36.8% decrease). Production by T cells decreased significantly by and respectively, on POD 1 [73]. The clinical significance of these changes is unclear.

7.3.4.3 CD31 Surface Marker/PECAM1

T-cells that are migrating from the circulation into tissue, presumably to participate in an immune response, have been shown to express on their surface the CD31 marker, also known as PECAM1 [74]. Inhibition or blockade of CD-31 prevents T-cell transendothelial migration [75]. In a study done by the authors' laboratory, open colorectal resection was associated with a decrease in the percentage of T-cells expressing CD-31 (CD3+CD31+) on POD 1 and POD 3 when compared to preoperative results. The laparoscopic patients did not exhibit a significant decrease from baseline at the same time points. Of note, an inverse correlation was noted between the percentage of CD31$^+$ T cells and the length of the abdominal incision which suggests that CD31 expression after surgery is related to the extent of abdominal wall trauma [76]. The clinical significance of this short lived decrease in CD31 expression, similar to many of the other transient immune parameter differences, is unclear.

7.3.4.4 Gene Expression and mRNA

A murine study that assessed T cell gene expression before and after laparotomy, CO_2 pneumoperitoneum, and anesthesia alone provides interesting data regarding the impact of both surgical methods. A microarray analysis was carried out on mRNA obtained from splenic T cells harvested from mice sacrificed 12 and 24 h after the surgical interventions. The goal was to determine whether surgery resulted in a change in gene expression. Microarrays of murine genes contain from 22,000 to 34,000 genes. Relative to the anesthesia control (AC) results 12 h after surgery, sham laparotomy resulted in notable alterations in 398 genes compared with 116 genes following pneumoperitoneum. At 24 h the differences between the two surgical methods were less marked, with gene expression alterations noted in 157 genes following laparotomy as opposed to 132 genes after pneumoperitoneum. The vast majority of the affected genes were upregulated after both types of surgery; a minority of genes was down regulated. Thus, 12 h after laparotomy there are notably more

T cell gene expression changes than after CO_2 pneumoperitoneum, however, at 24 h there is little difference between the two methods as regards to the number of expression changes [77].

7.4 Peritoneal Immunity

What is the impact of abdominal surgery on intraperitoneal immune function?

Peritoneal washings typically reveal a modest number of macrophages (<2,000/mL) which are the principal immune cells found in the abdomen [78]. Macrophages mediate the activation and amplification of T cell-specific responses via expression of MHC antigens. They are also capable of killing tumor cells in vitro and in vivo [79]. Macrophages are also capable of phagocytosis as well as generating and releasing a variety of cytokines and cytotoxic molecules. The list of surgery-related factors that may impact peritoneal macrophage function include:

- Length of the abdominal wall incision
- Organ manipulation
- CO_2 pneumoperitoneum
- Increased intra-abdominal pressure
- Decreased intra-abdominal temperature
- Desiccation
- Exposure to bacteria

Also of note, following traumatic insult, mast cells in the peritoneum (mesothelium) excrete histamine which increases vascular permeability resulting in complement and opsonins gaining access to the peritoneal cavity. Thus peritoneal fluid harvested postoperatively manifests some complement-mediated antibacterial activity.

There are a limited number of studies, mostly animal studies, comparing peritoneal macrophage function after open and laparoscopic surgery and the results are confusing and hard to interpret. Markers used to assess macrophage function perioperatively include MHC II expression, ex vivo in vitro production of nitric oxide, hydrogen peroxide, oxygen radicals, and cytokines such as IL-6 and TNF-α. In vivo studies that assess the clearance of bacteria or other pathogens after surgery have also been done. A quick review of two studies done to determine the response of peritoneal macrophages to infection illustrate why interpretation of the open vs. laparoscopic studies is difficult.

A murine model of peritonitis demonstrated that peritoneal macrophage expression of TNF-α and IL-1β mRNA expression increased 2.5- and 2-fold, respectively, within 6 h of cecal ligation and puncture and remained elevated for 24 h [80]. In a mouse model, both hypoxia and endotoxin injection into the peritoneum, resulted in significantly greater TNF-α.production as well as significantly lower prostaglandin E2 (PGE2) and Nitric Oxide production [81]. Activation does not lead to a uniform increase in production of cytokines but in selective production of a few proteins. Furthermore, different types of insult most likely result in different macrophage responses. In surgical studies the challenge is to determine what the desirable postoperative outcome is. The authors make the assumption that preservation of the preoperative response, in the absence of intra-abdominal infection, is probably the desired result.

A large animal study determined ex vivo peritoneal macrophage elaboration of TNF-α. and IL-6 in response to lipo-polysaccharide (LPS) stimulation. Three time points in the first 24 h after laparoscopic, hand-assisted or open nephrectomy were chosen. The macrophages in the open group secreted higher levels of IL-6 and TNF-α. than.the laparoscopic and hand-assisted group [82]. There were no differences noted between the latter two groups.

West et al. assessed in vitro murine peritoneal macrophage production of TNF-α. and IL-1 after LPS stimulation and incubation in CO_2 or room air. Macrophages incubated in CO_2 produced significantly less TNF-α and IL-1 [83]. Iwanaka et al. compared laparotomy, CO_2 pneumoperitoneum and gasless lifting methods in mice and evaluated postoperative production of TNF-α and nitric oxide by peritoneal macrophages. The macrophages in the open group produced significantly more of these proteins 24 h after surgery than the macrophages in the control group. No increases were noted with macrophages from the two minimally invasive groups. In another study it was noted that full laparotomy, mini-laparotomy, and CO_2 laparoscopy in rats were all associated with migration of circulating mononuclear cells into the peritoneal cavity. However, the open groups' peritoneal macrophages generated increased levels of nitric oxide when compared to the other two groups' results [84].

A fourth rodent study included an AC group in addition to a laparoscopic and open cecal resection group. Peritoneal macrophages were harvested 24 h after surgery and then stimulated in vitro after which TNF-α and

H_2O_2 (peroxide) levels were determined. In addition, peritoneal macrophage expression of surface MHC Class II proteins (rodent HLA-DR equivalent) was also assessed. With regard to TNF-α production, the macrophages in the open group released significantly more TNF-α than either of the other groups. However, the open group peritoneal macrophages generated significantly less H_2O_2 after stimulation than did the macrophages from the laparoscopic or the AC groups. Finally, open group macrophages expressed significantly less MHC Class II proteins than the other two groups. When the laparoscopic and AC results for these three parameters were compared, no differences were noted. These results suggest that, in some respect, open surgery stimulates peritoneal macrophages whereas it inhibits other functions. What can be said is that laparoscopic methods better preserve the baseline macrophage function as reflected by the AC group results.

The final rodent study evaluated the ability of rats to clear intraperitoneal *E. coli* after laparotomy and CO_2 insufflation. Significantly more *E. coli* were found 8 h after surgery in the CO_2 pneumoperitoneum group than in either the open or control group [85]. Although not evaluated in this study, it is assumed that peritoneal macrophages are responsible for the clearance of the bacteria.

These results suggest that after laparotomy, peritoneal macrophages are more readily stimulated as regards elaboration of TNF-α, IL-1, and nitric oxide. In addition, they are more capable of clearing intraperitoneal bacteria. It is possible that the CO_2 pneumoperitoneum used during laparoscopic surgery inhibits peritoneal macrophage function. However, peritoneal macrophages in the open group released less H_2O_2 and expressed less MHC Class II protein on their surface; thus, laparotomy is inhibitory in some respects. The clinical implications of these changes are uncertain. To date, significant differences in the rate of postoperative intraperitoneal infections have not been noted when comparing open and laparoscopic colectomy.

7.5 Anesthesia and Its Impact on the Immune Response

Major open and laparoscopic surgery is performed under general anesthesia. Although it is thought that tissue trauma is responsible for the majority of physiologic alterations noted after surgery, the type of anesthesia administered also has been shown to impact a variety of immune parameters. For example, nonsteroidal anti-inflammatory agents, phosphodiesterase inhibitors and opioids, all of which are commonly used during surgery, can alter blood cytokine levels perioperatively [86]. A study regarding Propofol and Fentanyl noted significant increases in blood levels of TNF-α, IL-1 β, and INF-γ 20 min after induction. This study also reported postinduction changes in the number of circulating lymphocytes; a significant increase in the percentage of T and B cells was noted in conjunction with a significant decrease in NK cells [87]. A small randomized study of women undergoing elective hysterectomy for nonmalignant disease assessed and compared the impact of the inhalation agents Isoflurane and nitrous oxide with the intravenous agents Alfentanil and Propofol on IL-1 β and IL-6, and cortisol and prolactin levels. The study results suggest that iv Alfentanil and Propofol was associated with lower IL-6 and cortisol levels postoperatively when compared to results after Isoflurane and nitrous oxide. No differences in prolactin or IL-1 β levels were noted between the two anesthetic approaches [88].

7.6 CO_2 Pneumoperitoneum and Its Effects on the Immune System

Although animal and human studies of a variety of different gases have been carried out, CO_2 remains the only gas to be used clinically throughout the world. In addition to its many other effects and attributes, the CO_2 pneumoperitoneum has been noted to affect the immune system.

A murine study assessed peritoneal macrophage as well as blood monocyte and neutrophil activity after CO_2 pneumoperitoneum, air pneumoperitoneum, or laparotomy. The air pneumoperitoneum and laparotomy groups, when compared to the CO_2 group, showed significantly greater release of TNF-α and superoxide by peritoneal macrophages and a decreased ability of macrophages to phagocytose Candida albicans. Significant LPS translocation across the gut into the peritoneal cavity and systemic circulation was noted in the air pneumoperitoneum and laparotomy groups but not the CO_2 group animals [61]. Gutt el al. used the carbon-clearance test, a well-established method of assessing the phagocytic activity of macrophages, in a murine study comparing open fundoplication, laparoscopic fundoplication with CO_2 pneumoperitoneum, and gasless laparoscopic fundoplication. Whereas phagocytosis was least suppressed in the gasless group ($t1/2 = 12.86$ min), in the CO_2 laparoscopy group moderate suppression was noted ($t1/2 = 16.1$ min). The greatest impairment of carbon clearance, however, was noted in the open surgery group ($t1/2 = 21.91$ min) [89]. Although there have been a fair number of studies demonstrating physiologic advantages of abdominal wall lifting methods, mainly by avoiding of CO_2 pneumoperitoneum, the method has not been widely utilized clinically. The exposure obtained is inferior and the lifting devices, which usually require separate incisions, are cumbersome and expensive. In the end, despite the evidence that CO_2 pneumoperitoneum has clear disadvantages, it remains the gas of choice.

7.7 Helium and Argon as Alternatives to CO_2 Pneumoperitoneum

Alternate gases that have been used for laparoscopy include argon, nitrous oxide, and helium. The nonabsorbable gases helium and argon do not result in hypercarbia and acidosis in contrast to CO_2. Nitrous oxide has never been widely utilized because of its combustibility and increased cost. Helium which offers some advantages over CO_2 is also not often utilized. Rodent studies which compared the above mentioned gases have documented that Helium or air insufflation avoid blood pH changes and do not result in the peritoneal macrophage inhibitory effects noted with CO_2 pneumoperitoneum. The lowered intra-abdominal pH, noted with CO_2 insufflation, may be responsible, at least in part, for the alterations in macrophage function. A murine study comparing laparotomy to helium and CO_2 pneumoperitoneum assessed the ability of the mice to clear intraperitoneal Listeria monocytogenes. Significantly lower bacterial clearance was noted in the laparotomy and CO_2 insufflation groups when compared to the helium pneumoperitoneum group [90]. As already mentioned, despite the demonstrated advantages of helium in animal studies it is not utilized clinically.

7.8 Surgery and Tumor Resistance

In comparing laparotomy, CO_2 insufflation, and anesthesia alone as controls in C3H/Hej mice subcutaneously injected with immunogenic mammary cancer cells (MC2), our group has demonstrated that, by a significant degree, tumors were more easily established and grew more aggressively after laparotomy than after CO_2 insufflation [91]. It is critical to note, however, that CO_2 pneumoperitoneum was also associated with increased tumor growth and establishment when compared to anesthesia alone. Similar results have been noted with other tumor cell lines and in different tumor models [47]. A murine lung metastasis study which compared laparotomy and CO_2 pneumoperitoneum to anesthesia alone found a stepwise increase in the number of surface lung metastases from the AC, to the CO_2 pneumoperitoneum, to the laparotomy group [92]. Similar results have been noted in murine studies wherein open and laparoscopic cecectomy have been compared. Tumor cell proliferation has been shown to be increased and apoptosis decreased after laparotomy [93].

Is the increased tumor growth noted in murine studies due to surgery-related immune-suppression?

Our group conducted one murine study which suggests that surgery-related immune-suppression is a contributor. Subcutaneous tumor growth was assessed after laparotomy and CO_2 pneumoperitoneum in both, immune-competent and immune-deficient nude mice. Whereas significantly larger tumors were noted in the open immune-competent mice, no differences in the tumor mass was noted when the open group was compared with the CO_2 pneumoperitoneum group. This suggested that the cell mediated immune-suppression associated with laparotomy in fact did contribute to the increased tumor growth noted in that group after surgery.

In humans, there are no data suggesting that surgery-related immune-suppression is associated with increased tumor growth in immune-competent patients.

7.9 Angiogenesis-Related Plasma Protein Changes

Although not related to immune function, recent findings regarding postoperative plasma levels of a number of proteins that play an important role in angiogenesis are worth noting. Angiogenesis is critical to both wound healing and tumor growth. Unlike the vast majority of blood proteins which, if altered after surgery, return to normal within a week, plasma levels of vascular-endothelial-growth-factor (VEGF),

Angiopoetin 2 (Ang2), Placental Growth Factor (PlGF), and soluble vascular cell adhesion molecule (VCAM) are significantly increased for 2–4 weeks after laparoscopic colon resection (LACR) [11, 82–84]. VEGF plays a critical early role in the formation of new blood vessels while Ang 2 and PlGF are important pro-angiogenic modulators which encourage VEGF-mediated angiogenesis [67]. Furthermore, plasma from the second and third postoperative weeks after minimally invasive colorectal resection significantly stimulates endothelial cell proliferation, migration, and invasion in vitro when compared to results obtained with preoperative plasma samples [56]. It is thought that these proangiogenic systemic protein concentration changes are related to wound healing. These results suggest that patients who harbor unrecognized tumor microfoci or viable tumor cells in the circulation after "curative" cancer resection are at risk for accelerated tumor growth or, possibly, the establishment of distant metastases during the first month after surgery. Although not directly related, the short duration early immune-suppressive changes may act together with the more persistent pro-angiogenic plasma compositional changes to collectively promote tumor growth during the first month after surgery.

7.10 Conclusion

With regard to local immune function in the peritoneal cavity it appears that CO_2 pneumoperitoneum is associated with some deleterious changes in macrophage function when studied in small animal models. It also appears that macrophages are more easily stimulated in vitro post harvest after open surgery. However, it must be noted that some studies show that open surgery is associated with deleterious macrophage changes such as decreased MHC Class II protein expression and decreased H_2O_2 elaboration. These results suggest that a patient undergoing laparoscopy should be at a disadvantage in regard to intra-abdominal infection. Clinically, increased rates of intra-abdominal abscesses or anastomotic leaks have not been noted in large randomized colectomy studies questioning the clinical significance of these basic science findings.

In general, from the viewpoint of systemic effects (blood protein levels, DTH response, etc.) CO_2 pneumoperitoneum and laparoscopic procedures are associated with less severe and usually shorter alterations than open surgical procedures.

What is the clinical ramification of the better preserved immune function that has been documented in animal studies?

There is no conclusive data linking preserved immune function to better outcome, however, there is some indirect data that can be interpreted to support this hypothesis. A recent review noted that, when compared to open surgery, laparoscopy was associated with lower mean rates of surgical site infections after cholecystectomy (1.1% vs. 4%), appendectomy (2% vs. 8%), colorectal resection (5% vs. 9.5%), and splenectomy (1.5% vs. 10%) [14]. Furthermore, a systematic Cochrane review of the colectomy literature noted a significantly lower rate of wound infections after laparoscopic resection when compared to open surgery [60]. A meta-analysis of the colorectal data made the same observation with regard to wound infections [61]. Laparoscopy has also been associated with lower rates of urinary tract infections after cholecystectomy (0.7% vs. 2%), colorectal resection (0.6% vs. 3%), and splenectomy (1% vs. 8%). This trend was also seen in regards to pulmonary infections after cholecystectomy (1.5% vs. 5%), appendectomy (0.3% vs. 3%), colorectal resection (4% vs. 9%), and splenectomy (10% vs. 15%). It should be noted that analysis of appendectomies showed higher rates of intra-abdominal abscess formation after laparoscopy [14]. Although by no means conclusive, these results do support the idea that preservation of immune function is associated with decreased rates of infection after surgery.

References

1. Ordemann, J., Jacobi, C.A., Schwenk, W., et al.: Cellular and humoral inflammatory response after laparoscopic and conventional colorectal resections. Surg. Endosc. **15**(6), 600–608 (2001)
2. Schietroma, M., Carlei, F., Mownah, A., et al.: Changes in the blood coagulation, fibrinolysis, and cytokine profile during laparoscopic and open cholecystectomy. Surg. Endosc. **18**(7), 1090–1096 (2004)
3. Wu, F.P., Sietses, C., von Blomberg, B.M., et al.: Systemic and peritoneal inflammatory response after laparoscopic or conventional colon resection in cancer patients: a prospective, randomized trial. Dis. Colon Rectum **46**(2), 147–155 (2003)
4. Bolufer, J.M., Delgado, F., Blanes, F., et al.: Injury in laparoscopic surgery. Surg. Laparosc. Endosc. **5**, 318–323 (1995)

5. Bruce, D.M., Smith, M., Walker, C.B., et al.: Minimal access surgery for cholelithiasis induces an attenuated acute phase response. Am. J. Surg. **178**(3), 232–234 (1999)
6. Dionigi, R., Dominioni, L., Benevento, A., et al.: Effects of surgical trauma of laparoscopic vs. open cholecystectomy. Hepatogastroenterology **41**(5), 471–476 (1994)
7. Grande, M., Tucci, G.F., Adorisio, O., et al.: Systemic acute phase response alter laparoscopic and open cholecystectomy. Surg. Endosc. **16**, 313–316 (2002)
8. Jakeways, M.S., Mitchell, V., Hashim, I.A., et al.: Metabolic and inflammatory responses after open or laparoscopic cholecystectomy. Br. J. Surg. **81**(1), 127–131 (1994)
9. Joris, J., Cigarini, I., Legrand, M., et al.: Metabolic and respiratory changes after cholecystectomy performed via laparotomy or laparoscopy. Br. J. Anaesth. **69**(4), 341–345 (1992)
10. Schietroma, M., Carlei, F., Cappelli, S., et al.: Effects of cholecystectomy (laparoscopic versus open) on PMN-elastase. Hepatogastroenterology **54**(74), 342–345 (2007)
11. Targarona, E.M., Pons, M.J., Balagué, C., et al.: Acute phase is the only significantly reduced component of the injury response after laparoscopic cholecystectomy. World J. Surg. **20**(5), 528–533 (1996)
12. Delgado, S., Lacy, A.M., Filella, X., et al.: Acute phase response in laparoscopic and open colectomy in colon cancer: randomized study. Dis. Colon Rectum **44**(5), 638–646 (2001)
13. Hildebrandt, U., Kessler, K., Plusczyk, T., et al.: Comparison of surgical stress between laparoscopic and open colonic resections. Surg. Endosc. **17**(2), 242–246 (2003)
14. Schwenk, W., Jacobi, C., Mansmann, U., et al.: Inflammatory response after laparoscopic and conventional colorectal resections - results of a prospective randomized trial. Langenbecks Arch. Surg. **385**(1), 2–9 (2000)
15. Targarona, E.M., Gracia, E., Garriga, J., et al.: Prospective randomized trial comparing conventional laparoscopic colectomy with hand-assisted laparoscopic colectomy: applicability, immediate clinical outcome, inflammatory response, and cost. Surg. Endosc. **16**(2), 234–239 (2002)
16. Braga, M., Vignali, A., Zuliani, W., et al.: Metabolic and functional results after laparoscopic colorectal surgery. Dis. Colon Rectum **45**(8), 1070–1077 (2002)
17. Sietses, C., Wiezer, M.J., Eijsbouts, Q.A., et al.: A prospective randomized study of the systemic immune response after laparoscopic and conventional Nissen fundoplication. Surgery **126**(1), 5–9 (1999)
18. Nguyen, N.T., Goldman, C.D., Ho, H.S., et al.: Systemic stress response after laparoscopic and open gastric bypass. J. Am. Coll. Surg. **194**(5), 557–566 (2002)
19. Hill, A.D., Banwell, P.E., Darzi, A., et al.: Inflammatory markers following laparoscopic and open hernia repair. Surg. Endosc. **9**(6), 695–698 (1995)
20. Baigrie, R.J., Lamont, P.M., Kwiatkowski, D., et al.: Systemic cytokine response after major surgery. Br. J. Surg. **79**, 757–760 (1992)
21. Cruickshank, A.M., Fraser, W.D., Burns, H.J., et al.: Response of serum interleukin-6 in patients undergoing elective surgery of varying severity. Clin. Sci. **79**, 161–165 (1990)
22. Berggren, U., Gordh, T., Grama, D., et al.: Laparoscopic versus open cholecystectomy: hospitalization, sick leave, analgesia, and trauma responses. Br. J. Surg. **81**, 1362 (1994)
23. Goodale, R.L., Beebe, D.S., McNevin, M.P., et al.: Hemodynamic, respiratory, and metabolic effects of laparoscopic cholecystectomy. Am. J. Surg. **166**, 533–537 (1993)
24. Kloosterman, T., von Blomberg, B.M., Borgstein, P., et al.: Unimpaired immune functions after laparoscopic cholecystectomy. Surgery **115**(4), 424–428 (1994)
25. Kuhry, E., Schwenk, W., Gaupset, R., et al.: Long-term outcome of laparoscopic surgery for colorectal cancer: a cochrane systematic review of randomised controlled trials. Cancer Treat. Rev. **34**(6), 498–504 (2008)
26. Maruszynski, M., Pojda, Z.: Interleukin 6(IL-6) levels in the monitoring of surgical trauma. A comparison of serum IL-6 concentration in patients treated by cholecystectomy via laparotomy or laparoscopy. Surg. Endosc. **9**, 882–885 (1995)
27. McMahon, A.J., O'Dwyer, P.J., Cruickshank, D.: Comparison of metabolic responses to laparoscopic and mini-laparotomy cholecystectomy. Br. J. Surg. **80**, 1255 (1993)
28. Ueo, H., Honda, M., Adachi, M.: et al Minimal increase in serum interleukin-6 levels during laparoscopic cholecystectomy. Am. J. Surg. **168**, 358–360 (1994)
29. Vander Velpen, G., Penninckx, F., Kerremans, R., et al.: Interleukin 6 and coagulation fibrinolysis fluctuation after laparoscopic and conventional cholecystectomy. Surg. Endosc. **8**, 1216 (1994)
30. Carter, J.J., Whelan, R.L.: The immunologic consequences of laparoscopy in oncology. Surg. Oncol. Clin. N. Am. **10**(3), 655–677 (2001)
31. Harmon, G.D., Senagore, A.J., Kilbride, M.J., et al.: Interleukin-6 response to laparoscopic and open colectomy. Dis. Colon Rectum **37**(8), 754–759 (1994)
32. Kirman, I., Poltaratskaia, N., Cekic, V., et al.: Depletion of circulating insulin-like growth factor binding protein 3 after open surgery is associated with high interleukin-6 levels. Dis. Colon Rectum **47**(6), 911–917 (2004)
33. Leung, K.L., Lai, P.B., Ho, R.L., et al.: Systemic cytokine response after laparoscopic-assisted resection of rectosigmoid carcinoma: a prospective randomized trial. Ann. Surg. **231**(4), 506–511 (2000)
34. Nishiguchi, K., Okuda, J., Toyoda, M., et al.: Comparative evaluation of surgical stress of laparoscopic and open surgeries for colorectal carcinoma. Dis. Colon Rectum **44**(2), 223–230 (2001)
35. Wichmann, M.W., Huttl, T.P., Winter, H., et al.: Immunological effects of laparoscopic vs open colorectal surgery. Arch. Surg. **140**, 692–697 (2005)
36. Hewitt, P.M., Ip, S.M., Kwok, S.P., et al.: Laparoscopic-assisted vs. open surgery for colorectal cancer: comparative study of immune effects. Dis. Colon Rectum **41**(7), 901–909 (1998)
37. Mehigan, B.J., Hartley, J.E., Drew, P.J., et al.: Changes in T cell subsets, interleukin-6 and C-reactive protein after laparoscopic and open colorectal resection for malignancy. Surg. Endosc. **15**(11), 1289–1293 (2001)
38. Tang, C.L., Eu, K.W., Tai, B.C., et al.: Randomized clinical trial of the effect of open versus laparoscopically assisted colectomy on systemic immunity in patients with colorectal cancer. Br. J. Surg. **88**(6), 801–807 (2001)
39. Collet, D., Vitale, G.C., Reynolds, M., et al.: Peritoneal host defenses are less impaired by laparoscopy than by open operation. Surg. Endosc. **9**(10), 1059–1064 (1995)

40. Jacobi, C.A., Ordemann, J., Zieren, H.U., et al.: Increased systemic inflammation after laparotomy vs. laparoscopy in an animal model of peritonitis. Arch. Surg. **133**(3), 258–262 (1998)
41. Glaser, F., Sannwald, G.A., Buhr, H.J., et al.: General stress response to conventional and laparoscopic cholecystectomy. Ann. Surg. **221**(4), 372–380 (1995)
42. Hammer, J.H., Nielsen, H.J., Moesgaard, F., et al.: Duration of postoperative immunosuppression assessed by repeated delayed type hypersensitivity skin tests. Eur. Surg. Res. **24**(3), 133–137 (1992)
43. Lennard, T.W., Shenton, B.K., Borzotta, A., et al.: The influence of surgical operations on components of the human immune system. Br. J. Surg. **10**, 771–776 (1995)
44. Allendorf, J.D., Bessler, M., Whelan, R.L., et al.: Better preservation of immune function after laparoscopic-assisted versus open bowel resection in a murine model. Dis. Colon Rectum **39**, 67–72 (1996)
45. Trokel, M.J., Bessler, M., Treat, M.R., et al.: Preservation of immune response after laparoscopy. Surg. Endosc. **8**, 1385–1387 (1994). discussion 1387–1388
46. Allendorf, J.D., Bessler, M., Whelan, R.L., et al.: Postoperative immune function varies inversely with the degree of surgical trauma in a murine model. Surg. Endosc. **11**(5), 427–430 (1997)
47. Gitzelmann, C.A., Mendoza-Sagaon, M., Talamini, M.A., et al.: Cell-mediated immune response is better preserved by laparoscopy than laparotomy. Surgery **127**(1), 65–71 (2000)
48. Whelan, R.L., Franklin, M., Holubar, S.D., et al.: Postoperative cell mediated immune response is better preserved after laparoscopic vs open colorectal resection in humans. Surg. Endosc. **17**(6), 972–978 (2003)
49. Kirman, I., Belizon, A., Balik, E., et al.: Perioperative sargramostim (recombinant human GM-CSF) induces an increase in the level of soluble VEGFR1 in colon cancer patients undergoing minimally invasive surgery. Eur. J. Surg. Oncol. **33**, 1169–1176 (2007)
50. Tjandra, J.J., Chan, M.K.: Systematic review on the short-term outcome of laparoscopic resection for colon and rectosigmoid cancer. Colorectal Dis. **8**(5), 375–388 (2006)
51. Eilber, F.R., Morton, D.L.: Impaired immunologic reactivity and recurrence following cancer surgery. Cancer **25**(2), 362–367 (1970)
52. Christou, N.V., Meakins, J.L., Gordon, J., et al.: The delayed hypersensitivity response and host resistance in surgical patients. 20 years later. Ann. Surg. **222**(4), 534–546 (1995)
53. Christou, N.V., Tellado-Rodriguez, J., Chartrand, L., et al.: Estimating mortality risk in preoperative patients using immunologic, nutritional and acute-phase response variables. Ann. Surg. **210**(1), 69–77 (1989)
54. Pietsch, J.B., Meakins, J.L.: Davis & Geck surgical essay. The delayed hypersensitivity response: clinical application in surgery. Can. J. Surg. **20**(1), 15–21 (1977)
55. Appel, S.H., Wellhausen, S.R., Montgomery, R., et al.: Experimental and clinical significance of endotoxin-dependent HLA-DR expression on monocytes. J. Surg. Res. **47**(1), 39–44 (1989)
56. Faist, E., Mewes, A., Strasser, T., et al.: Alteration of monocyte function following major injury. Arch. Surg. **123**(3), 287–292 (1988)
57. Hershman, M.J., Cheadle, W.G., Wellhausen, S.R., et al.: Monocyte HLA-DR antigen expression characterizes clinical outcome in the trauma patient. Br. J. Surg. **77**(2), 204–207 (1990)
58. Cheadle, W.G., Hershman, M.J., Wellhausen, S.R., et al.: HLA-DR antigen expression on peripheral blood monocytes correlates with surgical infection. Am. J. Surg. **161**(6), 639–645 (1991)
59. Decker, D., Schondorf, M., Bidlingmaier, F., et al.: Surgical stress induces a shift in the type-1/type-2 T-helper cell balance, suggesting down-regulation of cell-mediated and up-regulation of antibody-mediated immunity commensurate to the trauma. Surgery **119**(3), 316–325 (1996)
60. Bolla, G., Tuzzato, G.: Immunologic postoperative competence after laparoscopy versus laparotomy. Surg. Endosc. **17**(8), 1247–1250 (2003). Epub 2003 June 13
61. Watson, R.W., Redmond, H.P., McCarthy, J., et al.: Exposure of the peritoneal cavity to air regulates early inflammatory responses to surgery in a murine model. Br. J. Surg. **82**(8), 1060–1065 (1995)
62. Sandoval, B.A., Robinson, A.V., Sulaiman, T.T., et al.: Open versus laparoscopic surgery: a comparison of natural antitumoral cellular immunity in a small animal model. Am. Surg. **62**(8), 625–630 (1996). discussion 630-1
63. Da Costa, M.L., Redmond, P., Bouchier-Hayes, D.J.: The effect of laparotomy and laparoscopy on the establishment of spontaneous tumor metastases. Surgery **124**(3), 516–525 (1998)
64. Da Costa, M.L., Redmond, H.P., Bouchier-Hayes, D.J.: Taurolidine improves survival by abrogating the accelerated development and proliferation of solid tumors and development of organ metastases from circulating tumor cells released following surgery. J. Surg. Res. **101**(2), 111–119 (2001)
65. Griffith, J.P., Everitt, N.J., Lancaster, F., et al.: Influence of laparoscopic and conventional cholecystectomy upon cell-mediated immunity. Br. J. Surg. **82**(5), 677–680 (1995)
66. Leung, K.L., Tsang, K.S., Ng, M.H., et al.: Lymphocyte subsets and natural killer cell cytotoxicity after laparoscopically assisted resection of rectosigmoid carcinom. Surg. Endosc. **17**(8), 1305–1310 (2003)
67. Pollock, R.E., Lotzová, E., Stanford, S.D.: Mechanism of surgical stress impairment of human perioperative natural killer cell cytotoxicity. Arch. Surg. **126**(3), 338–342 (1991)
68. Ogawa, K., Hirai, M., Katsube, T., et al.: Suppression of cellular immunity by surgical stress. Surgery **127**(3), 329–336 (2000)
69. Walker, C.B., Bruce, D.M., Heys, S.D., et al.: Minimal modulation of lymphocyte and natural killer cell subsets following minimal access surgery. Am. J. Surg. **177**(1), 48–54 (1999)
70. Liang, J.T., Shieh, M.J., Chen, C.N., et al.: Prospective evaluation of laparoscopy-assisted colectomy versus laparotomy with resection for management of complex polyps of the sigmoid colon. World J. Surg. **26**(3), 377–383 (2002)
71. Perttilä, J., Salo, M., Ovaska, J., et al.: Immune response after laparoscopic and conventional Nissen fundoplication. Eur. J. Surg. **165**(1), 21–28 (1999)
72. Fujii, K., Sonoda, K., Izumi, K., et al.: T lymphocyte subsets and Th1/Th2 balance after laparoscopy-assisted distal gastrectomy. Surg. Endosc. **17**(9), 1440–1444 (2003)

73. Brune, I.B., Wilke, W., Hensler, T., et al.: Downregulation of T helper type 1 immune responseand altered pro-inflammatory and anti-inflammatory T cell cytokine balance followingconventional but not laparoscopic surgery. Am. J. Surg. **177**(1), 55–60 (1999)
74. Brezinschek, R.I., Oppenheimer-Marks, N., Lipsky, P.E.: Activated T cells acquire endothelial cell surface determinants during transendothelial migration. J. Immunol. **162**(3), 1677–1684 (1999)
75. Qing, Z., Sandor, M., Radvany, Z., et al.: Inhibition of antigen-specific T cell trafficking into the central nervous system via blocking PECAM1/CD31 molecule. J. Neuropathol. Exp. Neurol. **60**(8), 798–807 (2001)
76. Kirman, I., Cekic, V., Poltaratskaia, N., et al.: The percentage of CD31+ T cells decreases after open but not laparoscopic surgery. Surg. Endosc. **17**(5), 754–757 (2003)
77. Sylla, P., Nihalani, A., Whelan, R.L.: Microarray analysis of the differential effects of open and laparoscopic surgery on murine splenic T-cells. Surgery **139**(1), 92–103 (2006)
78. van Furth, R., Raeburn, J.A., van Zwet, T.I.: Characteristics of human mononuclear phagocytes. Blood **54**, 485–500 (1979)
79. Drysdale, B.E., Agarwal, S., Shin, H.S.: Macrophage-mediated tumoricidal activity: mechanisms of activation and cytotoxicity. Prog. Allergy **40**, 111–161 (1988)
80. McMasters, K.M., Cheadle, W.G.: Regulation of macrophage TNF alpha, IL-1 beta, and Ia (I-A alpha) mRNA expression during peritonitis is site dependent. J. Surg. Res. **54**(5), 426–430 (1993)
81. Arya, G., Garcia, V.F.: Hypoxia/reoxygenation affects endotoxin tolerance. J. Surg. Res. **59**(1), 13–16 (1995)
82. Novitsky, Y.W., Czerniach, D.R., Kaban, G.K., et al.: Immunologic effects of hand-assisted surgery on peritoneal macrophages: comparison to open and standard laparoscopic approaches. Surgery **139**(1), 39–45 (2006)
83. West, M.A., Hackam, D.J., Baker, J., et al.: Mechanism of decreased in vitro murine macrophage cytokine release after exposure to carbon dioxide: relevance to laparoscopic surgery. Ann. Surg. **226**(2), 179–190 (1997)
84. Jesch, N.K., Kuebler, J.F., Nguyen, H., et al.: Laparoscopy vc minilaparotoomy and full laparotomoy preserves circulatory but not peritoneal and pulmonary immune responses. J. Pediatr. Surg. **41**(6), 1085–1092 (2006)
85. Sare, M., Yesilada, O., Gürel, M., et al.: Effects of C02 insufflation on bacterial growth in rats with Escherichia coli-induced experimental peritonitis. Surg. Laparosc. Endosc. **7**(1), 38–41 (1997)
86. McBride, W.T., Armstrong, M.A., McBride, S.J.: Immunomodulation: an important concept in modern anaesthesia. Anaesthesia **51**(5), 465–473 (1996)
87. Brand, J.M., Frohn, C., Luhm, J., et al.: Early alterations in the number of circulating lymphocyte subpopulations and enhanced proinflammatory immune response during opioid-based general anesthesia. Shock **20**(3), 213–217 (2003)
88. Crozier, T.A., Müller, J.E., Quittkat, D., et al.: Effect of anaesthesia on the cytokine responses to abdominal surgery. Br. J. Anaesth. **72**(3), 280–285 (1994)
89. Gutt, C.N., Heinz, P., Kaps, W., et al.: The phagocytosis activity during conventional and laparoscopic operations in the rat. A preliminary study. Surg. Endosc. **11**(9), 899–901 (1997)
90. Chekan, E.G., Nataraj, C., Clary, E.M., et al.: Intraperitoneal immunity and pneumoperitoneum. Surg. Endosc. **13**(11), 1135–1138 (1999)
91. Allendorf, J.D., Bessler, M., Kayton, M.L., et al.: Increased tumor establishment and growth after laparotomy vs laparoscopy in a murine model. Arch. Surg. **130**(6), 649–653 (1995)
92. Shiromizu, A., Suematsu, T., Yamaguchi, K., et al.: Effect of laparotomy and laparoscopy on the establishment of lung metastasis in a murine model. Surgery **128**(5), 799–805 (2000)
93. Lee, S.W., Gleason, N., Blanco, I., Asi, Z.K., et al.: Higher colon cancer tumor proliferative index and lower tumor cell death rate in mice undergoing laparotomy versus insufflation. Surg. Endosc. **16**(1), 36–39 (2002)
94. Belizon, A., Balik, E., Horst, P., et al.: Persistent elevation of plasma vascular endothelial growth factor levels during the first month after minimally invasive colorectal resection. Surg. Endosc. **22**(2), 287–297 (2008)
95. Shantha Kumara, H.M.C., Yan, X., Herath, A.C.: Plasma soluble Vascular Adhesion Molecule-1 levels are persistently elevated during the first month after colorectal cancer resection. Accepted for presentation at SAGES WCES 12th Mtg (2010)
96. Shantha Kumara, H.M.C., Yan, X., Feingold, D.: Plasma Levels of Placental Growth Factor (PLGF), a proangiogenic protein, are elevated for 3 weeks after minimally invasive colorectal cancer resection. Accepted for presentation at SAGES WCES 12th Mtg (2010)
97. Shantha Kumara, H.M.C., Hoffman, A., Kim, I.Y., et al.: Colorectal resection, both open and laparoscopic-assisted, in patients with benign indications is associated with proangiogenic changes in plasma angiopoietin 1 and 2 levels. Surg. Endosc. **23**(2), 409–415 (2009)
98. Neufeld, G., Cohen, T., Gengrinovitch, S., et al.: Vascular endothelial growth factor (VEGF) and its receptors. FASEB J. **13**(1), 9–22 (1999)
99. Kumara, H.M., Feingold, D., Kalady, M., et al.: Colorectal resection is associated with persistent proangiogenic plasma protein changes: postoperative plasma stimulates in vitro endothelial cell growth, migration, and invasion. Ann. Surg. **249**(6), 973–977 (2009)
100. Boni, L., Benevento, A., Rovera, F., et al.: Infective complications in laparoscopic surgery. Surg. Infect. (Larchmt) **7**(Suppl 2), S109–S111 (2006)

Pneumoperitoneum and Its Effects on Malignancy

Alan T. Lefor and Atsushi Shimizu

8.1 Introduction

Over the past 2 decades, laparoscopy has emerged as a valuable tool in the diagnosis and management of many diseases in the realm of general surgery. For some conditions, laparoscopy has rapidly become the gold standard in treatment, relegating open surgery to a second line of therapy. The most obvious procedure in this category is laparoscopic cholecystectomy, which has afforded patients a dramatic decrease in length of hospital stay, increased comfort, and rapid return to employment.

The role of laparoscopy has expanded to include diagnosing, staging, treating, monitoring, and palliating a long list of malignancies. The early role of laparoscopy in the diagnosis of cancer was strictly visual. Intraabdominal masses were characterized visually, which gave a subjective impression as to their malignant potential. The use of laparoscopic biopsy forceps allows the diagnosis of malignancy by providing tissue specimens. Currently, laparoscopic ultrasound-guided biopsy techniques allow for the detection and biopsy of masses deep within solid organs such as the liver. Once a diagnosis is established, laparoscopic staging can identify unresectable disease, which often dramatically alters therapy. Originally used for staging disease in patients with lymphoma, laparoscopy now plays a role in excluding major abdominal resections when metastases are identified. For resectable disease, major laparoscopic resections ranging from splenectomy to complex pancreaticoduodenectomy have been described. After resection, tumor surveillance can be performed by direct observation, with carcinomatosis identified in second-look operations. In the case of unresectable disease or complications of advanced disease, laparoscopic procedures can provide palliation, for example, by relieving or bypassing bowel obstruction.

After an initial surge of enthusiasm, the use of laparoscopy for oncologic procedures was slowed for many reasons; the history of this is a study of the surgical mentality. Laparoscopy was used mainly by gynecologists in the United States until quite recently. The first report of a port-site recurrence described a patient with ovarian cancer undergoing diagnostic laparoscopy in 1978 [1]. Following the adoption of laparoscopic techniques by general surgeons in the late 1980s, many new procedures were attempted, and by the early 1990s, some surgeons were routinely performing laparoscopic colon resections in an attempt to provide their patients with the same benefits that follow laparoscopic cholecystectomy. In 1993, several case reports appeared describing the appearance of port-site recurrences at the site of trocar insertion following laparoscopic colon resections for cancer. These reports led to a rapid deceleration in the use of laparoscopy for patients with cancer. The surgical community responded with a widespread effort to investigate this in the laboratory and to determine the true incidence of port-site recurrences. Careful clinical studies were also initiated to investigate the true incidence of wound recurrences in open surgery, data which seemed to be sorely lacking. These observations also led to the initiation of a number of very well-designed prospective randomized multicenter trials to carefully study the role of laparoscopic resection in the treatment of patients with cancer, most notably, colon cancer.

A.T. Lefor (✉) and A. Shimizu
Department of Surgery, Center for Graduate Medical Education, Jichi Medical University, 3311-1 Yakushiji, Shimotsuke City, Tochigi, 329-0498, Japan
e-mail: alefor@jichi.ac.jp; ashimizu@jichi.ac.jp

In 1904, Halstead said "The hospital, the operating room, and the wards should be laboratories, laboratories of the highest order. And we know from experience that where this conception prevails, not only is the cause of higher education and of medical science best served, but also the welfare of the patient is best promoted. It remains with the teachers of medicine and surgery to make them so." In the true spirit of this statement, the history of laparoscopic colon cancer surgery shows that clinicians took a clinical observation, studied it, and then returned to the clinic with new approaches and the benefit of having objective data to refer to.

This chapter begins by reviewing available evidence about the effects of pneumoperitoneum on the whole patient with a malignancy. Following this, the effects of pneumoperitoneum on malignant cells are reviewed, including both in vitro and in vivo studies. The effects of the composition and pressure of the gas used to establish pneumoperitoneum is then reviewed, followed by a review of laboratory and clinical studies focusing specifically on port-site recurrences. Finally, the literature regarding approaches to the prevention of port-site recurrences is reviewed. In the simplest historical terms, the clinical and basic science related to the effects of pneumoperitoneum on malignancy is a direct result of studies of the clinical and basic science of port-site recurrences.

8.2 Effects of Pneumoperitoneum on the Whole Patient

An understanding of the effects of laparoscopy and pneumoperitoneum on malignancies begins with an understanding of the effects of the physiologic changes on the whole patient.

8.2.1 Deep Venous Thrombosis, Pulmonary Embolism, and Hypercoagulability

There have been a number of studies that have looked at the incidence of deep venous thrombosis after laparoscopic surgery. In addition, it is well known that patients with malignancy are often hypercoagulable compared to those without malignancy. These two statements raise concerns about increased risk for patients with malignancy who undergo laparoscopic surgery. Increased venous stasis has been demonstrated in clinical studies of patients undergoing laparoscopic cholecystectomy [2]. This finding has also been observed by others, who found a decrease in femoral blood flow velocity and an increase in femoral vein diameter with the establishment of pneumoperitoneum [3]. This finding was consistent with stasis because release of the pneumoperitoneum resulted in an increase in femoral vein blood flow. These findings were confirmed by Ido, using color flow Doppler studies [4].

The incidence of pulmonary embolism after laparoscopic surgery has been reported. In a review of 487 patients who underwent laparoscopic cholecystectomy, there were two clinically significant cases of pulmonary embolism despite heparin therapy [3]. Another retrospective review of 200 patients found a 1% incidence of clinically significant pulmonary embolism [5]. Data for DVT and/or pulmonary embolism were reported in the CLASSIC trial of laparoscopic resection of colon cancer [6] but not in the COST [7] or COLOR [8] trials. In the CLASSIC trial, there were two cases (2%) of deep venous thrombosis in the open surgery group and one (1%) in the laparoscopic group, which was not a significant difference ($p > .05$).

Results have shown that despite being minimally invasive, laparoscopic cholecystectomy induces a hypercoagulable state [9]. The induction of pneumoperitoneum causes the release of arginine vasopressin [10]. It has been postulated that the interaction of vasopressin with platelets may, in part, be responsible for the hypercoagulable state observed in patients who undergo a pneumoperitoneum [9]. Caprini evaluated postoperative hypercoagulability and DVT after laparoscopic cholecystectomy, and found significantly elevated hypercoagulability [11]. In light of all of these findings, it is recommended that surgeons minimize the head-up position and abdominal wall insufflation as much as possible to minimize the complications associated with hypercoagulability in these patients [9].

8.2.2 Systemic Immunity

Despite the reduction in local peritoneal inflammatory response, systemic immunocompetence appears better preserved after laparoscopic surgery than after open procedures. Some studies have shown significant decreases in the CD4 and CD8 cell counts in patients undergoing open cholecystectomy, and others have shown a derangement in the ratios of the T-cell subsets [12]. Vallina and Velasco studied peripheral lymphocyte populations in 11 patients undergoing laparoscopic cholecystectomy and found a transient decrease in the CD4 to CD8 ratio, with no difference in absolute CD4 and CD8 cell counts, followed by a return to the preoperative ratio within 1 week of surgery [13]. In a study of delayed-type hypersensitivity in sepsis, the death rate was 2.9% in patients with a normal delayed-type hypersensitivity response, whereas the death rate was 20.9% in anergic patients [14]. In prospective animal and human studies comparing laparotomy and laparoscopy, the laparotomy group showed a significantly sustained decrease in delayed-type hypersensitivity; the inference is thus that systemic cell-mediated immunity is better preserved with laparoscopy [15]. In animal studies, tumor inoculum implanted remotely from the abdomen showed greater growth after laparotomy than after laparoscopy.

The effects of pneumoperitoneum on cellular immunity are described above, and result in decreased release of C-reactive protein and IL-6 when compared to open surgery. The effects on macrophage function may represent a significant effect on local cellular immunity within the abdomen [16]. The effects of pneumoperitoneum may be contrasted with immune effects after VATS procedures in which CO_2 insufflation is not used. This may offer some advantages in regard to immune function when compared to laparoscopic procedures performed with CO_2 pneumoperitoneum [16]. Recent investigations have shown that postoperative leukocyte counts normalize earlier after laparoscopic resection of colon cancer than after open surgery and that HLA-DR expression is more reduced after open surgery compared to laparoscopic surgery [16]. However, the clinical importance of these observations remains unclear and will require further study to elucidate.

While parameters of systemic immunity seem to be better preserved after laparoscopic surgery compared to open surgery, the benefits of laparoscopic surgery may not be so obvious at the cellular level within the peritoneum [17]. The local immune environment has been shown to be modulated by the choice of insufflation gas as well as the pressure used. The impaired production of TNF-α by macrophages may inhibit their ability to successfully scavenge for cells liberated during laparoscopic surgery [17]. These studies underscore the fact that while laparoscopic surgery appears to maintain systemic immunity better than open surgery based on a number of measured parameters, the clinical significance of this remains unclear.

8.2.3 Central Nervous System

Much of what is known about the central nervous system effects of laparoscopy is derived from porcine models. In an intracranial pressure transduction study, CO_2, helium, and nitric oxide, all increased intracranial pressure equally [18]. The rise in intracranial pressure was independent of changes in acid–base balance and was thought to be secondary to increased intraabdominal pressure from the pneumoperitoneum. Despite the low morbidity shown in a single small retrospective study of patients with ventriculo-peritoneal shunts, caution is advised in patients with intracranial pathology [19].

8.2.4 Cardiac Effects

As the population ages, it is not uncommon to operate on older patients with cancer who also have significant medical comorbidities such as heart disease. It becomes imperative that the physiologic cardiovascular consequences of laparoscopic surgery be understood to prevent adverse results. The documentation of these effects in humans has been aided by the use of invasive and noninvasive devices. In a hemodynamic study carried out during laparoscopic colectomy for carcinoma, patients were monitored with arterial and pulmonary artery catheters along with transesophageal echocardiography [20]. The mean arterial pressure, central venous pressure, mean pulmonary artery pressure, pulmonary capillary wedge pressure, and systemic vascular resistance, all increased significantly. Cardiac index and ejection fraction decreased significantly, while heart rate remained relatively unchanged. To understand the physiologic consequences, Giebler et al. studied intraperitoneal laparoscopy and retroperitoneal laparoscopy in a pig model [21]. They found significant pressure gradients along the iliac veins and vena cava in the intraperitoneal group, which were absent in the retroperitoneal group. Also, airway pressures increased in the intraperitoneal group. It is likely that the decrease in cardiac function is the direct result of an interaction between decreased venous return and increased transmitted intrathoracic pressure.

8.2.5 Pulmonary Effects

In the usual clinical setting, the lungs remain a compliant organ. By manipulating ventilation, the anesthesiologist is able to prevent significant acid–base disturbances and keep the partial pressure of carbon dioxide (pCO_2) within the normal range. To understand the effects on an injured lung, a porcine adult respiratory distress syndrome model was used [22]. Following the induction of adult respiratory distress syndrome, animals were divided into two groups; one underwent laparoscopy and the other underwent conventional laparotomy. The laparoscopic group demonstrated significantly decreased pulmonary compliance compared with the laparotomy group, had a higher pCO_2, and was more acidotic. Despite the increase in pulmonary derangements caused by laparoscopy in animals with adult respiratory distress syndrome, overall cardiopulmonary function was preserved.

8.2.6 Visceral Effects

That visceral organs have diminished blood flow during insufflation with a variety of gases is well accepted. The magnitude of reduction can be significant, with reductions in flow of more than 30%. Often, the ischemia is mild, manifested by low urine output, but severe intestinal ischemia has also been observed in rare cases. The reduced blood flow has been attributed to a combination of factors, including direct vascular compression and reflexive neural pathways.

8.3 Effects of Pneumoperitoneum on Malignant Cells: *In Vitro* Studies

The reduction in postoperative pain, decreased healing time, and decreased adhesion formation after laparoscopic surgery may easily be attributed to the use of smaller incisions and avoidance of the need for retractors to hold incisions open for hours. However, patients who undergo laparoscopic splenectomy and then require an incision for removal of the intact specimen also note decreased pain in their incisions. Implicated in the beneficial effects of laparoscopy is the CO_2 gas that is commonly used to insufflate the abdominal wall. West et al. investigated the effect of different insufflation gases on murine peritoneal macrophage intracellular pH and correlated their use with alterations in lipopolysaccharide-stimulated inflammatory cytokine release [23]. Peritoneal macrophages were incubated for 2 h in air, helium, or CO_2, and the effect on tumor necrosis factor (TNF) level, Interleukin-1 level, and cytosol pH was determined. Macrophages incubated in CO_2 produced significantly less TNF and Interleukin-1 than those incubated in air or helium. In addition, exposure to CO_2, but not to air or helium, produced a marked acidification of the cytosol. These authors concluded that cellular acidification induced by peritoneal CO_2 insufflation contributes to the diminished local inflammatory response seen in laparoscopic surgery.

In another experiment, peritoneal macrophages harvested from volunteers were exposed to CO_2 under pressures similar to those used in laparoscopy and to a helium control environment [24]. This model showed a decrease in intraabdominal polymorphonuclear leukocyte function, as evidenced by a decrease in superoxide production. Also, the peritoneal macrophages secreted less TNF-α and Interleukin-1, and the activity of mitochondrial dehydrogenase became significantly impaired for up to 12 h after CO_2 exposure. It was also concluded that CO_2 was responsible for the decreased inflammation and pain after laparoscopy. In a randomized trial of laparoscopic versus conventional colon resections, Wu et al. measured levels of Interleukin-6, Interleukin-8, and TNF-α in patients undergoing colon resections for malignancy [25]. The laparoscopic group had significant reductions in serum Interleukin-6 and Interleukin-8 levels, whereas TNF-α was undetectable in both groups. These results confirm the attenuation of the acute-phase systemic response previously observed in clinical trials.

A common physiologic change during laparoscopy is the exposure of the abdominal contents to high intraabdominal pressures. Gutt et al. exposed cultures of two human tumor cell lines to 0-, 6-, and 12-mmHg CO_2 pressures [26]. The proliferation of colon carcinoma cells increased significantly as pressure increased, whereas the pancreatic carcinoma cells proliferated with CO_2 exposure independent of ambient pressure.

In an in vitro study, an increase in ambient pressure increased tumor adherence to matrix proteins; this effect was mitigated by administration of antibodies to the α_1-Integrin subunit [27]. In addition to altering the biologic characteristics of tumors so that they adhere to and invade tissues more readily, increased pressure also adversely affects the host barrier of normal mesothelial cells and thus decreases the natural defenses to tumor growth. One hour after laparoscopy was performed on mice, electron microscopy of the normal peritoneal surfaces revealed retraction and condensation of mesothelial cells [28]. Over the next 12 h, the intercellular clefts increased in size, exposing the basal membrane. In animals inoculated with tumor, the peritoneal surfaces rapidly became coated with malignant cells, which created widespread intraabdominal metastases that mimicked the carcinomatosis reported in humans after laparoscopy. In the control group exposed to pressure-less laparoscopy, tumor cells remained on top of intact mesothelial cells for a prolonged period before invading in a sporadic fashion. The growth of tumor remained localized to the port sites and lower abdomen, similar to the pattern of recurrences seen after open laparotomy. The effect of pressure is multifold:

- Induces tumor cells to grow larger
- Let tumor cells adhere better to other cells
- Allows tumor cells to penetrate more quickly

This not only leads to peritoneal host defense damage, but it has also been hypothesized to explain early carcinomatosis after laparoscopy.

Matrix metalloproteins (MMPs) are thought to be important in the invasiveness of tumor cells, and may contribute to the development of metastases. MMP inhibitors are being tested in clinical trials. Alterations in the expression of MMPs as well as the invasive capacity of tumor cells in a Matrigel-based invasion assay were evaluated in an in vitro study of a human colon adenocarcinoma cell line that was exposed to either CO_2 or helium to mimic laparoscopic surgery conditions [29]. This study showed significantly greater expression of MMPs in the cells exposed to both CO_2 and He compared to controls, with cells exposed to CO_2 having a significantly greater expression than cells exposed to He. A similar effect was seen in the cell invasion assay. Furthermore, by the addition of MMP inhibitors, the enhanced invasiveness was completely abrogated, with results returning to control values. Thus, the authors conclude that the laparoscopic environment may contribute to the dissemination of malignant cells in patients. They hypothesize that the common factor which leads to these changes may be hypoxia.

The adherence of tumor cells to mesothelial cells was studied in vitro, using conditions similar to laparoscopic surgery [30]. After exposing mesothelial cells in vitro to the pressure and conditions of a pneumoperitoneum, there was significant enhancement of adhesion of a tumor cell line to the mesothelial cells. This was paralleled by a significant increase in ICAM-1 expression by the mesothelial cells. By inhibiting ICAM-1 with an antibody, tumor cell adhesion was attenuated. These studies appear to be identifying some of the potential molecular effectors of the effects of pneumoperitoneum on tumor cells and the cells in their environment that may be responsible for the clinical phenomenon of port-site recurrences.

8.4 Effects of Pneumoperitoneum on Malignant Cells: *In Vivo* Studies

It has been suggested that insufflation itself may cause port-site recurrences by forcing viable cancer cells into the circulation, where they localize to sites of trauma (e.g. port sites) and form metastases. In an in vivo study, animals were injected with tumor cells intraperitoneally and then divided into three groups: control with an abdominal incision, insufflation with a 3-cm back incision, and back incision alone [31]. After sacrifice, animals with back incisions showed 0% with tumor implants on the back, while the control group had a 42% incidence of tumor implants in the midline wound. The distribution of intraabdominal disease was similar in all three groups. This study suggests that pneumoperitoneum does not promote hematogenous wound implantation of free intraperitoneal cancer cells.

In an in vivo model, rats underwent laparoscopy under 0-, 4-, and 16-mmHg pressure [32]. A colon adenocarcinoma cell line was injected intraperitoneally, and pneumoperitoneum was held for 60 min. On day 11, the rats were sacrificed and the volume of tumor was assessed. Rats that underwent higher pressure laparoscopy had a greater volume of tumor. In similar studies, other investigators have shown increased rates of metastases.

An area of controversy in the pathogenesis of port-site recurrences is the effect of pneumoperitoneum itself relative to the effect of tumor manipulation on their formation. In a study using a hamster tumor model, an established omental tumor was randomized to one of four groups (bivalve of the tumor, crush, strip, or excision), and then swept through the abdominal cavity with or without pneumoperitoneum [33]. The results showed no effect of the presence of pneumoperitoneum on wound implants, and these investigators conclude that tumor implantation at trocar sites is due to spillage of tumor during manipulation and not to pneumoperitoneum.

The effect of pneumoperitoneum on tumor cells in the portal vein during laparoscopic surgery was investigated in a rabbit model [34]. Tumor cells were inoculated in the portal vein immediately before establishment of CO_2 pneumoperitoneum or laparotomy alone. On day 17, the animals were sacrificed and the number of nodules in the liver evaluated. In this model, animals in the pneumoperitoneum group had significantly ($p<.01$) more nodules than the laparotomy group.

Adhesion molecules may play a role in the formation of metastases, and have been studied in vivo to parallel the in vitro work described above. In a murine model, tumor cells were administered via intrasplenic injection, and the animals divided into three groups: CO_2 peritoneum, open laparotomy, and anesthesia alone [35]. Seven days later, the livers were evaluated for tumor load, and significantly more tumor nodules were seen in the pneumoperitoneum group compared to the other two groups. In a parallel experiment, the CO_2 pneumoperitoneum group also showed significantly higher expression of ICAM-1 and TNF-α mRNA in the liver. Other molecules are also implicated in the mechanism of tumor dissemination. In a nude mouse model, human colon adenocarcinoma was implanted in the cecum, and animals underwent laparotomy alone, CO_2 pneumoperitoneum, or anesthesia alone [36]. This model resulted in significantly more nodules of peritoneal dissemination after laparotomy than after CO_2 pneumoperitoneum or anesthesia alone. The laparotomy group also had decreased expression of E-cadherin mRNA in the tumors. Integrin and CD44 may also play a role in this complex process. In a murine model of port-site recurrences, antiintegrin and anti-CD44 antibody decreased both the number and weight of port-site recurrences in the presence of hyaluronic acid [37]. The significance of these interesting findings will require further experiments.

The effect of laparoscopic surgery on the formation of lung metastases was evaluated in a murine model [38]. After undergoing anesthesia alone, open cecectomy, or laparoscopic cecectomy, mice received a tail-vein injection of tumor cells and the resulting numbers of pulmonary tumor nodules were evaluated. This experiment showed significantly more tumor nodules in the animals that underwent open surgery compared to those that underwent laparoscopic surgery, and the authors propose that this may be due to greater immunosuppression after open surgery compared to laparoscopic surgery.

8.5 Effect of the Insufflation Gas: Composition and Pressure – *In Vitro* and *In Vivo* Studies

Another component of routine laparoscopy is use of the insufflation gas CO_2. In tissue culture experiments, CO_2 (in comparison to helium and air) increased ovarian carcinoma cell growth by 52%; however, in in vivo studies, CO_2 had no impact on tumor growth and metastases [39]. The cecal wall of rats was inoculated via a 1-cm abdominal incision with 2 million viable tumor cells [39]. Two weeks later, the rats were randomly assigned to laparoscopy or laparotomy. In the laparoscopy group, a standard 5-mm port was inserted, and the abdominal cavity was insufflated for 30 min with CO_2. The laparotomy group underwent a midline 4-cm incision, which remained open for 30 min. Four weeks after the second procedure, tissues were examined histologically and grossly. There was no difference between groups in liver metastases, lung metastases, nodal metastases, wound/port recurrences, or cecal tumor weight. A criticism of the study is that animals underwent two operations, which confounds the results and conclusion. Because of the numerous conflicting results of in vitro and in vivo studies, the specific effect of CO_2 on tumor cells and their ability to form metastases still remains unknown.

In a study of tumor cell adhesion and growth, a rat transitional cell carcinoma cell-line was exposed to CO_2 at pressures varying from 0 to 15 mmHg and at concentrations varying from 5% to 15% (in air) by volume [40]. This experiment showed a significant decrease in tumor cell adhesion after CO_2 insufflation, and an increase in cell growth, apoptosis, and necrosis for the first 24 h, followed by a steady decline. Concentrations of CO_2 greater than 5% inhibited cell growth only for the first 48 h. Insufflation pressure had a greater effect on inhibiting tumor growth than did CO_2 concentration. It was concluded that CO_2 has a toxic effect on transitional cell carcinoma and inhibits cell adhesion and growth.

In another study using transitional cell carcinoma, using an in vitro model, tumor cell adhesion and growth were measured after insufflation with CO_2, N_2, and He at three different pressures (0, 10, and 15 mmHg) [40]. These investigators found that the tumor adhesion rate was lowest with CO_2 and highest with N_2. Higher gas pressures resulted in decreased adhesion rates in CO_2 and He, but increased adhesion in N_2. While tumor cell proliferation was increased in CO_2 and He for the first 24 h, with a subsequent decrease, proliferation showed enhancement in N_2 at all pressures studied. Apoptosis and necrosis were higher in He than in CO_2 or N_2. Overall, these investigators conclude that the type of gas and pressure of insufflation significantly affects cell adhesion and tumor growth.

In a rat model, animals were injected with hepatocellular carcinoma and then underwent resection of the tumor by open laparotomy or laparoscopic resection with pneumoperitoneum using air, CO_2, or helium [41]. A control group received anesthesia alone. Tumor recurrence was significantly less in animals undergoing laparoscopic resection using helium insufflation compared to air or CO_2 insufflation. They also concluded that exposure to room air (laparotomy) resulted in stimulation of tumor recurrence and metastasis.

In a murine model, the effect of gasless laparoscopy was compared to laparotomy and CO_2 pneumoperitoneum with regard to the growth of experimentally induced liver metastases [42]. Metastases were induced by intraportal injection of a colon cancer cell line, and the animals divided into four groups (CO_2 pneumoperitoneum, laparotomy, gasless laparoscopy, and control). Fourteen days later, the hepatic tumor load was evaluated. While tumor growth was enhanced by laparotomy and CO_2 pneumoperitoneum, animals that underwent gasless laparoscopy had tumor growth similar to that observed in control animals. The authors conclude that gasless laparoscopy better preserves host defenses than laparotomy or CO_2 pneumoperitoneum. In a similar study from the same laboratory, the effect of insufflation pressure was evaluated using the same model, using radiolabeled tumor cells. They found that higher insufflation pressure (15 mmHg) led to more accumulation of tumor cells in the liver than lower (5 and 10 mmHg) insufflation pressures and controls.

The cause of the controversy concerning tumor cell biology under laparoscopic conditions is multifactorial. During laparoscopy, abdominal contents, including malignant cells, are exposed to changes in homeostasis. The effects of these changes have been studied mainly in animal models, and controversy exists regarding which species and tumor model most represents human biology. Furthermore, a review of existing studies shows that the results vary depending on many factors, and are not easily combined to a single statement of effect. At this time, most clinical laparoscopy is performed using carbon dioxide pneumoperitoneum at routine pressures of 10–15 mmHg.

8.6 Clinical Studies of the Effect of Pneumoperitoneum on Tumor Cells

Intraoperative peritoneal lavage was performed in a study of 36 patients undergoing laparoscopic resection of colon cancer and 45 patients undergoing conventional open resections [43]. Lavage was performed just after entry into the abdominal cavity and just before closing. Malignant cells were not detected in the CO_2 filtrate gas. The incidence of positive cytology was 33% in the prelavage in both groups, and in the postlavage, it was 8.33% in the laparoscopic group and 11.1% in the open surgery group. Thus, in this study, pneumoperitoneum was shown not to affect tumor cell dissemination and seeding.

In humans, radiolabeled red blood cells injected into the bed of the gallbladder during standard laparoscopic cholecystectomy migrated to port sites, even though the specimen were removed using a protective bag [44]. In the gasless laparoscopic group, no radioactivity was detected at the port sites. During laparoscopy for benign and malignant diseases, Ikramuddin attached a saline suction trap to filter the pneumoperitoneum effluent. Normal mesothelial cells were identified in the benign group while two patients out of 15 with malignancies had large numbers of malignant cells in the trap [45]. These two patients had carcinomatosis during the initial laparoscopic procedure; one of them went on to develop port-site metastasis.

Pneumoperitoneum and degree of tumor burden are two independent factors for the development of port-site metastases.

8.7 Port-site Recurrence: Laboratory Studies

8.7.1 Aerosolization of Tumor Cells

One theory of the pathogenesis of port-site recurrences is that the constant flow of gas used to create a pneumoperitoneum seeds the port site through the constant exposure to aerosolized tumor cells. Hewett et al., using an in vivo pig model, inserted radiolabeled tumor cells into the peritoneum. As observed by gamma camera, tumor cells traveled throughout the abdominal cavity faster in animals with pneumoperitoneum [46]. In a later complex study, Hewett's group inserted radiolabeled human colon cancer cells into the peritoneal cavity of pigs. Ports were placed and pneumoperitoneum established. After 2 h, the ports were removed, and the port sites were excised and examined [47]. The study examined the effects of two variables, tumor burden and insufflation pressure. Insufflation pressure was 0, 4, 8, or 12 mmHg. With increased tumor burden (more than 2.5×10^6 cells), tumor became detectable at the port sites. In the second portion of the study, as insufflation pressure increased, less tumor was identified at the port sites. The intraoperative manipulation of the tumor using laparoscopic instruments, thought to enhance tumor dispersion, has also been shown to lead to increased rates of port-site recurrences [48]. It appears that

- Aerosolization caused by pneumoperitoneum,
- Aerosolization caused by tumor manipulation, and
- Tumor burden itself are important factors for the development of port-site recurrences. The amount of tumor required to cause port-site recurrences in humans is currently unknown.

8.7.2 Impact of Abdominal Wall Trauma

Other investigators looked at abdominal wall trauma as a factor promoting the development of port-site recurrences. In a scanning electron microscopy study, tumor cells were injected into the abdomen of rats, followed by the placement of ports and 20 min of laparoscopy [49]. The rats were sacrificed on day 0, 3, or 8, and the port sites were examined under an electron microscope. Immediately after laparoscopy on day 0, the peritoneal lining was noted to have been peeled away, subperitoneal tissue was exposed, and inflammatory cells with tumor cells were present in the underlying damaged tissues. On day 3, the peritoneal wound was covered by regenerative and immature mesothelial cells with a scattering of malignant cells. The subperitoneal surfaces and muscular defects were replaced by granulation tissue. On day 8, a small macroscopic tumor nodule, completely covered by a layer of mesothelial cells and consisting of numerous cancer cells, was found to have invaded the damaged muscular layer of the port site. The peritoneum was completely intact in the surrounding areas of damage. Tissue trauma, whether by repeated insertions of a port or devitalization by crushing, appears to provide a medium for tumor adherence, invasion, and growth.

While the aerosolization of tumor cells has been implicated in the formation of port-site recurrences, experimental data is not consistent. In an in vivo rat model using paired animals connected by a plastic tube, the abdominal cavity of one animal was injected with a tumor innoculum and then insufflated with CO_2, with the gas passing from one animal to the next through the conecting tube [50]. These investigators found a limited growth of tumor only in animals that received a large tumor inoculum and concluded that aerosolization of tumor is not of major relevance in the pathogenesis of port-site recurrences.

8.7.3 Type of Wound Closure

The impact of the method of wound closure on the formation of wound site recurrences has also been evaluated in an experimental study. Using a rat model, tumors were grown and then transplanted to an intraabdominal location, in control animals and animals that underwent a 60 min CO_2 pneumoperitoneum [51]. The wounds were closed in three different ways: skin only, skin/fascia, and skin/fascia/peritoneum. There were no differences observed in tumor implantation comparing the pneumoperitoneum and no pneumoperitoneum groups for any of the closure methods. However, the rate of tumor implantation was higher in the skin closure only group vs. closure of all three layers. These data show that while pneumoperitoneum did not affect port-site recurrence rates, the method of wound closure may have an effect.

8.7.4 Port Placement

In an experiment to evaluate the effect of port placement, rabbits were divided into three groups: CO_2 pneumoperitoneum with insertion of nine trocars, insertion of nine trocars alone, or nine abdominal incisions in a control group [52]. The experiment was conducted three days after intraperitoneal inoculation of tumor cells. The frequency of wound implantation was similar in the pneumoperitoneum group and the trocar alone group, and was greater than the control group although it missed statistical significance ($p=.06$). This study suggests that the presence of a trocar may be a factor in the development of port-site recurrences, but that pneumoperitoneum does not appear to be a factor.

8.7.5 Port Composition

Brundell et al. studied the effects of different port compositions, and the removal and replacement of ports to mimic typical laparoscopy [53]. Significantly more tumor cells adhered to metal ports than to plastic ports. The removal and replacement of a port resulted in significantly more tumor deposition in the wound than if the port was left in situ for the duration of the procedure. They concluded that, to minimize risks, the use of plastic ports that are secured to prevent dislodgement is mandatory.

8.7.6 Immunosuppression Theory

Other investigators have put forward an immunosuppression theory of the development of port-site recurrences. Local peritoneal inflammatory changes are clearly demonstrated with laparoscopy; however, there is no consensus as to the significance of these changes.

Table 8.1 Tumor cell dissemination in laparoscopic surgery for cancer: Possible causes

Causes for tumor cell dissemination
Adverse effects of CO_2 gas on malignant cells
• Enhances growth
• Increases cell adhesion to surrounding tissues
Dispersion of cells by insufflated gas
Tumor spillage from manipulation and instrumentation
Tumor spillage at extraction site
Immunosuppressive effect of pneumoperitoneum
Excessive manipulation of the tumor
Stage of tumor

Some of the overall physiologic and immunologic changes that occur are discussed in Sect. 8.2.

Table 8.1 briefly outlines some of the causes that have been suggested for port-site recurrences. The exact clinical significance of these factors remains elusive at this time.

8.8 Port-site Recurrences: Clinical Studies

Once they were alerted to the phenomenon, investigators sought to know the true incidence of port-site recurrences. Although several small, early series indicated that port-site recurrences occurred in up to 21% of patients, before implicating the laparoscopic method itself, the incidence of wound recurrences after laparotomy had to be established [54]. Hughes et al. reviewed data for 1,603 patients with colon carcinoma and found a total recurrence rate of 0.8%. Recurrences consisted of 11 cases in the laparotomy scar and 5 in the stoma or drain site [55]. Reilly et al. reviewed 1,711 laparotomy cases and found a 0.6% recurrence rate [56]. From these large retrospective studies, the wound recurrence rate in open colon resections is estimated to be less than 1%.

Early reports of port-site recurrences after laparoscopic surgery for colorectal carcinoma were discouraging; however, later reports showed such recurrences to be an uncommon phenomenon. Results for a series of 480 patients in the American Society of Colon and Rectal Surgeons laparoscopic registry showed a port-site recurrence rate of 1.1% [57]. In 2001, Zmora and

Table 8.2 Impact of laparoscopy on colo-rectal cancer: Multicenter trials

	Patients (*n*)	Laparoscopic resection *n* (#wound recurrences)	Open resection *n* (#wound recurrences)
COST trial[7]	863	435 [2]	428 [1]
COLOR trial[8]	1,082	536 (pending)	546 (pending)
CLASSIC trial[6]	737	484 (pending)	253 (pending)

Weiss performed a meta-analysis of laparoscopic colorectal resections for carcinoma, including only studies that involved more than 50 patients [58]. This step was taken to eliminate bias in reports from surgeons early in the learning process. Of 1,737 patients, they identified 17 (0.6%) with port-site recurrences. Unfortunately, many of the early studies were not prospective and nonrandomized, and had a short follow-up period. Despite these limitations, the results compare favorably with those of prospective randomized studies. Lacy et al. published the results of a randomized prospective trial involving 219 patients and found only one port-site metastasis in 106 patients after colectomy [59]. Large series have also shown low rates of port-site metastasis after laparoscopic surgery for upper gastrointestinal malignancies. In a prospective study of laparoscopic procedures involving placement of 4,299 ports, 0.79% of port sites developed recurrences at times ranging from 15 days to 17 months after surgery [60]. Wound recurrence for open procedures was reported to be 0.86%. A preponderance of patients with port-site metastases and wound recurrences had an advanced stage of disease at initial presentation, which allowed the authors to conclude that port-site or wound recurrence is a marker of advanced disease. One particular upper gastrointestinal malignancy, gallbladder carcinoma, continues to be associated with a high incidence of port-site recurrences. In an international survey of 117,840 cholecystectomies for presumed benign disease, 409 nonapparent gallbladder cancers were identified, and wound recurrence occurred in 70 (17.1%) of the cases [61].

In larger series, port-site recurrences occurred in association with advanced disease at initial presentation; however, numerous cases have been reported in patients with early disease in a relatively short period of time after surgery. The occurrences in patients with early disease, such as Stage I colon cancer, have been associated with carcinomatosis and adverse outcomes.

When examining the evidence regarding the incidence of port-site recurrences, perhaps the most important clinical data is from three major prospective randomized trials that have recently reported their results. The importance of this data stems, in part, from the fact that these trials were designed because of the initial concern about port-site recurrences and laparoscopic resection of colon cancer. These three trials include the COST trial [7], the COLOR trial [6], and the CLASSIC trial [8]. Data for the CLASSIC and COLOR trials regarding port-site recurrences are pending at this time, but it is important to mention these two well-designed and conducted trials. The port-site recurrence data for the COST trial shows a similar incidence of port-site recurrences, with a $p=.50$. Meta-analyses of port-site recurrence rates have consistently shown rates less than 1% in numerous studies, a rate similar to that seen in open resections of colon cancer [62] (Table 8.2).

Port-site recurrences have been reviewed specifically in cases of urologic surgery [63]. There were nine cases described in clinical and experimental studies that were reviewed by these authors. They identified a number of etiologic factors including natural behavior of the disease, host immune status, local wound factors, factors related to the laparoscopic conduct of the procedure (e.g. aerosolization of tumor cells, type of gas used, insufflation, desufflation, etc.) and technical skills of the surgeon and operating team.

8.9 Port-site Recurrence: Prevention

It is difficult to design scientifically based strategies to prevent that for which we do not know the exact cause. Such is the case with strategies to prevent port-site recurrences. Yet, some authors have tried to make a reasonable best-guess for ways to prevent port-site recurrences. The quick reference guide demonstrates some interventions to minimize these causes. Many of these are in the category of good basic surgical care, and serve as reminders of the importance of basic procedures. The references are included in this table to facilitate further review, and do not constitute a "vote" by the authors on best practices. Most authors seem to concur that surgical technique is the greatest factor contributing to this phenomenon.

After recognizing the problem of port-site recurrences, several investigators attempted to mitigate factors leading to the development of port-site recurrences. A simple procedural change would be to use plastic bags to remove specimens; however, it has already been shown that aerosolized cells adhere to ports and port sites. To eliminate the effects of pneumoperitoneum, gasless laparoscopy has been recommended, but port-site recurrences have been reported even under these conditions. The studies that investigated changing the insufflation gas to helium or some other agent often generated conflicting results. Wu et al. excised the wound during surgery, but this did not completely eliminate port-site recurrences [64]. Moreover, excising port sites enlarges the wound and thus eliminates one of the purported advantages of laparoscopy – small wounds.

After carefully reviewing nine cases of port-site recurrences in urologic oncology procedures, Tsivian and Sidi recommend the following measures to help prevent port-site recurrences [63]:

- Sufficient technical preparation of the operating team
- Avoidance of laparoscopic surgery when ascites is present
- Trocar fixation
- Avoidance of gas leakage
- Minimal tumor handling
- Cautious consideration of morcellating the tumor
- Use of a protective bag for tumor extraction
- Irrigation of instruments, trocars, and wound sites with povidone-iodine
- Suturing of wounds ≥10 mm

Curet emphasizes the importance of adequate training and experience of the surgeon and the surgical team [1]. Decreased handling of the tumor is an important component of this overall goal. Poor surgical technique is highlighted as a common thread in reviews of port-site recurrences and must be avoided. Extraction sites must be protected to avoid direct tumor implantation. The counsel of senior surgeons is also suggested for those with less experience. This review also highlights the importance of basic oncologic principles such as high ligation of vasculature. Jacobi et al. review a large number of studies designed to evaluate methods of minimizing port-site recurrences [65]. They make no specific recommendations, however, about which approaches should be used in clinical practice. The use of topical agents has undergone some study. In a rat model, investigators used topical oxaloplatin at trocar sites after a CO_2 pneumoperitoneum was established and tumor cells inoculated [66]. They found no significant differences in tumor recurrence at the port site ($p=0.1$) although there was a trend toward lower incidence in the treatment group (37%) compared to the control group (68%). This study demonstrates some of the difficulties with the use of animal models to study this important clinical phenomenon. In a hamster model of pancreatic carcinoma, animals underwent CO_2 pneumoperitoneum after induction of a pancreatic tumor [67]. At the end of the procedure, the abdomen was irrigated with saline, octreotide, or taurolidine. Results showed a decrease in the number of liver metastases in the groups irrigated with taurolidine and octreotide compared to the saline group. There were no port-site recurrences in the taurolidine group, but both the saline group (36.8%) and the octreotide group (37.5%) had evidence of port-site recurrences. Further study of this novel approach is indicated.

A comprehensive review of approaches to prevent port-site recurrences was conducted by Balli and colleagues [68]. They report an 8 year experience with 320 cases of laparoscopic resection of colorectal cancer, with an average of 54 month follow-up. They report no instances of port-site recurrences in their series. This study reviews the possible effects of carbon dioxide pneumoperitoneum, the process of tumor resection, and actions after resection. They state that there are six steps to follow as a routine including:

- Trocar fixation
- Minimal tumor handling
- High vascular ligation
- Intraoperative colonoscopy with intraluminal irrigation using 5% povidone-iodine
- Specimen isolation using a bag
- Irrigation of the peritoneal cavity and trocar sites with a tumoricidal solution (povidone-iodine)

This review presents a reasonable set of recommendations to follow that may help reduce the incidence of port-site metastases.

8.10 Conclusion

Laparoscopy is a procedure that sparked renewed interest in the late 1980s. Because of advances in video imaging, optics, and instrumentation; its application has been profound. Pioneers have now applied this technique to all aspects of oncologic surgery, including diagnosis, staging, therapy, and palliation. There are a large number of effects of laparoscopic surgery on the patient, some of which are especially important in the management of patients with cancer. The wide range of laboratory and clinical studies that have been done to evaluate the range of these effects is testimony to their importance. The widespread application of laparoscopy to the resection of tumors was delayed by literature suggesting that these patients were at high risk of recurrent disease. Due to the conduct of carefully designed trials, we now know that the risk of port-site recurrences is similar to that with open surgery for colon cancer, at less than 1%. The exact mechanism by which port-site recurrences occur is unclear at this time, and represents the outcome of a multifactorial process involving complex interactions of surgical technique, tumor cell biology, host biology, and the pneumoperitoneum. Further study may eventually elucidate the details, but currently, there are a number of reasonable recommendations to help prevent the phenomenon of port-site recurrences that reflect the state of our knowledge at this time.

In 1994, a volume appeared entitled "The Future of Laparoscopy in Oncology," just after the appearance of multiple anecdotal reports of port-site recurrences. In this volume, Wexner emphasized a very important point [69]:

> Assume that a patient could undergo a laparoscopic colectomy as an outpatient, with no pain, no incision, and no ileus and could return to work immediately. In this ideal setting, the question of paramount importance is "Would the patient trade cure and long-term survival for improved short-term recovery?" The answer must be a resounding "no." The surgical community must insist that science prevails and that prospective randomized trials be performed to answer the question of acceptability for the cure of cancer.... We must approach the application of the laparoscope to the cure of (colorectal) malignancy with cautious and critical enthusiasm to fulfill the most important part of the Hippocratic Oath: Primum non nocere – first, do no harm.

These words are as true today as they were in 1994, and should continue to guide future investigations of the effects of pneumoperitoneum and laparoscopy on malignant cells, and more importantly, on our patients.

Quick Reference Guide

Interventions to minimize the formation of Port-site Recurrences

Intervention	Reference
Use helium, nitrogen, or ambient room air	
Avoid sudden loss of pneumoperitoneum and desufflation with trocars in place	[1],[50],[63],[68]
Avoid excessive manipulation of the tumor	[1],[63],[68]
Use protected tumor extraction (plastic bag)	[1],[63],[68]
Irrigate the abdomen with tumoricidal solutions	[1],[68]
Avoid laparoscopic Surgery when ascites is present	[63]
Trocar Fixation	[1],[63],[68],[53]
Povidone iodine irrigation of instruments, trocars and wound sites	[1],[63],[68]

References

1. Curet, M.J.: Port site metastases. Am. J. Surg. **187**(6), 705–712 (2004)
2. Beebe, D.S., McNevin, M.P., Crain, J.M., et al.: Evidence of venous stasis after abdominal insufflation for laparoscopic cholecystectomy. Surg. Gynecol. Obstet. **176**, 443–447 (1993)
3. Jorgensen, J.O., Lalak, N.J., North, L., et al.: Venous stasis during laparoscopic cholecystectomy. Surg. Laparosc. Endosc. Percutan. Tech. **4**, 128–133 (1994)
4. Ido, K., Suzuki, T., Kimura, K., et al.: Lower extremity venous stasis during laparoscopic cholecystectomy as assessed using color Doppler ultrasound. Surg. Endosc. **9**, 310–313 (1995)
5. Mayol, J., Vincent-Hamlin, E., Sarmiento, J.M., et al.: Pulmonary embolism following laparoscopic cholecystectomy: report of two cases and review of the literature. Surg. Endosc. **8**, 214–217 (1994)
6. Guillou, P.J., Quirke, P., Thorpe, H., et al.: Short term endpoints of conventional versus laparoscopic assisted surgery in patients with colorectal cancer (MRC CLASSIC trial): muticentre randomized controlled trial. Lancet **365**, 1718–1726 (2005)

7. COST study group: a comparison of laparoscopically assisted and open colectomy for coloncancer. NEJM **350**, 2050–2059 (2004)
8. COLOR Study Group: Laparoscopic surgery versus open surgery for colon cancer: short-term outcomes of a randomized trial. Lancet Oncol. **6**, 477–484 (2005)
9. Jakub, J., Greene, F.L.: Pneumoperitoneum in cancer. In: Rosenthal, R., Friedman, R.L., Phillips, E.H. (eds.) The pathophysiology of pneumo-peritoneum. Springer, New York (1998)
10. Punnnonen, R., Viinamaki, O.: Vasopressin release during laparoscopy: role of increased intra-abdominal pressure. Lancet **1**, 175–6 (1982)
11. Caprini, J.A., Arcelus, J.I., Laubach, M., et al.: Postoperative hypercoagulability and deep venous thrombosis after laparoscopic cholecystectomy. Surg. Endosc. **9**, 304–309 (1995)
12. Hansborough, J.F., Bender, E.M., Zapata-Sirvent, R., et al.: Altered helper and suppressor lymphocyte populations in surgical patients: a measure of postoperative immunosuppression. Am. J. Surg. **148**, 303 (1984)
13. Vallina, V.L., Velasco, J.M.: The influence of laparoscopy on lymphocyte subpopulations in the surgical patient. Surg. Endosc. **10**, 481 (1996)
14. Christou, N.V., Meakins, J.L., Gordon, J., et al.: The delayed hypersensitivity response and host resistance in surgical patients 20 years later. Ann. Surg. **222**, 534 (1995)
15. Allendorf, J.D., Bessler, M., Whelan, R.L., et al.: Better preservation of immune function after laparoscopic assisted vs open bowel resection in a murine model. Dis. Colon Rectum **39**, 67 (1996)
16. Ng, C.S.H., Whelan, R.L., lacy, A.M., Yim, A.P.C.: Is minimal access surgery for cancer associated with immunologic benefits? World J. Surg. **29**, 975–981 (2005)
17. Gupta, A., Watson, D.I.: Effect of laparoscopy on immune function. Br. J. Surg. **88**(10), 1296–1306 (2001)
18. Schob, O.M., Allen, D.C., Benzel, E.: A comparison of the pathophysiologic effects of carbon dioxide, nitrous oxide, and helium pneumoperitoneum on intracranial pressure. Am. J. Surg. **172**, 248 (1996)
19. Jackman, S.V., Weingart, J.D., Kinsman, S.L., et al.: Laparoscopic surgery in patients with ventriculoperitoneal shunts: safety and monitoring. J. Urol. **164**, 1352 (2000)
20. Harris, S.N., Ballantyne, G.H., Luther, M.A., et al.: Alterations of cardiovascular performance during laparoscopic colectomy: a combined hemodynamic and echocardiographic analysis. Anesth. Analg. **83**, 482 (1996)
21. Giebler, R.M., Kabatnik, M., Stegan, B.H., et al.: Retroperitoneal and intraperitoneal CO_2 insufflation have markedly different cardiovascular effects. J. Surg. Res. **68**, 153 (1997)
22. Greif, W.M., Forse, A.: Cardiopulmonary effects of the laparoscopic pneumoperitoneum in a porcine model of ARDS. Am. J. Surg. **177**, 216 (1999)
23. West, M.A., Hackam, D.J., Baker, J., et al.: Mechanism of decreased in vitro murine macrophage cytokine release after exposure to carbon dioxide. Ann. Surg. **226**, 179 (1997)
24. Kopernik, G., Avinoach, E., Grossman, Y., et al.: The effect of a high partial pressure of carbon dioxide environment on metabolism and immune functions of human peritoneal cells – relevance to carbon dioxide pneumoperitoneum. Am. J. Obstet. Gynecol. **179**, 1503 (1998)
25. Wu, F., Sietses, C., Blomberg, B., et al.: Systemic and peritoneal inflammatory response after laparoscopic or conventional colon resection in cancer patients. Dis. Colon Rectum **46**, 147 (2003)
26. Gutt, N.C., Kim, Z.G., Hollander, D., et al.: CO_2 environment influences the growth of cultured human cancer cells dependent on insufflation pressure. Surg. Endosc. **15**, 314 (2001)
27. Basson, M.D., Yu, C.F., Herden-Kirchoff, O., et al.: Effects of increased ambient pressure on colon cancer cell adhesion. J. Cell. Biochem. **78**, 47 (2000)
28. Volz, J., Koster, S., Spacek, Z., et al.: The influence of pneumoperitoneum used in laparoscopic surgery on an intraabdominal tumor growth. Cancer **86**, 770 (1999)
29. Paraskeva, P.A., Ridgway, P.F., Jones, T., Smith, A., Peck, D.H., Darzi, A.W.: Laparoscopic environmental changes during surgery enhance the invasive potential of tumours. Tumour Biol. **26**(2), 94–102 (2005)
30. Ziprin, P., Ridgway, P.F., Peck, D.H., Darzi, A.W.: Laparoscopic enhancement of tumour cell binding to the peritoneum is inhibited by anti-intercellular adhesion molecule-1 monoclonal antibody. Surg. Endosc. **17**(11), 1812–1817 (2003)
31. Hofstetter, W., Ortega, A., Chiang, M., Brown, B., Paik, P., Youn, P., Beart, R.W.: Abdominal insufflation does not cause hematogenous spread of colon cancer. J. Laparoendosc. Adv. Surg. Tech. A **10**(1), 1–4 (2000)
32. Witich, P., Steyerber, E.W., Simons, S.H., et al.: Intraperitoneal tumor growth is influenced by pressure of carbon dioxide pneumoperitoneum. Surg. Endosc. **14**, 817 (2000)
33. Halpin, V.J., Underwood, R.A., Ye, D., Cooper, D.H., Wright, M., Hickerson, S.M., Connett, W.C., Connett, J.M., Fleshman, J.W.: Pneumoperitoneum does not influence trocar site implantation during tumor manipulation in a solid tumor model. Surg. Endosc. **19**(12), 1636–1640 (2005)
34. Ishida, H., Murata, N., Yamada, H., Nakada, H., Takeuchi, I., Shimomura, K., Fujioka, M., Idezuki, Y.: Pneumoperitoneum with carbon dioxide enhances liver metastases of cancer cells implanted into the portal vein in rabbits. Surg. Endosc. **14**(3), 239–242 (2000)
35. Izumi, K., Ishikawa, K., Tojigamori, M., Matsui, Y., Shiraishi, N., Kitano, S.: Liver metastasis and ICAM-1 mRNA expression in the liver after carbon dioxide pneumoperitoneum in a murine model. Surg. Endosc. **19**(8), 1049–1054 (2005). Epub 2005 May 12
36. Takeuchi, H., Inomata, M., Fujii, K., Ishibashi, S., Shiraishi, N., Kitano, S.: Increased peritoneal dissemination after laparotomy versus pneumoperitoneum in a mouse cecal cancer model. Surg. Endosc. **18**(12), 1795–1799 (2004). Epub 2004 Oct 26
37. Hirabayashi, Y., Yamaguchi, K., Shiraishi, N., Adachi, Y., Saiki, I., Kitano, S.: Port-site metastasis after CO_2 pneumoperitoneum: role of adhesion molecules and prevention with antiadhesion molecules. Surg. Endosc. **18**(7), 1113–1117 (2004)
38. Carter, J.J., Feingold, D.L., Kirman, I., Oh, A., Wildbrett, P., Asi, Z., Fowler, R., Huang, E., Whelan, R.L.: Laparoscopic-assisted cecectomy is associated with decreased formation of postoperative pulmonary metastases compared with open cecectomy in a murine model. Surgery **134**(3), 432–436 (2003)

39. Lecuru, F., Agostini, A., Camatte, S., et al.: Impact of pneumoperitoneum on tumor growth. Surg. Endosc. **16**, 1170 (2002)
40. Tan, B.J.: Is carbon dioxide insufflation safe for laparoscopic surgery? A model to assess the effects of carbon dioxide on transitional-cell carcinoma growth, apoptosis, and necrosis. J. Endourol. **20**(11), 965–969 (2006)
41. Schmeding, M., Schwalbach, P., Reinshagen, S., Autschbach, F., Benner, A., Kuntz, C.: Helium pneumoperitoneum reduces tumor recurrence after curative laparoscopic liver resection in rats in a tumor-bearing small animal model. Surg. Endosc. **17**(6), 951–959 (2003)
42. Ishida, H., Hashimoto, D., Takeuchi, I., Yokoyama, M., Okita, T., Hoshino, T.: Liver metastases are less established after gasless laparoscopy than after carbon dioxide pneumoperitoneum and laparotomy in a mouse model. Surg. Endosc. **16**(1), 193–196 (2002)
43. Jingli, C., Rong, C., Rubai, X.: Influence of colorectal laparoscopic surgery on dissemination and seeding of tumor cells. Surg. Endosc. **20**(11), 1759–1761 (2006)
44. Cavina, E., Goletti, O., Molea, N., et al.: Trocar site tumor recurrences: may pneumoperitoneum be responsible? Surg. Endosc. **12**, 1294 (1998)
45. Ikramuddin, S., Lucas, J., Ellison, C., et al.: Detection of aerosolized cells during carbon dioxide laparoscopy. J. Gastrointest. Surg. **2**, 580 (1998)
46. Hewett, P.J., Texler, M.L., Anderson, D., et al.: In vivo real time analysis of intraperitoneal radiolabeled tumor cell movement during laparoscopy. Dis. Colon Rectum **42**, 868 (1999)
47. Brundell, S.M., Tucker, K., Brown, B., et al.: Variables in the spread of tumor cells to trocars and port sites during operative laparoscopy. Surg. Endosc. **16**, 1413 (2002)
48. Mathew, G., Watson, D.I., Rofe, A.M., et al.: Wound metastases following laparoscopic and open surgery for abdominal cancer. Br. J. Surg. **83**, 1087 (1996)
49. Hirabayashi, Y., Yamaguchi, K., Shiraishi, N., et al.: Development of port site metastasis after pneumoperitoneum: a scanning electron microscopy study. Surg. Endosc. **16**, 864 (2002)
50. Wittich, Ph, Marquet, R.L., Kazemeier, G., Bonjer, H.J.: Port site metastases after CO_2 laparoscopy: is aerosolization of tumor cells a pivotal factor? Surg. Endosc. **14**, 189–192 (2000)
51. Burns, J.M., Matthews, B.D., Pollinger, H.S., Mostafa, G., Joels, C.S., Austin, C.E., Kercher, K.W., Norton, H.J., Heniford, B.T.: Effect of carbon dioxide pneumoperitoneum and wound closure technique on port site tumor implantation in a rat model. Surg. Endosc. **19**(3), 441–447 (2005)
52. Ishida, H., Murata, N., Yamada, H., et al.: Influence of trocar placement and CO_2 pneumoperitoneum on port site metastasis following laparoscopic tumor surgery. Surg. Endosc. **14**, 193–197 (2000)
53. Brundell, S., Tsopelas, C., Chatterton, B., et al.: Effect of port composition on tumor cell adherence. Dis. Colon Rectum **46**, 637 (2003)
54. Berends, F.J., Kazemier, G., Bonjer, H.J., et al.: Subcutaneous metastases after laparoscopic colectomy. Lancet **344**, 58 (1994)
55. Hughes, E.S., McDermontt, F.T., Poligless, A.L., et al.: Tumor recurrence in the abdominal wall scar tissue after large bowel cancer surgery. Dis. Colon Rectum **26**, 571 (1983)
56. Reilly, W.T., Nelson, H., Schroeder, G., et al.: Wound recurrence following conventional treatment of colorectal cancer. A rare but perhaps underestimated problem. Dis. Colon Rectum **39**, 200 (1996)
57. Vukasin, P., Ortega, A.E., Greene, F.L., et al.: Wound recurrence following laparoscopic colon cancer resection: results of the American society of colon and rectal surgeons laparoscopic registry. Dis. Colon Rectum **39**, S20 (1996)
58. Zmora, O., Weiss, E.: Trocar site recurrence in laparoscopic surgery for colorectal cancer, myth or real concern? Surg. Oncol. Clin. N. Am. **10**, 625 (2001)
59. Lacy, A.M., Garcia-Valdecasas, J.C., Delgado, S., et al.: Laparoscopy assisted colectomy versus open colectomy for treatment of non-metastatic colon cancer: a randomised trial. Lancet **359**, 2224 (2002)
60. Shoup, M., Brennan, M.F., Karpeh, M.S., et al.: Port site metastasis after diagnostic laparoscopy for upper gastrointestinal tract malignancies: an uncommon entity. Ann. Surg. Oncol. **9**, 632 (2002)
61. Paolucci, V., Schaeff, B., Schneider, M., et al.: Tumor seeding following laparoscopy: international survey. World J. Surg. **23**, 989 (1999)
62. Cera, S.M., Wexner, S.D.: Minimally invasive treatment of colon cancer. Cancer J. **11**, 26–35 (2005)
63. Tsivian, A., Sidi, A.A.: Port site metastases in urological laparoscopic surgery. J. Urol. **169**, 1213–1218 (2003)
64. Wu, J.S., Guo, L.W., Ruiz, M.B., et al.: Excision of trocar sites reduces tumor implantation in an animal model. Dis. Colon Rectum **41**, 1107 (1998)
65. Jacobi, C.A., Bonjer, H.J., Puttick, M.I., et al.: Oncologic implications of laparoscopic and open surgery. Surg. Endosc. **16**, 441–445 (2002)
66. Tai, Y.S., Abente, F.C., Assalia, A., Ueda, K., Gagner, M.: Topical treatment with oxaliplatin for the prevention of port-site metastases in laparoscopic surgery for colorectal cancer. JSLS **10**(2), 160–165 (2006)
67. Wenger, F.A., Kilian, M., Braumann, C., et al.: Effects of taurolidine and octreotide on port site and liver metastases after laparoscopy in an animal model of pancreatic cancer. Clin. Exp. Metastasis **19**, 169–173 (2002)
68. Balli, J.E., Franklin, M.E., Almeida, J.A., et al.: How to prevent port-site metastases in laparoscopic colorectal surgery. Surg. Endosc. **14**, 1034–1036 (2000)
69. Wexner, S., Cohen, C.: Laparoscopic colectomy for malignancy: advantages and limitations. In: Wexner, S.D. (ed.) The future of laparoscopy in oncology. Surg. Oncol. Clin. N. Am. **3**, 637–643 (1994)

9 Laparoscopy in the Elderly

Michael Ujiki and Nathaniel Soper

9.1 Introduction

The evolution and dissemination of laparoscopy has occurred at a good time. The population is aging and current estimates are that by the year 2050, 31% of the population will be over 65 years of age [1]. The aging population will challenge the healthcare industry in many ways. It is predicted that healthcare expenditures will triple and Medicare expenses will account for almost 10% of the gross domestic product [2]. For surgeons, elderly patients pose a challenge because age is an independent predictor of postoperative complications and length of stay [3]. Compared to younger patients, the elderly have a higher prevalence of chronic diseases, pulmonary and cardiovascular comorbidities, and less reserve, and therefore do not tolerate the stress of surgery and surgical complications as well. In addition, postoperative pain together with limited mobility puts elderly patients at higher risk for certain common postsurgical complications, such as deep venous thrombosis and pneumonia (Table 9.1).

Fortunately, technological developments, better training, and an improved understanding of the physiological effects of laparoscopy have led to a wider breadth of operations that can be performed with minimal access techniques. Multiple studies have demonstrated that minimally invasive techniques result in reduced postoperative pain and therefore a lesser need for narcotic pain medications, earlier ambulation, and shorter periods of ileus. Given the proven benefits of minimally invasive surgery, its application among the growing group of elderly patients may diminish the potential stress put on the healthcare industry. For the oncologic surgeon, this is even more relevant since cancer is primarily a disease of the elderly [4].

9.2 Epidemiology of Aging and Cancer

Recent demographic studies have shown that the proportion of elderly patients in industrialized countries continues to increase due to a longer average life span and progressive reduction in birth rates [5]. Between 1960 and 1994, the population of those older than 85 years grew 274% [6]. By 2050, the average life expectancy is predicted to be 86.4 years for males and 92.3 years for females [1]. It is estimated that once 65, the mean life expectancy is an additional 17 years, and once 85, an additional 6 years [7]. Projections are that by 2050 the US population will be over 416 million, with 4 million over 100 years of age, 30 million over 85 years of age, and nearly 97 million over 65 years of age [1].

The probability of developing a malignancy during one's lifetime is 38% for females and 45% for males [8]. At least 50% of malignancies are diagnosed in patients older than 65 years [9]. Estimates are that by 2050 there will be four times the number of cancer patients older than 85 years [10]. Though death due to cardiac-related disease has decreased, death related to cancer has increased over 5% between 1973 and 1999, and some

M. Ujiki
Pritzker School of Medicine, University of Chicago,
NorthShore University HealthSystem, 2650 Ridge Ave,
Evanston, IL 60201, USA
e-mail: mujiki@northshore.org

N. Soper (✉)
Departement of Surgery, Northwestern University Feinberg
School of Medicine, 251 E. Huron St, Galter 3-150, Chicago,
IL 60611, USA
e-mail: nsoper@nmh.org

Table 9.1 US population projections for 2050

Age group	Projected population
Total us population	416,000,000
>65 years	97,000,000
>85 years	30,000,000
>100 years	4,000,000

predict that cancer will soon become the leading cause of death [11]. Cancer is a disease of the elderly and as the elderly population expands, surgeons will be faced with caring for more and more elderly patients with cancer.

9.3 Pathophysiological Changes in the Elderly

Surgeons, including those trained in minimal access techniques, must have a significant amount of insight into the physiological changes accompanied with age in order to provide state-of-the-art care. The aging process in general is associated with a gradual loss of reserve capacity which manifests itself in periods of stress, such as with surgery, chemotherapy, or radiation [12]. This gradual diminution in reserve and functional capacity is exacerbated by the physiologic effects on the body caused by malignancy and has a direct impact on the choice of cancer therapy. In addition, it is unusual for a cancer patient older than 65 years of age to present without comorbidities, the most common of which include hypertension, diabetes, atherosclerosis, chronic obstructive pulmonary disease, and osteoarthritis [13–15].

9.3.1 Cardiovascular

The leading cause of postoperative mortality in surgical patients older than 80 years is myocardial infarction [16]. Over half of all postoperative morbidity and mortality is related to the cardiovascular system [17]. One reason for this is a higher prevalence of cardiovascular disease in the elderly. Intimal hyperplasia of the coronary arteries is strongly associated with age [18, 19]. Age is also accompanied by effects on the conduction system characterized by fibrosis, calcifications, and a decrease in the number of sino-atrial pacemaker cells [20].

A reduced threshold for calcium overload lowers the threshold for arrhythmias, a not uncommon complication after surgery, particularly for thoracic disease [21]. Beta-adrenergic responsiveness decreases, limiting the maximum achievable heart rate needed during periods of stress [22]. Progressive loss of myocytes and reciprocal increase in myocyte volume occurs in both ventricles leading to increased wall thickness, stiffness, and decreased compliance [23]. Older patients, even with normal systolic function preoperatively, progressively lose the ability to increase cardiac output and are more dependent on preload. However, cardiac reserve is reduced and decreased contractility impairs the response to increased afterload, which ultimately results in an increased risk of congestive heart failure [24, 25].

9.3.2 Pulmonary

The elderly exhibit decreased respiratory reserve due to changes that affect pulmonary mechanics, respiratory musculature, gas exchange, and pulmonary vasculature. Decreased diaphragmatic strength, calcification of intercostal cartilage, and atrophy of the intercostal muscles lead to increased chest wall rigidity, decreased elastic recoil, and decreased respiratory muscle strength [26–29]. This manifests itself through decreased forced expiratory volume and vital capacity, as well as an increase in functional residual volume. The surface area available for gas exchange decreases 15% by age 70 [30]. This is not helped by the fact that the alveolar basement membrane thickens with age leading to decreased diffusion capabilities [31]. The result of these changes is a ventilation–perfusion mismatch and decrease in responsiveness to changes in blood gas levels [32]. Impaired airway protective reflexes place elderly patients at increased risk for aspiration in an already functionally compromised patient. Lastly, impaired ciliary function, coupled with the above poor mechanics, leaves the elderly with an increased risk of atelectasis and postoperative pulmonary infections.

9.3.3 Renal

Cortical tissue loss begins after age 50, and by age 70 more than half of the original nephron complements may be lost [33, 34]. The elderly have a blunted ability to reabsorb and secrete solutes owing in part to tubular senescence [35, 36]. They are left susceptible to electrolyte and acid–base disorders for which younger patients are better able to compensate. Glomerular capillaries are lost with age which results in a 1 mL/min/year decrease in glomerular filtration after age 40 [37, 38]. The elderly are therefore left with a low filtration reserve and decreased ability to concentrate urine, and are more prone to ischemic or nephrotoxic insults with subsequent renal failure. Lastly, the juxtaglomerular apparatus produces less renin with age resulting in a blunted response to aldosterone [39].

9.3.4 Gastrointestinal

Intestinal motility decreases with age due to prolongation of the migrating motor complex, slower propagation velocity, and a prolonged postprandial state [40]. Even in the most proximal portions of the gastrointestinal tract, improper motility based on a failure to coordinate reflexes can lead to dysphagia and aspiration. In terms of absorptive capacity, a decrease in the height of small bowel villi results in a decrease in surface area available for absorption after age 60 [41]. The potential for malnutrition is therefore incredibly high for an elderly patient in a hypermetabolic state due to cancer and recent surgery. In addition, the size of the liver steadily decreases after age 50 and may fail to increase its synthetic and metabolic function under hypermetabolic states [42, 43].

9.3.5 Endocrine

In women, aging is associated with decreased estrogen resulting in loss of its cardio-protective effect [44]. In men, testosterone levels have been shown to decrease with age leading to anemia, muscle atrophy, and osteoporosis [44]. An age-related decrease in thyroid function has been seen [45]. The adrenal gland has been found to have a decreased ability to respond to stress leading to less capacity to regulate pulse, blood pressure, pH, and oxygen [44]. Arguably the most important endocrine effect in the surgical patient, however, is the progressive impairment of glucose tolerance [46].

Some have shown a 45% rate of impaired glucose tolerance in those over 80 compared to those younger than 30 years [47]. This difference appears to be due to enhanced insulin resistance rather than decreased insulin secretion [48].

9.3.6 Immunological

Immune function has an age-related decline characterized by impairment of T-cell-mediated immunity and increased susceptibility to infections [49]. Response to IL-2 and natural killer cell activity has also been found to be impaired, which is a significant issue in elderly patients with a malignancy [50]. Surgical trauma has been found to lead to alterations in immune function as well, but some have found minimal access surgery to cause less pronounced perturbations in immune function [51].

9.3.7 Musculoskeletal

Changes in body fat distribution and muscle mass may affect response to drug therapy in general and to anesthetic drugs in particular [52]. As total body water is reduced there is a reduction in the volume of distribution of water-soluble drugs. When coupled with decreased renal clearance, higher levels of water-soluble non-depolarizing muscle relaxants can occur resulting in prolonged effects. Similarly, with age, total body fat is increased and the distribution of lipid-soluble drugs is also increased resulting in prolonged effects [53].

9.3.8 Neurological

There is some evidence that elderly patients with decreased cognitive ability have worse surgical outcomes [54]. Cortical atrophy has been repeatedly demonstrated to progress with age and is associated with dementia and a lower threshold for postoperative delirium [55–57]. It follows then that the decreased requirement for narcotic use in the postoperative period, as seen after laparoscopy, should benefit this group of

Table 9.2 Physiologic changes in the elderly

	Physiologic changes with age
Cardiovascular	↑Coronary intimal hyperplasia, ↑fibrosis of pacemaker system, ↓threshold for arrhythmia, ↓beta adrenergic responsiveness, ↓ventricular wall compliance, ↑risk of CHF
Pulmonary	↓Forced expiratory volume, ↓vital capacity, ↑functional residual volume, ↓surface area for gas exchange, ↓airway protection reflexes
Renal	↑Cortical tissue loss, ↓ability to resorb/secrete, ↓number of glomerular capillaries, ↑sensitivity to ischemic or nephrotoxic insults
Gastrointestinal	↓Intestinal motility, ↓absorptive capacity
Endocrine	↓Estrogen/testosterone, ↓thyroid function, ↓adrenal responsiveness, ↓glucose tolerance
Immunologic	↓T-cell-mediated immunity, ↓response to IL-2
Musculoskeletal	↓Total body water, ↑total body fat
Neurologic	↑Cortical atrophy, ↓threshold for delirium, ↓cerebral circulation

patients. Moreover, the elderly may not tolerate the potential side effects of narcotic medications, such as hypoxia, hypercapnia, or hypotension, as well as their younger counterparts. Older patients are also more susceptible to hypothermia due to a less than vigorous vasoconstrictive response to cold stimuli [58]. Lastly, cerebral circulation and oxygen consumption decline with age resulting in an increased risk of cerebrovascular accidents [59–61] (Table 9.2)

9.4 Minimally Invasive Management of Selected Cancers in the Elderly

There has been concern that the onco-geriatric population does not receive potentially curative treatment, even when a malignancy is diagnosed in the early stages [11, 62]. It has been shown, however, that older patients sustain similar benefits as younger patients when the same treatment modalities are used [63, 64]. Even elderly patients with incurable cancers live longer and enjoy better quality of life if surgery is instituted rather than supportive care alone [65–67]. The hesitancy among primary care physicians and surgeons to recommend surgery to elderly patients is based upon fears that those patients will suffer complications related to the surgery as well as deterioration in quality of life. Fortunately, minimally invasive techniques show promise in lowering morbidity, mortality, and concerns over quality of life postoperatively. Trepidation about the appropriateness of minimally invasive techniques for potentially curable malignancies has stimulated a plethora of recent studies to address this question.

9.4.1 Lung Cancer

In the Western world, lung cancer is the leading cause of cancer-related deaths in people older than 65 years [68]. Video-assisted thoracic surgery (VATS) has resulted in decreased recovery time and fewer complications in the elderly without compromising the oncologic principles of adequate resection [69–71]. A matched case-control study comparing VATS and thoracotomy in patients over 70 years with early-stage cancer revealed fewer and overall reduced severity of complications, along with a shorter stay in those undergoing the minimally invasive approach [72]. Even in patients over 80 years, VATS has shown acceptable morbidity, mortality, and survival rates [73, 74].

9.4.2 Esophageal Cancer

Esophageal cancer is a disease of the elderly and its incidence in patients older than 70 years has steadily been increasing [75]. It has already been shown that age should not be a limiting factor in using an aggressive surgical approach for esophageal cancer since morbidity, mortality, and survival appear similar across all age groups [75–77]. It follows then that a minimally invasive approach should benefit the elderly even more. Luketich and colleagues recently summarized their experience with minimally invasive esophagectomy and found no mortalities, acceptable morbidity, and reduced length of stay in patients older than 75 years with esophageal cancer [78].

Table 9.3 Advantages of minimally invasive surgery

Minimally invasive approach	Advantages
Video-assisted thoracic surgery (VATS)	Complication severity, hospital stay
Minimally invasive esophagectomy	Length of stay
Minimally invasive gastrectomy	Complication severity, hospital stay
Minimally invasive colectomy	Ileus, hospital stay, complication rate

9.4.3 Gastric Cancer

Cancer of the stomach is an uncommon malignancy of the young and peaks in incidence around age 70 [79]. Surgery is the treatment modality of choice regardless of age with similar outcomes between young and old [80]. Singh and colleagues reported their gastrectomy experience in patients older than 75 and found that the minimally invasive technique offered equivalent oncologic integrity in the short term but with superior safety and economy when compared to the open approach [81]. Similarly, a group from Japan found that even though their cohort of elderly patients presented with significantly more comorbidities, the overall 5-year survival rates were not significantly different between a matched younger cohort when undergoing laparoscopic-assisted gastrectomy [82].

9.4.4 Colorectal Cancer

There is probably no study more elegantly designed to address the appropriateness of laparoscopy in patients with malignant disease than the Clinical Outcomes of Surgical Therapy (COST) trial that evaluated laparoscopic versus open colectomy [83]. Though it does not specifically address elderly patients, it is one of the only prospective randomized studies with sufficient power to prove that laparoscopic colectomy is not inferior to open colectomy for the surgical treatment of colon cancer.

Other studies evaluating laparoscopic colectomy in elderly patients have generally shown an earlier resumption of diet, shorter length of stay, and fewer complications [84, 85]. Law's group presented 65 versus 89 patients over 70 who underwent laparoscopic versus open colectomy, and though the cohorts were equal in terms of premorbid conditions, the laparoscopic group experienced less postoperative morbidity, an earlier return of bowel function, and earlier discharge [85]. Person and colleagues compared laparoscopic and open colectomies in elderly and young patients and found that the elderly who undergo laparoscopy have significantly shorter length of stay and fewer complications compared to the elderly who undergo open colectomy, and suggested that laparoscopy should be considered in all patients regardless of age [86] (Table 9.3).

9.5 Surgical Approach to the Aging Patient

9.5.1 Preoperative Management

9.5.1.1 Preoperative Assessment of Cancer in the Elderly (PACE)

The minimally invasive oncologic surgeon must first learn to provide adequate cancer care to each patient regardless of age. He or she must diligently approach each elderly patient with an individualized plan of care that begins with assessing surgical risk. Multiple tools have been developed to quantify the degree of sickness and overall patient health, but one of the more promising tools is the Preoperative Assessment of Cancer in the Elderly (PACE), which is aimed specifically at onco-geriatric surgical candidates and has already proven feasible and well-accepted by patients [87, 88]. PACE uses already validated instruments including the Mini-Mental State exam, activities of daily living, American Society of Anesthesiologists physical status, and Eastern Cooperative Oncology Group Performance Status. Validation trials are still under way, but the bottom line is that risk must be individualized and then discussed in detail with the patient.

9.5.1.2 Postoperative Support System

The minimally invasive oncologic surgeon must next assess the support system available postoperatively for the patient. Not only are the elderly more likely to have difficulty with independent daily activities, but the absence of spouses or other family members is commonplace. One could theorize that without proper support systems, outcomes would be affected. Anticipation of postoperative needs, such as rehabilitation, skilled nursing, and home caregivers, allows the elderly patient to have more time and better means to make arrangements in the preoperative setting.

9.5.1.3 Medical Needs

Many postoperative medical needs are best met in the preoperative setting. For example, many ostomy nurses can offer better education and recommendations to both the patient and the surgeon when involved prior to the creation of the stoma. Patients undergoing pancreatic resections that may result in diabetes are often better prepared when an endocrinology consultation is obtained in the preoperative period. Lastly, the specialty of geriatrics has expanded significantly in order to meet the needs of the growing elderly population. A preoperative consultation with a geriatrician would likely improve care in the postoperative setting in many cases.

9.5.1.4 Adjuvant/Neo-adjuvant Therapy and Its Toxicity

Any surgeon who deals with oncology must be familiar with the toxicity profiles of other adjuvant modalities. For example, the ability to provide a hepatic resection through minimal access techniques for a patient with colorectal metastases who has undergone neo-adjuvant therapy does not protect the patient from complications relating to the chemotherapeutic effects on the remaining liver.

9.5.1.5 Preexisting Medical Conditions

It is imperative that the elderly oncologic patient's condition be optimized preoperatively. Obtaining a nutrition consult can be critical in improving the malnourished state of onco-geriatric patients and result in a better surgical outcome. Assessment of immunization status and education on smoking cessation can have a positive impact. Intravascular fluid depletion in surgical patients, particularly elderly ones, is common in the perioperative period. It is therefore important that close attention be paid to the hydration status of the elderly patient preoperatively, intraoperatively, and postoperatively. Obtaining tests related to comorbidities, such as pulmonary and cardiac function, not only assesses risk but also aids in understanding which therapies can optimize the existing conditions going into major surgery.

9.5.2 Intraoperative Management

Prior to inducing general anesthesia, it is essential to remember that elderly patients, in general, have decreased reserves. Thus, prevention of adverse events such as aspiration, dehydration, and fluid overload are important in obtaining good outcomes. Early after the introduction of laparoscopy, concerns over the physiologic effects of pneumoperitoneum led some to feel that age was a contraindication to laparoscopic surgery. Fortunately, we now have enough experience and more results from well-designed studies to understand the physiologic changes caused by pneumoperitoneum and the means to prevent its direct complications. Pulmonary effects of pneumoperitoneum include a decrease in functional residual capacity and lung compliance, increase in peak airway pressure, hypercapnia, and acidemia. Most patients are not significantly adversely affected; however, because elderly patients present with a higher incidence of pulmonary comorbidities and decreased pulmonary reserve, the aged patient may not tolerate these effects as well as younger individuals. Adjustments in minute ventilation and peak end expiratory pressure can usually obviate these effects.

Pneumoperitoneum influences preload, afterload, and cardiac contractility. In general, venous return is decreased due to the mechanical effects of a higher intra-abdominal pressure and this can lead to a state similar to congestive heart failure. It is easy to mistake oliguria in these circumstances as being caused by dehydration, and then overload the patient with fluid.

9.5.3 Postoperative Management

It is important that the minimally invasive oncologic surgeon does not treat patients in the same way as one would after a major open operation. Aggressive fluid resuscitation is necessary after major open abdominal surgery, but third space fluid will be less after laparoscopy due to less insensible loss and a decreased stress response. The deleterious effects of raising afterload in the elderly patient have already been discussed. Conversely, the elderly have a low renal filtration reserve and are therefore more sensitive to ischemic or nephrotoxic insults if fluid balance is not maintained. Be wary of potentially nephrotoxic medications and resume baseline medications as soon as possible in order to restore baseline homeostasis. Encouraging pulmonary toilet is crucial in the elderly due to already weakened intercostal muscles and a weakened diaphragm. Fortunately, abdominal muscles are better able to compensate for this effect after laparoscopy than following laparotomy. As after any major surgery, electrolyte imbalances are common in the elderly and must be watched closely and corrected if present to avoid complications such as arrhythmias, ileus, and respiratory failure. Tight glucose control may lead to better outcomes and the elderly generally have worse glucose tolerance. Increase mobility as soon as possible, obtaining physical and occupational therapy consults as necessary. The advantages of minimally invasive surgery in terms of earlier mobilization cannot be stressed enough.

9.5.3.1 Role of Adjuvant Therapy

Most malignancies are treated with a combination of therapeutic modalities. Elderly patients benefit from adjuvant therapy as much as the young and it is crucial that oncologic surgeons offer these modalities remembering that age alone is not a risk factor for complications from chemotherapy and radiation. The physiologic changes associated with aging can be compensated for without affecting efficacy while still decreasing the toxicity. Reduced doses or less toxic regimens may be required, and hemopoietic growth factors may be useful. Another advantage of minimally invasive techniques is that fewer complications and quicker recovery mean a higher percentage of patients can be offered adjuvant therapies in a timely fashion.

Lastly, it is important that surgeons educate referring physicians as to their outcomes in order to alleviate the fear of referring elderly patients for potentially curative surgery [89]. Many primary physicians were not trained in the era of minimal access surgery and may not be as aware of the potential benefits afforded the elderly patient.

9.6 Future Trends

As the validation trials for objective stratification of predicted postoperative morbidity and mortality come to a close, it will improve the number of onco-geriatric patients that can successfully undergo potentially curative surgery. The expansion of minimal access techniques to all solid organ cancers has already begun. Currently there are no published trials that focus on minimally invasive hepato-biliary surgery in the elderly, but these are certain to come in the near future and may even include encouraging results from laparoscopically applied radiofrequency ablation. Endoscopic techniques for early esophageal cancers such as endoscopic mucosal resection or radiofrequency ablation may prove to be as effective as resection with much less morbidity. Transanal endoscopic microsurgery has already gained momentum in treating early cancers and long-term results may show similar oncologic benefit with much less morbidity than perineal or low anterior resections. No one can ignore the new popularity of natural orifice techniques and their application to malignant conditions may be a possibility in the future. In terms of adjuvant therapies, more trials that include elderly patients will likely take place that will give oncologists a better idea of how to tailor therapies to the geriatric population. Finally, research will continue to give us answers as to the pathophysiology of malignancies to allow earlier treatment with less morbid procedures.

Quick Reference Guide

1. Understand the physiology of aging
2. Assess postoperative risk preoperatively in each individual patient
3. Assess the availability of postoperative support systems preoperatively
4. Obtain preoperative tests to assess baseline functions of each individual patient
5. Based on the above, optimize the patient's status preoperatively
   - Nutrition
   - Cardiopulmonary
   - Immunizations
6. Understand the physiologic effects of pneumoperitoneum and its impact on the elderly
7. Manage perioperative fluid status appropriately
8. Tailor pharmaceuticals to the elderly patient
9. Refer for adjuvant therapy, remembering that the elderly will have similar benefits compared to young patients
10. Educate primary care physicians about surgical outcomes

References

1. Day, J.C.: Population projections of United States, age, sex, race, and Hispanic origin: 1995–2050. In: Series P25-1130 US Government printing office, Washington, DC (1996)
2. Lee, R., Miller, T.: An approach to forecasting health expenditures, with application to the US medicare system. Health Serv. Res. **37**, 1365–1386 (2002)
3. Polanczyk, C.A., Marcantonlo, E., Goldman, L., et al.: Impact of age on perioperative complications and length of stay in patients undergoing noncardiac surgery. Ann. Intern. Med. **134**, 637–643 (2001)
4. Simmonds, M.A.: Cancer statistics, 2003: further decrease in mortality rate, increase in persons living with cancer. CA Cancer J. Clin. **53**, 4 (2003)
5. Ramesh, H., Jain, S., Audisio, R.A.: Implications of aging in surgical oncology. Cancer J. **11**, 488–494 (2005)
6. Bureau of the census. Sixty-five Plus in the United States: Statistical Brief 95. Available at: http://www.census.gov/apsd/www/statbrief/sb95_8.pdf
7. Historical statistics of the United States: Washington DC: US dept of commerce, bureau of the census, national center for health statistics, department of health and human services (2000)
8. Jemal, A., Murray, T., Samuels, A., et al.: Cancer statistics. CA Cancer J. Clin. **53**, 5–26 (2003)
9. Yancik, R.: Population aging and cancer: a cross-national concern. Cancer J. **11**, 437–441 (2005)
10. Lowenfels, A.: Improving outcomes of major abdominal surgery in elderly patients. 91st American college of surgeons (2005)
11. Monson, K., Litvak, D.A., Bold, R.J.: Surgery in the aged population: surgical oncology. Arch. Surg. **138**, 1061–1067 (2003)
12. Evers, B.M., Townsend Jr., C.M., Thompson, J.C.: Organ physiology of aging. Surg. Clin. North Am. **74**, 23–39 (1994)
13. Yancik, R., Havlik, R.J., Wesley, M.N., et al.: Cancer and comorbidity in older patients: a descriptive profile. Ann. Epidemiol. **6**, 399–412 (1996)
14. Yancik, R., Ganz, P.A., Varricchio, C.G., Conley, B.: Perspectives on comorbidity and cancer in older patients: approaches to expand the knowledge base. J. Clin. Oncol. **19**, 1147–1151 (2001)
15. Ogle, K.S., Swanson, G.M., Woods, N., et al.: Cancer and comorbidity: redefining chronic diseases. Cancer **88**, 653–663 (2000)
16. Djokovic, J.L., Hedley-Whyte, J.: Prediction of outcome of surgery and anesthesia in patients over 80. JAMA **242**, 2301–2306 (1979)
17. Gerson, M.C., Hurst, J.M., Hertzberg, V.S., et al.: Prediction of cardiac and pulmonary complications related to elective abdominal and non-cardiac thoracic surgery in geriatric patients. Am. J. Med. **88**, 101–107 (1990)
18. Lidman, D.: Histopathology of human extremital arteries throughout life: including measurements of cystolic pressures in ankle and arm. Acta Chir. Scand. **148**, 575–580 (1982)
19. Banks, J., Booth, F.V., MacKay, E.H.: The physical properties of human pulmonary arteries and veins. Clin. Sci. Mol. Med. **55**, 477–484 (1978)
20. Bharati, S., Lev, M.: Pathologic changes of the conduction system with aging. Cardiol. Elder. **2**, 152–160 (1994)
21. Hano, O., Bogdanov, K.Y., Sakai, M., et al.: Reduced threshold for myocardial cell calcium intolerance in the rat heart with aging. Am. J. Physiol. **269**(suppl 5, pt 2), H1607–H1612 (1995)
22. Lakatta, E.G.: Cardiovascular reserve capacity in healthy older humans. Aging **6**, 213–223 (1994)
23. Olivetti, G., Melissari, M., Capasso, J.M., et al.: Cardiomyopathy of the aging human heart: myocyte loss

23. and reactive cellular hypertrophy. Circ. Res. **68**, 1560–1568 (1991)
24. Fleg, J.L., O'Connor, F., Gerstenblith, G., et al.: Impact of age on the cardiovascular response to dynamic upright exercise in healthy men and women. J. Appl. Physiol. **78**, 890–900 (1995)
25. Martinez-Selles, M., Garcia Robles, J.A., Prieto, L., et al.: Heart failure in the elderly: age-related differences in clinical profile and mortality. Int. J. Cardiol. **102**, 55–60 (2005)
26. Turner, J.M., Mead, J., Wohl, M.E.: Elasticity of human lungs in relation to age. J. Appl. Physiol. **25**, 664–671 (1968)
27. Knudson, R.J., Lebowitz, M.D., Holberg, C.J., et al.: Changes in the normal maximal expiratory flow-volume curve with growth and aging. Am. Rev. Respir. Dis. **127**, 725–734 (1983)
28. Polkey, M.I., et al.: The contractile properties of the elderly human diaphragm. Am. J. Respir. Crit. Care Med. **155**(5), 1560–1564 (1997)
29. Tolep, K., Kelsen, S.G.: Effect of aging on respiratory skeletal muscles. Clin. Chest Med. **14**, 363–378 (1993)
30. Thurlbeck, W.M., Angus, G.E.: Growth and aging of the normal human lung. Chest **67**(2 suppl), 3S–6S (1975)
31. D'Errico, A., Scarani, P., Colosimo, E., et al.: Changes in the alveolar connective tissue of the ageing lung: an immunohistochemical study. Virchows Arch. A Pathol. Anat. Histopathol. **415**, 137–144 (1989)
32. Sorbini, C.A., Grassi, V., Solinas, E., et al.: Arterial oxygen tension in relation to age in healthy subjects. Respiration **25**, 3–13 (1968)
33. Zawada Jr., E.T., Horning, J.R., Salem, A.G.: Renal fluid electrolyte and acid base problems during surgery in the elderly. In: Katlic, M.R. (ed.) Geriatric surgery. Urban & Scwarzenberg, Baltimore (1990)
34. Dunnill, M.S., Halley, W.: Some observations on the quantitative anatomy of the kidney. J. Pathol. **110**, 113–121 (1973)
35. Epstein, M.: Renal physiologic changes with age. Colo: PSG Publishing, Littleton (1985)
36. Lubran, M.M.: Renal function in the elderly. Ann. Clin. Lab. Sci. **25**, 122–133 (1995)
37. Brenner, B.M., Meyer, T.W., Hostetter, T.H.: Dietary protein intake and the progressive nature of kidney disease: the role of hemodynamically mediated glomerular injury in the pathogenesis of progressive glomerular sclerosis in aging, renal ablation, and intrinsic renal disease. N Engl. J. Med. **307**, 652–659 (1982)
38. Ryan, J., Zawada, E.: Renal function and fluid and electrolyte balance. Springer, Inc., New York (2001)
39. Weidmann, P., De Myttenaere-Bursztein, S., Maxwell, M.H., et al.: Effect on aging on plasma rennin and aldosterone in normal man. Kidney Int. **8**, 325–333 (1975)
40. Huseby, E., Engedal, K.: The patterns of motility are maintained in the human small intestine throughout the process of aging. Scand. J. Gastroenterol. **27**, 397–404 (1992)
41. Adkins, R.B., Marshall, B.A.: Anatomic and physiologic aspects of aging. In: Adkins, R.B., Scott, H.W. (eds.) Surgical care for the elderly. Lippincott-Raven Publishers, Philadelphia (1998)
42. Salem, S.A., Rajjayabun, P., Shepard, A.M., et al.: Reduced induction of drug metabolism in the elderly. Age Ageing **7**, 68–73 (1978)
43. Koruda, M.J., Sheldon, G.F.: Surgery in the aged. Adv. Surg. **24**, 293–331 (1991)
44. Aalami, O.O., Fang, T.D., Song, H.M., et al.: Physiological features of aging persons. Arch. Surg. **138**, 1068–1076 (2003)
45. Sirota, D.K.: Thyroid function and dysfunction in the elderly: a brief review. Mt. Sinai J. Med. **47**, 126–131 (1980)
46. Perry, H.M.: The endocrinology of aging. Clin. Chem. **45**, 1369–1376 (1999)
47. McConnell, J.G., Buchanan, K.D., Ardill, J., et al.: Glucose tolerance in the elderly: the role of insulin and its receptor. Eur. J. Clin. Invest. **12**, 55–61 (1982)
48. Barbieri, M., Rizzo, M.R., Manzella, D., et al.: Age-related insulin resistance: is it an obligatory finding? The lesson from healthy centenarians. Diabetes Metab. Res. Rev. **17**, 19–26 (2001)
49. Effros, R.B.: Ageing and the immune system. Novartis Found. Symp. **235**, 130–149 (2001)
50. Naliboff, B.D., Benton, D., Solomon, F., et al.: Immunological changes in young and old adults during brief laboratory stress. Psychosom. Med. **53**, 121–132 (1991)
51. Sylla, P., Kirman, I., Whelan, R.L.: Immunological advantages of advanced laparoscopy. Surg. Clin. N. Am. **85**, 1–18 (2005)
52. McLesky, C.H.: Anesthesia for the geriatric patient. In: Barash, P.G., Cullen, F., Stoelting, R.K. (eds.) Clinical anaesthesia. JB Lippincott, Philadelphia (1992)
53. Buxbaum, J.L., Schwartz, A.J.: Perianesthetic considerations for the elderly patient. Surg. Clin. North Am. **74**, 41–58 (1994)
54. Goodwin, J.S., Samet, J.M., Hunt, W.C.: Determinants of survival in older cancer patients. J. Natl. Cancer. Inst. **88**, 1031–1038 (1996)
55. Coffey, C.E., Lucke, J.F., Saxton, J.A., et al.: Sex differences in brain aging: a quantitative magnetic resonance imaging study. Arch. Neurol. **55**, 169–179 (1998)
56. Coffey, C.E., Saxton, J.A., Ratcliff, G., et al.: Relation of education to brain size in normal aging: implications for the reserve hypothesis. Neurology **53**, 189–196 (1999)
57. Long, D.M.: Aging in the nervous system. Neurosurgery **17**, 348–354 (1985)
58. Smolander, J.: Effect of cold exposure on older humans. Int. J. Sports Med. **23**, 86–92 (2002)
59. Yamaguchi, T., Kanno, I., Uemura, K.: Reduction in regional cerebral metabolic rate of oxygen during human aging. Stroke **17**, 1220–1228 (1986)
60. Dastur, D.: Cerebral blood flow and metabolism in normal human aging, pathologic aging, and senile dementia. J. Cereb. Blood Flow Metab. **5**, 1–9 (1985)
61. Fazekas, J., Alivan, R., Bessman, A.: Cerebral physiology of the aged. Am. J. Med. Sci. **223**, 245–257 (1952)
62. Audisio, R.A., Bozzetti, F., Gennari, R., et al.: Surgical management of elderly cancer patients: recommendations of SIOG surgical task force. Eur. J. Cancer **40**, 926–938 (2004)
63. Sargent, D.J., Goldberg, R.M., Jacobson, S.D., et al.: A pooled analysis of adjuvant chemotherapy for resected colon cancer in elderly patients. N Engl. J. Med. **345**, 1091–1097 (2001)
64. Neugut, A.I., Fleischauer, A.T., Sundararajan, V., et al.: Use of adjuvant chemotherapy and radiation therapy for rectal

cancer among the elderly: a population-based study. J. Clin. Oncol. **20**, 2643–2650 (2002)
65. Langer, C.J.: Elderly patients with lung cancer: biases and evidence. Curr. Treat. Options Oncol. **3**, 85–102 (2002)
66. Honecker, F., Kohne, C.H., Bokemeyer, C.: Colorectal cancer in the elderly: is palliative chemotherapy of value? Drugs Aging **20**, 1–11 (2003)
67. Fata, F., Mirza, A., Craig, G., et al.: Efficacy and toxicity of adjuvant chemotherapy in elderly patients with colon carcinoma: a 10-year experience of the Geisinger medical center. Cancer **94**, 1931–1938 (2002)
68. Cangemi, V., Volpino, P., D'Andrea, N., et al.: Lung cancer surgery in elderly patients. Tumori **82**, 237–241 (1996)
69. Jaklitsch, M.T., Pappas, E.A., Bueno, R.: Thoracoscopic surgery in elderly lung cancer patients. Crit. Rev. Oncol. Hematol. **49**, 165–171 (2004)
70. Kirby, T.J., Mack, M.J., Landreneau, R.J., et al.: Lobectomy-video-assisted thoracic surgery versus muscle-sparing thoracotomy: a randomized trial. J. Thorac. Cardiovasc. Surg. **109**, 997–1002 (1995)
71. McKenna Jr., R.J., Wolf, R.K., Brenner, M., et al.: Is lobectomy by video-assisted thoracic surgery an adequate cancer operation? Ann. Thorac. Surg. **66**, 1903–1908 (1998)
72. Cattaneo, S.M., Park, B.J., Wilton, A.S., et al.: Use of video-assisted thoracic surgery for lobectomy in the elderly results in fewer complications. Ann. Thorac. Surg. **85**, 231–235 (2008)
73. Mun, M., Kohno, T.: Video-assisted thoracic surgery for clinical stage I lung cancer in octogenarians. Ann. Thorac. Surg. **85**, 406–411 (2008)
74. Koren, J.P., Bocage, J.P., Geis, W.P., et al.: Major thoracic surgery in octogenarians: the video-assisted thoracic surgery (VATS) approach. Surg. Endosc. **17**, 632–635 (2003)
75. Thomas, P., Doddli, C., Neville, P., et al.: Esophageal cancer in the elderly. Eur. J. Cardiothorac. Surg. **10**, 941–946 (1996)
76. Ellis Jr., F.H., Williamson, W.A., Heatley, G.J.: Cancer of the esophagus and cardia: does age influence treatment selection and surgical outcomes? J. Am. Coll. Surg. **187**, 345–351 (1998)
77. Alexiou, C., Beggs, D., Salama, F.D., et al.: Surgery for oesophageal cancer in elderly patients: view from Nottingham. J. Thorac. Cardiovasc. Surg. **116**, 545–553 (1998)
78. Perry, Y., Fernando, H.C., Buenaventura, P.O.: Minimally invasive esophagectomy in the elderly. JSLS **6**, 299–304 (2002)
79. Young, J.L., Percy, C.L., Aj, A.: Surveillance, epidemiology, and end results: incidence and mortality data 1973–1977. US printing office 66 (1981)
80. Saidi, R.F., Bell, J.L., Dudrick, P.S.: Surgical resection of gastric cancer in elderly patients: is there a difference in outcome. J. Surg. Res. **118**, 15–20 (2004)
81. Singh, K.K., et al.: Laparoscopic gastrectomy for gastric cancer: early experience among the elderly. Surg. Endosc. **22**(4), 1002–1007 (2008)
82. Mochiki, E., Ohno, T., Kamiyama, Y., et al.: Laparoscopy-assisted gastrectomy for early gastric cancer in young and elderly patients. World J. Surg. **29**, 1585–1591 (2005)
83. Fleshman, J., Sargent, D.J., Green, E., et al.: Laparoscopic colectomy for cancer is not inferior to open surgery ased on 5-year data from the COST study group trial. Ann. Surg. **246**, 655–664 (2007)
84. Stewart, B.T., Stitz, R.W., Lumley, J.W.: Laparoscopically assisted colorectal surgery in the elderly. Br. J. Surg. **86**, 938–941 (1999)
85. Law, W.L., Chu, K.W., Tung, P.H.: Laparoscopic colorectal resection: a safe option for elderly patients. J. Am. Coll. Surg. **195**, 768–773 (2002)
86. Person B, Cera SM, Sands DR, et al (2007) Do elderly patients benefit from laparoscopic colorectal surgery? Surg Endosc 24:epub ahead of print
87. Riccardo, A.A., Roberto, G., Koki, S., et al.: Preoperative assessment of cancer in elderly patients: a pilot study. Supp. Cancer Ther. **1**, 55–60 (2003)
88. Ramesh, H.S., Pope, D., Gennari, R., et al.: Optimising surgical management of elderly cancer patients. World J. Surg. Oncol. **3**, 17–31 (2005)
89. Weber, D.M.: Laparoscopic surgery: an excellent approach in elderly patients. Arch. Surg. **138**, 1083–1088 (2003)

10 Transluminal Surgery: Is There a Place for Oncological Procedures?

Patricia Sylla and David W. Rattner

10.1 Introduction

Minimally invasive procedures performed through percutaneous, endoscopic, and endovascular access routes have changed the management of a variety of malignancies. Natural orifice transluminal endoscopic surgery (NOTES) is a novel access route to the peritoneal and thoracic cavities utilizing transvisceral incisions and flexible endoscopes to perform surgical procedures. NOTES appears to be feasible and preliminary clinical experience with NOTES is accumulating rapidly. Although few studies have described the use of NOTES in the oncologic setting, based on published data in humans and swine, it seems that NOTES has potential applications in cancer patients including diagnostic peritoneoscopy, thoracoscopy and mediastinoscopy, lymph node resection, gastro-jejunostomy, solid organ resection, and intestinal resection. In spite of this potential, there are currently few data to support the superiority or even equivalence of NOTES to current surgical therapy. Additional data and clinical experience with NOTES will be required before definite conclusions can be drawn regarding future applications of NOTES in oncology.

P. Sylla and D.W. Rattner (✉)
Department of Surgery, Massachusetts General Hospital,
15 Parkman Street, WACC 460, Boston, MA 02114, USA
e-mail: psylla@partners.org; drattner@partners.org

10.2 The Era of Minimally Invasive Techniques

Advances in dynamic imaging combined with technological innovations have enabled percutaneous, endoscopic, and endovascular procedures to replace more invasive surgical procedures. These minimally invasive approaches have decreased the morbidity of many interventions and are often performed under conscious sedation in the ambulatory setting. Minimally invasive techniques have been particularly beneficial in oncology, especially for tissue diagnosis, cancer staging, and more recently for the surgical treatment of early-stage malignancies. Whether or not NOTES will have as big an impact as laparoscopic and thoracoscopic surgery did over the last two decades is an exciting question to ponder.

The breakthroughs achieved with endoscopic, endoluminal, and advanced laparoscopic techniques are bridging expertise from multiple disciplines including radiology, endoscopy, and surgery, and allow complex diagnostic and therapeutic procedures to be performed through smaller incisions, puncture sites, or no incisions at all. It follows that endoscopic transluminal access to a body cavity, although not new conceptually, represents the next logical step in procedural innovation with the ultimate goal of completely eliminating the need for skin incisions.

10.3 NOTES: Revolutionary or Evolutionary?

Routine endoscopic procedures such as percutaneous endoscopic gastrostomy (PEG) and endoscopic transgastric drainage of pancreatic pseudocysts require the intentional perforation of a visceral organ. In these procedures, the perforation is maintained with a tube or stent for therapeutic purposes and does not typically require closure. While these procedures technically fall under the category of transluminal or transvisceral intra-abdominal access, NOTES refers to using this perforation as the primary access route to perform a procedure using flexible endoscopes. Transvaginal peritoneoscopy has been performed to diagnose pelvic pathology since it was first described in 1902. Traditionally, perforation of the gastrointestinal (GI) tract during an endoscopic procedure mandated a laparotomy to repair the perforation. At the turn of the current century, several reports described successful endoscopic clip repair of a sphincterotomy-related duodenal perforation [1] and endoscopic clip closure and omental patch of full-thickness gastric perforations following endoscopic mucosal resection (EMR) of gastric neoplasms in seven patients [2]. Separate from these reports, several series of hybrid transvaginal surgery have been reported in the gynecologic literature. Gynecologists have combined culdoscopy with laparoscopy to improve visualization, assist in retraction and dissection of pelvic and abdominal structures, and facilitate specimen extraction [3]. More recently, laparoscopy and transvaginal endoscopy were combined to perform additional procedures such as nephrectomy in swine [4]. In 2004, transluminal endoscopy was actively sought as a primary access route to a body cavity to perform a range of diagnostic and therapeutic procedures. Kalloo et al. described transgastric endoscopic access to the peritoneal cavity with liver biopsy in a survival and non-survival swine model [5]. Shortly thereafter, Rao and Reddy demonstrated the feasibility and therapeutic potential of NOTES in humans by performing transgastric appendectomy and tubal ligation. The term NOTES was subsequently coined to describe endoscopic transvisceral approach to perform surgical procedures (Fig. 10.1). The ensuing enthusiasm among gastroenterologists and surgeons alike was reminiscent of that from the early laparoscopic reports. Relative to open and laparoscopic procedures, transluminal endoscopic procedures could eliminate wound infections and incisional hernias with both improved cosmetic results and reduced postoperative pain from the lack of skin incisions. Other potential advantages of NOTES include easier access to intra-abdominal organs in morbidly obese patients and more direct access to

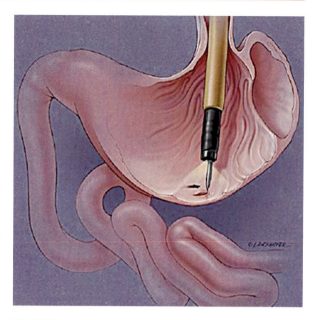

Fig. 10.1 Transgastric access to the peritoneal cavity with creation of a gastrostomy using a needle-knife inserted through a flexible endoscope. (Reprinted from [26], p. 6. With permission by Elsevier)

retroperitoneal structures, thereby avoiding extensive soft tissue and abdominal dissection. In addition, if completed entirely endoscopically, NOTES could theoretically be performed under conscious sedation in the ambulatory setting with significant decrease in length of hospital stay and hospitalization-related morbidity and costs.

10.4 Natural Orifice Surgery Consortium for Assessment and Research (NOSCAR)

In an effort to prevent the premature application of this emerging technique which safety and efficacy are still largely unproven, experts from both the American Society of Gastrointestinal Endoscopy (ASGE) and the Society of American Gastrointestinal and Endoscopic Surgeons (SAGES) created the Natural Orifice Surgery Consortium for Assessment and Research (NOSCAR) whose goal is to oversee NOTES-related research and ensure that standard practice guidelines based on results from laboratory and clinical investigations are developed and enforced

Table 10.1 Potential barriers to clinical practice of NOTES [6]

Access to the peritoneal cavity
Gastric (intestinal closure)
Prevention of infection
Development of suturing device
Development of anastomotic (non-suturing) device
Spatial orientation
Development of a multitasking platform to accomplish procedures
Control of intraperitoneal hemorrhage
Physiologic untoward events
Training other providers

to ensure patient safety (www.noscar.org). As outlined in a NOSCAR white paper published in 2006, in order to achieve this goal, a number of challenges have been outlined that need to be resolved before NOTES can be routinely and safely performed in humans (Table 10.1) [6]. Among these challenges, safe, expeditious and reliable endoscopic creation and closure of viscerotomies to access a body cavity is one of the most difficult and crucial steps. Other challenges include the prevention of infection, management of complications, difficulties with spatial orientation, and the development of endoscopic suturing and anastomotic devices as well as a multitasking platform (Table 10.1) [6].

Over the last 3 years, over 30 NOTES-related studies have been published consisting mostly of case reports and short series on the feasibility or short-term outcomes of a variety of procedures, with additional publications focused on the development and testing of novel endoscopic devices (Table 10.2).

10.5 NOTES: Current Experience in Animal Models and Human Applications

While access through natural orifices for NOTES includes transesophageal, transgastric, transcolonic, transrectal, transvesical, and transvaginal routes, the most commonly investigated access in these reports has been the transgastric route. The primary body cavity accessed through NOTES is the abdominal cavity, although access to the thoracic cavity and mediastinum for diagnostic and therapeutic applications is also under active investigation. The majority of NOTES studies were conducted in survival and non-survival swine models, with some reports in human cadavers. In addition to Rao and Reddy's yet unpublished series on transgastric appendectomy and tubal ligation, only four case reports and two case series in humans have been published (Table 10.3). These include laparoscopy-assisted transvaginal cholecystectomy in two patients, as well as transgastric peritoneoscopy in one patient and transvesical peritoneoscopy in another patient (Table 10.3). In the two largest series published to date, Hazey et al. prospectively compared transgastric peritoneoscopy with or without biopsy to standard diagnostic laparoscopy in the evaluation of pancreatic cancer resectability [38]. Tsin et al. published a retrospective series of 100 combined laparoscopic and culdoscopic procedures including appendectomy, cholecystectomy, oophorectomy, salpingectomy, ovarian cystectomy, and myomectomy [3].

Existing data on the feasibility, safety profile, and short-term outcomes of NOTES procedures are still sparse, and drawing conclusions regarding the future of NOTES is premature (Table 10.2). While a few groups with extensive endoscopic expertise and prior laboratory experience have been able to make the transition from the laboratory to the clinical setting, only a limited number of NOTES procedures have been performed in highly selected patients (Table 10.3). The widespread applicability of NOTES is currently limited by a number of challenges, most of which were outlined in the NOSCAR white paper. The major rate-limiting factor in NOTES' widespread applicability is related to the lack of specialized equipment required to perform these procedures. While it is difficult at this time to foresee which NOTES procedures have the most potential usefulness and clinical applicability, there are a number of possible advantages to NOTES in the management of cancer.

10.6 NOTES and Oncology

Advantages of NOTES over open and laparoscopic surgery in the oncologic setting include the same benefits as for other types of surgical procedures such as reduced postoperative pain, recovery time, wound

Table 10.2 Published NOTES studies in animals (cadaver studies not included)

NOTES procedure	Author	Access	Number acute, survival	Endoscope	Enterostomy closure	Other	Complications
Peritoneoscopy	Kalloo [5]	TG	12,5	SCUE	Clips	Liver biopsies	Microabscess (2)
	Lima [7]	TVe	3,3	5-mm ureteroscope	Not closed (catheter)		None
	Rentschler [8]	TG	1,0	Mobile endoluminal robot	Endoclip, endoloop		None
	Kantsevoy [9]	TG	12,0	SCUE	Not closed		None
	Onders [10]	TG	8,0	SCUE	Not closed (PEG)	Biopsies, LOA	None
	Fong [11]	TC	0,6	DCUE	Clips, endoloop, prototype		None
	Wilhelm [12]	TC	3,5	SCUE, TEM proctoscope	Pursestring, linear stapler		None
Thoracoscopy	Lima [13]	TVe	0,6	5-mm ureteroscope	Not closed (catheter)		None
Mediastinoscopy	Sumiyama [14]	TE	0,4	SCUE with EMR cap	Clips (mucosal)	SEMF	Pleural injury (1)
Lymphadenectomy	Fritscher-Ravens [15]	TG, EUS	6,0	SC echoendoscope	Suturing device		Incomplete (2/6)
Gastro-jejunostomy	Kantsevoy [16]	TG	0,2	SCUE	N/A		None
	Kantsevoy [17]	TG	11,0	Colonoscope	N/A		None
	Bergstrom [18]	TG	6,6	DCUE	N/A		None
Gastric reduction	Kantsevoy [19]	TG	4,0	DCUE	Not closed		None
Cholecystectomy	Park [20]	TG, +/-lap	8,8	DCUE x2	Endoscopic suturing	Cholecysto-gastrostomy	None
	Pai [21]	TC	0,5	Sigmoidoscope, DCUE	Endoop, endoclip		Sepsis (1)
	Scott [22]	TVa	4,0	SCUE, MAGS	Sutures		Incomplete (2/4)
	Sumiyama [23]	TG	0,6	DCUE with EMR cap, scope	Clip, tissue anchor (mucosal closure)		Death (2), Sepsis (2)
	Rolanda [24]	TG, TVe	7,0	5-mm ureteroscope, DCUE	Not closed		Bleeding (1), Bile leak (1)

Procedure	Author	Size (cm)	Access	Scope	Closure	Other	Complications
Splenectomy	Kantsevoy [25]	6,0	TG	DCUE	Not closed		None
Distal pancreatectomy	Matthes [26]	6,0	TG	DCUE	Clips		Bleeding (1)
	Ryou [27]	3,2	TC, TVa	Sigmoidoscope, DCUE, R-scope	Endoloop (colon), vagina not closed	CO_2 (Veress)	None
Nephrectomy	Gettman [4]	4,2	TVa, lap	Flexible cystoscope	Sutures		None
	Clayman [28]	1,0	TVa, lap	DCUE, Transport multilumen platform	Not closed		None
Tubal ligation	Jagannath [29]	0,5	TG	DCUE	Not closed		None
Partial hysterectomy	Merrifield [30]	0,5	TG	SCUE, DCUE	Endoclips		Sepsis (1), Abscess (1)
Oophorectomy	Wagh [31]	3,3	TG	DCUE	Endoclips	Peritoneoscopy	None
Tubectomy	Wagh [32]	0,6	TG	SCUE, DCUE	Endoclips		None
Diaphragm pacing, stimulation	Onders [33]	4,0	TG	SCUE	Not closed (PEG)		None
Ventral hernia repair	Hu [34]	2,0	TG	DCUE	Endoclips		None
	Fong [35]	3,2	TC	DCUE	Endoloops, Endoclips	CO_2 (Veress), Mesh fixation	None

SCUE single-channel endoscope, *DCUE* dual-channel endoscope, *SEMF* submucosal endoscopy with a mucosal flap, *EMR* endoscopic mucosal resection, *MAGS* magnetic anchoring and guidance system, *LOA* lysis of adhesions, *Lap* laparoscopic-assisted, *EUS* endoluminal ultrasound-assisted, *TG* transgastric, *TC* transcolonic, *TE* transesophageal, *TVa* transvaginal, *TVe* transvesical

Table 10.3 Published clinical NOTES studies

NOTES procedure	Author	Access	N	Endoscope	Enterostomy closure	Other	Complications
Peritoneoscopy	Marks [36]	TG	1	SCUE	Not closed (PEG)	PEG rescue	None
	Gettman [37]	TVe	1	Ureteroscope	Suture closure		None
	Hazey [38]	TG	10	SCUE	Not closed	Lap-peritoneoscopy	Understaging pancreatic cancer (1)
Cholecystectomy	Bessler [39]	TVa, lap	1	Suture closure	Suture closure		None
	Marescaux [40]	TVa, lap	1	Suture closure	Suture closure		None
Appendectomy Myomectomy Oophorectomy Salpingectomy	Tsin [3]	Culdo-laparoscopy TVa, lap	100	Suture closure	Suture closure	Liver biopsy Cholecystectomy	Drug-related fever (1)

SCUE single-channel endoscope, *DCUE* dual-channel endoscope, *Lap* laparoscopic-assisted, *PEG* percutaneous endoscopic gastrostomy, *TG* transgastric, *TVa* transvaginal, *TVe* transvesical

infections, and incisional hernias, as well as reduced overall surgical trauma. Reduced surgical trauma may have significant immunologic benefits in cancer patients. Numerous experimental studies have demonstrated that laparotomy, when compared with CO_2 pneumoperitoneum or anesthesia alone, is associated with increased tumor establishment and growth [41–44]. In a murine model, tumor-cell proliferation was increased and apoptosis decreased after laparotomy [45]. The underlying mechanism for these effects may include laparotomy-related inhibition of cell-mediated immune function [46]. Although no studies on the effects of NOTES on immune function have been published, it is an area under active investigation. By avoiding skin incisions, NOTES may be associated with better preservation of cell-mediated immunity and overall improved immune function.

Only one clinical study on the applicability of NOTES in patients with malignancy has been published to date [38]. Given the overall limited clinical experience with NOTES and the need for rigorous assessment of the feasibility and safety of these procedures prior to their application, more data are needed to ascertain the potential impact of NOTES in cancer patients. Published data on NOTES with respect to specific types of procedures may have potential applications in the oncologic setting. Therefore, a close review of these studies with regard to technique, access, outcomes, and complications might help identify procedures that are better suited for and may have significant impact on the surgical management of cancer patients.

10.7 NOTES: Current Applications

10.7.1 Peritoneoscopy

In 2004, Kalloo et al. described transgastric endoscopic peritoneal exploration with liver biopsy in 12 acute and 5 survival experiments in swine [5]. This procedure involved creating a gastrotomy using needle-knife cautery, inserting a guide wire, and dilating the gastrostomy with a balloon followed by insertion of a flexible upper endoscope into the abdominal cavity. Intraperitoneal microabscesses were noted on necropsy 14 days postoperatively [5]. Two subsequent reports in swine confirmed the feasibility of transgastric endoscopic access to the peritoneal cavity with excellent visualization and the ability to perform biopsies. In these reports, the gastrostomy was either left open in acute experiments [9], closed with endoclips [5], or managed by leaving a PEG tube in place [10]. While transgastric endoscopic access has been the most common form of transluminal access for peritoneoscopy and other NOTES procedures, factors limiting widespread application of transgastric access include difficulties in achieving reproducible and secure gastrostomy closure. In an attempt to resolve issues related to scope manipulation and orientation, a prototype mobile endoluminal robot was described in one acute swine experiment and inserted transgastrically under esophagogastroduodenoscopy (EGD) control to perform peritoneoscopy. Following exploration of the abdominal cavity, the robot was retracted into the stomach and the gastrostomy was closed with endoloops and clips without complications [8].

Other transvisceral routes have been explored. Transcolonic endoscopic peritoneoscopy was described in two separate reports in 3 acute and 11 survival experiments in swine [11, 12]. Peritoneal access was achieved successfully through an anterior colotomy in both reports with [12] or without [11] the use of a transanal endoscopic microsurgery (TEM) rectoscope serving as an overtube and performed either by direct puncture [11] or by using ultrasound combined with intraperitoneal instillation of fluid to identify a safe entry site for insertion of a double-channel endoscope [12]. The colotomies were closed using endoclips, endoloops, a prototype closure device [11], or a linear stapler [12], with good outcomes in all animals after 10 or 14 survival days. Transvesical endoscopic peritoneoscopy with liver biopsy was also performed in three acute and five 14-day survival experiments in swine using a 5.5 mm overtube and cystoscope inserted through the dome of the bladder [7]. The vesicotomy site was left open and a catheter was left in place for 4 days to drain the bladder without adverse outcomes [7]. Regardless of the type of transluminal approach, these reports, although limited in number of animals and long-term follow-up, suggest that NOTES peritoneoscopy is feasible with good outcomes in swine survival models.

Three recent clinical reports have described NOTES peritoneoscopy in a total of 12 patients [36–38]. Peritoneal access was achieved transgastrically in two reports [36, 38] and transvesically in one [37]. Transgastric endoscopic peritoneoscopy was performed at the bedside in one neurologically impaired patient in the intensive care unit, whose gastrostomy tube had been dislodged 3 days following insertion [36]. The PEG tube was visualized and repositioned using the endoscope inserted through the preexisting gastrostomy without complications. Incidental transvesical peritoneoscopy was also reported in a patient in whom endoscopic placement of a suprapubic catheter under laparoscopic visualization prior to robotic prostatectomy was attempted [37]. A flexible ureteroscope was advanced through the vesicotomy thereby providing access to the peritoneal cavity. Although placement of the suprapubic catheter was not possible, this approach provided visualization of the peritoneal cavity with no complications [37]. Most recently, in the first report to date of NOTES performed in patients with a malignancy, Hazey et al. evaluated and compared transgastric endoscopic peritoneoscopy using a single-channel diagnostic gastroscope to standard diagnostic laparoscopy in patients with pancreatic cancer with respect to the ability to determine tumor resectability [38]. Ten patients underwent diagnostic laparoscopy followed by transgastric endoscopic peritoneoscopy with or without tissue biopsy performed by an endoscopist blinded to the findings of the laparoscopy. Findings and outcomes with respect to the decision to proceed with resection versus palliation were compared between each approach. The authors pointed out several shortcomings in the design of the study [38]. Transgastric peritoneal access was obtained under direct laparoscopic visualization through a single transabdominal port in order to ensure safe anterior gastric wall puncture, which is a deviation from a pure NOTES procedure. In addition, the gastrostomy created did not require closure since it was incorporated in the distal gastrectomy specimen for the Whipple procedure or in the gastrojejunostomy for palliation [38]. The operative time required for NOTES was more than twice that required for the laparoscopic approach (24.8 vs. 12.3 min) and both procedures were performed under general anesthesia. However, there was good correlation between each approach in findings, leading to the decision to proceed with resection versus palliation in nine of ten patients [38]. Due to difficulties with spatial orientation, endoscopic visualization of all quadrants was incomplete and biopsies of suspicious lesions within the peritoneum were unsuccessful in four and two patients respectively, although these limitations did not impact final staging. Interestingly, the authors found that visualization of the anterior abdominal wall with the endoscope was superior to that from standard laparoscopy [38].

In addition to these reports of successful transvesical and transgastric peritoneoscopy in carefully selected patients, culdoscopy, which consists of visualizing pelvic and abdominal organs through a posterior vaginal colpotomy, has been routinely performed since 1902 when it was first described by Von Ott [47]. With the introduction of the fiber-optic culdoscope in the 1960s, flexible culdoscopy became an important tool for the diagnosis and treatment of pelvic pathology [48]. Applications have ranged from peritoneoscopy, biopsies, tubal ligation, and resection of endometrial implants [48]. More recently, laparoscopy and culdoscopy have been combined to perform a wider range of more complex pelvic procedures [49]. Culdoscopy is currently performed through an incision in the posterior vaginal wall into the cul-de-sac with insertion of a cannula and flexible endoscope with or without laparoscopic visualization with later transvaginal closure of the colpotomy [49]. In their series, Tsin et al. reported that among the 100 combined laparoscopic and transvaginal pelvic and abdominal procedures performed over 7 years, no surgical complications were noted [49]. However, prior to being performed under laparoscopic visualization, culdoscopy was associated with complications related to limited visualization such as uterine or bowel perforation [48]. While this approach is clearly successful, a hybrid approach is still required to ensure safety.

Despite limitations related to transvaginal access including the need for laparoscopic assistance and limitations to transgastric access including difficult spatial orientation with retroflexion and gastrostomy closure, transluminal peritoneoscopy is a promising minimally invasive alternative that can be performed safely and with good results. Assuming that adequate gastrostomy and colotomy closure can be performed, the potential advantages of this approach include the ability to be performed in the ambulatory setting or bedside under sedation, to be included in the outpatient staging work-up of patients with pancreatic cancer or other malignancies, and to perform complex procedures in critically ill patients who might not tolerate more aggressive procedures. This would not only allow patients with locally advanced disease or who are critically ill to avoid unnecessary surgery and general anesthesia, but would also reduce postoperative pain, recovery time, and the cost of hospitalization and shorten the interval to adjuvant therapy.

10.7.2 Thoracoscopy and Mediastinoscopy

Thoracoscopy has become the mainstay approach for the management of a variety of benign thoracic pathologies. Video-assisted thoracic surgery (VATS) is currently the standard approach for diagnostic procedures and treatment of benign pulmonary and pleural-based lesions. Prospective [50] and randomized controlled studies [51, 52] have documented reduced postoperative pain, pulmonary dysfunction, and shorter length of hospital stay following thoracoscopy relative to thoracotomy for the management of pulmonary nodules [52], recurrent pneumothorax [50], and lung biopsy [51]. Although thoracoscopy has become the standard of care for the management of benign lung pathology and biopsies, the routine use of VATS in the management of lung cancers is controversial. Thoracoscopy still requires several incisions through the chest wall associated with significant incisional pain and complications related to the insertion of ports such as intercostal neuritis, pulmonary herniation through port sites, conversion to thoracotomy, pulmonary parenchymal or diaphragm injury, liver laceration, and prolonged air leak [53]. There are significant theoretical advantages to performing thoracic procedures through NOTES in the oncologic setting, particularly for diagnosing and staging lung cancer and in the evaluation and tissue confirmation of metastatic disease. One group investigated the feasibility and outcomes of transluminal endoscopic thoracoscopy using transvesical access in six survival experiments in swine [13]. After cystoscopy and the creation of a vesicotomy through the dome of the bladder, a 5 mm ureteroscope was advanced over a wire and overtube into the peritoneal cavity. Transdiaphragmatic thoracoscopy and lung biopsy were performed through a small incision made in the diaphragm with the ureteroscope, ensuring to maintain a pressure-controlled CO_2 pneumothorax. Procedures were successfully completed in all animals with no complications over the 15 survival days [13]. This study demonstrates several advantages of a transvesical approach to the chest including relatively sterile access, access to both the abdominal and thoracic cavity through a single lumen, excellent visualization by maintaining a straight line of vision with the scope, and complete healing of the vesicotomy without formal closure. In addition, because of the proximity of the scope to the mediastinum and pericardium, this approach may be useful in the treatment of pericardial effusion and malignant pleural effusions. It is, however, limited by the size of the endoscope that can be introduced through the bladder. Another group described transesophageal access to the posterior mediastinum by first raising a mucosal flap with the endoscope, creating a 10 cm-long submucosal tunnel, and using cap EMR to create a myotomy through the muscularis propria to enter the posterior mediastinum [14]. In three survival experiments using swine, the authors reported great visualization of the vagal nerve trunks, descending aorta, posterior pericardium, and good outcomes during the 14 survival days with clips applied at the mucosal puncture site [14]. These preliminary studies on the use of NOTES for transvesical and other types of transluminal access to the thoracic cavity and mediastinum suggest potential applications beyond thoracoscopy and mediastinoscopy including mediastinal or hilar node sampling, drainage of malignant effusions, pleurodesis, lung wedge resection, and other advanced procedures that could potentially be performed in the endoscopy suite or at the bedside under conscious sedation.

10.7.3 Lymph Node Biopsy

Several studies have demonstrated the safety and effectiveness of transesophageal endoscopic ultrasound (EUS)-guided fine-needle aspiration (FNA) and transbronchial needle aspiration of hilar and mediastinal lesions to assist in lung cancer staging [54] or to drain mediastinal abscess or hematoma [55]. Several studies have documented that EUS-FNA was more accurate and had a higher predictive value than positron emission tomography (PET) or computed tomography (CT) scan for detecting posterior mediastinal lymphadenopathy in lung cancer patients [56–58]. Theoretical advantages of NOTES in this setting include the ability to remove an unlimited number of nodes and to resect a node in its entirety rather than sampling it with more accurate microscopic assessment and cancer staging. In a recent study, EUS-guided transgastric endoscopic lymph node resection was described in acute swine experiments using an enchoendoscope to locate, puncture, anchor, and resect a target lymph node transgastrically with endoscopic suture closure of the gastrostomy. The full sequence of transgastric lymph node resection was successful in two of six animals [15]. The same group recently described their experience with transesophageal endoscopic mediastinoscopy using endoscopic ultrasound for the selection of an appropriate esophageal puncture site in two acute and seven long-term survival studies using swine. In addition to mediastinoscopy, endoscopic mediastinal lymph node removal, saline injection into the myocardium, and pericardial fenestration were performed with no adverse outcomes at 6 weeks postoperatively [59]. Although preliminary, these studies demonstrate that transesophageal access may be incorporated in lung cancer staging and may have additional diagnostic and therapeutic cardiothoracic applications. Although no additional experimental or clinical data on NOTES lymph node harvest in the abdomen have been published, previous published data on peritoneoscopy with or without liver biopsy suggest that abdominal, pelvic, and retroperitoneal lymphadenectomy, performed completely endoscopically or under laparoscopic or either ultrasonographic guidance, is feasible through a variety of transluminal access routes.

10.7.4 Gastro-jejunostomy

Creation of GI anastomoses is an essential step in the restoration of intestinal continuity following resection for benign disease or malignancy or for bypassing an obstructed intestinal segment. Intracorporeally sutured and stapled anastomoses can be fashioned entirely laparoscopically or with laparoscopic assistance through small incisions, but are still associated with incisional pain and substantial risks of wound infection and port-site hernias. Anastomoses completed endoscopically in the setting of NOTES would prevent incision-related complications and when performed to palliate gastric outlet obstruction (GOO) from unresectable gastric, duodenal, or pancreatic malignancy, NOTES has the potential advantage of reducing morbidity associated with extensive open surgery and improving the quality of life of relatively immunosupressed, nutritionally depleted, and terminal cancer patients.

Endoscopic enteral and biliary stenting of GOO and obstructive jaundice respectively have become the first line of treatment for palliating unresectable pancreatic cancer and are associated with less morbidity relative to surgical bypass and chemotherapy. Although surgical gastro-jejunostomy is the standard of care for palliating GOO, it is associated with relatively high morbidity and mortality in cancer patients. Laparoscopic gastro-jejunostomy is a less invasive alternative associated with reduced pain, shorter length of hospital stay, and faster return to normal activity than open gastro-jejunostomy in patients with GOO from unresectable gastric cancer [60, 61]. However, laparoscopic gastro-jejunostomy has not been consistently associated with significant reduction in morbidity relative to open surgical bypass [60, 62]. Endoscopic enteral stenting using self-expandable metal stents (SEMS) has been increasing in popularity, particularly for end-stage cancer patients with short life expectancy and high surgical risk. In addition, SEMS can be performed under conscious sedation, and several studies have demonstrated that SEMS are associated with shorter procedure time, faster resumption of oral intake [63, 64], and shorter hospital stay [62]. However, the rate of successful stent placement varies across studies from 77.3% [64] to 92% [65]. In patients with longer life expectancy, stent placement was associated with more frequent recurrence of obstructive symptoms than open gastro-jejunostomy [62]. Given the limitations of SEMS, open and laparoscopic gastro-jejunostomy in palliating end-stage cancer patients with GOO, endoscopically and translumenally completed gastro-jejunostomy would in theory alleviate the morbidity associated with skin incisions and from stent migration or occlusion.

Endoscopic gastro-jejunal anastomosis was successfully performed and described in three experimental studies in swine comprising a total of 17 acute and 8 survival animals. Transgastric access to the peritoneum was achieved with the gastroscope and used to grasp a loop of jejunum, which was then pulled into the stomach through the gastrostomy and sutured in position using a prototype suturing device (Fig. 10.2) [16, 18]. This approach, although successful, was initially limited by the fact that the gastro-jejunal anastomosis was completed after pulling a random loop of jejunum [16, 18]. In a later study using 11 animals, this technical limitation was overcome by combining the use of an endoscopic transilluminator and fluoroscopy for the precise localization of a target loop of jejunum in preparation for anastomosis [17]. These studies demonstrate that transgastric gastro-jejunostomy is feasible and potentially safe in swine. With the continued development of specialized equipment such as endoscopic suturing and stapling devices, transilluminators, and other endoscopic markers, a wide range of GI anastomoses might be achievable for palliation and to complement primary oncologic resections.

10.7.5 Solid Organ Resection in Animal Models

To date, solid organ resection using NOTES has been reported in experimental studies, predominantly in swine, and include splenectomy, distal pancreatectomy, nephrectomy, cholecystectomy, hysterectomy, and oophorectomy (Table 10.1). Of these, only NOTES cholecystectomy has been performed in humans. Although not described in the setting of malignancy, all of these procedures have potential oncologic applications.

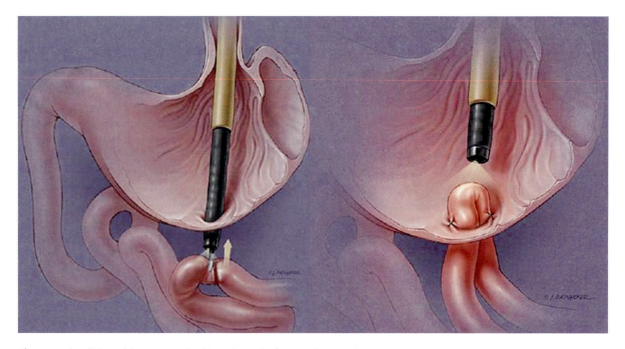

Fig. 10.2 Small bowel loop grasped with endoscopic forceps through the gastrostomy in preparation for gastro-jejunostomy. (Reprinted from [26], p. 6. With permission by Elsevier)

10.7.5.1 Splenectomy

In acute experiments conducted in six swine, NOTES splenectomy was performed using endoscopic transgastric access to the upper abdomen, retroflexing the endoscope to visualize the spleen, and ligating splenic vessels with endoloops and clips [25]. The specimens were extracted transgastrically after substantially enlarging the gastrostomy, which was not closed [25]. This demonstration of feasibility is probably not directly translatable to humans. A human splenectomy would likely be a hybrid procedure involving a stapler or other device to provide secure hemostasis of the large splenic vessels.

10.7.5.2 Distal Pancreatectomy

Distal pancreatectomy was described in three acute and two survival experiments using transcolonic access for endoscopic dissection of the pancreas with transvaginal access for insertion of a computer-assisted linear stapler [27]. The anterior colotomy was closed with an endoloop and the vagina was not closed. Through this dual-port approach, endoscopic distal pancreatectomy was technically feasible with animals placed in a prone position and resulted in no postoperative complications during the 14-day survival period [27]. As with the prior description of a swine splenectomy, several significant modifications are likely to be necessary prior to attempting this on humans. Combined transrectal and transvaginal access probably carries a substantial risk of creating a rectovaginal fistula. An alternative technique was described in six acute experiments with swine placed in the right lateral decubitus position. Distal pancreatectomy was successfully completed transgastrically using an endoloop to secure the pancreatic remnant and clips to close the gastrostomy [26]. With the exception of one animal in whom a splenic laceration resulted in 250 cc of blood loss, no other complications were noted [26]. The authors of both reports emphasized the significant advantage of transluminal endoscopic access to dissection of the pancreas. Division and mobilization of the gastrocolic omentum and division of the splenocolic ligament was not required for distal pancreatectomy with excellent exposure of the pancreas with the endoscope inserted either transgastrically or transvaginally in animals in either a prone or right lateral decubitus position [26, 27].

10.7.5.3 Nephrectomy

Dual-port access was also used to perform NOTES nephrectomy in six acute swine experiments using transgastric and transvesical access [66]. Dual endoscopic access permitted greater flexibility in dissection and retraction to complete the procedures. Although ligation of renal vessels required both an ultrasonic device and clips to achieve hemostasis, right and left nephrectomies were technically feasible in this model with excellent exposure of retroperitoneal structures through this approach. The main limitation of the procedure was extraction of the specimen [66].

10.7.5.4 Partial Hysterectomy, Salpingectomy, and Oophorectomy

Transgastric partial hysterectomy was described in five survival swine experiments using an endoloop and polypectomy snare for retraction and resection and endoclips for closure of the gastrostomy [30]. Outcomes of this survival study included a septic complication in one animal related to incomplete closure of the gastrostomy. Transgastric salpingectomy and oophorectomy was described by Wagh in three acute and nine survival swine experiments with endoclip closure of the gastrostomy with no adverse events [31, 32]. These studies again demonstrate the feasibility of NOTES organ or partial organ resection and the importance of achieving adequate and secure closure of the viscerotomy.

10.7.5.5 Conclusion

Overall, these experimental studies of NOTES organ resection in swine demonstrate the feasibility of using single or dual transluminal access to perform endoscopic procedures ranging in complexity from oophorectomy to distal pancreatectomy and nephrectomy. The importance of developing new devices such as endoscopic staplers, sealing, and morcellation devices to permit safe completion of these procedures and safe extraction of specimens is particular emphasized. These procedures all have potential applications in the oncologic setting, but more experimental and clinical data are needed.

With the exception of transvaginal cholecystectomy described in swine and humans, other NOTES abdominal solid organ resection with potential oncologic applications include transvaginal hysterectomy, oophorectomy, and salpingectomy performed with laparoscopic assistance in humans as previously described (Table 10.2) [3]. These procedures were performed using three 3-mm transabdominal laparoscopic ports and a 12-mm vaginal port used in combination for insufflation, endoscopic visualization, retraction, dissection, morcellation, and specimen extraction with successful completion of all procedures and no surgical complications [3].

10.7.6 Intestinal Resection

Although intestinal resection has not yet been described in an experimental or clinical setting, a recently published feasibility study in three human cadavers described radical sigmoid resection using TEM [67]. TEM is typically performed through a 4-cm-wide rectoscope connected to a magnifying optical lens and camera, a CO_2 insufflator to establish pneumorectum, through which long dissecting instruments can be introduced. TEM has been used since 1982 to perform mucosal and full-thickness excision of rectal lesions including adenomas, strictures, carcinoid tumors, and T1 rectal cancer not otherwise accessible endoscopically or transanally due to location or size. In this preliminary study, TEM was used to enter the presacral space through a full-thickness incision through the rectal wall with circumferential resection of the sigmoid colon and mesentery using the rectoscope as an overtube to facilitate retraction and exposure [67]. The length of the dissecting instruments limited the proximal extent of colonic dissection to the proximal sigmoid. Following colonic mobilization, the specimen was pulled out through the anus, transected, and anastomosed to the rectum using a circular stapler. Given the integrity of the specimen and its mesentery, this study suggests that this approach might be useful as an alternative to open or laparoscopic rectosigmoid resection in the clinical setting provided that adequate vascular control, length of colon resection, and anastomosis can be achieved. Long-term survival data will be required to evaluate outcomes of this promising approach for colorectal resection before it can be considered for colorectal cancer resections [67].

10.8 Optimal Access to NOTES

10.8.1 Trans-gastric Route

Regarding access for transluminal surgery, based on the available data, the optimal approach remains unclear. Since the introduction of NOTES, transgastric endoscopic access has remained the most popular type of transluminal access due to the relative ease of access and limited risk of intra-abdominal contamination. However, one of the limiting factors to widespread application of transgastric NOTES procedures as reflected in the experimental data has been difficulties related to gastrostomy closure. The use of a gastrostomy tube [10], endoscopic clips with or without endoloops [30], prototype endoscopic suturing and plicating devices [20, 68, 69] or linear staplers [70], or no formal closure [29] has been described with limited experience. With the exception of critically ill patients and/or patients with an existing gastrostomy tube in whom closure of NOTES gastrostomy with a PEG tube can be achieved with minimal morbidity [36], the consensus remains that extensive laboratory training is needed before transgastric endoscopic intra-abdominal or intrathoracic procedures can be routinely performed in humans. At present, all human NOTES procedures should be performed under the scrutiny of an Institutional Review Board (IRB). Additional difficulties specific to transgastric access include the lack of a stable platform for scope manipulation and difficulties with spatial orientation during retro-flexion of the endoscope required to visualize upper abdominal structures.

10.8.2 Trans-vesical Route

To address concerns related to gastrostomy closure, endoscopic access through the bladder was proposed as a relatively sterile transluminal alternative where closure might not even be required. Transvesical access to the peritoneal and thoracic cavity, however, was achieved using a 5.5-mm endoscope which would not accommodate tools needed to perform more complex procedures [13].

10.8.3 Trans-esophageal Route

Transesophageal access with or without submucosal endoscopy and mucosal flap was also described as an alternative that only requires simple mucosal closure [14, 59]. This approach was described to gain access to the posterior mediastinum in an experimental model [14, 59]. However, this type of access is limited in scope to cardiothoracic applications and carries significant risk of mediastinal contamination.

10.8.4 Transvaginal Route

Transvaginal access has recently been described with NOTES transvaginal cholecystectomy having been performed successfully in several female patients with the addition of one or more laparoscopic ports [39, 40]. Transvaginal access has the advantage of a relatively safe entry site with limited risk of adjacent organ injury and potential bacterial contamination, and of a relatively easy closure which alleviates concerns regarding viscerotomy closure. This approach is limited, however, by the fact that it can only be performed in female patients and raises concerns regarding long-term effects of transvaginal access such as dyspareunia. In addition, all transvaginal procedures performed in the setting of NOTES thus far have been performed with laparoscopic assistance [21, 39] or in combination with other types of transluminal access [27].

10.8.5 Trans-colonic Route

Transcolonic NOTES has been described in few reports, mainly due to concerns related to fecal contamination of the abdominal cavity. Transcolonic peritoneoscopy ($N=11$) [11, 12] and cholecystectomy ($N=5$) [24] have been published in several reports with peritonitis occurring in one animal (9%) following an unsuccessful attempt at complete closure of the anterior colotomy [21].

10.8.6 Dual-port Access

Finally, dual-port access has been recently described as a technique that could eliminate the need for laparoscopic assistance and optimize endoscopic visualization and organ retraction to perform complex surgical tasks. Dual transvaginal and transcolonic access was used to perform endoscopic distal pancreatectomy, using the colonic access for dissection and the vaginal access for stapling of the pancreas [27]. Combined transgastric and transvesical endoscopic access was used to perform cholecystectomy in seven [21] and nephrectomy in six [66] acute swine experiments. The procedures, which included both right and left nephrectomy, could be completed by alternating ports for retraction and dissection of the renal hilum.

10.8.7 Conclusion

Overall, there are several important benefits and disadvantages to each type of transluminal access and if complex procedures including oncologic procedures are to be performed using "pure" NOTES, multiluminal access might be better suited. Data from experimental studies on solid organ resection identified several issues that may play an important role in the selection of the optimal type of transluminal access for oncologic NOTES including the method of specimen extraction and the availability of specialized endoscopic bags and morcellation devices.

10.9 Final Remarks

Since the original description of transgastric peritoneoscopy in swine and the first clinical reports of transgastric endoscopic appendectomy in 2004, NOTES has generated tremendous interest from gastroenterologists and surgeons and stimulated extensive research to investigate the feasibility and outcomes of

NOTES for a wide range of surgical applications. Most experimental studies published consist of case reports and series with short-term survival data. While NOTES has significant advantages over open and laparoscopic procedures related to the lack of skin incisions, considerable experience is still needed to establish optimal transluminal access, optimize viscerotomy closure, develop endoscopic equipment specialized to perform NOTES procedures, and anticipate NOTES-specific complications in order to prevent and treat them effectively. Concerns for patient safety in the face of incomplete experimental data and limited clinical experience as highlighted by NOSCAR should result in strict regulation of the clinical application of NOTES through the IRB. Five published reports to date have described initial clinical experience with select NOTES procedures and one report has specifically investigated and confirmed the safety and feasibility of NOTES peritoneoscopy in the evaluation of pancreatic cancer resectability relative to diagnostic laparoscopy. Based on this report and other published experimental and clinical NOTES experience, a wide range of procedures of increasing complexity can be achieved safely and might have potential applications in oncologic resections. Additional experience including long-term survival data in experimental oncologic models and clinical data will be needed before definite conclusions on the feasibility and safety of NOTES in oncology can be established.

References

1. Baron, T.H., Gostout, C.J., Herman, L., et al.: Hemoclip repair of a sphincterotomy-induced duodenal perforation. Gastrointest. Endosc. **52**, 566–568 (2000)
2. Tsunada, S., Ogata, S., Ohyama, T., et al.: Endoscopic closure of perforations caused by EMR in the stomach by application of metallic clips. Gastrointest. Endosc. **57**, 948–951 (2003)
3. Tsin, D.A., Columbero, L.T., Lambeck, J., et al.: Minilaparoscopy-assisted natural orifice surgery. JSLS **11**, 24–29 (2007)
4. Gettman, M.T., Lotan, Y., Napper, C.A., et al.: Transvaginal laparoscopic nephrectomy: development and feasibility in the porcine model. Urology **59**, 446–450 (2002)
5. Kalloo, A.N., Singh, V.K., Jagannath, S.B., et al.: Flexible transgastric peritoneoscopy: a novel approach to diagnostic and therapeutic interventions in the peritoneal cavity. Gastrointest. Endosc. **60**, 114–117 (2004)
6. Rattner, D., Kalloo, A., ASGE/SAGES Working Group: ASGE/SAGES Working Group on natural orifice translumenal endoscopic surgery. Surg. Endosc. **20**, 329–333 (2005)
7. Lima, E., Rolanda, C., Pogo, J.M., et al.: Transvesical endoscopic peritoneoscopy: a novel 5 mm port for intra-abdominal scarless surgery. J. Urol. **176**, 802–805 (2006)
8. Rentschler, M.E., Dumpert, J., Platt, S.R., et al.: Natural orifice surgery with an endoluminal mobile robot. Surg. Endosc. **21**, 1212–1215 (2007)
9. Kantsevoy, S.V., Jagannath, S.B., Niiyama, H., et al.: A novel safe approach to the peritoneal cavity for per-oral transgastric endoscopic procedures. Gastrointest. Endosc. **65**, 497–500 (2007)
10. Onders, R.P., McGee, M.F., Marks, J., et al.: Natural orifice transluminal endoscopic surgery (NOTES) as a diagnostic tool in the intensive care unit. Surg. Endosc. **21**, 681–683 (2007)
11. Fong, D.G., Pai, R.D., Thompson, C.C., et al.: Transcolonic endoscopic abdominal exploration: a NOTES survival study in a porcine model. Gastrointest. Endosc. **65**, 312–318 (2007)
12. Wilhelm, D., Meining, A., von Delius, S., et al.: An innovative, safe and sterile sigmoid access (ISSA) for NOTES. Endoscopy **39**, 401–406 (2007)
13. Lima, E., Henriques-Coelho, T., Rolanda, C., et al.: Transvesical thoracoscopy: a natural orifice Transluminal endoscopic approach for thoracic surgery. Surg. Endosc. **21**, 854–858 (2007)
14. Sumiyama, K., Gostout, C.J., Rajan, E., et al.: Transesophageal mediastinoscopy by submucosal endoscopy with mucosal flap safety valve technique. Gastrointest. Endosc. **65**, 679–683 (2007)
15. Fritscher-Ravens, A., Mosse, C.A., Ikeda, K., et al.: Endoscopic transgastric lymphadenectomy by using EUS for selection and guidance. Gastrointest. Endosc. **63**, 302–306 (2006)
16. Kantsevoy, S.V., Jagannath, S.B., Niiyama, H., et al.: Endoscopic gastrojejunostomy with survival in a porcine model. Gastrointest. Endosc. **62**, 287–292 (2005)
17. Kantsevoy, S.V., Niiyama, H., Jagannath, S.B., et al.: The endoscopic transilluminator: an endoscopic device for identification of the proximal jejunum for transgastric endoscopic gastrojejunostomy. Gastrointest. Endosc. **63**, 1055–1058 (2006)
18. Bergstrom, M., Ikeda, K., Swain, P., et al.: Transgastric anastomosis by using flexible endoscopy in a porcine model (with video). Gastrointest. Endosc. **63**, 307–312 (2006)
19. Kantsevoy, S.V., Hu, B., Jagannath, S.B., et al.: Technical feasibility of endoscopic gastric reduction: a pilot study in a porcine model. Gastrointest. Endosc. **65**, 510–513 (2007)
20. Park, P.O., Bergstrom, M., Ikeda, K., et al.: Experimental studies of transgastric gallbladder surgery: cholecystectomy and cholecystogastric anastomosis (videos). Gastrointest. Endosc. **61**, 601–606 (2005)
21. Pai, R.D., Fong, D.G., Bundga, M.E., et al.: Transcolonic endoscopic cholecystectomy: a NOTES survival study in a porcine model (with video). Gastrointest. Endosc. **64**, 428–434 (2006)
22. Scott, D.J., Tang, S.J., Fernandez, R., et al.: Completely transvaginal NOTES cholecystectomy using magnetically anchored instruments. Surg. Endosc. **21**, 2308–2316 (2007)

23. Sumiyama, K., Gostout, C.J., Rajan, E., et al.: Transgastric cholecystectomy: transgastric accessibility to the gallbladder improved with the SEMF method and a novel multibending therapeutic endoscope. Gastrointest. Endosc. **65**, 1028–1034 (2007)
24. Rolanda, C., Lima, E., Pego, J.M., et al.: Third-generation cholecystectomy by natural orifices: transgastric and transvesical combined approach (with video). Gastrointest. Endosc. **65**, 111–117 (2007)
25. Kantsevoy, S.V., Jagannath, S.B., Vaughn, C.A., et al.: Transgastric endoscopic splenectomy. Surg. Endosc. **20**, 522–525 (2006)
26. Matthes, K., Yusuf, T.E., Willingham, F.F., et al.: Feasibility of endoscopic transgastric distal pancreatectomy in a porcine animal model. Gastrointest. Endosc. **66**, 762–766 (2007)
27. Ryou, M., Fong, D.G., Pai, R.D., et al.: Dual-port distal pancreatectomy using a prototype endoscope and endoscopic stapler: a natural orifice transluminal endoscopic surgery (NOTES) survival study in a porcine model. Endoscopy **39**, 881–887 (2007)
28. Clayman, R.V., Box, G.N., Abraham, J.B., et al.: Rapid communication: transvaginal single-port NOTES nephrectomy: initial laboratory experience. J. Endourol. **21**, 640–644 (2007)
29. Jagannath, S.B., Kantsevoy, S.V., Vaughn, C.A., et al.: Peroral transgastric endoscopic ligation of fallopian tubes with long-term survival in a porcine model. Gastrointest. Endosc. **61**, 449–453 (2005)
30. Merrifield, B.F., Wagh, M.S., Thompson, C.C.: Peroral transgastric organ resection: a feasibility study in pigs. Gastrointest. Endosc. **63**, 693–697 (2006)
31. Wagh, M.S., Merrifield, B.F., Thompson, C.C.: Endoscopic transgastric abdominal exploration and organ resection: initial experience in a porcine model. Clin. Gastroenterol. Hepatol. **3**, 892–896 (2005)
32. Wagh, M.S., Merrifield, B.F., Thompson, C.C.: Survival studies after endoscopic transgastric oophorectomy and tubectomy in a porcine model. Gastrointest. Endosc. **63**, 473–478 (2006)
33. Onders, R., McGee, M.F., Marks, J., et al.: Diaphragm pacing with natural orifice transluminal endoscopic surgery: potential for difficult-to-wean intensive care unit patients. Surg. Endosc. **21**, 475–479 (2007)
34. Hu, B., Kalloo, A.N., Chung, S.S., et al.: Peroral transgastric endoscopic primary repair of a ventral hernia in a porcine model. Endoscopy **39**, 390–393 (2007)
35. Fong, D.G., Ryou, M., Pai, R.D., et al.: Transcolonic ventral wall hernia mesh fixation in a porcine model. Endoscopy **39**, 865–869 (2007)
36. Marks, J.M., Ponsky, J.L., Pearl, J.P., et al.: PEG "rescue": a practical NOTES technique. Surg. Endosc. **21**, 816–819 (2007)
37. Gettman, M.T., Blute, M.L.: Transvesical peritoneoscopy: initial clinical evaluation of the bladder as a portal for natural orifice Transluminal endoscopic surgery. Mayo Clin. Proc. **82**, 843–845 (2007)
38. Hazey, J.W., Narula, V.K., Renton, D.B., et al.: Natural-orifice transgastric endoscopic peritoneoscopy in humans: initial clinical trial. Surg. Endosc. **22**, 16–20 (2008)
39. Bessler, M., Stevens, P.D., Milone, L., et al.: Transvaginal laparoscopically assisted endoscopic cholecystectomy: a hybrid approach to natural orifice surgery. Gastrointest. Endosc. **66**, 1243–1245 (2007)
40. Marescaux, J., Dallemagne, B., Perretta, S., et al.: Surgery without scars: report of transluminal cholecystectomy in a human being. Arch. Surg. **142**, 823–826 (2007)
41. Allendorf, J.D., Bessler, M., Kayton, M.L., et al.: Increased tumor establishment and growth after laparotomy vs laparoscopy in a murine model. Arch. Surg. **130**, 649–653 (1995)
42. Lee, S.W., Southall, J.C., Allendorf, J.D., et al.: Tumor proliferative index is higher in mice undergoing laparotomy vs. CO_2 pneumoperitoneum. Dis. Colon Rectum **42**, 477–481 (1999)
43. Shiromizu, A., Suematsu, T., Yamaguchi, K., et al.: Effect of laparotomy and laparoscopy on the establishment of lung metastasis in a murine model. Surgery **128**, 799–805 (2000)
44. Southall, J.C., Lee, S.W., Allendorf, J.D., et al.: Colon adenocarcinoma and B-16 melanoma grow larger following laparotomy vs. pneumoperitoneum in a murine model. Dis. Colon Rectum **41**, 564–569 (1998)
45. Lee, S.W., Gleason, N., Blanco, I., et al.: Higher colon cancer tumor proliferative index and lower tumor cell death rate in mice undergoing laparotomy versus insufflation. Surg. Endosc. **16**, 36–39 (2002)
46. Allendorf, J.D., Bessler, M., Horvath, K.D., et al.: Increased tumor establishment and growth after open vs laparoscopic surgery in mice may be related to differences in postoperative T-cell function. Surg. Endosc. **13**, 233–235 (1999)
47. Von Ott, D.: Die Beleuchtung der Bauchhohle (Ventroskopie) als Mehode bei Vaginaler Coeliotomie. Abl. Gynakol. **231**, 817–823 (1902)
48. Paulson, J.D., Ross, J.W., El-Sahwi, S.: Development of flexible culdoscopy. J. Am. Assoc. Gynecol. Laparosc. **6**, 487–490 (1999)
49. Da, T., Columbero, L.T., Mahmood, D., et al.: Operative culdolaparoscopy: a new approach combining operative culdoscopy and minilaparoscopy. J. Am. Assoc. Gynecol. Laparosc. **8**, 438–441 (2001)
50. Waller, D.A., Forty, J., Morritt, G.N.: Video-assisted thoracoscopic surgery versus thoracotomy for spontaneous pneumothorax. Ann. Thorac. Surg. **58**, 372–376 (1994)
51. Ayed, A.K., Raghunathan, R.: Thoracoscopy versus open lung biopsy in the diagnosis of interstitial lung disease: a randomized controlled trial. J. R. Coll. Surg. Edinb. **45**, 159–163 (2000)
52. Santambrogio, L., Nosotti, M., Bellaviti, N., et al.: Videothoracoscopy versus thoracotomy for the diagnosis of the indeterminate solitary pulmonary nodule. Ann. Thorac. Surg. **59**, 868–870 (1995)
53. Solaini, L., Prusciano, F., Bagioni, P. et al.: Video-assisted thoracic surgery (VATS) of the lung. Analysis of intraoperative and postoperative complications over 15 years and review of the literature. Surg. Endosc. **22**, 298–310 (2008)
54. Larsen, S.S., Vilmann, P., Krasnik, M., et al.: Endoscopic ultrasound guided biopsy performed routinely in lung cancer staging spares futile thoracotomies: preliminary results from a randomised clinical trial. Lung Cancer **49**, 377–385 (2005)
55. Fritscher-Ravens, A., Sriram, P.V., Pothman, W.P., et al.: Bedside endosonography and endosonography-guided fine-needle

aspiration in critically ill patients: a way out of the deadlock? Endoscopy **32**, 425–427 (2000)
56. Eloubeidi, M.A., Cerfolio, R.J., Chen, V.K., et al.: Endoscopic ultrasound-guided fine needle aspiration of mediastinal lymph node in patients with suspected lung cancer after positron emission tomography and computed tomography scans. Ann. Thorac. Surg. **79**, 263–268 (2005)
57. Fernandez-Esparrach, G., Gines, A., Belda, J., et al.: Transesophageal ultrasound-guided fine needle aspiration improves mediastinal staging in patients with non-small cell lung cancer and normal mediastinum on computed tomography. Lung Cancer **54**, 35–40 (2006)
58. Fritscher-Ravens, A., Bohuslavizki, K.H., Brandt, L., et al.: Mediastinal lymph node involvement in potentially resectable lung cancer: comparison of CT, positron emission tomography, and endoscopic ultrasonography with and without fine-needle aspiration. Chest **123**, 442–451 (2003)
59. Fritscher-Ravens, A., Patel, K., Ghanbari, A., et al.: Natural orifice transluminal endoscopic surgery (NOTES) in the mediastinum: long-term survival animal experiments in transesophageal access, including minor surgical procedures. Endoscopy **39**, 870–875 (2007)
60. Al-Rashedy, M., Dadibhai, M., Shareif, A., et al.: Laparoscopic gastric bypass for gastric outlet obstruction is associated with smoother, faster recovery and shorter hospital stay compared with open surgery. J. Hepatobiliary Pancreat. Surg. **12**, 474–478 (2005)
61. Choi, Y.B.: Laparoscopic gatrojejunostomy for palliation of gastric outlet obstruction in unresectable gastric cancer. Surg. Endosc. **16**, 1620–1626 (2002)
62. Jeurnink, S.M., van Eijck, C.H., Steyerberg, E.W., et al.: Stent versus gastrojejunostomy for the palliation of gastric outlet obstruction: a systematic review. BMC Gastroenterol. **7**, 18 (2007)
63. Del Piano, M., Ballare, M., Montino, F., et al.: Endoscopy or surgery for malignant GI outlet obstruction ? Gastrointest. Endosc. **61**, 421–426 (2005)
64. Maetani, I., Akatsuka, S., Ikeda, M., et al.: Self-expandable metallic stent placement for palliation in gastric outlet obstructions caused by gastric cancer: a comparison with surgical gastrojejunostomy. J. Gastroenterol. **40**, 932–937 (2005)
65. Mosler, P., Mergener, K.D., Brandabur, J.J., et al.: Palliation of gastric outlet obstruction and proximal small bowel obstruction with self-expandable metal stents: a single center series. J. Clin. Gastroenterol. **39**, 124–128 (2005)
66. Lima, E., Rolanda, C., Pego, J.M., et al.: Third-generation nephrectomy by natural orifice transluminal endoscopic surgery. J. Urol. **178**, 2648–2654 (2007)
67. Whiteford, M.H., Denk, P.M., Swanstrom, L.L.: Feasibility of radical sigmoid colectomy performed as natural orifice Transluminal endoscopic surgery (NOTES) using transanal endoscopic microsurgery. Surg. Endosc. **21**, 1870–1874 (2007)
68. McGee, M.F., Marks, J.M., Onders, R.P., et al.: Complete endoscopic closure of gastrostomy after natural orifice transluminal endoscopic surgery using the NDO plicator. Surg. Endosc. **22**, 214–220 (2008)
69. Mellinger, J.D., MacFadyen, B.V., Kozarek, R.A., et al.: Initial experience with a novel endoscopic device allowing intragastric manipulation and placation. Surg. Endosc. **21**, 1002–1005 (2007)
70. Magno, P., Giday, S.A., Dray, X., et al.: A new stapler-based full-thickness transgastric access closure: results from an animal pilot trial. Endoscopy **39**, 876–880 (2007)

Part II

Special Topics: Cancer of the Esophagus and the Gastro-Esophageal Junction

11 Cancer of the Esophagus and the Gastroesophageal Junction: Two-cavity Approach

Christopher R. Morse, Omar Awais, and James D. Luketich

11.1 Introduction

The incidence of esophageal cancer has been increasing by approximately 10% per year in the United States [1]. Approximately 15,000 people are diagnosed with esophageal cancer each year and 14,000 are expected to die from it [2]. Because of the propensity of esophageal cancer to metastasize early and the often advanced stage of the disease at the time of diagnosis, the survival rate has improved only slightly, from 6% to 15%, over the last 3 decades [2–4] Ninety-five percent of all esophageal cancers are either squamous cell carcinoma (SCC) or adenocarcinoma. For most of the last century, SCC comprised the vast majority of esophageal cancers and esophageal adenocarcinomas were considered extremely uncommon. However, over the past 2 decades, the incidence of adenocarcinoma has increased dramatically in Western countries, becoming the most predominant histologic type in the United States [5, 6]. The two forms of esophageal cancer differ in a number of features as smoking and alcohol are major predisposing factors for SCC, while Barrett's esophagus, obesity, and, possibly, GERD are the risk factors for adenocarcinoma, but their treatments strategies are similar [7].

C.R. Morse
Division of Thoracic Surgery Massachusetts
General Hospital/Harvard Medical School 55 Fruit St.,
Boston, MA 02114, USA

O. Awais and J.D. Luketich (✉)
Division of Thoracic and Foregut Surgery, Heart, Lung and Esophageal Surgery Institute, Department of Cardiothoracic Surgery, University of Pittsburgh Medical Center Health System, UPMC Cancer Centers, UPMC Presbyterian, Digestive Disorders Center,
200 Lothrop Street, Pittsburgh, PA, USA
e-mail: luketichjd@upmc.edu

11.2 Anatomy of the Esophagus

The esophagus includes cervical, thoracic, and abdominal segments and travels through the posterior mediastinum to join the stomach via the esophageal hiatus of the diaphragm. It is accompanied along its course by the anterior and posterior vagal trunks. The esophagus is a muscular tube, approximately 25cm long, and lacks a serosal layer. It is lined with squamous epithelium and transitions from striated muscle to smooth muscle in its decent through the thoracic cavity. The blood supply of the esophagus is segmental, with limited overlap, but the lymphatic anatomy is rich in intramural, extramural, and transmural lymphatic channels, allowing for rapid spread of esophageal cancer from an early localized tumor to metastatic disease.

11.3 Most Commonly Performed Resections

Surgical resection remains the primary treatment modality for resectable esophageal cancer, and transhiatal esophagectomy or Ivor Lewis esophagogastrectomy are the two most commonly performed operations.

A *transhiatal esophagectomy* is performed through

- Midline abdominal incision
- Blunt dissection of the thoracic esophagus through the esophageal hiatus
- A gastric pull-up
- Cervical esophagogastric anastomosis

An *Ivor Lewis esophagectomy* is performed through

- Upper midline abdominal incision
- Mobilization and creation of the gastric conduit
- Right thoracotomy with dissection and removal of the thoracic esophagus
- Construction of an intrathoracic esophagogastric anastomosis

Both transhiatal and Ivor Lewis esophagectomy are complex operations that have considerable morbidity and mortality in the range of 6–7% in experienced centers [8]. However, in a national review, the mortality rate from esophagectomy ranges from 8% in high-volume centers to as much as 23% in low-volume centers [9].

11.4 Role of Laparoscopy in Esophageal Cancer

Laparoscopy has become the standard approach in the treatment of a variety of benign esophageal diseases, such as reflux and achalasia. This shift has been driven by a consistent observation that minimally invasive surgery is associated with equal efficacy, less pain, and an earlier return to work as compared to open surgery. An open approach is still the standard of care for patients with esophageal cancer, because of concerns that minimally invasive surgery may not be equivalent in terms of nodal clearance and completeness of resection and may not have a measurable impact on morbidity.

We would argue, though, that minimally invasive esophagectomy (MIE) is associated with less morbidity and mortality than the open approach [10] Two of the more frequent complications following esophagectomy are pneumonia and pulmonary failure; with pneumonia carrying a 20% mortality risk. The avoidance of synchronous laparotomy and thoracotomy incisions may reduce the incidence of these complications. Although no randomized studies have been performed, our experience and that of others suggests that MIE is associated with a lower rate of complications and mortality than that following open esophagectomy.

11.5 Evolution of Minimally Invasive Techniques in Esophageal Surgery

The minimally invasive approach to esophagectomy was initially a hybrid operation consisting of thoracoscopy with esophageal mobilization to reduce the respiratory morbidity associated with a right thoracotomy [11, 12]. Thoracoscopic esophageal mobilization, however, still required a standard midline laparotomy for construction of the gastric conduit in combination with gastric pull-up, and construction of a cervical esophagogastric anastomosis. Alternatively, another hybrid technique for esophagectomy was described with laparoscopic construction of the gastric conduit followed by a right thoracotomy for removal of the thoracic esophagus and construction of an intrathoracic anastomosis [13, 14]. These two hybrid approaches to esophagectomy utilized minimally invasive techniques, but required either a thoracotomy or laparotomy.

In 1995, Depaula described 48 patients who underwent a laparoscopic transhiatal esophagectomy predominantly for end stage megaesophagus secondary to Chagas disease. Their approach consisted of laparoscopic construction of the gastric conduit followed by laparoscopic mobilization of the mediastinal esophagus through the esophageal hiatus. A neck incision was performed for construction of an esophagogastric anastomosis. Only two patients were converted to an open esophagectomy [15]. Two years later, Swanstrom described 9 patients with small tumors, benign strictures, and Barrett's esophagus who underwent minimally invasive transhiatal esophagectomy [16]. Subsequently in 1998, Luketich et al. reported the combined thoracoscopic and laparoscopic approach to esophagectomy [17]. Our early technique consisted of thoracoscopic esophageal mobilization, followed by laparoscopic construction of the gastric conduit, gastric pull-up, and a neck anastomosis (Table 11.1). In 1999, a minimally invasive Ivor Lewis technique was reported by Watson et al, who described the laparoscopic construction of a gastric conduit, followed by thoracoscopic esophagectomy with the construction of an intrathoracic esophagogastric anastomosis [22] (Table 11.2).

The benefit of the minimally invasive Ivor Lewis approach is that it avoids a neck incision, thereby lowering the likelihood of a recurrent laryngeal nerve injury. Initially, our operation was a hybrid,

Table 11.1 Thoracoscopic and laparoscopic esophagectomy with cervical anastomosis: Outcomes in selected series

	Year	n	Mean OR time (min)	Median hospital stay (day)	Mortality 30 day (%)	Leak rate (%)	Conversion rate (%)
Watson et al. [18]	2000	7	265[a]	12	0	28.5	14.3
Nguyen et al. [19]	2003	46	350	8	4.3	4.3	2.2
Luketich et al. [10]	2003	222	–	7	1.4	11.7	7.2
Collins et al. [20]	2006	25	350	9	4	12	8
Leibman et al. [21]	2006	25	330[a]	11	0	8	8

OR operative time, – data not available

[a]Median value

Table 11.2 Laparoscopic and thoracoscopic Jvor Lewis esophagectomy: Outcomes in selected series

	Year	n	Mean OR time (min)	Mean hospital stay (day)	Mortality 30 day (%)	Leak rate (%)	Conversion rate (%)
Watson et al. [22]	1999	2	255	10	0	0	0
Nguyen et al. [23]	2001	1	450	8	0	0	0
Kunisaki et al. [24]	2004	15	544	29.6	0	13.3	–
Bizekis, et al. [25][a]	2006	35	–	7	6%	6%	2%

OR operative time, – data not available

[a]15 patients underwent minithoracotomy and were analyzed separately

encompassing laparoscopy with a right mini thoracotomy. As our experience grew, we began to perform the operation totally minimally invasively. We have performed close to 250 minimally invasive Ivor Lewis esophagectomies. The operative details are similar to the three-hole approach, except that we start the operation with laparoscopic construction of the gastric conduit, followed by right VATS.

11.6 Nonsurgical Management of Esophageal Cancer

For superficial cancers of the esophagus and high-grade dysplasia (HGD), the standard of care has been esophagectomy [26, 27]. However, endoscopic approaches such as photodynamic therapy (PDT) and endoscopic mucosal resection as definitive therapy for HGD and superficial cancers have become increasingly popular. These techniques are appropriate only for patients who have a small risk of lymph node metastases. PDT induces cell death with the injection of a photosensitizing agent and exposure of light at an appropriate wavelength via an endoscope. Long-term tumor control has been achieved in small numbers of patients treated with PDT (with or without EMR), but experience is limited [28, 29]. With endoscopic mucosal resection (EMR), neoplastic epithelium is excised rather than ablated and an understanding of the efficacy of EMR for management of superficial esophageal cancer is still evolving. Although randomized trials are not yet available, in appropriately selected patients, the success rate with EMR may be comparable to that with surgical therapy, but with potentially fewer complications. EMR is occasionally used in conjunction with PDT to allow for the treatment of larger lesions [26, 30].

Recently, two randomized trials directly compared chemoradiation alone to chemoradiation followed by surgery [31, 32]. Both studies failed to demonstrate better survival with esophagectomy, although both did show better locoregional control with surgery. Important to note is the fact that the pathology in both series were either exclusively or predominantly SCC. When examined closely, these studies suggest that patients who undergo esophagectomy after chemoradiation have better locoregional control and a similar quality of life. Thus, surgery remains the preferred treatment approach for clinically resectable esophageal cancer, particularly for adenocarcinoma, as there is little data regarding nonsurgical management.

11.7 Staging of Esophageal Cancer

11.7.1 Noninvasive Staging Modalities

Preoperative evaluation of a patient for MIE is no different than that for a patient undergoing an open procedure. The two primary issues are whether a patient is resectable, and whether the patient has sufficient cardio-pulmonary reserve to tolerate the operation. Staging of esophageal cancer at our center includes

- Upper endoscopy
- Endoscopic ultrasound (– EUS)
- Computed tomography (CT) scanning
- PET scanning

Upper endoscopy is performed to identify the proximal and distal extent of the tumor, which may have an impact on the type of procedure; this is often done in the operating room at the time of the operation. The primary benefit of EUS is to determine the degree of invasion of the esophageal wall by tumor. Patients with T3 or N1 disease are usually treated with induction chemotherapy prior to esophagectomy. CT imaging is useful to determine the presence of bulky nodal disease within the abdomen. Bulky disease limited to the celiac nodal basin does not preclude esophagectomy, provided there is significant response to induction therapy. Finally, PET scanning, along with CT imaging, is primarily used to rule out distant metastatic disease which would preclude esophagectomy. We have not found PET particularly helpful in identifying periesophageal nodal disease as activity within these nodes is often obscured by the primary tumor.

11.7.2 Invasive Staging – Laparoscopy

A final staging modality often used at our center is laparoscopy. Typically, patients undergo laparoscopy at the time of placement of an infusaport for induction chemotherapy. We have found laparoscopy to be a simple and safe method to identify abdominal metastases to the liver or peritoneum that may not be seen on CT imaging. In addition, the presence of bulky nodal disease can be assessed by laparoscopy and confirmed by biopsy. For these patients, additional radiation therapy may be added to the neoadjuvant treatment plan. Laparoscopy can usually be completed within 30 min, and patients can be discharged on the same day.

11.8 Other Preoperative Considerations

Patients with a significant tobacco history should also undergo pulmonary function testing. In addition, the majority of patients with locally advanced cancer will have some degree of dysphagia and weight loss prior to diagnosis. Dysphagia often will improve with induction therapy. If the patient has severe dysphagia, we will place a jejunostomy tube during laparoscopic staging, although this has not been common practice at our institution. We strongly discourage the placement of either an esophageal stent or percutaneous gastrostomy tube for any patient who may be an operative candidate. Esophagectomy may still be performed in these situations, although it will render an already technically challenging procedure even more complex.

11.9 Surgical Management of Esophageal Cancer

11.9.1 Abdominal Dissection

11.9.1.1 Patient Positioning and On-table Endoscopy

The patient is initially positioned supine and is intubated with a double-lumen endotracheal tube. We proceed with an on-table endoscopy to assess tumor location and extension, both proximally and distally (on to the cardia of the stomach). The suitability of the stomach as a gastric conduit is also evaluated. If the tumor and the preoperative evaluation are favorable for resection, we start with the laparoscopic abdominal portion of the operation.

11.9.1.2 Operating Room Set-up and Trocar Placement

The surgeon remains on the right side while the assistant is positioned to the patients left side. Five abdominal ports are used for the gastric mobilization. A set of four 5-mm trocars and one 10- to 12-mm trocar is usually sufficient. The camera port is inserted above the umbilicus to the left of the midline and is usually a 5-mm trocar. Mirroring the camera port, we place a 10- to 12-mm trocar at the same level to the right of the midline. This trocar is used for the stapling device. The working ports, 5-mm trocars, are inserted in the subcostal area, two on the right side and one on the left. If necessary, a sixth trocar is added to facilitate retraction and creation of the gastric conduit. The initial port is placed via an open technique, while the remaining ports are placed under direct visualization. (Fig. 11.1)

11.9.1.3 Diagnostic Laparoscopy and Decision about Resectability

After an initial inspection of the peritoneal surfaces and the liver to rule out any metastatic disease, the gastro hepatic omentum is opened. The left gastric vascular pedicle is identified and the celiac nodes are examined. If there are any enlarged nodes suspicious for metastatic implants, they are dissected out and sent for frozen section analysis. If the nodes are not worrisome or return negative on frozen section, then we proceed with resection.

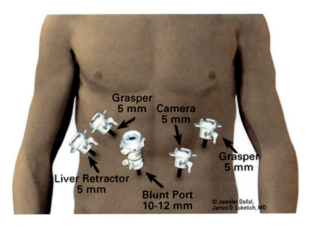

Fig. 11.1 Minimally invasive esophagectomy – two-cavity approach: Port placement for abdominal dissection

11.9.1.4 Mobilization of the Gastric Fundus

The right crus is dissected free, mobilizing the lateral aspect of the esophagus. The dissection is then carried anteriorly and superiorly on top of the esophagus, mobilizing the anterior hiatus. The dissection is continued toward the left crus in order to mobilize the fundus of the stomach. We attempt not to completely divide the phrenoesophageal ligament until the conclusion of laparoscopy as this allows for the maintenance of pneumoperitoneum. After creating a retroesophageal window by completing the dissection of the inferior aspect of the right crus, attention is turned to the gastrocolic omentum.

11.9.1.5 Mobilization of the Greater Curvature

By carefully retracting the antrum of the stomach, a window is created in the greater omentum, allowing access to the lesser sac. This is done while carefully preserving the right gastroepiploic vessels. The dissection is carried along the greater curvature of the stomach until the end of the gastroepipoloic arcade is reached. The short gastric vessels are taken either with ultrasonic shears (Ultrasonix, Hamonic scalpel) or the LigaSure™ device (Valleylab). Occasionally, clips are used to control large short gastric vessels.

11.9.1.6 Retrogastric Dissection

With the greater curvature mobilized, the fundus of the stomach is rotated toward the patient's right shoulder, exposing the retrogastric attachments. These are dissected free until the left gastric artery and vein are encountered. The retrogastric attachments are also divided toward the hiatus, completely mobilizing the fundus and the distal esophagus.

11.9.1.7 Mobilization of the Gastric Antrum

The mobilization of the stomach is then taken back toward the pyloro-antral region where the dissection must be meticulous. An injury to the gastroepiploic arcade or the gastroduodenal artery renders the gastric conduit unusable. There are significant retroantral and periduodenal adhesions that need to be divided to allow for adequate length of the gastric conduit to reach into the chest. As we have transitioned to an intrathoracic anastomosis, we have noted that an extensive Kocher maneuver is not necessary. The pylorus is considered adequately mobilized when it reaches the right crus without tension.

11.9.1.8 Dissection of Left Gastric Artery and Vein

Once the stomach is completely mobilized, the left gastric artery and vein are divided with an Endo GIA stapler, vascular load (USSC, Norwalk, CT). This is done by approaching the vascular pedicle from the lesser curvature. It is important to clear the pedicle completely off all nodal tissue and swipe all celiac nodes toward the specimen. Once the pedicle is divided, the distal esophagus, the gastric fundus, and antrum should be completely mobile.

11.9.1.9 Creation of the Gastric Conduit

The gastric conduit is created prior to the completion of the pyloroplasty and placement of the jejunostomy feeding tube. This sequence provides time to assess the viability of the conduit prior to bringing it into the chest. The first step in creating the gastric conduit is one firing of a vascular staple load across the vessels on the lesser curvature, but not onto the gastric antrum. The 10/12-mm right midclavicular port is changed to a 15-mm port to allow for the placement of a 4.8-mm Endo GIA stapler. An additional 12-mm port is placed in the right lower quadrant to assist with the creation of the gastric conduit. During this step, it is important to have the first assistant grasp the tip of the fundus along the greater curvature and gently stretch it toward the spleen, while a second grasper is placed at the antrum, with a slight downward retraction being applied. These two maneuvers put the stomach on a slight stretch and assist in creating a straight staple line. The staple line should parallel the gastroepiploic arcade. Initially, using 4.8-mm staple loads, the stomach is divided across the antrum with the goal of creating a conduit of 5- to 6-cm width (Fig. 11.2).

Early in our experience, we discovered a significant increase in gastric tip necrosis and anastomotic leaks with a conduit of only 3- to 4-cm width.

11.9.1.10 Division of the Antrum and Fundus

Once the antrum is divided, the right mid clavicular port is changed back to a 10/12-mm port and the fundus is divided using stapler loads of 3.5-mm heights. The graspers are readjusted as the fundus is divided, again to keep the stomach on stretch. If there is any concern about extension of tumor into the gastric cardia, a wider margin will be obtained in this region. It has not been our practice to routinely oversew the staple line. The right gastric vessels are preserved (Fig. 11.3).

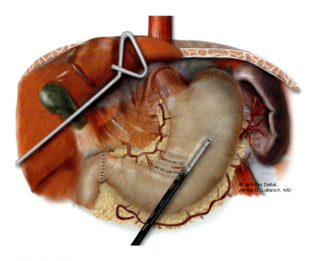

Fig. 11.2 Minimally invasive esophagectomy – two-cavity approach: Creation of gastric conduit-division of antrum

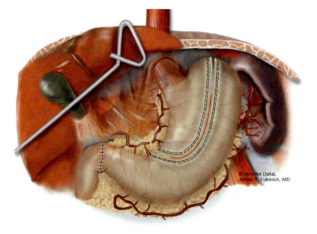

Fig. 11.3 Minimally invasive esophagectomy – two-cavity approach: Creation of gastric conduit-division of fundus

11.9.1.11 Pyloroplasty – Heinecke-mikulicz

Next a pyloroplasty is performed. Stay sutures are placed at the superior and inferior aspect of the pylorus (Fig. 11.4). Once the pylorus has been placed on stretch, we perform a full thickness pyloromyotomy with ultrasonic shears (Fig. 11.5). The pyloroplasty is closed in a Heineke-Mikulicz fashion, using interrupted sutures with the endostich device (USSC, Norwalk, CT) (Fig. 11.6 and Fig. 11.7). This usually requires three or four stitches. At the conclusion of the abdominal portion of the operation, the pyloroplasty will be covered with omentum. In our experience, a laparoscopic pyloromyotomy is difficult to perform.

11.9.1.12 Placing of a Feeding Jejunostomy

Using a needle catheter kit, a 5 or 7 Fr feeding jejunostomy is placed (Compat Biosystems, Minneapolis, MN) in the left lower quadrant. By reflecting the transverse colon anterior and cephelad, the ligament of Treitz is easily identified. A limb of jejunum of 30- to 40-cm length is chosen and tacked to the abdominal wall, using the endostich device. The additional port

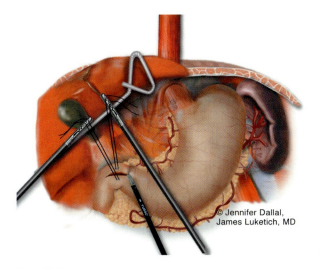

Fig. 11.4 Minimally invasive esophagectomy – two-cavity approach: Pyloroplasty-opening of pylorus in between stay sutures using harmonic scalpel

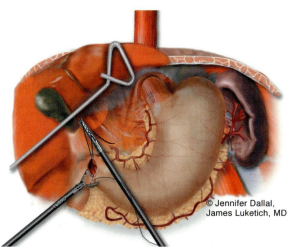

Fig. 11.6 Minimally invasive esophagectomy – two-cavity approach: Pyloroplasty Heineke-Mikulicz using the endo-stitch device

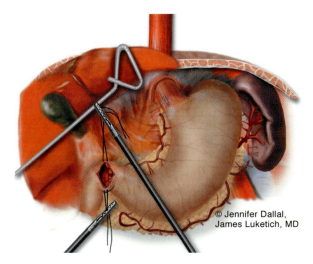

Fig. 11.5 Minimally invasive esophagectomy – completed pyloromyotomy

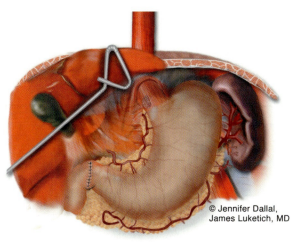

Fig. 11.7 Minimally invasive esophagectomy – two-cavity approach: Completed Heineke-Mikulicz pyloroplasty

placed in the right lower quadrant aids in this step. A needle and then a guidewire are passed into the jejunum under laparoscopic vision. Proper placement of the catheter is confirmed by observing distension of the jejunum as air is insufflated through the needle catheter. The jejunum surrounding the feeding tube is then tacked to the abdominal wall using several additional endostitches.

11.9.1.13 Maintaining Rotation of the Conduit

Finally, using an endostitch, the most superior portion of the gastric conduit is anchored to the specimen (Fig. 11.8). This stitch helps to maintain correct orientation of the gastric conduit as it is delivered into the chest. The laparoscopic portion of the procedure is completed by dividing the phrenoesophageal membrane. The crus are also assessed to determine if a stitch should be placed to avoid herniation of the conduit into the chest.

11.9.2 Thoracic Dissection

11.9.2.1 Operating Room Set-up and Trocar Placement

The patient is turned to the left lateral decubitus position for the throacoscopic mobilization of the esophagus and creation of the intrathoracic anastomosis. The operating surgeon stands on the right side of the table facing the patient's back. The assistant surgeon is positioned on the left side of the operating table. A total of five thoracoscopic ports are used. A 10-mm camera port is placed in the seventh or eighth intercostal space, just anterior to the midaxillary line. A 10-mm working port is placed at the eighth or ninth intercostal space, dorsal to the posterior axillary line. This port usually accommodates the surgeon's right hand. A 10-mm port is placed in the anterior axillary line in the fourth intercostal space, through which a fan shaped retractor holds the lung anteriorly to expose the esophagus. A 5-mm port is placed just anterior to the tip of the scapula and is used for retraction. A final port is placed at the sixth rib at the anterior axillary line for the suction device and is important in creating the anastomosis (Fig. 11.9).

11.9.2.2 Retraction of the Diaphragm

The initial step is placing a retracting suture through the central tendon of the diaphragm, which is brought out through the anterior chest wall at the level of the insertion of the diaphragm through a 1-mm stab incision. This suture retracts the diaphragm inferiorly, and allows visualization of the gastroesophageal junction.

11.9.2.3 Medial Dissection and Mobilization of the Subcarinal Node Package

Dissection in the chest begins by dividing the inferior pulmonary ligament. By dividing the inferior pulmonary

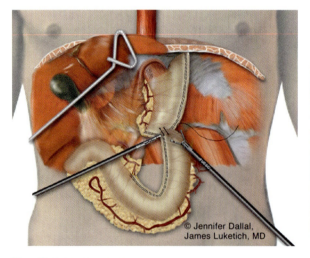

Fig. 11.8 Minimally invasive esophagectomy – two-cavity approach: Preservation of the right gastric vessels; preparation of conduit for pull up

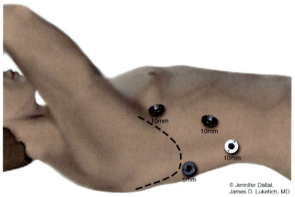

Fig. 11.9 Minimally invasive esophagectomy – two-cavity approach: Port placement for thoracic dissection

ligament, it is important to get directly onto the pericardium as it marks the medial aspect of the dissection. The inferior pulmonary vein is retracted anteriorly and the dissection is carried along the pericardium mobilizing the subcarinal lymph nodes. During the mobilization of the subcarinal nodes, the membranous wall of the right mainstem bronchus is at risk and should therefore be clearly identified. After complete dissection of the subcarinal space, the left mainstem bronchus should be identified. The subcarinal nodal package remains with the specimen and is removed later.

11.9.2.4 Dissection of the Azygos Vein

The pleura is then opened along the hilum up to the level of the azygos vein. The parietal pleura is opened above the azygos vein. After complete circumferential dissection, we divide the azygos vein with a vascular load of the Endo GIA stapler.

11.9.2.5 Lateral Dissection and Thoracic Duct

Attention is then turned to mobilizing the lateral aspect of the pleura overlying the esophagus. The pleura is opened carefully so as to avoid injury to the thoracic duct and the underlying aorta. We do not routinely resect the thoracic duct with the specimen. Any tissue suspicious for branches of the thoracic duct or aorto-esophageal vessels is clipped before being divided with ultrasonic shears. The extent of the lateral dissection reaches from the azygos vein to the GE junction and the deep margin of the dissection is marked by the contra lateral pleura, which is occasionally entered, especially in the setting of a bulky tumor.

11.9.2.6 Positioning of the Conduit and Completion of Dissection

With the esophagus mobilized medially and laterally, the specimen is pulled into the chest with the attached gastric conduit. It is extremely important that the gastric tube remains properly oriented with the staple line facing the lateral chest wall at all times. The stitch is cut between the specimen and the conduit and the specimen is retracted anteriorly and superiorly. The dissection continues posteriorly to completely mobilize the esophagus off the contra lateral pleura. As mentioned, the subcarinal nodes should remain with the specimen. When dissecting the esophagus above the level of the azygos vein, the left vagus is routinely divided and the dissection plane moves to the wall of the esophagus. This helps to avoid injury to the recurrent laryngeal nerve. We do not routinely harvest lymph nodes above the azygos vein.

11.9.3 Esophagogastric End-to-side Anastomosis

With the esophagus completely mobilized, the inferior, lateral port is enlarged to approximately 3 cm and a wound protector is placed. The esophagus is transected using Endo Shears at a level appropriate for the tumor. The specimen is removed through the wound protector and sent for pathologic analysis of the margins. The anvil of a 28-mm EEA stapler is placed in the proximal esophagus and secured with a purse string suture. A second purse string suture is placed to further secure the anvil and incorporate any mucosal defects into the staple donut. The gastric conduit is then pulled up to the apex of the chest and the ultrasonic shears are used to open up the tip of the gastric conduit along the staple line. The EEA stapler gun is placed through the posterior, inferior port site which had been enlarged and is inserted into the conduit. The spike is brought out along the greater curvature of the gastric conduit and is connected with the anvil (Fig. 11.10).

Prior to creating the anastomosis, we carefully ascertain the amount of conduit that will lie in the chest. It is a common mistake to bring an excess amount of stomach into the chest in an effort to minimize tension on the anastomosis. This excess conduit will often assume a sigmoid curve above the diaphragm and may lead to significant problems with gastric emptying. In addition, ensuring proper orientation of the stomach is critical at this point of the procedure. The spike of the stapler and the anvil are now docked and the stapler fired, creating a circular end-to-side esophagogastric anastomosis. Ideally, the anastomosis lies approximately at the level of the azygos vein. The gastrostomy, through which the stapler was placed, is stapled close with an articulating linear Endo GIA stapler.

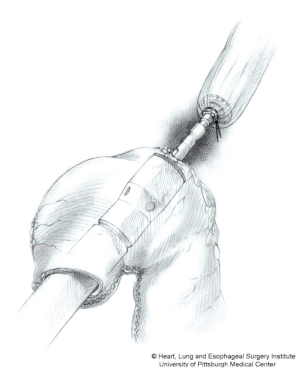

Fig. 11.10 Minimally invasive esophagectomy – two-cavity approach: Esophagogastric end-to-side anastomosis

11.9.4 Drain Placement and Wound Closure

A 28 Fr chest tube is left in the right hemithorax and a Jackson-Pratt (JP) drain is placed by the anastomosis. The potential space between the conduit and the right crus of the diaphragm is closed with a single interrupted stitch to prevent delayed herniation. We routinely perform intercostal nerve blocks with a long-acting analgesic for postoperative pain control. A nasogastric tube is left across the anastomosis, with the tip positioned at the level of the diaphragm. All wounds are closed with 4/0 subcuticular absorbable running suture. Fascial defects are closed with 2/0 PDS. Most patients are extubated in the operating room after bronchoscopy demonstrates an intact membranous wall of the right mainstem bronchus.

11.9.5 Postoperative Management

Postoperatively, the patients routinely spend 12–24 h in the ICU and are transferred to the regular floor after uneventful recovery. Tube feedings are started on the second postoperative day and advanced to target by postoperative day 3. A barium swallow is obtained on the fourth or fifth day postsurgery. If there is no leak on fluoroscopy, we remove the chest tube and start the patient on clear liquids, with a maximal amount of 1–2 oz/h. The patients are routinely discharged on the fifth or sixth day postsurgery. Prior to discharge, the JP drain is pulled back slightly. Follow-up is done in the clinic in 2 weeks.

11.10 Conclusion

Minimally invasive Ivor Lewis esophagectomy requires advanced skills in laparoscopy and thoracoscopy. Multiple single institution reports demonstrate safety, feasibility, and comparable survival when compared with traditional esophagectomy. The added benefit of decreased postoperative pain, fewer pulmonary complications, and decreased length of stay makes this approach attractive. Multiinstitutional trials (ECOG 2202) are presently underway to further document potential advantages of this approach to esophagectomy.

11.11 Future Trends

With renewed interest among medical oncologists to treat patients with chemoradiation alone, the techniques of esophagectomy must be refined. As cited above, two recent papers on squamous cell cancer of the esophagus lend some support to this practice. Furthermore, in recent guidelines, the National Comprehensive Cancer Network considers definitive chemoradiation to be an acceptable alternative to esophagectomy. With these challenges, it is incumbent on esophageal surgeons to refine the technique of esophagectomy in order to offer therapy with lower morbidity, improved survival, and decreased length of stay when compared with traditional esophagectomy. With minimally invasive approaches to esophageal resections we are beginning to achieve many of these objectives.

As we continue to push the envelope, robotic surgery, although still in its infant stage, will further enhance our precision in performing esophagectomies.

With the ability to work in tight working spaces and the added degree of freedom, the ergonomic difficulties of VATS can be eliminated [33]. Although early reports indicate longer operative times, robotic esophagectomy has been performed using the Ivor Lewis [34] and transhiatal approach [35]. Clearly, the advantages of the robot are more evident in the transhiatal approach due to limitation of working space. The feasibility of robotic esophagectomy has to be further studied as our experience grows.

Quick Reference Guide

1. Preoperative evaluation includes
   - Computed tomography imaging (CT)
   - Endoscopic ultrasound (EUS)
   - Positron emission tomography imaging (PET)
   - On-table endoscopy to evaluate tumor extension
2. Creation of the gastric conduit requires
   - Careful preservation of the gastroepiploic artery
   - The arcade must not be injured during the gastric mobilization
3. Adequate mobilization of the stomach and pylorus is essential for adequate conduit length. The pylorus should reach the right crus when completely mobilized
4. All celiac nodes should be dissected and swept up with the specimen prior to dividing the left gastric artery and vein
5. Proper orientation of the conduit when it is tacked to the specimen is important, as the conduit cannot come into the chest twisted
6. The margins of the dissection in the chest include:
   - Pericardium
   - Contra lateral pleura
   - Aorta and thoracic duct
   - We do not routinely take the thoracic duct as part of the specimen
7. When dissecting above the azygos vein, it is important to stay directly on the wall of the esophagus so as not to injure the recurrent laryngeal nerve
8. No excess gastric conduit should be pulled into the chest for the esophagogastric anastomosis as this can lead to redundant stomach in the chest and cause significant symptoms
9. An epidural catheter is not routinely used and intercostal rib blocks are placed at the conclusion of the chest portion of the procedure
10. Tube feedings are started on postoperative day 2 and a barium swallow is obtained on postoperative day 4–5 prior to starting oral intake

References

1. Jemal, A., et al.: Cancer statistics, 2003. CA Cancer J. Clin. **53**(1), 5–26 (2003)
2. Jemal, A., et al.: Cancer statistics, 2007. CA Cancer J. Clin. **57**(1), 43–66 (2007)
3. Eloubeidi, M.A., et al.: Temporal trends (1973-1997) in survival of patients with esophageal adenocarcinoma in the United States: a glimmer of hope? Am. J. Gastroenterol. **98**(7), 1627–1633 (2003)
4. Enzinger, P.C., Mayer, R.J.: Esophageal cancer. N. Engl. J. Med. **349**(23), 2241–2252 (2003)
5. Daly, J.M., Karnell, L.H., Menck, H.R.: National Cancer Data Base report on esophageal carcinoma. Cancer **78**(8), 1820–1828 (1996)
6. Younes, M., et al.: Incidence and survival trends of esophageal carcinoma in the United States: racial and gender differences by histological type. Scand. J. Gastroenterol. **37**(12), 1359–1365 (2002)
7. Engel, L.S., et al.: Population attributable risks of esophageal and gastric cancers. J. Natl. Cancer Inst. **95**(18), 1404–1413 (2003)
8. Kelsen, D.P., et al.: Chemotherapy followed by surgery compared with surgery alone for localized esophageal cancer. N. Engl. J. Med. **339**(27), 1979–1984 (1998)
9. Birkmeyer, J.D., et al.: Hospital volume and surgical mortality in the United States. N. Engl. J. Med. **346**(15), 1128–1137 (2002)
10. Luketich, J.D., Rivera, M.A., et al.: Minimally invasive esophagectomy: outcomes in 222 patients. Ann. Surg. **238**, 486–495 (2003)
11. Cuschieri, A., Shimi, S., Banting, S.: Endoscopic oesophagectomy through a right thoracoscopic approach. J. R. Coll. Surg. Edinb. **37**(1), 7–11 (1992)
12. Collard, J.M., et al.: En bloc and standard esophagectomies by thoracoscopy. Ann. Thorac. Surg. **56**(3), 675–679 (1993)
13. Jagot, P., et al.: Laparoscopic mobilization of the stomach for oesophageal replacement. Br. J. Surg. **83**(4), 540–542 (1996)
14. Bonavina, L., et al.: A laparoscopy-assisted surgical approach to esophageal carcinoma. J. Surg. Res. **117**(1), 52–57 (2004)
15. DePaula, A.L., et al.: Laparoscopic transhiatal esophagectomy with esophagogastroplasty. Surg. Laparosc. Endosc. **5**(1), 1–5 (1995)
16. Swanstrom, L.L., Hansen, P.: Laparoscopic total esophagectomy. Arch. Surg. **132**(9), 943–947 (1997). discussion 947-9

17. Luketich, J.D., et al.: Minimally invasive approach to esophagectomy. JSLS **2**(3), 243–247 (1998)
18. Watson, D.I., Jamieson, G.G., Devitt, P.G.: Endoscopic cervico-thoraco-abdominal esophagectomy. J. Am. Coll. Surg. **190**(3), 372–378 (2000)
19. Nguyen, N.T., et al.: Thoracoscopic and laparoscopic esophagectomy for benign and malignant disease: lessons learned from 46 consecutive procedures. J. Am. Coll. Surg. **197**(6), 902–913 (2003)
20. Collins, G., et al.: Experience with minimally invasive esophagectomy. Surg. Endosc. **20**(2), 298–301 (2006)
21. Leibman, S., et al.: Minimally invasive esophagectomy: short- and long-term outcomes. Surg. Endosc. **20**(3), 428–433 (2006)
22. Watson, D.I., Davies, N., Jamieson, G.G.: Totally endoscopic Ivor Lewis esophagectomy. Surg. Endosc. **13**(3), 293–297 (1999)
23. Nguyen, N.T., et al.: Minimally invasive Ivor Lewis esophagectomy. Ann. Thorac. Surg. **72**(2), 593–596 (2001)
24. Kunisaki, C., et al.: Video-assisted thoracoscopic esophagectomy with a voice-controlled robot: the AESOP system. Surg. Laparosc. Endosc. Percutan. Tech. **14**(6), 323–327 (2004)
25. Bizekis, C., et al.: Initial experience with minimally invasive Ivor Lewis esophagectomy. Ann. Thorac. Surg. **82**(2), 402–406 (2006). discussion 406–7
26. Fujita, H., et al.: Optimum treatment strategy for superficial esophageal cancer: endoscopic mucosal resection versus radical esophagectomy. World J. Surg. **25**(4), 424–431 (2001)
27. Westerterp, M., et al.: Outcome of surgical treatment for early adenocarcinoma of the esophagus or gastro-esophageal junction. Virchows Arch. **446**(5), 497–504 (2005)
28. Pech, O., et al.: Long-term results of photodynamic therapy with 5-aminolevulinic acid for superficial Barrett's cancer and high-grade intraepithelial neoplasia. Gastrointest. Endosc. **62**(1), 24–30 (2005)
29. Overholt, B.F., Panjehpour, M., Halberg, D.L.: Photodynamic therapy for Barrett's esophagus with dysplasia and/or early stage carcinoma: long-term results. Gastrointest. Endosc. **58**(2), 183–188 (2003)
30. Peters, F.P., et al.: Endoscopic treatment of high-grade dysplasia and early stage cancer in Barrett's esophagus. Gastrointest. Endosc. **61**(4), 506–514 (2005)
31. Stahl, M., et al.: Chemoradiation with and without surgery in patients with locally advanced squamous cell carcinoma of the esophagus. J. Clin. Oncol. **23**(10), 2310–2317 (2005)
32. Bedenne, L., et al.: Chemoradiation followed by surgery compared with chemoradiation alone in squamous cancer of the esophagus: FFCD 9102. J. Clin. Oncol. **25**(10), 1160–1168 (2007)
33. Bodner, J., Wykypiel, H., et al.: First experience with the da Vinci trademark operating robot in thoracic surgery. Eur. J. Cardiothorac. Surg. **25**, 844–851 (2004)
34. Melvin, W., Needleman, B., et al.: Computer enhanced robotic telesurgery: initial experience in foregut surgery. Surg. Endosc. **16**, 1790–1792 (2002)
35. Horgan, S., Berger, R., et al.: Robotic-assisted minimally invasive transhiatal esophagectomy. Am. Surg. **69**, 624–669 (2003)

Cancer of the Esophagus and the Gastroesophageal Junction: Transhiatal Approach

Lee Swanstrom and Michael Ujiki

12.1 Introduction

The treatment options for esophageal precancers and cancers are undergoing an evolution and change at a rate almost equal to the rapid increase of these diseases in the population. At the same time, there has been a general decrease in referrals for radical surgery, largely due to general nihilism about its success rate as a cure, high morbidity and mortality rates, and a perception that there is a poor quality of life in the patient population who do survive. In many institutions, the majority of esophageal cancer patients are never seen by a surgeon unless there are complications. Ironically, surgery remains the only chance for a definitive cure of invasive cancers in spite of improvements in chemotherapy and radiation treatment. Equally ironic is the fact that improvements in surgical technique and postoperative surgical care, as well as the movement toward volume concentration of procedures, has led to a dramatic decrease in the mortality of esophagectomy while, on the other hand, improving 5-year survival rates dramatically. Series survival rates for radical en bloc esophagectomy of 50% are reported and institutional 5-year survivals with multimodal therapy including surgery are >25%.

L. Swanstrom (✉) and M. Ujiki
Division of Gastrointestinal and Minimally Invasive Surgery, Department of Surgery, University of Oregon Health Sciences, 1040 North West 22nd Avenue Suite 560, Portland, OR 97210, USA
e-mail: lswanstrom@aol.com; mujiki@northshore.org

12.2 Minimally Invasive Esophagectomy: Why?

Arguments for consideration of a minimally invasive approach to esophageal cancers hinge primarily on perceptions that it will improve the morbidity and quality of life profile of surgery while at the same time maintaining the oncologic principles of a radical resection. There is indeed, increasing evidence in the literature that minimally invasive esophagectomy (MIE) is safe and does not compromise oncologic outcomes. There is, however, little yet that truly defines any improvements in quality of life aside from a shorter hospital stay. Still, the psychological impact of interventions cannot be minimized and patients uniformly prefer a less invasive option when surgery is considered. From the surgeon's standpoint, the ability to offer a less morbid option for resection can be a marketing advantage when it comes to building a surgery-based esophageal cancer program. It is not uncommon at some institutions that most esophageal cancer patients are not seen by a surgeon, because the referring physicians feel that an open esophagectomy is a "fate worse than death." These same physicians are often much more likely to refer for a "laparoscopic" intervention as it is "not really 'surgery'." These arguments carry special weight when dealing with premalignant or very early cancers, occurring in a younger population with a good prognosis and where an extremely morbid procedure can seem especially devastating.

12.3 Esophageal Resection: Which Approach to Choose?

The esophageal surgery world remains divided on the relative merits of different operative approaches. While it is generally accepted that a transhiatal resection is a good way to treat Barrett's/high-grade dysplasia (HGD) and intramucosal lesions, transhiatal resection remains controversial for curative resections of higher-grade cancers. In spite of decades of experience and studies, this question remains unanswered with epidemiologic studies showing no survival advantage of one approach over the other and yet selected case series showing that extended resections may offer some survival benefit. Most centers, ours included, tailor the approach to the disease and particular patient. Early disease, distal disease, and high-risk patients are ideally suited for a laparoscopic transhiatal approach. Benefits are a decrease in operative blood loss, postoperative morbidity, and hospital stay.

12.4 Overview of the Literature: New Life for the Transhiatal Approach

Esophagectomy remains one of the most technically challenging surgical procedures despite the development of many advances over the last several decades. Postoperative morbidity and mortality rates after esophagectomy are some of the highest of all general surgical procedures performed. With the evolution of minimally invasive techniques, the hope has been that these rates would decrease. Some have indeed proved this to be true, but questions remain as to which minimally invasive technique offers the best oncologic advantage [1].

The laparoscopic transhiatal approach was first introduced in 1995 by DePaula and has since proven safe, feasible, and effective without sacrificing oncologic principles in many small retrospective reviews [2–6]. In general, these studies have shown mortality rates of 0–5.1%, morbidity rates around 25–30%, and adequate lymph node harvests. Technically, however, the limited workspace does make the mediastinal lymph node dissection challenging and could theoretically result in improper staging and neo-adjuvant therapy planning. This fact has led some experienced esophageal surgeons to abandon the approach for the minimally invasive transthoracic method [7]. The transhiatal approach, on the other hand, has several advantages in a group of patients that in general are elderly, malnourished, and often stricken with pulmonary comorbidities:

- No need for repositioning
- No need for selective intubation
- Less operative time
- Less pulmonary complications
- Less surgical trauma

In general, studies comparing the open transhiatal approach to the transthoracic approach have failed to show an advantage of one approach over the other in terms of survival. Chang et al. identified over 800 patients through the Surveillance Epidemiology and End Results (SEER) data base and found lower operative mortality (6.7% vs. 13.1%) for transhiatal esophagectomy with no survival advantage for either procedure [8]. Utilizing the Nationwide Inpatient Sample Database, Connors and colleagues compared outcomes of over 17,000 patients and found no difference in terms of postoperative morbidity and mortality [9]. They did find, however, that hospital volume (>10 procedures/year) resulted in significantly better outcomes, no matter which approach was used. A prospective study of 945 patients through the National Surgical Quality Improvement Program (NSQUIP) also showed no difference in morbidity and mortality between the two procedures [10] In the only prospective randomized study performed, 220 patients were randomized and the transhiatal group experienced a lower postoperative morbidity with no survival advantage for either group, though there was a trend toward longer survival for the transthoracic group [11].

No prospective randomized studies comparing minimally invasive transhiatal to the transthoracic approach are published, but a few recent retrospective comparisons exist. Dapri et al. compared the transhiatal approach with the minimally invasive three-hole approach utilizing the prone position and found that complications and survival were similar [12]. If compared to laparoscopic gastric mobilization and open thoracotomy, the minimally invasive transhiatal approach results in less operative time, shorter stay in the intensive care unit, and shorter length of stay in hospital, with comparable survival [13]. Bottger and colleagues compared all three minimally invasive techniques (transhiatal, thoracoscopic, and laparoscopic mobilization/thoracotomy) and found that morbidity, mortality, and number of lymph nodes harvested were not significantly different [14]. While the debate goes on, the evolution of the transhiatal technique continues. Jobe et al. recently published the results of their inversion technique and found it safe and effective, while others are researching the possible benefits of robotics during the mediastinal part of the dissection [15, 16]. Though both techniques appear promising, more experience with transhiatal techniques along with better technology figure to improve a challenging but gratifying technique.

12.5 Surgical Management of Esophageal Cancer

12.5.1 The PORTLAND Approach

A thorough preoperative evaluation is essential. The patient needs to be in the best physical shape possible as this surgery represents a major physiological "hit." We routinely perform a two-stage procedure:

- *Stage I* – Staging laparoscopy with
  - D2 node dissection
  - Division of the left gastric artery
  - Placement of a feeding jejunostomy for invasive cancers
- *Stage II* – Resection of the disease

This allows a period of nutritional supplementation if the patient is malnourished from the disease or after neo-adjuvant therapy before she/he undergoes resection.

12.5.1.1 Stage I: Staging Laparoscopy

Patient Positioning and Trocar Placement

The patient is placed supine and arms are tucked. We routinely use a configuration of five trocars, one 1-mm and four 5-mm ports and place them in the same pattern that will be used for the resection later on. Exploration of all the peritoneal surfaces is performed and biopsies taken of any suspicious lesion. Laparoscopic ultrasound will be used if any liver lesions are noted. If there is no gross evidence of extraesophageal disease, attention is turned to a formal lymph node dissection (Fig. 12.1).

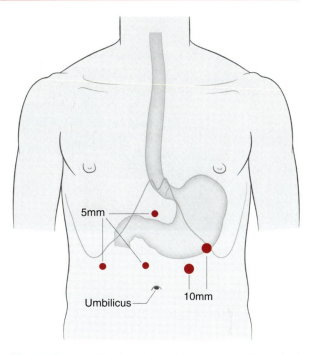

Fig. 12.1 Minimally invasive esophagectomy – Transhiatal approach: Port placement. (Drawing by Hippmann GbR, Schwarzenbruck, Germany)

Lymphadenectomy and Division of Left Gastric Artery

The left lobe of the liver is lifted up with an atraumatic liver retractor and the stomach is retracted to the patient's left side by the assistant surgeon. The hepatogastric ligament is dissected widely, extending from the porta hepatis to the right crus. Starting at the common bile duct, all nodal tissue between

- Portal vein
- Inferior vena cava
- Common hepatic artery is teased up and resected using ultrasonic scissors. The final extent of this dissection is usually the celiac nodal package, dissection of which will expose the base of the left gastric artery (Fig. 12.2).

We divide the left gastric artery with an endoscopic vascular stapler for two reasons

- Removal of the celiac node package
- Induction of ischemia, for preconditioning of the gastric conduit

All node packets are labeled and removed with impermeable tissue capture bags.

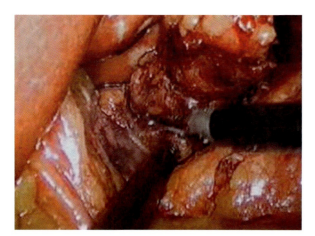

Fig. 12.2 Minimally invasive esophagectomy – Transhiatal approach: Exposure of the para-celiac lymph nodes and left gastric artery

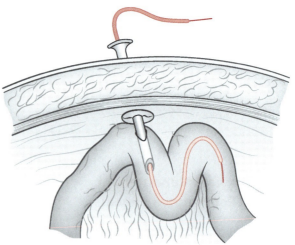

Fig. 12.3 Minimally invasive esophagectomy – Transhiatal approach: Laparoscopic placement of a feeding jejunostomy. (Drawing by Hippmann GbR, Schwarzenbruck, Germany)

Laparoscopic Feeding Jejunostomy

Now we turn our attention to the feeding tube placement. A 5-mm camera is used through one of the right-sided ports. The ligament of Treitz is identified and the jejunum is run for 30 cm. An absorbable suture is placed at the antimesenteric border of the target bowel loop which will be tacked to the anterior abdominal wall. Three additional sutures are placed to fix a 2×2 cm area of the chosen bowel loop to the abdominal wall. Before we tie the last suture, we place a Seldinger needle to access the bowel percutaneously. Injected air confirms intraluminal placement. A guide wire is inserted through the needle followed by a 12 French dilator/peel-away sheath (Fig. 12.3). The last placed suture is now tied to seal the bowel wall firmly to the parietal peritoneum. A 12 French catheter is inserted and the peel-away sheath removed. The feeding tube is securely sutured in place. The patient is discharged the next day and tube feedings arranged if needed. Pathology results will determine the timing of further treatment

- Chemo-radiation if the lymph nodes are positive
- Primary resection for node-negative disease

12.5.1.2 Stage II: Esophagectomy

Laparoscopic transhiatal esophagectomy (LTE) is a 4–8-h procedure. Hypothermia prevention, DVT prophylaxis, and appropriate invasive monitoring lines are crucial. A second surgical team, to save time and to prevent fatigue, performs the cervical dissection and anastomosis. Experienced anesthesia and a dedicated nursing team insure optimal outcomes.

Patient Positioning and Trocar Placement

The patient is placed on a split-leg operating table with the legs spread. Footplates are positioned to bear weight when the patient is in reverse Trendelenburg. The left arm is padded and tucked, the right arm stays extended. The head will be turned to the right to facilitate the cervical anastomosis. The port configuration is exactly the same as for staging laparoscopy and includes a 10-mm camera port, a 12-mm epigastric port, and three 5-mm ports. If staging was not done separately it is performed now.

Mobilization of the Greater and Lesser Curvature

The left lobe of the liver is retracted anteriorly with an atraumatic instrument which is then attached to a table-mounted holder. The greater curvature is first mobilized starting at the antrum and working cephalad (Fig. 12.4). Care is taken to stay wide of the epiploic arcade which can be difficult in obese patients where the artery is not easily visible. If there is doubt as to its location, laparoscopic Ultrasound/Doppler should be used as injury to the arcade is disastrous. Ultrasonic scissors or bipolar sealing devices work well for this step of the dissection. We avoid grasping the vascular pedicle or the stomach wall at the greater curvature and use blunt retraction

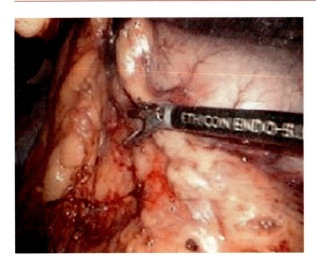

Fig. 12.4 Minimally invasive esophagectomy – Transhiatal approach: Mobilization of the greater curvature of the stomach

instead. This dissection is continued cephalad until the left crus is exposed. Distally, wide dissection is continued toward the duodenum, separating the transverse colon and allowing the duodenum to be mobilized. Medial duodenal mobilization (Kocherization) is performed as needed. The pylorus should then be grasped and elevated. This part of the dissection is finished if it reaches the right crus. The lesser curvature is mobilized by widely dividing the hepato-gastric ligament to expose the right crus. The left gastric artery is divided if it has not already been done.

12.6 Creation of the Gastric Conduit

An EndoGIA, with a 3.8-mm green load, is inserted through the epigastric port. The first firing is perpendicular across the antrum toward the greater curvature. Subsequent firings are parallel to the greater curvature and create a 3-cm conduit with the blood supply based on the carefully preserved epiploic arcade. Tube creation is terminated 5 cm below the distal tumor margin to allow for a safe margin.

12.6.1 Transhiatal and Lower Mediastinal Dissection

The mediastinum is accessed by dividing the phrenoesophageal membrane circumferentially. Mediastinal dissection then proceeds along the mediastinal pleura, aorta, and pericardium up to and under the azygos vein keeping the entire lymphatic tissue with the specimen.

12.6.2 Cervical and Upper Mediastinal Dissection

This is started in the meantime by the second team. A transverse collar incision is made and the sternocleidomastoid muscle is mobilized and retracted laterally. The esophagus is isolated and a Penrose drain placed around it. Circumferential dissection is continued distally and the vagal trunks are divided at the distal extent of this dissection. Upper mediastinal dissection of the esophagus is performed using a lubricated sponge on a long curved clamp. Care must be taken to avoid injury to the membranous trachea during this dissection. With the laparoscope inserted into the mediastinum, the sponge stick can be observed and safe dissection assured.

12.6.3 Specimen Extraction

Once mobilization from above and below is completed and the cervical esophagus is transected low in the neck, the specimen can be removed via the neck or through a small incision in the upper abdomen. In either case, the specimen should be placed in an impermeable retrieval bag to avoid wound contamination and cancer spillage.

12.6.4 The Inversion Extraction Technique

For very distal and early stage cancers, we favor an inversion extraction technique to complete the upper mobilization as it is quick and efficacious. This is accomplished by passing a nasogastric tube through an esophagotomy made at the site of the cervical anastomosis. It is advanced until stopped at the distal tip of the transected stomach. The tube is securely fixed to the stomach by a heavy transmural suture. Slow steady withdrawal of the tube through the neck is initiated while holding the proximal stomach in place. This results in an imbrication of the stomach into the esophagus. Progressive withdrawal inverts the entire

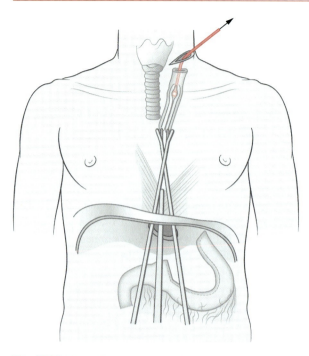

Fig. 12.5 Minimally invasive esophagectomy – Transhiatal approach: The inversion technique for specimen removal. (Drawing by Hippmann GbR, Schwarzenbruck, Germany)

esophagus as the specimen is withdrawn from the esophagotomy site. If needed, the esophagus can be followed with an extralong laparoscope and instruments to divide any attachments resisting the withdrawal of the specimen (Fig. 12.5).

12.7 Pull Up of the Gastric Conduit

Once the specimen is removed, a 20 French chest tube is passed from the neck into the abdomen. The gastric conduit is attached to the end of the tube with a heavy suture. As it is pulled up through the mediastinum, care must be taken to avoid any twisting or trauma to the vascular pedicle. Ideally, the conduit is long enough to permit excision of the proximal tip and still allow approximately 2 cm of tubularized gastric tube to lie below the hiatus.

12.8 Cervical Anastomosis

It can be performed by any of the traditional methods, stapled or hand sewn. If there is some redundant length of the conduit, we tend to use a functional side-to-side

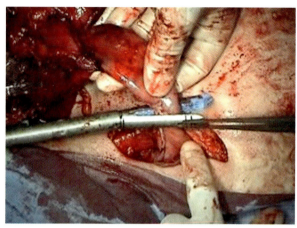

Fig. 12.6 Minimally invasive esophagectomy – Transhiatal approach: Cervical anastomosis double stapling technique

stapled anastomosis. We do not hesitate to do a single layer hand-sewn anastomosis if the conduit is short or the neck too deep to pull the ends up for proper stapler placement (Fig. 12.6). A nasogastric tube is placed into the gastric pouch before completing the anastomosis and a closed suction drain left adjacent to the esophagus as the wound is closed in layers.

12.9 Fundoplication

Abdominally, the hiatus is loosely closed and, when possible, a Dor anterior fundoplication as an antireflux mechanism is created by folding the antrum up to the rim of the hiatus. If not done previously a feeding jejunostomy is placed at that point. The abdomen is lavaged and a closed suction drain brought out through one of the port sites (Fig. 12.7).

12.10 Postoperative Management

Postoperatively, the patient is brought to the ICU for observation if significant comorbidities exist. In all other cases, the patients are transferred to the regular surgical floor. The drains are closely monitored and the output checked for amylase daily. An additional contrast upper GI is obtained if the amylase becomes elevated. The nasogastric tube is kept to suction for

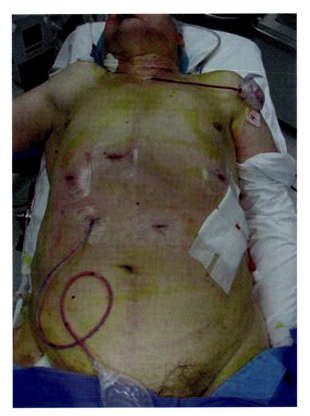

Fig. 12.7 Minimally invasive esophagectomy – Transhiatal approach: Completion of a laparoscopic transhiatal esophagectomy

3 days and then a routine upper GI study will be performed. If the study is normal a diet is started. The drains are removed immediately prior to discharge. The patient's diet is advanced to a pureed diet which they are kept on for 2-weeks post discharge. Tube feedings via the jejunostomy are started on postoperative day 2 and the patient usually goes home with supplemental night time feedings for 2–4 weeks.

12.11 Future Trends

There is a steady and persistent growth in interest in less invasive esophageal cancer treatments. Many of these therapies are endoscopic based, both flexible and laparo/thoracoscopic. These are alternative therapies that may replace many traditional open surgical approaches (Table 12.1).

12.11.1 Staging Laparoscopy: Yes or No?

Laparoscopy and/or thoracoscopy has been shown to be highly accurate as a staging modality to determine resectability. Its use has been adopted by the majority of major cancer centers although, whether it is done as an outpatient stand-alone procedure or as part of a planned definitive operation remains variable and is determined by institutional policies and surgeons preference.

12.11.2 Endoluminal Treatment of Early Cancers and Barret's Dysplasia

The treatment of Barrett's dysplasia and tumors confined to the superficial mucosa is just entering into a paradigm change that will probably mostly eliminate surgical resection for this stage of the disease. Ablative treatments like photodynamic therapy and endoscopic thermal ablation never achieved wide-spread use due to their side effects, difficulty to apply, and variable response. With the arrival of catheter-based radiofrequency ablation, which has proven to be a simple and reproducible method to treat Barrett's dysplasia, this is rapidly changing (Fig. 12.8). If long-term studies confirm initial results of complete ablation and genetic down regulation, this modality will probably eliminate the need for esophagectomy for dysplastic Barrett's in most instances. The issue of nodular Barrett's dysplasia or carcinoma in situ is more controversial because of the difficulty to accurately stage these patients, the decreased efficacy of ablation, and the possibility of extraesophageal spread. While esophagectomy should be considered as the "gold standard" today, radical surgery is losing ground to local treatment with endoscopic submucosal dissection (ESD) and ablation, if high resolution EUS does not show deeper invasion or nodal spread. This trend toward endoscopic treatment will undoubtedly increase as staging imagery improves and as genetic markers for risk profiling mature. If esophagectomy is performed for very early cancers, it is incumbent on the surgeon to perform it in the least invasive manner possible. Although not widely performed as of yet, laparoscopic vagal sparing esophagectomy is probably the procedure that offers the best post resection quality of life for these patients.

For truly invasive cancers, formal esophagectomy is still the best treatment for those who can tolerate the

Table 12.1 Esophageal malignancy: Evolution of surgical treatment

	Open procedure	Minimally invasive alternative
Dysplastic Barrett's	Transhiatal esophagectomy	• Laparoscopic esophagectomy • Endoscopic mucosal resection • Radiofrequency ablation
Early cancer (cis – T1)	Esophagectomy	• Laparoscopic esophagectomy • Endoscopic mucosal resection (EMR)
Staging a patient	Exploratory laparotomy Exploratory thoracotomy	• EUS • PET/CT • Laparoscopy • Thoracoscopy
Invasive cancer	Esophagectomy en-bloc	• Definitive chemo/radiation • Laparoscopic resection • Thoracoscopic resection
Stage 4 cancer	Palliative open resection	• Stenting • Photodynamic ablation • Minimally invasive resection

Cis carcinoma in situ

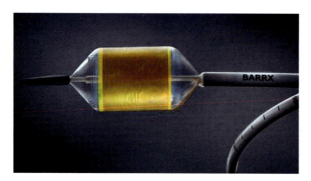

Fig. 12.8 Minimally invasive esophagectomy – Transhiatal approach: Radiofrequency catheter for ablation of Barrett's dysplasia (With permission by Barxx Medical, Sunnyvale, CA, USA)

surgical trauma. Because of its perceived lesser morbidity, definitive chemo-radiation will be an increasingly popular alternative to surgery even though it is only palliative. The challenge is to replicate the results of the best open practices using the endoscope. This is possible as has been demonstrated for colorectal cancer, but will require education, perseverance, and proof. Currently, en-bloc excisions are probably the most definitive cancer treatment. Formal node dissection is possible using the laparoscope and thoracoscope but is currently not widely practiced. It may actually be possible to perform transhiatal en-bloc node dissection using the laparoscope but this is not yet proven. Until such proof, laparoscopic transhiatal resection is best reserved for very early distal cancers.

Quick Reference Guide

1. **Patient positioning**

    - Split leg table with legs apart
    - Assure very good padding because of the length of the procedure
    - Table placed in 30° reverse Trendelenburg to allow maximum exposure

2. **Trocar placement**

    - Ports should be placed relatively low, slightly above the umbilicus

- Extralong instruments will be used (45 cm) to allow both mobilization of the greater curvature/duodenum as well as the upper and transhiatal dissection

3. **"No-touch" technique**
   Should be applied throughout the procedure as much as possible. In particular, the greater curvature vascular pedicle and the area of the stomach that will be used as the gastric interposition should never be directly grasped and blunt retraction used instead

4. **Duodenal mobilization, or Kocherization**
   Proceeds until the pylorus can be grasped and easily reaches the right crus

5. **Lymphadenectomy**
   A D-2 node dissection is routinely performed (unless done previously during the laparoscopic staging). The Porta hepatis, paracaval, and celiac nodes are removed as a separate packet. It is also possible, during the laparoscopic part, to perform a nodal dissection of the lower mediastinum. These nodes are left attached to the esophagus!

6. **Left gastric artery**
   - Best *mobilized* from beneath the stomach, with the assistant retracting the stomach upwards
   - Best *divided* from the lesser curvature using an EndoGIA with a white vascular load

7. **Creation of the gastric conduit**
   - Start from the greater curvature and use sequential firings of green stapler loads The first firing from the epigastric port is perpendicular across the antrum
   - We prefer a narrow gastric tube (3 cm) for its long-term function
   - We do not routinely oversaw the staple line

8. **Mediastinal mobilization**
   - This is the most tedious and difficult portion of the case!
   - Upper dissection is done with a sponge stick via the neck incision
   - Distal and small tumors are removed through the neck by inverting the proximal stomach into the esophagus

9. **Cervical anastomosis**
   - Can be performed hand sewn or stapled
   - Leak rates are similar between the two techniques
   - We perform the double staple technique of Orranger if possible

10. **Pyloroplasty**
    Is not routinely added as it contributes to troublesome bile regurgitation later

Much like a pylorus sparing Whipple however, one must be prepared for a period of delayed gastric emptying and we always add a feeding jejunostomy during the staging or primary surgery

References

1. Nguyen, N.T., Follette, D.M., Lemoine, P.H., Roberts, P.F., Goodnight, J.E.: Minimally invasive IVOR Lewis esophagectomy. Ann. Thorac. Surg. **72**, 593–596 (2001)
2. DePaula, A.L., Hashiba, K., Ferreira, E.A., DePaula, R.A., Grecco, E.: Laparoscopic transhiatal esophagectomy with esophagogastroplasty. Surg. Laparosc. Endosc. **5**, 1–5 (1995)
3. Swanstrom, L., Hansen, P.: Laparoscopic total esophagectomy. Arch. Surg. **132**, 943–949 (1997)
4. Avital, S., Zundel, N., Szomstein, S., Rosenthal, R.: Laparosocpic Transhiatal esophagectomy for esophageal cancer. Am. J. Surg. **190**(1), 69–74 (2005)
5. Tinoco, R., El-Kadre, L., Tinoco, A., Rios, R., Sueth, D., Pena, F.: Laparoscopic transhiatal esophagectomy: outcomes. Surg. Endosc. **21**(8), 1284–1287 (2007)
6. Sanders, G., Borie, F., Hussin, E., Blanc, P.M., Di Mauro, G., Claus, C., Millat, B.: Minimally invasive Transhiatal esophagectomy: lessons learned. Surg. Endosc. **21**, 1190–1193 (2007)
7. Luketich, J.D., Alveolo-Rivera, M., Buenaventura, P.O., Christie, N.A., McCaughan, J.S., Litle, V.R., Schauer, P.R., Close, J.M., Fernando, H.C.: Minimally invasive esophagectomy: outcomes in 222 patients. Ann. Surg. **238**, 486–495 (2003)
8. Chang, A.C., Ji, H., Birkmeyer, N.J., et al.: Outcomes after Transhiatal and transthoracic esophagectomy for cancer. Ann. Thorac. Surg. **85**, 424–429 (2008)
9. Connors, R.C., Reuben, B.C., Neumayer, L.A., Bull, D.A.: Comparing outcomes after transthoracic and Transhiatal esophagectomy: a 5-year prospective cohort of 17, 395 patients. J. Am. Coll. Surg. **205**(6), 735–740 (2007)
10. Rentz, J., Bull, D.A., Harpole, D., et al.: Transthoracic versus Transhiatal esophagectomy: a prospective study of 945 patients. J. Thorac. Cardiovasc. Surg. **125**, 1114–1120 (2003)
11. Hulscher, J.B., Van Sandick, J.W., De Boer, A.G., et al.: Extended transthoracic resection compared with limited Transhiatal resection for adenocarcinoma of the esophagus. N. Engl. J. Med. **347**, 1662–1669 (2002)
12. Dapri, G., Himpens, J., Cadiere, G.B.: Minimally invasive esophagectomy for cancer: laparoscopic Transhiatal procedure or thoracoscopy in prone position followed by laparoscopy. Surg. Endosc. **22**(4), 1060–1069 (2008). 2007 epub Dec 11
13. Benzoni, E., Terrosu, G., Bresadola, V., Uzzau, A., Intini, S., Noce, L., Cedolini, C., Bresadola, F., DeAnna, D.: A com-

parative study of the transhiatal laparoscopic approach versus laparoscopic gastric mobilisation and right open transthoracic esophagectomy for esophageal cancer management. J. Gastrointest. Liver Dis. **16**(4), 395–401 (2007)
14. Bottger, T., Terzic, A., Muller, M., Rodehurst, A.: Minimally invasive Transhiatal and transthoracic esophagectomy. Surg. Endosc. **21**, 1695–1700 (2007)
15. Jobe, B.A., Kim, C.Y., Minjarez, R.C., et al.: Simplifying minimally invasive Transhiatal esophagectomy with the inversion approach. Arch. Surg. **141**, 857–866 (2006)
16. Galvani, C.A., Gorodner, M.V., Moser, F., Jacobsen, G., Chretien, C., Espat, N.J., Donahue, P., Horgan, S.: Robotically assisted laparoscopic transhiatal esophagectomy. Surg. Endosc. **22**, 188–195 (2008)

Part III
Special Topics: Cancer of the Stomach

Laparoscopic Distal Gastrectomy – *LADG*

13

Mutter Didier, O.A. Burckhardt, and Perretta Silvana

13.1 Introduction

Open gastrectomy with D2 lymph node dissection is currently the standard surgical procedure for the management of advanced gastric cancer. The laparoscopic approach to this disease has not yet been widely accepted since it is considered technically difficult. These technical difficulties apply mostly to D2 lymphadenectomy. However, despite a longer operative time [1], the combination of good laparoscopic experience with a significant learning curve in cases of gastrectomy, allows an advanced team to perform laparoscopic gastrectomy for gastric cancer effectively with surgical results and outcomes that are favorable for the patient [2].

13.2 Indications for Laparoscopic Distal Gastrectomy

Laparoscopic distal gastrectomy is indicated in patients presenting with histologically proven adenocarcinoma of the stomach. Laparoscopic distal gastrectomy with D2 lymph node dissection is indicated in patients with T2 N0 and T1 N1 gastric cancer [3]. Laparoscopic distal gastrectomy can also be advocated for the treatment of gastrointestinal stromal tumors. In these cases, D2 lymph node dissection is not performed [4].

13.3 Lymph Node Dissection and the Japanese Classification

Lymph node dissection will be performed in a standard manner and will follow a classic outline. Each lymph node station will be numbered according to the Japanese classification of gastric carcinoma (Fig. 13.1). Stations No. 1 to No. 6 are perigastric lymph nodes, while stations No. 7, No. 8a, No. 9, No. 11p, 12a, and

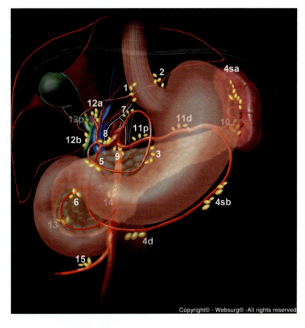

Fig. 13.1 Lymph node stations according to the Japanese classification of gastric carcinoma

M. Didier (✉), O.A. Burckhardt, and P. Silvana
Digestive and Endocrine Surgery, IRCAD-EITS Institute,
University Hospital Strasbourg, 1 Place de l'Hôpital,
67091 Strasbourg, France
e-mail: didier.mutter@ircad.fr

No. 14 are second row lymph nodes. These are located along the left gastric artery, the common hepatic artery, the celiac trunc, and the proximal half of the splenic artery, the proper hepatic artery, and the surface of the superior mesenteric vein [5].

13.4 Sentinel Lymph Node Mapping

Several authors have promoted sentinel node mapping during laparoscopic distal gastrectomy for gastric cancer [5]. The feasibility and accuracy of this mapping has also been demonstrated. Two milliliters of liquid radioisotope or 2% patent blue are injected endoscopically into the submucosal layer surrounding the primary tumor. Sentinel nodes are defined as nodes stained by the blue dye within 5–10 min of the dye injection. Such sentinel node mapping appears to be an accurate diagnostic tool in the detection of lymph node metastases in patients with early stage gastric cancer. This method does not seem to have been validated in advanced cancers [5].

13.5 Surgical Technique

13.5.1 Patient Positioning

The surgical procedure is performed under general anesthesia and orotracheal intubation. A naso-gastric tube is placed in order to remove any fluid present in the stomach. The patient is placed on the operating table in split leg technique in a 10–20° reverse Trendelenburg position. The left arm is kept for the anesthesiologist and will not be tucked [6, 7]. The team consists of the main surgeon standing between the patient's legs and two assistant surgeons, one on each side of the patient. Finally, two monitors allow the assistants to face the operating image (Fig. 13.2).

13.5.2 Instruments Required

Gastric surgery requires atraumatic graspers, hooks, and scissors linked to an electro-surgical device for

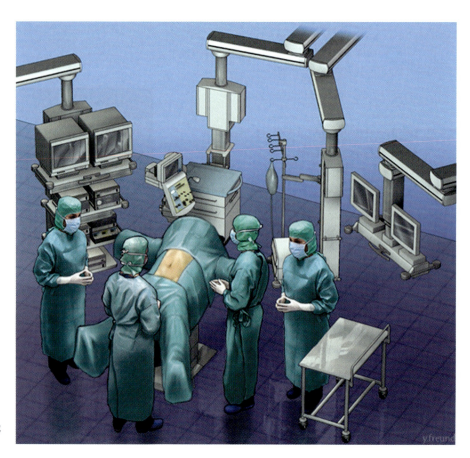

Fig. 13.2 Patient positioning and operating room setup

monopolar and bipolar cautery, an irrigation/suction device, as well as an extraction bag for the removal of the specimen at the end of the surgical procedure. Clips are used for hemostasis. The dissection can be performed with ultrasonic dissectors (Autosonix™ – Covidien) or with an automatic bipolar electrocautery system (Ligasure™ – Covidien). These types of dissectors allow to significantly shorten the operative time. Linear stapling devices are used to cut the stomach and duodenum and to perform the anastomosis. Needle holders and stitches are required for the closure of the introduction enterotomy of the staplers into the bowel.

13.5.3 Trocar Placement

The procedure is conventionally performed with a set of five ports placed in a semicircular configuration. The pneumoperitoneum is created following open insertion of the first trocar at the umbilicus. A 12-mm port is placed in order to allow the introduction of clips and staplers. The intraoperative working pressure is set at 12 mmHg. Further, trocars are inserted under direct vision. After insertion of the first port at the umbilicus, two 10-mm ports are placed in the left and right midclavicular line 2 cm above the umbilicus and a 5-mm trocar below the left costal margin in the right midclavicular line. If necessary, we place a fifth port at the level of the xiphoid process (Fig. 13.3).

13.6 Typical Distal Gastrectomy: The Steps

13.6.1 Step I: Diagnostic Laparoscopy

The abdominal cavity is explored to confirm the feasibility of the laparoscopic approach, which is taken when the following three points are assured:

- Lack of significant adhesions
- Good exposure
- Operability in cases of cancer by exclusion of metastatic disease

We determine the extent of the resection and use clips or superficial electrocautery burns to outline all landmarks.

13.6.2 Step II of the Procedure

- Mobilization of the stomach
- Dissection of lymph nodes along the vascular supply of the stomach
- Division of the duodenum

The mobilization of the stomach starts with opening the lesser sac. A grasper introduced through the left subcostal port brings the omentum into the operative field. The gastro-colic ligament is divided at a distance of 3 cm from the gastro-omental vascular supply in order to harvest all the lymph nodes along these vessels. Lymph node station 4d and 4sb stay with the specimen and the dissection is carried on progressively from right to left (Clips 13.1 and 13.2). We use ultrasonic dissectors or, alternatively, the Ligasure device. The

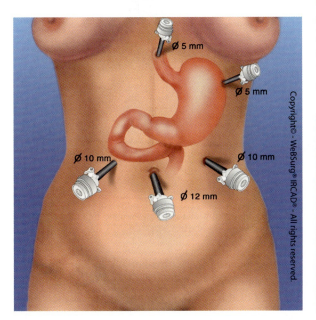

Fig. 13.3 Trocar placement

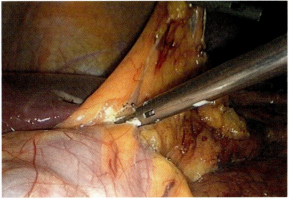

Clip 13.1 Division of the gastro-colic ligament (case 1)

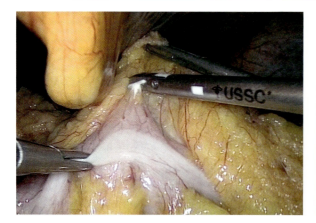

Clip 13.2 Division of the gastro-colic ligament (case 2)

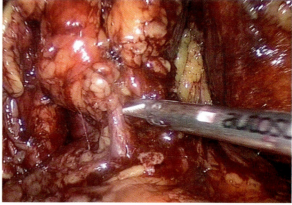

Clip 13.4 Dissection of the right gastro-omental vessels (case 2)

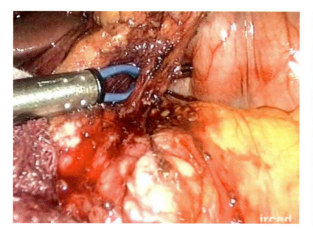

Clip 13.3 Dissection of the right gastro-omental vessels and of the inferior side of the proximal duodenum (case 1)

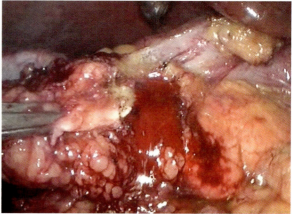

Clip 13.5 Vascular lesions on the right gastro-omental vessels

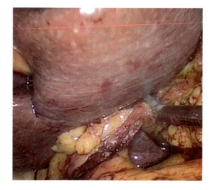

Clip 13.6 Dissection of the gastro-hepatic ligament up to the hepatic common artery (case 2)

dissection is continued until we obtain exposure of the left gastro-omental vessels below the spleen. These vessels are controlled with the Ligasure device or divided between clips and represent the dissection of the lymph node station 4sb. The dissection is then conducted from left to right and towards the pylorus. The right gastro-omental vein is exposed and divided, followed by the right gastro-omental artery, in order to dissect the infrapyloric lymph node station No. 6. (Clips 13.3 and 13.4) The key of this dissection lies in the presentation of the stomach. Good superior traction allows placing tension on the gastro-omental vessels in order to clearly identify them. This dissection may be difficult in adipose patients and can result in hemorrhage that is difficult to control, occasionally leading to conversion to an open procedure. (Clip 13.5) Ideally, a very small bipolar cautery helps at this point, but ultrasonic dissectors can be used as an alternative. Once the right gastro-omental vessels are divided, the pylorus and proximal duodenum are dissected at their posterior aspect.

After incising the gastro-hepatic ligament and the hepato-duodenal ligament, the proper hepatic artery, a branch of the common hepatic artery, is identified. Lymph nodes located at the left border of the proper hepatic artery correspond to station No. 12a and are cleared during the exposure of this vessel (Clips 13.6

13 Laparoscopic Distal Gastrectomy – LADG

Clip 13.7 Dissection of the gastro-hepatic ligament up to the hepatic common artery (case 1)

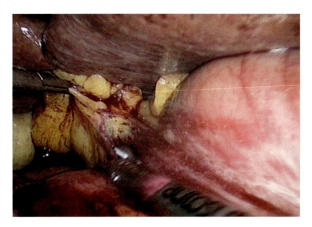

Clip 13.9 Posterior dissection and division of the duodenum (case 2)

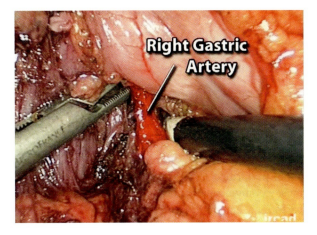

Clip 13.8 Division of the right gastric artery

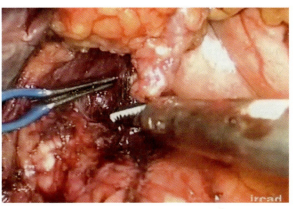

Clip 13.10 Posterior dissection and division of the duodenum (case 1)

and 13.7). The exposure of these structures requires the retraction of the left lobe of the liver using an atraumatic retractor placed either through the left subcostal trocar or through a port placed in the epigastrium. The right gastric artery is now identified and dissected completely, which removes the suprapyloric lymph nodes corresponding to station No. 5. We then divide this vessel at its root between clips with a posterior approach from behind the pylorus (Clip 13.8).

The inferior and superior border of the duodenum is then freed and can be divided with a linear stapler introduced through the left latero-umbilical port (Clips 13.9 and 13.10). A blue cartridge is used and the dissection performed 0.5-cm distal to the pylorus. The distal part of the stomach is grasped and lifted cephalad. This maneuver exposes the common hepatic artery, which is dissected towards the trunk of the splenic artery. This represents the dissection of the lymph node station 8 (Clip 13.11).

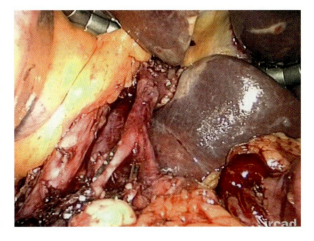

Clip 13.11 Dissection of the common hepatic artery

Clear identification of the celiac trunk and the origin of the hepatic and splenic arteries is necessary in order to avoid any injury to these vessels. The left gastric vein is completely dissected before being controlled by clips and then divided.

13.6.3 Step III: Further Dissection of the Left Gastric Artery

The trunk is dissected and its surrounding lymph nodes, station No. 7, are removed. Lymph node station No. 9, around the celiac trunk, is also dissected while paying attention to the celiac vagal branch, which heads to the celiac node traveling just behind the left gastric artery. The left gastric artery is divided between clips (Clip 13.12). Complete freeing up of the lesser omentum allows resection of the right pericardial lymph node station No. 1 and of the lymph nodes of the lesser curvature corresponding to station No. 3. At this point in the procedure, the dissection is completed and the stomach can be divided. Graspers introduced through the trocars in the right and left subcostal region present the specimen. The stapler is brought in through the left latero-umbilical port. Two to three firings of a green 60-mm load are required to divide the stomach (Clip 13.13).

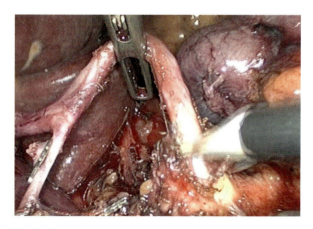

Clip 13.12 Lymphadenectomy of nodal stations 7, 8, and 9

"En bloc" resection of the stomach and its lymph nodes is now completed. The stomach with its dissected perigastric lymph nodes is placed in a retrieval bag and left in the upper part of the abdominal cavity. It will be removed at the end of the procedure through a mini laparotomy.

13.6.4 Step IV: Creation of the Gastro-jejunal Anastomosis

13.6.4.1 Different Techniques

- Ante-colic
- Trans-mesocolic
- Intra-corporeal
- Extra-corporeal

We perform the anastomosis completely intra-corporeal. Another option is to extract the specimen through a 5–6-cm mini-laparotomy and to create the anastomosis extracorporeal. A smaller laparotomy can also be used to extract the specimen with the anastomosis being performed laparoscopically. This is one of the most common approaches. The anastomosis can be performed ante-colic which is the easiest way chosen by many authors [7]. The trans-mesocolic route is another option, more difficult, but preferred by our group. The stomach will be exposed by suspension to the abdominal wall, using two sutures, which helps creating the anastomosis (Clip 13.14). For this technique, a suture with a straight needle is introduced through the abdominal wall, in front of one side of

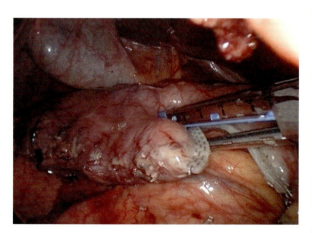

Clip 13.13 Division of the stomach

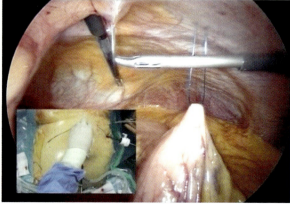

Clip 13.14 Exposure of the stomach by trans-abdominal suspension

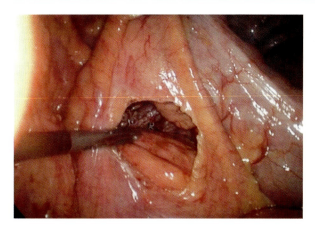

Clip 13.15 Trans-mesocolic route and approximation of the stomach to the mesocolon

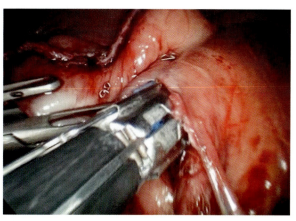

Clip 13.16 Gastro-jejunal anastomosis, closure of the mesocolic window and extraction of the specimen (case 1)

the gastric remnant. The stitch is placed full thickness through the stomach and brought out close to its entry point. Tension on this suture, combined with a second suture placed on the other side of the stomach, allows to expose the posterior aspect of the stomach. Another technical variant would be in approximating the gastric stump at the mesocolic window by placing three sutures, hence improving the exposure for the anastomosis (Clip 13.15).

13.6.4.2 Creation of Anastomosis

We place the camera in the subcolic area. We identify the point where we will open the small bowel, which is exactly 40 cm after the ligament of Treitz. The small bowel is opened using scissors. The stomach is opened at the left side of the anastomotic line. A stapler is inserted through the latero-umbilical port and its jaws are introduced into the small bowel and the stomach, in order to perform an anisoperistaltic anastomosis. Two firings with 45-mm blue cartridges are used (Clips 13.16 and 13.17). The resulting enterotomy is closed with a running suture (Polysorb 2/0 – Covidien). The mesocolic as well as the mesenteric windows are closed with a running suture. If necessary, the quality of the anastomosis can be controlled endoscopically or by injecting methylene blue into the stomach through the previously placed naso-gastric tube.

The specimen is finally extracted either through an enlargement of the umbilical incision or through a suprapubic incision.

The postoperative management is the same as in traditional open surgery.

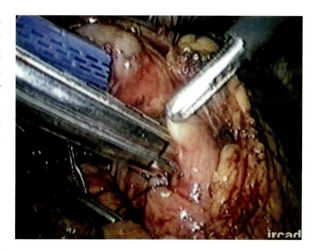

Clip 13.17 Gastrojejunal anastomosis (case 2)

13.7 Results and Complications

Patients who are candidates for a laparoscopic distal gastrectomy usually present with tumors located in the middle and lower part of the stomach. An uneventful procedure takes between 2 and 4 h. It is not associated with a higher mortality since it does not pose a specific vascular risk. Several intraoperative complications have been described in the literature, which are usually due to incorrect handling of the instruments: colon perforation, liver perforation, and splenic laceration [8].

Conversion to open surgery will be necessary when the quality of the dissection does not appear to be totally safe, or in case of a hemorrhage which cannot be controlled laparoscopically. The conversion rate is at around 5%.

Postoperative complications are the same as those observed in classic gastrectomies, including postoperative intra-abdominal bleeding. The most feared complication is a duodenal stump leak which can be treated conservatively, if it is well drained.

Late complications are gastric outflow obstruction and gastric motility disorders that lead to impaired food intake and reflux. Dietary modifications may solve those problems most of the time and revisional surgery is seldom necessary.

Long-term complications are due to peptic ulcers and, potentially, cancers 5 years after the surgical procedure at the gastric stump. Those outcomes are unpredictable and their surgical treatment remains a difficult challenge.

13.8 Conclusion

Laparoscopic distal gastrectomy with D2 lymph node dissection is safe for an experienced team with advanced laparoscopic skills and results in equivalent oncological outcomes. This technique is well-standardized and offers the same long-term results as other more traditional approaches. Several teams suggest using a surgical robot to perform this resection [9]. They demonstrate that a robot can be used to complete this surgical procedure, but the use of a robot does not show significant benefits in outcomes. As well, several teams suggest performing transvaginal NOTES gastrectomies, but keep in mind that NOTES surgery remains a very complex procedure despite promising initial results [10].

Quick Reference Guide

1. Position patient in split leg technique, with surgeon standing between the legs
2. Instrumentations:
   - Use of atraumatic graspers is crucial
   - Automatic bipolar electrocautery systems like Ligasure™ shorten operative time and secure hemostasis
   - Linear staplers are used to transect the stomach (60 mm green), the duodenum (45 mm blue), and to perform the anastomosis (45 mm blue)
3. As a first step perform a staging laparoscopy to rule out T4 disease
4. Consider Sentinel lymph node mapping in early stage cancer
5. Mobilization of stomach and lymph node dissection
   - Start by dividing the gastro-colic ligament and dissecting along the gastro-omental vessels below the spleen
   - Now turn dissection from left to right towards the pylorus. Gastro-omental vein and artery are divided to gain access to infra-pyloric lymph nodes
   - Clear lymph nodes to the left border of the main hepatic artery by retraction of the left lobe of the liver
   - Divide right gastric artery at its root
6. Divide the duodenum using a linear stapler with a 45-mm blue cartridge
7. Identification of celiac trunk and origin of hepatic and splenic artery is crucial to avoid any injury to these structures
   - Left gastric vein is now divided
   - Lymph node dissection is completed around celiac trunk
   - Left gastric artery is now divided
8. The stomach is now divided using a linear stapler with 60-mm green cartridges
9. Specimen is placed in a retrieval bag
10. Perform an anisoperistaltic anastomosis:
    - Open small bowel using scissors
    - Open stomach to the left of the staple line using scissors
    - Two firings of the 45mm linear stapler (blue cartridge) must be applied in order to anastomose the bowel with the stomach
    - The stapler's introduction enterotomy is closed with a running suture (Polysorb 2/0)
    - Close the mesocolic and mesenteric windows
11. The specimen is extracted through an umbilical or suprapubic incision

Acknowledgments The authors thank Guy Temporal and Richard Bastier for reviewing the manuscript.

References

1. Miura, S., Kodera, Y., Fujiwara, M., Ito, S., Mochizuki, Y., Yamamura, Y., Hibi, K., Ito, K., Akiyama, S., Nakao, A.: Laparoscopy-assisted distal gastrectomy with systemic lymph node dissection: a critical reappraisal from the viewpoint of lymph node retrieval. J. Am. Coll. Surg. **198**, 933–938 (2004)
2. Lee, S.I., Choi, Y.S., Park, D.J., Kim, H.H., Yang, H.K., Kim, M.C.: Comparative study of laparoscopy-assisted distal gastrectomy and open distal gastrectomy. J. Am. Coll. Surg. **202**, 874–880 (2006)
3. Tokunaga, M., Hiki, N., Fukunaga, T., Nohara, K., Katayama, H., Akashi, Y., Ohyama, S., Yamaguchi, T.: Laparoscopy-assisted distal gastrectomy with D2 lymph node dissection following standardization – a preliminary study. J. Gastrointest. Surg. **13**, 1058–1063 (2009)
4. Silberhumer, G.R., Hufschmid, M., Wrba, F., Gyoeri, G., Schoppmann, S., Tribl, B., Wenzl, E., Prager, G., Laengle, F., Zacherl, J.: Surgery for gastrointestinal stromal tumors of the stomach. J. Gastrointest. Surg. **13**(7), 1213–1219 (2009)
5. Orsenigo, E., Tomajer, V., Di Palo, S., Albarello, L., Doglioni, C., Masci, E., Viale, E., Staudacher, C.: Sentinel node mapping during laparoscopic distal gastrectomy for gastric cancer. Surg. Endosc. **22**, 118–121 (2008)
6. Mayers, T.M., Orebaugh, M.G.: Totally laparoscopic Billroth I gastrectomy. J. Am. Coll. Surg. **186**, 100–103 (1998)
7. Seshadri, P.A., Mamazza, J., Poulin, E.C., Schlachta, C.M.: Technique for laparoscopic gastric surgery. Surg. Laparosc. Endosc. Percutan. Tech. **9**, 248–252 (1999)
8. Bo, T., Zhihong, P., Peiwu, Y., Feng, Q., Ziqiang, W., Yan, S., Yongliang, Z., Huaxin, L.: General complications following laparoscopic-assisted gastrectomy and analysis of techniques to manage them. Surg. Endosc. **23**(8), 1860–1865 (2009)
9. Song, J., Kang, W.H., Oh, S.J., Hyung, W.J., Choi, S.H., Noh, S.H.: Role of robotic gastrectomy using da Vinci system compared with laparoscopic gastrectomy: initial experience of 20 consecutive cases. Surg. Endosc. **23**, 1204–1211 (2009)
10. Nakajima, K., Nishida, T., Takahashi, T., Souma, Y., Hara, J., Yamada, T., Yoshio, T., Tsutsui, T., Yokoi, T., Mori, M., Doki, Y.: Partial gastrectomy using natural orifice translumenal endoscopic surgery (NOTES) for gastric submucosal tumors: early experience in humans. Surg. Endosc. Apr 9 (2009)

Laparoscopic Total Gastrectomy – *LATG*

Seigo Kitano, Norio Shiraishi, Koji Kawaguchi, and Kazuhiro Yasuda

14.1 Introduction

Many diagnostic modalities for gastric cancer have been developed in the recent past and mass screenings have become popular in Japan. This is thought to have contributed to an increased incidence of early gastric cancer (EGC). EGC now accounts for over 50% of the total incidence of gastric cancer. For the treatment of EGC, minimally invasive therapies, such as laparoscopic and endoscopic procedures, have been adopted [1–3].

It was in 1991 when the first laparoscopy-assisted distal gastrectomy (LADG) for EGC was performed in Japan [4]. Since then, laparoscopic surgeons have made efforts to establish safe and standardized LADG techniques and to clarify the feasibility and oncologic accuracy of LADG for EGC. The number of patients who have undergone LADG has rapidly increased in Asian countries, and many studies have shown that LADG for EGC can achieve the same oncological results when compared to an open procedure. LADG has become the treatment of choice for ECG worldwide.

With the development of new surgical instruments and advanced laparoscopic gastrectomy (LG) techniques, and with accumulating evidence of its advantages, the indications for LG have spread in two directions. LADG with extended lymph node dissection has been applied to advanced cancer confined to the gastric wall without preoperative evidence of lymph node metastasis [5, 6]. Laparoscopic-assisted total gastrectomy (LATG) and laparoscopic-assisted proximal gastrectomy (LAPG) have each been applied to EGC located in the proximal stomach [7].

In this chapter, the indications for, techniques of, and current status of LATG for gastric cancer are described.

14.2 Indications

The gastrectomy method and the extent of lymph node dissection are selected according to the location and size of the gastric cancer. The location, size, and depth of the cancer are determined preoperatively with a barium swallow study and an upper endoscopy. After completion of preoperative workup, the procedure necessary to completely remove local cancer is chosen.

LATG is used for cancers in which the oral margin is located in the upper third of the stomach. Although these cancers, theoretically, include not only proximal cancers but also advanced cancers, LATG is currently limited to early cancers and cancers confined to the proper muscularis layer without preoperative evidence of lymph node metastasis. The reasons for this limitation are technical difficulties and undetermined oncologic accuracy.

Early cancers include

- Cancers confined to the upper third of the stomach
- Cancers with lateral type spread

Among patients with early cancer, the incidence of lymph node metastasis is low: 2–5% in cases where the cancer is confined to the mucosa and 15–20% in

---

S. Kitano (✉), N. Shiraishi, K. Kawaguchi, and K. Yasuda
Department of Surgery I, Oita University Faculty of Medicine,
Oita 879-5593, Japan
e-mail: kitano@oita-med.ac.jp

cases where the submucosal layer is involved [8]. Endoscopic therapies such as mucosal resections (EMR) and endoscopic submucosal dissections (ESD) have become popular in Asian countries. The indication for ESD is a well-differentiated carcinoma confined to the mucosal layer or a well-differentiated carcinoma (size <3 cm) with slight invasion into the submucosal layer but without vascular invasion [9]. LATG is used to treat early cancers that are not suitable for EMR or ESD because of their size or depth of invasion. Endoscopic removal would be technically difficult in these cases.

There are several reports pertaining to lymph node metastasis in cases of advanced cancer confined to the upper third of the stomach [10, 11]. The incidence of microscopic lymph node metastasis among gastric cancer patients without serosal exposure of the cancer or without macroscopic lymph node metastasis is low. When LATG is performed, perigastric lymph nodes and lymph nodes along the common hepatic artery are dissected. Therefore, EGC and gastric cancer confined to the proximal stomach but invading the proper muscularis layer can be removed completely performing an LATG.

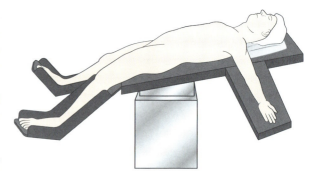

Fig. 14.1 Patient positioning for LATG. (Drawing by Hippmann GbR, Schwarzenbruck, Germany)

14.3 Surgical Technique

14.3.1 Patient Positioning

The patient is placed supine in a slight 10° reverse Trendelenburg position on the operating table. After general anesthesia is induced and gastric tube and Foley catheter are inserted, the patient's legs are abducted. The surgeon stands on the patient's right side, and the camera assistant stands between the patient's abducted legs. The first assistant stands on the patient's left side, and the second assistant stands on the surgeon's left side (Fig. 14.1).

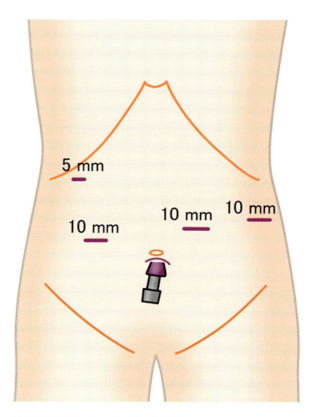

Fig. 14.2 Port placements for LATG

14.3.2 Trocar Placement

A vertical subumbilical incision of 1 cm is made and a Hassan trocar inserted. All trocars are inserted under direct vision. The abdomen will be insufflated with CO_2 to a pressure of 10 mmHg. Two 10-mm working ports are placed above the level of the camera trocar, to the right and left of the umbilicus. A 10-mm trocar, used by the first assistant, is then inserted into the left lateral abdomen. An additional 5-mm trocar, which will be alternatively used by the primary surgeon or second assistant, is placed in the right upper quadrant (Fig. 14.2).

14.3.3 Dissection of the Greater Omentum and Gastro-splenic Ligament

Under laparoscopic vision, the greater omentum and gastro-colic ligament are opened near the middle of the body of the stomach using laparoscopic ultrasonic coagulation shears (LCS). The opening is extended toward the inferior pole of the spleen (Fig. 14.3). During this step, the assistant grasps and lifts the greater omentum or gastro-colic ligament up to expose the operative field. The left gastro-epiploic vessels can be identified near the inferior pole of the spleen. These vessels are gently divided between clips and with ultrasonic coagulation. The gastro-splenic ligament is then dissected with LCS. Any bleeding and injury to the spleen should be avoided at this point (Fig. 14.4).

14.3.4 Division of the Right Gastro-epiploic Vessels

Dissection of the greater omentum and gastro-colic ligament is now extended toward the infra-pyloric area. In the infra-pyloric area, the greater omentum and gastro-colic ligament are dissected layer by layer, and the surface of the pancreatic head is exposed. The right gastro-epiploic vein is identified on the surface of the pancreatic head. The right gastro-epiploic vein is clipped and then divided. The assistant grasps and lifts the antrum cephalad. With this maneuver, the anterior surface of the pancreas and the gastroduodenal artery are easily found. The root of the right gastro-epiploic artery is exposed and divided using clips and ultrasonic coagulation (Fig. 14.5). Thus, peri-gastric lymph nodes along the greater curvature and infra-pyloric lymph nodes are dissected.

14.3.5 Dissection of the Lesser Omentum and Division of the Right Gastric Vessels

The second assistant lifts the left lobe of the liver up using a snake retractor. The lesser omentum is dissected starting from the left side of the hepatoduodenal ligament toward the right side of the esophago-cardial junction. The first assistant then grasps and lifts the right gastric vessels and isolates them. The avascular plane above the duodenal bulb is opened, and the lesser omentum along the right gastric vessels incised. This

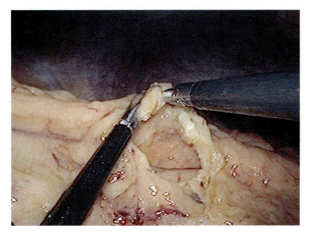

Fig. 14.3 Dissection of the greater omentum

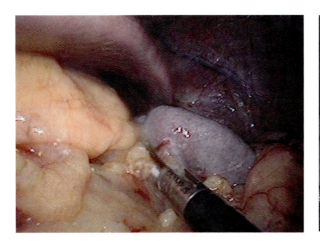

Fig. 14.4 Dissection of the gastrosplenic ligament

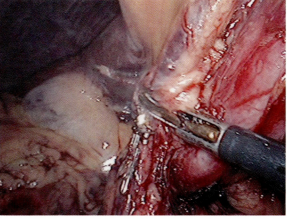

Fig. 14.5 Dissection of the right gastroepiploic artery

allows us to easily identify the roots of the vessels. The right gastric vessels are clipped and divided with LCS. At the completion of this step, the supra-pyloric lymph nodes are dissected en-bloc.

14.3.6 Transection of the Duodenum

Roux-en-Y reconstruction is the most popular method after LATG as well as after open total gastrectomy. The first assistant lifts the antrum of the stomach cephalad and the duodenal bulb is skeletonized circumferentially. Preferably, this step is done 'cold' in order to avoid any injury to the duodenum. The transected line is at the level of the duodenal bulb and we use a linear stapler for this. It is important to prevent bleeding at the cut line and to prevent injury to surrounding structures such as the hepatoduodenal ligament and liver.

14.3.7 Division of the Left Gastric Vessels

To identify the roots of the left gastric vessels, the gastropancreatic ligament is stretched out by the first assistant using a forceps. The peritoneum along the anterior border of the right crus of the diaphragm and the peritoneum along the anterior surface of the pancreas are incised. The roots of the left gastric vessels are easily isolated and divided between clips. Ultrasonic coagulation is used to dissect the lymph nodes along the left gastric artery (Fig. 14.6).

14.3.8 Dissection of Lymph Nodes Along the Common Hepatic Artery

To obtain better exposure of the operative field, the first assistant retracts the pancreas downward and the surgeon lifts the connective tissue containing the lymph nodes up. A longitudinal incision is made in the peritoneum along the anterior surface of the pancreas and the lymph nodes along the hepatic artery are dissected upward using LCS.

14.3.9 Division of the Posterior Gastric Artery and Transection of the Esophagus

After the gastro-diaphragmatic ligament is divided and the distal stomach lifted upward, the roots of the posterior gastric vessels, separated from the splenic artery, are identified. The posterior gastric vessels are clipped and divided. Remaining connective tissue between the stomach and the crus of the diaphragm is now dissected and the anterior and posterior branches of the vagus nerve are divided with ultrasonic coagulation. After complete dissection of the area around the abdominal esophagus, we transect the esophagus using a linear stapler. The proximal cut end has to be at the upper part of the esophago-cardial junction in order to include the entire cardia (Fig. 14.7).

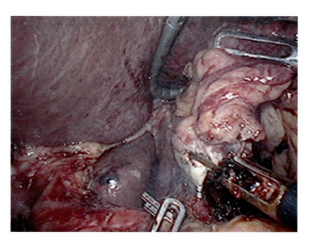

Fig. 14.6 Dissection of the left gastric artery

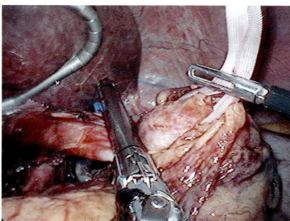

Fig. 14.7 Transection of the esophagus

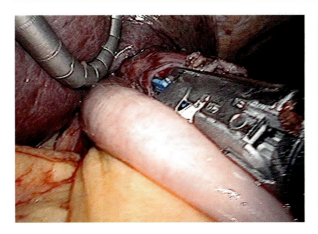

Fig. 14.8 Esophago-jejunostomy using a linear stapler to create the backwall of the anastomosis

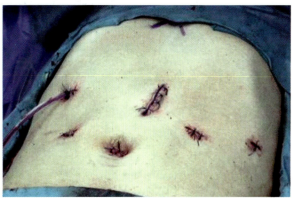

Fig. 14.9 The operative wounds after LATG

14.3.10 Mini-laparotomy, Roux-en-Y Reconstruction and Braun's Anastomosis

A 5-cm mini-laparotomy is made in the upper midline of the abdomen and a wound protector is inserted. The entire resected specimen, stomach and lymph nodes en-bloc, is exteriorized through this mini-laparotomy. After partial exteriorization of the small bowel, we identify the ligament of Treitz and transect the jejunum with a linear stapler 40 cm downstream. We create a jejuno-jejunostomy (Y-anastomosis) as a functional end-to-end anastomosis extracorporeal.

14.3.11 Esophago-jejunostomy

Pneumoperitoneum is reestablished laparoscopically and a side-to-side esophago-jejunostomy is performed intracorporeal with a linear cutter for the backwall (Fig. 14.8). The resulting enterotomy is hand-sewn laparoscopically to prevent anastomotic stenosis.

14.3.12 Irrigation, Drainage, and Wound Closure

After the abdominal cavity is irrigated with copious amounts of warm saline, the operative field is checked for complete hemostasis. A closed-suction drain is placed near the esophago-jejunostomy, and the operative wounds are closed in standard fashion (Fig. 14.9).

14.4 Present Status of LATG in Japan

The Japanese Society of Endoscopic Surgery (JSES) conducts a nationwide survey of endoscopic surgeries every 2 years since 1992. Although LATG is not as popular as LADG, the number of LATGs is increasing gradually in Japan. According to the 10th nationwide JSES survey (2010), a total of 35,000 laparoscopic gastrectomies were performed for cancer between 1991 and 2009. These surgeries included 26,033 (75%) LADGs at 423 institutions and 3,216 (9%) LATGs at 260 institutions (Fig. 14.10). In conjunction with an LADG, peri-gastric lymph node dissection (D1, D1+α) was performed at 80 (19%) institutions and extended lymph node dissection (D1+β, D2) at 335 (79%) (Fig. 14.11).

14.5 Complications and Technical Difficulties

14.5.1 Intra- and Postoperative Complications of LADG and LATG

Intraoperative and postoperative complication rates, according to the national JSES survey, are shown in Table 14.1. The LATG postoperative complication rate

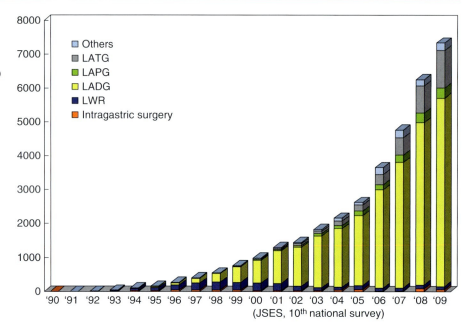

Fig. 14.10 Laparoscopic surgery for gastric cancer in Japan (Japanese Society of Endoscopic Surgery [JSES], 10th nationwide survey 2010)

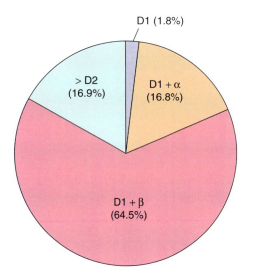

Fig. 14.11 Lymph node dissection in LATG (Japanese Society of Endoscopic Surgery [JSES], 10th nationwide survey 2010)

decreased remarkably from 51.3% at the time of the sixth national survey (2002) to 21.8% at the time of the tenth national survey, and it is now comparable to that of LADG. The most frequent postoperative complications were anastomotic leaks and anastomotic stenosis. The intraoperative complication rate for LATG remains higher than that of LADG. Frequent intraoperative complications are bleeding and injury to other organs.

14.5.2 Methods for Reconstruction for the Esophago-jejunostomy in LATG

There are few reports about the method of reconstruction after LATG, including [12, 13].

- Roux-en-Y reconstruction
- Jejunal interposition
- Jejunal pouch interposition

Postoperative complications occurred most frequently when a classical esophago-jejunostomy was performed. To decrease the incidence of complications after LATG, several modalities in creating an esophago-jejunostomy have been developed (Fig. 14.12). In a standard esophago-jejunostomy, a circular or linear stapler is used. If the anastomosis is performed with a circular stapler it is done through a mini-laparotomy. In general, there are two types of side-to-side esophago-jejunostomies commonly used laparoscopically, using a linear stapler:

- Anisoperistaltic side-to-side esophago-jejunostomy
- Isoperistaltic side-to-side esophago-jejunostomy

It still remains unclear which reconstruction method is superior in terms of patients' quality of life and postoperative complications.

Table 14.1 Complication rates associated with LADG/LATG (Japanese Society of Endoscopic Surgery [JSES], 10th nationwide survey 2010)

	National survey (year)	Sixth (2002)	Seventh (2004)	Eighth (2006)	Ninth (2008)	Tenth (2010)
LADG						
	Intraoperative	2.9%	3.5%	1.6%	1.7%	1.1%
	Postoperative	15.5%	14.3%	10.9%	8.2	7.5%
LATG						
	Intraoperative	0%	0.8%	2.5%	2.7%	2.7%
	Postoperative	51.3%	28.9%	7.1%	17.8	21.8%

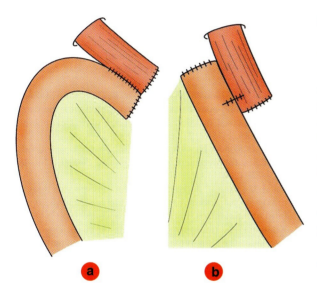

Fig. 14.12 Two different types of Esophago-jejunostomy. (**a**) Anisoperistaltic (antiperistaltic) side-to-side esophago-jejunostomy and (**b**) isoperistaltic side-to-side esophago-jejunostomy

14.6 Evaluation of Clinical Outcomes After LATG

To our knowledge, there are only a few reports regarding clinical outcomes after LATG. Tanimura et al. analyzed the results of 72 LATGs and showed that LATG is safe and oncologically feasible for T1 or T2 gastric cancers [14]. Usui et al. conducted a case-control study and showed that LATG is suitable for EGC and has the advantage of a shorter recovery time when compared with open total gastrectomy [15]. Further clinical studies to clarify the safety and oncologic feasibility of LATG are needed.

14.7 Conclusions

Since 1991 EGC has been treated laparoscopically, either performing LADG or LATG. Particular in Asian countries, LADG seems to be the standard for EGC. LATG is not yet common because of the small number of ECG providing an indication for the procedure and because of its technical challenges. As the indications for LG have expanded to advanced gastric cancer and laparoscopic techniques developed, the use of LATG has clearly increased. In the near future we will have to

- Establish standard techniques for LATG
- Verify the advantages of LATG using a minimally invasive approach
- Evaluate the oncologic accuracy of LATG

Quick Reference Guide

1. Patient is placed in a supine position, legs abducted. The surgeon stands on the right side of the patient.
2. A set of 5 trocars is used: one Hassan, three 10-mm, and one 5-mm trocar.
3. Vessels:
   - The greater omentum and gastro-colic ligament are divided to gain access to the gastro-epiploic vessels near the inferior pole of the spleen. Vessels are divided using clips
   - Exposure of the right gastro-epiploic artery at the root and division with clips; lymph node dissection along the greater curvature and infra-pyloric

- Opening of the lesser omentum and isolation of right gastric vessels above the duodenal bulb
4. Transection of the duodenum using a linear stapler.
5. Dissection of the lymph nodes along the common hepatic artery
    - Retract pancreas downward
    - Lift up the lymph node package at the anterior surface of the pancreas
6. Lift the stomach cephalad, identify the roots of the posterior gastric vessels, clip, and divide.
7. Clear the abdominal esophagus of all connective tissue and transect with a linear stapler. Make sure to include the entire esophago-cardial junction. Divide the main trunk of the posterior and anterior vagal nerve.
8. Insertion of a wound protector through a 5-cm mini-laparotomy in the upper midline and retrieval of the specimen.
9. Anastomosis:
    - Creation of an end-to-end functional jejuno-jejunostomy 40-cm downstream of ligament of Treitz, extra-corporeal
    - Reestablishing of the pneumoperitoneum and creation of a side-to-side esophago-jejunostomy, intracorporeal
        – Backwall: linear stapler
        – Anterior wall: hand sewn laparoscopically
10. Perform an *anisoperistaltic* anastomosis:
    - Place a closed suction drain near the esophago-jejunostomy.

References

1. Shiraishi, N., Yasuda, K., Kitano, S.: Laparoscopic gastrectomy with lymph node dissection for gastric cancer. Gastric Cancer **9**, 167–176 (2006)
2. Ono, H., Kondo, H., Gotoda, T., et al.: Endoscopic mucosal resection for treatment of early gastric cancer. Gut **48**, 225–229 (2001)
3. Shiraishi, N., Adachi, Y., Kitano, S., et al.: Indication for and outcome of laparoscopy-assisted Billroth-I gastrectomy. Br. J. Surg. **86**, 541–544 (1999)
4. Kitano, S., Iso, Y., Moriyama, M., et al.: Laparoscopy-assisted Billroth I gastrectomy. Surg. Laparosc. Endosc. **4**, 146–148 (1994)
5. Tanimura, S., Higashino, M., Fukunaga, Y., et al.: Laparoscopic distal gastrectomy with regional lymph node dissection for gastric cancer. Surg. Endosc. **19**, 1177–1181 (2005)
6. Uyama, I., Sugioka, A., Fujita, J., et al.: Laparoscopic total gastrectomy with distal pancreatosplenectomy and D2 lymphadenectomy for advanced gastric cancer. Gastric Cancer **2**, 230–234 (1999)
7. Tanimura, S., Higashino, M., Fukunaga, Y., et al.: Laparoscopic gastrectomy with regional lymph node dissection for upper gastric cancer. Gastric Cancer **6**, 64–68 (2003)
8. Yasuda, K., Shiraishi, N., Suematsu, T., et al.: Rate of detection of lymph node metastasis is correlated with the depth of submucosal invasion in early stage gastric carcinoma. Cancer **85**, 2119–2123 (1999)
9. Ono, H., Kondo, H., Gotoda, T., et al.: Endoscopic mucosal resection for treatment of early gastric cancer. Gut **48**, 225–229 (2001)
10. Katai, H., Sano, T., Fukugawa, T., et al.: Prospective study of proximal gastrectomy for early gastric cancer in the upper third of the stomach. Br. J. Surg. **90**, 850–853 (2003)
11. Kitamura, K., Yamaguchi, T., Nishida, S., et al.: The operative indications for proximal gastrectomy in patients with gastric cancer in the upper third of the stomach. Surg. Today **27**, 993–998 (1997)
12. Mochiki, E., Kamimura, H., Haga, N., et al.: The technique of laparoscopically assisted total gastrectomy with jejunal interposition for early gastric cancer. Surg. Endosc. **16**, 540–544 (2001)
13. Omori, T., Nakajima, K., Endo, S., et al.: Laparoscopy assisted total gastrectomy with jejunal pouch interposition. Surg. Endosc. **20**, 1497–1500 (2006)
14. Tanimura, S., Higashi, M., Fukunaga, Y., et al.: Laparoscopic gastrectomy with regional lymph node dissection for upper gastric cancer. Br. J. Surg. **94**, 204–207 (2006)
15. Usui, S., Yoshida, T., Ito, K., et al.: Laparoscopy-assisted total gastrectomy for early gastric cancer: comparison with conventional open total gastrectomy. Surg. Laparosc. Endosc. Percutan. Tech. **15**(6), 309–314 (2005)

Endoluminal Procedures for Early Gastric Cancer

15

Brian J. Dunkin and Rohan Joseph

15.1 Introduction

Gastric cancer is the second leading cause of cancer death in the world and the leading cause in Japan. Countries in Central and South America as well as the former Soviet Union also have high death rates from gastric cancer. Fortunately, the incidence of gastric cancer in the USA has been steadily declining over the last 6 decades. In the 1940s gastric cancer was the third leading cause of death from cancer in the USA, but in 2007 the incidence declined to its current level of the 7th leading cause and 14th most common cancer overall [1].

The high incidence and prevalence of gastric cancer in Japan led to the development of a nationwide screening program to detect it at an earlier stage. In 1983, Japan began screening all individuals aged 40 or older for gastric cancer using photofluoroscopy [2]. This led to a substantial increase in the detection of this malignancy in its early and more treatable stages. The term "early gastric cancer" (EGC) was coined to describe these early forms of gastric cancer confined to the mucosa or submucosa only, regardless of lymph node status [3]. As a result of their screening program, the incidence of detecting EGC in Japan rose from 10.3% in the 1960s to as high as 60% today [4].

Because of the lower incidence of gastric cancer in the USA, screening programs are not cost-effective as they are in Japan. As a result, gastric cancer in the U.S.A. is usually diagnosed in its advanced stage with few treatment options and poor survival. Even so, 10% of gastric cancers diagnosed in the USA are EGC, and if high risk individuals underwent proper evaluation with esophagogastroduodenoscopy (EGD) this percentage would be higher.

15.2 Risk Factors for Gastric Cancer

People at high risk for developing gastric cancer are those with

- Pernicious anemia
- Gastric ulcer
- Chronic atrophic gastritis
- Intestinal metaplasia in the stomach
- A surgical history of
  - Vagotomy
  - Partial gastric resection
  - Gastroenterostomy

In addition, all patients over the age of 40 who suffer from dyspepsia should undergo an EGD since there is a 1 in 50 chance of gastric cancer in this group [5].

15.3 Rational for Endoscopic Resection of Early Gastric Cancer (EGC)

The traditional treatment for EGC has been gastric resection with lymphadenectomy resulting in 5-year survival rates of over 90% in Japan and Europe [6]. Retrospective analysis of the pathology specimens from these cases coupled with long term outcome data demonstrated that the risk of lymph node involvement

B.J. Dunkin (✉) and R. Joseph
Department of Surgery, Methodist Institute for Technology, Innovation and Education (MITIE), 6550 Fannin Street, SM 1661A, Houston, TX 77030, USA
e-mail: bjdunkin@tmhs.org

in the majority of EGC cases was negligible [7]. As a result, practitioners in Japan began to consider endoscopic resection as a possible less invasive treatment for EGC. Endoscopic resection of sessile polyps in the colon was first described by Deyhle et al. in 1973 [8]. This technique was first applied to elevated EGC lesions in Japan in 1974 [8]. The technique then progressed to a revolutionary endoscopic mucosal resection (EMR) technique called "strip-off biopsy" in 1984 [9]. Strip biopsy was designed to harvest more complete mucosal specimens from the stomach for more accurate staging of the malignancy and to guide therapy. EMR has become an accepted modality for excising EGC, but it is limited in the ability to achieve en bloc resection for lesions greater than 20 mm in dimension. Larger lesions must then be removed piecemeal which can lead to incomplete removal and higher local recurrence rates [4]. These limitations of EMR led to the development of a new endoscopic procedure which utilized novel cutting devices for submucosal dissection of larger specimens en bloc. First described in 2000, it has been termed endoscopic submucosal dissection (ESD) [4].

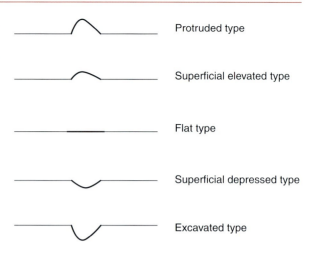

Fig. 15.1 Early gastric cancer: Macroscopic appearance

most frequent dye used in the stomach and colon [7]. Combining chromoendoscopy with high magnification video endoscopes may further enhance mucosal details thus better delineating the features and extent of EGC and possibly increasing the completeness of endoscopic resection [7].

15.4 Selecting Patients for Endoscopic Resection of EGC

15.4.1 Endoscopic Staging

In order to properly select patients for endoscopic resection of EGC, the Japanese have developed a very comprehensive staging system. In fact, the International and Japanese Gastric Cancer Associations recommend that EGC lesions be described very precisely, both endoscopically and pathologically [10]. On endoscopy, the number and size of the lesions along with the tumor location must be described. In addition, the macroscopic appearance of the lesion should be described as shown in Fig. 15.1 [10].

15.4.1.1 Chromoendoscopy

Abnormal areas of gastric mucosa may be better delineated by staining them with dye – a technique called chromoendoscopy. Indigo carmine (0.5–1.0%) is the

15.4.1.2 Endoscopic Ultrasound

Radiologic imaging has been used to try to differentiate EGC from deeper gastric cancer. Kwee et al. report a comprehensive review of the literature examining the accuracy of endoscopic ultrasound (EUS) to accurately predict depth of gastric cancer [11]. Unfortunately, they found that most published studies of this modality include a very heterogeneous group of patients and utilize different ultrasound techniques, making it impossible to determine if EUS can accurately differentiate between mucosal and deeper gastric cancers.

15.4.1.3 Virtual Gastroscopy

Virtual gastroscopy using three-dimensional computer tomography has also been tested for accuracy in evaluating gastric cancer but, like EUS, early work in this area examines a very heterogeneous group of tumors and does not demonstrate improved accuracy over EUS [12].

15.4.2 Pathologic Staging

Mucosal lesions removed endoscopically should be pinned on a flat corkboard and the size, shape, and orientation of the margins recorded, followed by fixation in formalin. The fixed material is then sectioned at 2 mm intervals and the following features recorded:

- Histological type
- Largest dimension
- Presence or absence of
  - Ulceration
  - Lymphatic invasion
  - Vascular invasion

If the vertical margin is clear, the depth of invasion is recorded as well using the dimensions described in Fig. 15.2 [7]. The depth of submucosal invasion is recorded in microns (sm1 < 500 μm, sm2 ≥ 500 μm).

15.5 Indications for Endoscopic Resection of EGC

15.5.1 Standard Indications

In 1998, prior to the advent of ESD, the Japanese Gastric Cancer Association (JGCA) recommended the following criteria for selecting patients for endoscopic resection of their EGC [3]:

- Well or moderately differentiated adenocarcinoma
- Cancer confined to the mucosa only
- Lesion < 20 mm in greatest dimension
- No endoscopic evidence of ulceration

Using these accepted criteria, the incidence of lymph node metastasis is only 0.36% [13].

15.5.2 Extended Indications

These strict criteria led to many patients having surgical resection of their EGC despite a low risk of lymph node metastasis. In 2000, Gotoda et al. published a report comparing 3,016 intramucosal EGCs with 2,249 submucosal tumors from patients who had surgical resection of EGC. They found that the best predictor of lymph node metastasis was the presence of lymphatic or vascular involvement [14]. Based on this work, extended criteria were suggested as appropriate for endoscopic resection of EGC. These guidelines were accepted by the JGCA and published in 2004 although it was recommended that they be applied only as part of a clinical trial [15].

Extended guidelines for endoscopic resection of EGC are

1. Well or moderately differentiated adenocarcinoma with no lymphatic or vascular invasion (Table 15.1)
   - Mucosa (m1, m2, m3) or superficial submucosa (sm1 < 500 μm), no ulcer

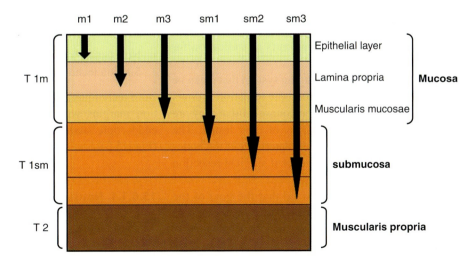

Fig. 15.2 Early gastric cancer: Histopathological classification: m1 – confined to epithelial layer, m2 – invasion of lamina propria, m3 – invasion of muscularis mucosa, sm1 – invasion into upper one-third of submucosa, sm2 – invasion into middle one-third of submucosa, sm3 – invasion into lower one-third of submucosa

Table 15.1 Extended guidelines for resection of EGC. Well differentiated adenocarcinoma with no lymphatic or vascular invasion

Depth of invasion	Ulcer	Size	Treatment
Mucosa (m1, m2, m3) or superficial submucosa (sm1 < 500 μm)[a]	No	Any	Resect endoscopically, en bloc if possible
Mucosa (m1, m2, m3) or superficial submucosa (sm1 < 500 μm)[a]	Yes	≤3 cm	Resect endoscopically, en bloc if possible
Mucosa (m1, m2, m3) or superficial submucosa (sm1 < 500 μm)[a]	Yes	>3 cm	Surgical resection

[a] See Fig. 15.2 for definition of "m" levels

Table 15.2 Extended guidelines for resection of EGC. Poorly differentiated adenocarcinoma with no lymphatic or vascular invasion

Depth of invasion	Ulcer	Size	Treatment
Mucosa (m1, m2, m3) or superficial submucosa (sm1 < 500 μm)[a]	No	≤2 cm	Resect endoscopically, en bloc if possible
Mucosa (m1, m2, m3) or superficial submucosa (sm1 < 500 μm)[a]	Yes	>2 cm	Surgical resection

[a] See Fig. 15.2 for definition of "m" levels

- Any size
- Resect en bloc if possible
- Mucosa (m1, m2, m3) or superficial submucosa (sm1 < 500 μm), with ulcer
  - ≤3 cm
  - Resect en bloc if possible
2. Undifferentiated adenocarcinoma with no lymphatic or vascular invasion (Table 15.2)
   - Mucosa (m1, m2, m3) or superficial submucosa (sm1 < 500 μm), no ulcer
     - ≤2 cm
     - Resect en bloc if possible

These extended criteria recommendations continue to evolve. Studies like that of Ishikawa et al. suggest that ulcerated lesions should be confined to less than 20 mm and that any submucosal invasion is an indication for surgical resection [16].

It is also clear from this staging system that it can be completed only after the endoscopic resection is done. As a result, patients should be counseled that they are undergoing an excisional biopsy of their lesion. The final pathologic evaluation will determine if the endoscopic resection was adequate, or if surgical resection will be required as a next step.

It should also be emphasized that the goal of the first endoscopic resection of EGC is complete en bloc removal of the lesion. Oda et al. have shown that ESD achieves a higher curative resection rate than EMR (73.6% vs. 61.1%) and a higher residual and recurrent tumor free 3-year survival (97.6% vs. 92.5%). [4] The authors speculate that a one-piece resection with negative tumor margins is responsible for these improved results using ESD. Takanaka et al. have confirmed this finding [17].

15.6 Techniques for Endoscopic Resection of EGC

15.6.1 Endoscopic Mucosal Resection (EMR)

There are two main methods of performing EMR:

- Nonsuction technique (lift-and-cut)
- Suction technique (suck-and-cut)

Both techniques begin by marking the planned resection margins with brief bursts of cautery using an endoscopic snare with the wire minimally deployed (Fig. 15.3).

15.6.1.1 Nonsuction Technique – *"Lift-and-cut"*

The original strip-off biopsy technique described by Tada et al. in 1984 utilized a lift-and-cut technique

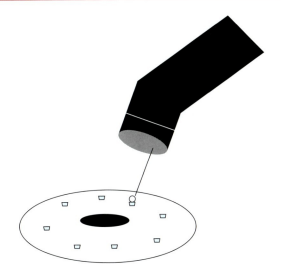

Fig. 15.3 Marking of resection margin with a snare

of the bleb [19], and Indigo carmine (0.004%) is often added to the injectate to stain the submucosa and provide a better evaluation of the depth of resection. Submucosal injection can also be used to determine if a lesion is appropriate for endoscopic resection. Lack of elevation of a lesion with submucosal injection indicates deep submucosal involvement and is a relative contraindication to proceeding with EMR [7].

The strip-off biopsy technique is performed with a double-channel gastroscope. After creating the submucosal elevation, the lesion is grasped with a rat-tooth forceps that has been passed through an open polypectomy snare. The forceps lifts the lesion and the snare is pushed down around its base and resection ensues. This procedure has been simplified so that it can be accomplished with a standard single-channel gastroscope by simply elevating with submucosal injection and then snaring free-hand with the polypectomy snare.

(Fig. 15.4) [18]. All of these techniques begin with the creation of a submucosal bleb to elevate the lesion off the submucosa and decrease the risk of perforation. This injection was originally done with saline, but other solutions have been used to gain better results. Epinephrine can be added to decrease bleeding. Hypertonic saline (3.75% NaCl), 20% dextrose, or sodium hyaluronate are used to improve the development and maintenance

15.6.1.2 Suction Technique – "Suck-and-cut"

In this method, the lesion is aspirated into a cap attached to the tip of the endoscope to elevate it off the muscularis propria, with or without submucosal injection, and then resected. The most common methods

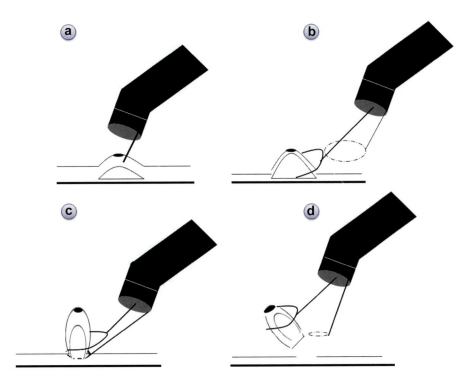

Fig. 15.4 Endoscopic mucosal resection: "*Lift-and-Cut*" technique. (**a**) Submucosal injection to lift mucosa, (**b**) lesion lifted by forceps passed through an open snare, (**c**) snare tightened around the lesion, and (**d**) excision with diathermy

utilize either a cap (EMR-C) or a band ligating device (EMR-L) fitted on the end of the endoscope. For EMR-C (Fig. 15.5), a specialized cap is fitted to the end of the endoscope providing a chamber for aspiration of mucosa. Typically the lesion is elevated with a submucosal injection and a crescent shaped snare is mounted into the distal inner rim of the cap. The lesion is then aspirated into the cap and the snare tightened around its base. The snared "pseudopolyp" is then pushed outside the cap and excised with monopolar energy. The special EMR caps come in various sizes and shapes, the largest of which is 18 mm in diameter.

When performing EMR-L (Fig. 15.6), submucosal injection may not be required. This technique utilizes a variceal band ligator to ligate the mucosal lesion and create a pseudopolyp. The banded tissue is then simply snare excised either above or below the band (Figs. 15.7 and 15.8).

Both EMR-C and EMR-L are limited in their capacity to accomplish en bloc resection. The maximum diameter amenable to one-piece excision is approximately 20 mm. If multiple resections are required, they should be accomplished at the initial setting if possible to optimize the submucosal lift which will not be readily attainable once scar tissue has formed.

15.6.2 Endoscopic Submucosal Dissection (ESD)

ESD allows for larger en bloc resections and proceeds in a fashion completely different from EMR. The procedure begins by marking the periphery of the lesion with small cautery burns using the tip of a snare. A margin of at least 5 mm is planned and marks are placed approximately every 2 mm (Fig. 15.9). A submucosal injection is then accomplished around the periphery of the lesion utilizing a solution such as sodium hyaluronate so that the elevation will persist throughout the procedure (Fig. 15.10). The submucosal solution is often stained with 0.004% Indigo carmine. A circumferential incision is then made to isolate the lesion using an ESD electrosurgical knife (Fig. 15.11). There are a number of ESD knifes to choose from:

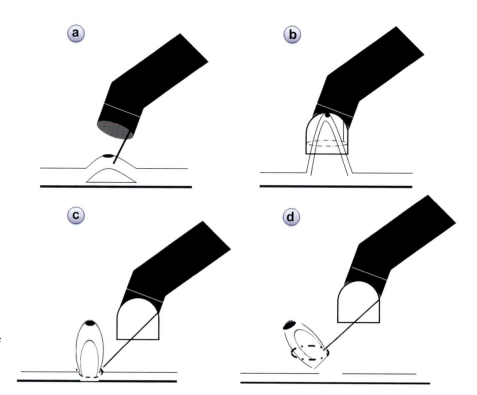

Fig. 15.5 Endoscopic mucosal resection: Suction cap – (EMR-C). (**a**) Submucosal injection to lift mucosa, (**b**) suction of lesion into cap and encircling by the snare, (**c**) snare tightened around the lesion, and (**d**) excision with diathermy

Fig. 15.6 Endoscopic mucosal resection: Band ligator – (EMR-L). (**a**) Endoscope with mounted EMR band ligator, (**b**) suction of lesion into band ligator, (**c**) banded lesion snared above or below band, and (**d**) excision with diathermy

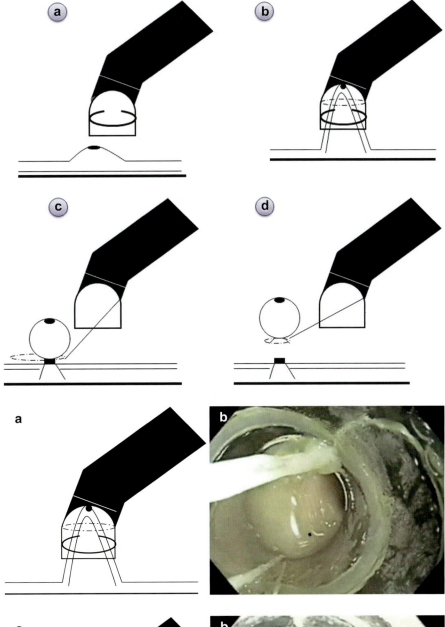

Fig. 15.7 Endoscopic mucosal resection: Band ligator – (EMR-L). Suction of lesion into band ligator. (**a**) Suction cap, (**b**) tissue suctioned into cap

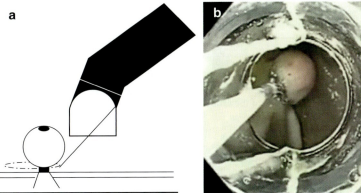

Fig. 15.8 Endoscopic mucosal resection: Band ligator – (EMR-L). Banded lesion snared above or below band. (**a**) Snare, (**b**) snare around base of lesion

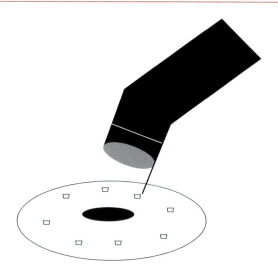

Fig. 15.9 Endoscopic submucosal dissection (ESD). Marking of planned resection margin

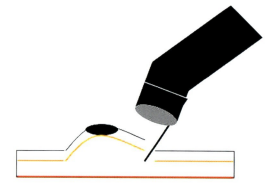

Fig. 15.11 Endoscopic submucosal dissection (ESD). Mucosal incision using a needle knife

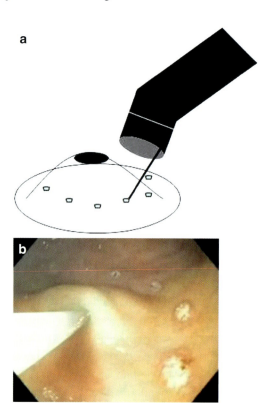

Fig. 15.10 Endoscopic submucosal dissection (ESD). Submucosal injection around the periphery of the lesion

- *Needle knife* (Fig. 15.12)
  First used for ESD by Hirao et al. in 1988. This knife has a fine tip and small contact area which allows sharp incision [20]. Because of its sharp nature, it can easily cause perforation if not controlled carefully. Mucosal incisions are usually begun with a needle knife, but then a switch is made to a protected tip knife to minimize the risk of perforation.

- *IT Knife* (Fig. 15.12)
  The insulated tip knife is a needle knife with the tip covered by a ceramic ball. This blunt, nonthermal tip reduces the risk of perforation. A second generation IT knife has a conducting surface on the bottom of the ball tip to allow for better tissue division when drawing back on the knife.

- *Hook knife* (Fig. 15.13)
  This is a needle knife with the distal 1 mm of the tip bent at a right angle. The knife also rotates for optimal positioning.

- *Flex knife* (Fig. 15.13)
  This knife has a rounded tip made of a twisted wire like a snare. Its length can be adjusted as needed. The shaft of the catheter is flexible with a thickened tip that acts as a tissue stop to minimize the chance of perforation.

- *Triangle tip knife* (Fig. 15.13)
  This knife has a triangular conductive tip that facilitates cutting mucosa. This knife was designed to be used for all parts of the ESD procedure.

Once the circumferential incision is complete, additional solution is injected into the submucosa in the center to obtain a more complete lift. One of the ESD knives is then used to excise the lesion in the submucosal plane (Figs. 15.14 and 15.15). Meticulous hemostatis is critical in order to facilitate visualization, and the lesion is often positioned opposite the ground to utilize gravity to clear the field. An electrosurgical hemostatic forceps (Fig. 15.16) may be useful to maintain hemostasis. A transparent hood is often mounted on the end of the endoscope to facilitate visualization and dissection into the submucosal plane.

15.7 Complications

15.7.1 Bleeding

Bleeding and perforation are the two most common serious complications of EMR and ESD. Bleeding is the most frequent complication and can occur at the time of the procedure or later (0–30 days afterward). Intraprocedure bleeding can usually be controlled using a combination of diathermy and endoscopic clips. Delayed bleeding, manifest by hematemesis or melena, usually occurs within 12 h of the procedure and is an indication for urgent repeat endoscopy. The incidence of bleeding post endoscopic resection of EGC varies from 1.5% to 24% depending on how it is defined. Oda et al. in a review of 714 resections had only one patient (0.1%) require a blood transfusion post EMR [4].

15.7.2 Perforation

Perforation is the most feared complication of EMR and ESD with rates of approximately 1% and 3% respectively [21]. Perforations recognized at the time of occurrence are often managed with endoscopic clip closure. Perforations as large as 25 mm have been closed using an omental patch held in place by endoscopic clips [22]. Patients with symptomatic pneumoperitoneum from the perforation have the air removed by needle aspiration. Post clip closure, these patients receive nasogastric tube decompression, empiric broad spectrum antibiotics, high dose acid suppression therapy, and frequent clinical reevaluation. Signs of worsening overall condition or generalized peritonitis are indications for operative exploration and repair. Oda et al. managed 16 perforations in 714 endoscopic resection patients with clip closure only. None required surgical exploration [4].

15.8 Postprocedure Management

In the short term, patients are placed on double dose proton pump inhibitors and carafate to aid healing of the resected site. EGC is frequently associated with synchronous lesions and, even after complete endoscopic resection, metachronous lesions can occur. As a result, a post resection endoscopic surveillance program is important. Two studies have demonstrated that

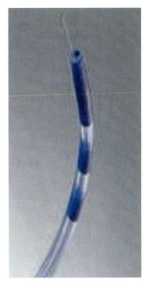
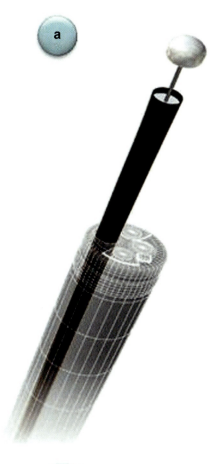

Fig. 15.12 ESD knives (courtesy of Olympus©). (**a**) Needle knife, (**b**) insulated tip knife. (With permission by Olympus America Inc, PA, USA)

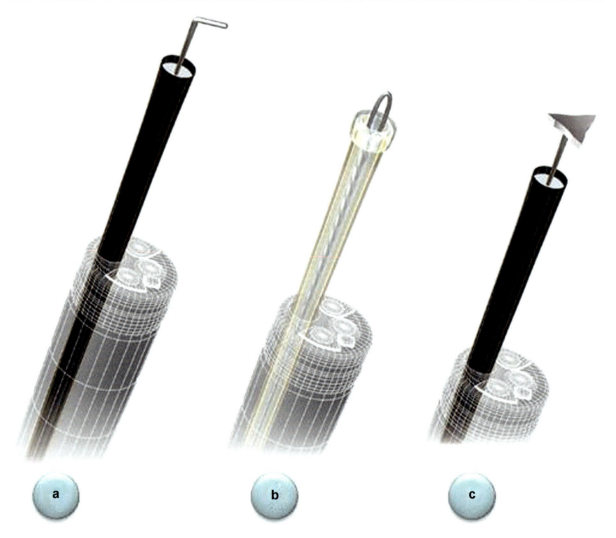

Fig. 15.13 ESD knives (courtesy of Olympus©). (**a**) Hook knife, (**b**) flex knife, and (**c**) triangle tip knife. (With permission by Olympus America Inc, PA, USA)

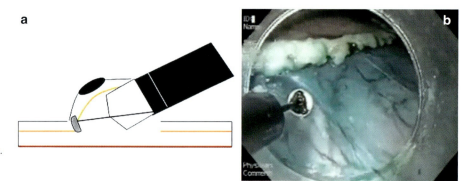

Fig. 15.14 Endoscopic submucosal dissection (ESD). Submucosal dissection using an IT knife

Fig. 15.15 Endoscopic submucosal dissection (ESD). Completion of dissection and resection

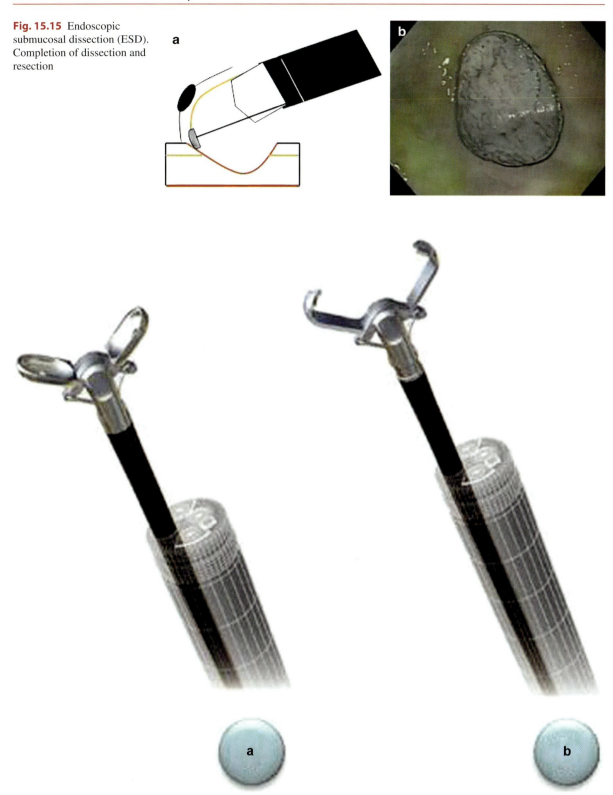

Fig. 15.16 Hemostatic forceps (courtesy of Olympus©). (**a**) *Hotbite* hemostatic forceps and (**b**) *hotclaw* hemostatic forceps. (With permission by Olympus America Inc, PA, USA)

Table 15.3 Outcomes for endoluminal procedures in EGC – Reference summary

Outcomes	Study design	Reference
EMR has a disease specific 5 and 10-year survival rates of 99% making it the procedure of choice for well differentiated mucosal EGC <2 cm	Retrospective study of 131 patients followed for 18 years after en bloc EMR for small, well differentiated EGC	Uedo et al. [23]
Endoscopic Techniques (EMR and ESD) offer a 3-year tumor-free survival and overall survival rates of 94.4% and 99.2% respectively. ESD further affords the advantage of higher one piece resections and reducing local recurrences	Multicenter retrospective study of EGC in 655 patients meeting the following criteria; (a) Well or moderately differentiated adenocarcinoma (b) Depth of penetration into mucosa or less than 500 μm into submucosa (sm1) (c) Nonulcerated lesions irrespective of size, or less than 30 mm if ulcerated	Oda et al. [4]

annual endoscopic examinations are adequate to allow for early diagnosis and endoscopic treatment of synchronous or metachronous lesions while preserving the function of the stomach [7].

15.9 Outcomes

In 2005 Uedo et al. published their long-term outcomes for endoscopic resection of small (<20 mm) differentiated mucosal EGC lesions and compared them to surgical resection [23]. They demonstrated disease-specific 5- and 10-year survival rates of 99%. These types of results have led to EMR being the procedure of choice for managing small, differentiated mucosal EGC in Japan (Table 15.3).

For expanded criteria, the results for endoscopic resection of EGC in initial retrospective studies are encouraging. Oda et al. report a 100% 3 year disease specific survival rate and an overall 94.4% residual-free/recurrence-free rate. ESD also resulted in significantly higher (97.6%) residual-free/recurrence-free rates than EMR (92.5%) [4]. A prospective, phase II trial investigating the use of ESD to treat expanded indications for EGC has been initiated in Japan (JCOG 0607). This will be the first study to report 5-year outcomes from prospectively collected data and should clarify the utility of using ESD as the definitive therapy from treating EGC in patients with expanded indications.

It has been shown that ESD is safe when used in elderly patients with EGC who have poor performance status [7]. ESD has also been shown to be useful in treating recurrent lesions in patients who have had prior EMR [7].

15.10 Summary

EGC constitutes a distinct subgroup of patients with disease localized to the mucosa or submucosa regardless of lymph node involvement. Endoluminal therapies (EMR and ESD) have clearly demonstrated excellent overall and disease free survival with negligible morbidity as compared to surgical procedures. However, optimal criteria for patient selection will form the backbone of successful outcomes and long term data supporting ESD for extended criteria are still forthcoming.

In the meantime it will be imperative to educate patients that should the pathology from their endoscopy suggest deeper invasion a surgical procedure will be necessary.

Quick Reference Guide

Endoscopic Mucosal Resection (EMR)

1. Mark the margins of the area of interest with small cautery burns using the edge of a snare which is minimally deployed
2. When using the "Lift and Cut" or "Suction Cap" (EMR-C) techniques, submucosal injection is performed to elevate the lesion. Submucosal injection is not required while performing EMR-L. Failure of elevation of the lesion with submucosal injection is a relative contraindication to EMR as this indicates deeper extension of the tumor
3. A solution which maintains the bleb for a longer time is preferred and epinephrine may also be added to decrease bleeding

4. This elevated submucosal bleb may be steadied with a rat tooth forceps and directly snared when performing the "Lift-and-Cut Technique"
5. Alternately, during EMR-C and EMR-L the lesion is aspirated into the suction cap to create a pseudopolyp over which a snare is passed and tightened
6. The pseudopolyp is then excised with brief bursts of cautery
7. Perform multiple resections of the lesion at the initial setting itself, should en bloc resection not be possible

Endoscopic Submucosal Dissection (ESD)

1. Mark the periphery of the lesion with small cautery burns using the edge of a snare at intervals of 2 mm and with a margin of 5 mm from the edge of the lesion
2. The submucosa of the lesion is injected with sodium hyaluronate mixed with 0.004% indigo carmine dye to create a bleb, which will persist during the procedure. The indigo carmine stains the submucosa and clues the operator to the depth of resection
3. Further injections may be performed as needed during the procedure
4. A needle knife or triangle tip knife is used to incise the mucosa and gain access to the submucosa. A triangle tip knife or IT knife is then used to make a circumferential incision around the lesion over the areas marked by cautery burns.
5. After the mucosal incision the submucosa may be injected further to obtain a more complete lift
6. The needle knife is exchanged for an IT knife whose blunt insulated tip reduces the risk of perforation. Alternatively another preferred knife may be used
7. The dissection is carried out in the submucosal plane until the lesion is completely free from the underlying surface
   Positioning the lesion inferiorly by manipulating the scope's dials facilitates the dissection
8. Be vigilant for bleeding and manage this with available hemostatic devices
9. If a perforation is detected at the end of the procedure, it may be managed by endoscopic clips. Monitor the patient for any signs of peritonitis

References

1. Cabebe, E.C., Mehta, V.K., Fisher, G.: Gastric cancer. In: Perry, M.C., Talavera, F., Movsas, B., McKenna, R., Harris, J.E. (eds.) (2007) http://www.emedicine.com/med/TOPIC845.HTM
2. Hamashima, C., Shibuya, D., Yamazaki, H., et al.: The Japanese guidelines for gastric cancer screening. Jpn. J. Clin. Oncol. **38**, 259–267 (2008)
3. Japanese Gastric Cancer Association: Japanese classification of gastric carcinoma. Gastric Cancer **1**, 10–24 (1998). 2nd English edition
4. Oda, I., Saito, D., Tada, M., et al.: A multicenter retrospective study of endoscopic resection for early gastric cancer. Gastric Cancer **9**, 262–270 (2006)
5. Hallissey, M.T., Allum, W.H., Jewkes, A.J., et al.: Early detection of gastric cancer. BMJ **301**, 513–515 (1990)
6. Oliveira, J.F., Ferrão, H., Furtado, E., et al.: Early gastric cancer: report of 58 cases. Gastric Cancer **1**, 51–56 (1998)
7. Larghi, A., Waxman, I.: State of the art on endoscopic mucosal resection and endoscopic submucosal dissection. In: Waxman, I., Lightdale, C.J. (eds.) Gastrointest Endoscopy. Clin. N. Am. Endosurg, pp. 441-469. Saunders Philadelphia, Pennsylvania (2007)
8. Deyhle, P., Largiader, F., Penny, P.: A method for endoscopic electroresection of sessile colonic polyps. Endoscopy **5**, 38–40 (1973)
9. Takenaka, R., Kawahara, Y., Okada, H., et al.: Risk factors associated with local recurrence of early gastric cancers after endoscopic submucosal dissection. Gastrointest. Endosc. **68**(5), 887–894 (2008)
10. Larghi, A., Waxman, I.: Endoscopic mucosal resection: a treatment of neoplasia. In: Kochman, M.L., Shah, J.N. (eds.) Gastrointestinal Endoscopy. Clin. N Am. Endosc. Oncol. (2005), pp. 431–454. Saunders Philadelphia, Pennsylvania
11. Kwee, R.M., Kwee, T.C.: The accuracy of endoscopic ultrasonography in differentiating mucosal from deeper gastric cancer. Am. J. Gastroenterol. **103**, 1–9 (2008)
12. Bhandari, S., Shim, C.S., Kim, J.H., et al.: Usefulness of three-dimensional, multidetector row CT (virtual gastroscopy and multiplanar reconstruction) in the evaluation of gastric cancer: a comparison with conventional endoscopy, EUS, and histopathology. Gastrointest. Endosc. **59**(6), 619–626 (2004)
13. Yamao, T., Shirao, K., Ono, H., et al.: Risk factors for lymph node metastasis from intramucosal gastric carcinoma. Cancer **77**(4), 597–598 (1996)
14. Gotoda, T., Yanagisawa, A., Sasako, M., et al.: Incidence of lymph node metastasis from early gastric cancer: estimation with a large number of cases at two large centers. Gastric Cancer **3**, 219–225 (2000)
15. Japanese Gastric Cancer Association: Treatment guidelines for gastric cancer in Japan (in Japanese), 2nd edn. Kanehara, Tokyo (2004)
16. Ishikawa, S., Togashi, A., Inoue, M., et al.: Indications for EMR/ESD in cases of early gastric cancer: relationship between histological type, depth of wall invasion, and lymph node metastasis. Gastric Cancer **10**, 35–38 (2007)
17. Tanaka, M., Ono, H., Hasuike, N., et al.: Endoscopic submucosal dissection of early gastric cancer. Digestion **77**(suppl 1), 23–28 (2008)

18. Tada, M., Shimada, M., Murakami, F., et al.: Development of strip-off biopsy (in Japanese with English abstract). Gastroenterol. Endosc. **26**, 833–839 (1984)
19. Fujishiro, M., Yahagi, N., Kashimura, K., et al.: Comparison of various submucosal injection solutions for maintaining mucosal elevation during endoscopic mucosal resection. Endoscopy **36**, 579–583 (2004)
20. Hirao, M., Masuda, K., Asanuma, T., et al.: Endoscopic resection of early gastric cancer and other tumors with local injection of hypertonic saline-epinephrine. Gastrointest. Endosc. **34**(3), 264–269 (1988)
21. Ida, K., Nakazawa, S., Yoshino, J., et al.: Multicentre collaborative prospective study of endoscopic treatment of early gastric cancer. Dig. Endosc. **16**, 295–302 (2004)
22. Tsunada, S., Ogata, S., Ohyama, T., et al.: Endoscopic closure of perforations caused by EMR in the stomach by application of metallic clips. Gastrointest. Endosc. **57**(7), 948–951 (2003)
23. Uedo, N., Ishii, H., Tatsuta, M., et al.: Long-term outcomes after endoscopic mucosal resection for early gastric cancer. Gastric Cancer **9**, 88–92 (2006)

Part IV

Special Topics: Small Bowel

Laparoscopic Management of Small Bowel Tumors

Miguel Burch, Brian Carmine, Daniel Mishkin, and Ronald Matteotti

16.1 Introduction

Historically, small bowel tumors have been diagnosed at advanced stages because of lack of clear clinical symptoms. This resulted in potentially difficult operations at an advanced disease stage and was associated with a grim prognosis [1–3]. Until lately, the small bowel was a black box, whose contents could not be easily or reliably studied due to a lack of adequate instrumentation. With the next generation of endoscopes and applying diagnostic laparoscopies, the small bowel has become examinable in a less invasive and more accurate fashion. This has allowed for earlier diagnosis of disease and better prognosis for the patient.

Minimally invasive surgery has been applied widely to intra-abdominal malignancies with similar oncological outcome when compared to open surgery. Several studies, especially addressing colorectal tumors, have shown equivalent outcomes in terms of survival, recurrence rates, and number of lymph nodes harvested [4, 5].

Anastomosing small bowel laparoscopically has become a routine and successful practice in many surgical departments. This is in large part due to the routine performance of laparoscopic bariatric procedures at high-volume centers and therefore increased experience with advanced laparoscopic skills. Leak rates at the gastro-jejunostomy site are minimal, with many centers reporting rates as low as 1% [6, 7]. Leaks and obstructions at the jejuno-jejunostomy site have been rarely reported [8]. Thus, performing a diagnostic laparoscopy with added small bowel resection and intracorporeal anastomosis was a logical next step.

16.2 Epidemiology

Small bowel tumors are rare entities of the gastrointestinal tract. They account for less than 3% of all malignant bowel tumors despite the fact that the small bowel accounts for 90% of the gastrointestinal tract mucosa (Table 16.1). Data have been mainly collected as a single institution series over the last decades, making it difficult to develop definitive treatment algorithms, but allowing some understanding of risk factors and demographics of the affected population.

Small bowel tumors have a slight predominance in males. More than 50% of patients with malignant small bowel tumors are in their seventh decade of life.

Primary malignant neoplasms of the small bowel are more commonly found in individuals with certain predisposing conditions such as familial adenomatous polyposis (FAP), Crohn's disease, or Peutz-Jeghers syndrome. In the absence of such diagnoses, if a malignant small bowel lesion is identified, distant metastasis should be ruled out.

Approximately 10% of small bowel tumors are asymptomatic and discovered incidentally. Patients with small bowel malignancies usually present with a spectrum of vague symptoms, like abdominal pain, nausea,

M. Burch (✉)
Department of Surgery, Cedars Sinai Medical Center,
8635 W. 3rd Street, Suite 650W, Los Angeles,
CA, USA
e-mail: burchm@cshs.org

B. Carmine and D. Mishkin
Department of Surgery, Boston University School of Medicine,
Boston Medical Center, 715 Albany Street, Boston,
MA, USA
e-mail: brian.carmine@bmc.org

R. Matteotti
Surgical Oncologist/Minimally Invasive Surgeon,
263 Osborn Street, Philadelphia, PA 19128, USA
e-mail: ronald.matteotti@gmail.com

and weight loss. Hemorrhage, anemia, and a palpable abdominal mass are less common. Because of these vague symptoms, many small bowel tumors are misdiagnosed as irritable bowel syndrome or even somatic manifestations of psychiatric disorders. As such, they are often identified at an advanced stage [1]. Different types of small bowel tumors have a characteristic distribution throughout the intestine. This often helps to narrow down the list of differential diagnoses (Fig. 16.1).

16.3 Malignant Small Bowel Tumors

16.3.1 Adenocarcinoma

Adenocarcinoma represents the most common primary malignant small bowel tumor, accounting for 80–90% of small bowel malignancies, and 40% of all small intestine tumors. Eighty percent of these tumors

Table 16.1 Distribution, characteristics and prevalence of small bowel tumors

	Histology	Cell of origin	Distribution	Prevalence[a]	Notes
Benign	Leiomyoma	Smooth muscle cell	Equally	30–40%	
	Adenoma	Brunner's gland	Duodenum, proximal Jejunum	<2%	25% harbor malignancy
	Hamartoma	Mesenchyma	Jejunum, Ileum	<2%	Frequent in Peutz-Jeghers syndrome
	Hemangioma	Vasculature	Jejunum, Ileum	<2%	
	Lipoma	Adipocyte	Equally	<1%	
Malignant	Adenocarcinoma	Brunner's gland	Duodenum, proximal Jejunum	40–45%	More common in Crohn's, FAP, Peutz-Jeghers
	Carcinoid	Enterochromaffin cell	Throughout; Appendix and rectum most common	<1%	
	Lymphoma	Lymph node	Stomach (60%), Small bowel (30%)	<1%	
	GIST	Interstitial cell of Cajal	Throughout; Stomach and duodenum most common	2%	
	Metastasis	Any cell	Throughout	>90%	

[a] Numbers correlate with the prevalence of primary small bowel tumors, but >90% are metastatic with a distant primary source

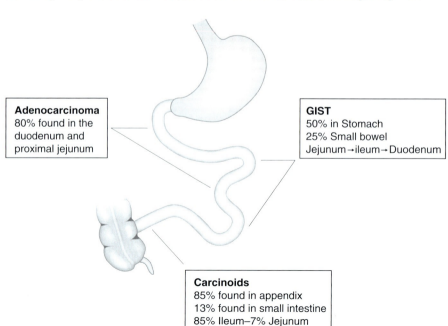

Fig. 16.1 Relative distribution of the three most common primary small bowel malignancies.
(Drawing by Hippmann GbR, Schwarzenbruck, Germany)

Adenocarcinoma
80% found in the duodenum and proximal jejunum

GIST
50% in Stomach
25% Small bowel
Jejunum→ileum→Duodenum

Carcinoids
85% found in appendix
13% found in small intestine
85% Ileum–7% Jejunum

are located in the duodenum and proximal jejunum. Originating from the bowel mucosa, they tend to present initially with obstructive symptoms. If located in the periampullary region of the duodenum, they may even present with obstructive jaundice or pancreatitis. The only curative therapy remains surgical resection. These lesions are more common in patients with long-term mucosal injury such as Crohn's disease and long-standing celiac sprue. These lesions, on initial radiological work up, present themselves often as apple core-type lesions [2].

16.3.2 Carcinoid Tumor

Small bowel carcinoids originate from enterochromaffin cells located in the crypts of Lieberkuhn (Fig. 16.2). These cells are neuroendocrine in origin and are involved in the amine precursor uptake and decarboxylation (APUD) system, thus making them capable of secreting functionally active polypeptides resulting in the carcinoid syndrome. In general, these tumors, even though pathologically malignant, follow an indolent course. One autopsy study showed that the rate of detection of a carcinoid tumor during an autopsy was 2,000 times greater than the annual incidence in a living population. This further suggests slow growth. Carcinoid tumors tend to occur later in life, with a mean age of 60 at presentation, and exhibit a slight predominance in males. When symptomatic, carcinoids present with obstruction, pain, or carcinoid syndrome. This syndrome is a constellation of vasomotor, cardiac, and gastrointestinal symptoms caused by substances released by the tumor. These factors include serotonin, histamine, kallikrein, bradykinin, and prostaglandins. The syndrome usually occurs after the primary tumor has metastasized to the liver or lung and therefore allows the secreting peptides to enter the systemic circulation. In the event the tumor is still confined to the small bowel, most of these substances are delivered to the liver via the portal circulation and are metabolized [3].

The prognosis of a carcinoid tumor is dependent on the size of the lesion, and the size corresponds to the metastatic potential of the primary lesion. Tumors less than 1 cm in size have around 20% incidence of metastasis to regional lymph nodes and beyond, whereas tumors 1–2 cm or greater than 2 cm in size have metastatic incidences of 70% and 90%, respectively. These observations guide surgical strategy. Smaller lesions may be adequately treated with local excision; larger lesions often require regional lymphadenectomy and potential hepatic resection if metastatic disease is present. In the event of widely metastatic disease, the therapy aims to relieve symptoms and is mainly palliative. This subset of patients may be managed medically or with a variety of ablative strategies, especially to control the tumor burden in the liver [9].

16.3.3 Non-hodgkin's Lymphoma (NHL)

Ten to fifteen percent of all Non-Hodgkin's Lymphoma (NHL) present as a primary gastrointestinal tumor. A large number of these tumors are low grade lymphomas arising from mucosa-associated lymphoid tumors (MALT), and are strongly associated with *H. pylori* infection. Celiac sprue, HIV, Epstein–Barr infection, and prolonged immunosuppresion are also predisposing conditions for GI lymphomas [10].

Typically, the stomach is the most common gastrointestinal site, followed by the small bowel in 30% of patients. Eighty percent of gastrointestinal NHL are of the B-cell variant, while the remainder are either T-cell or indeterminate in origin. Eradication of *H. pylori* often results in regression or cure of these tumors if located in the stomach; however, MALT'omas in the small bowel should be resected.

Multiple histologic subsets of these tumors exist. The most common subtype is diffuse large-cell lymphoma, followed by B-cell subtypes such as immunoproliferative small intestinal disease (IPSID), alpha

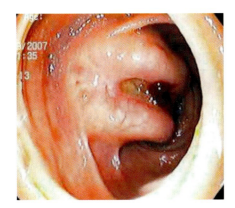

Fig. 16.2 Carcinoid tumor: endoscopic appearance

heavy-chain disease, and Mediterranean lymphoma. These latter conditions are associated with severe malabsorption and poor prognosis, though IPSID has shown comparable regression to MALT'omas if *H. pylori* is eradicated.

Treatment of these lesions is usually surgical when disease is isolated, though this represents less than 30% of patients. Adjuvant chemotherapy is a key component of treatment, and NHL is the only primary small bowel malignancy with proven response to adjuvant therapy. As with most cancers, the most important consideration when determining prognosis is the stage of the disease at the time of first presentation. In children, Burkitt's B-cell lymphoma is the most common tumor of the small bowel and is far more sensitive to adjuvant chemotherapy than counterparts in the adult population even when given following limited surgical resection.

16.3.4 GIST

Mesenchymal tumors of the small bowel are generally divided into two categories:

Those that are common to soft tissue tumors found elsewhere in the body

- Lipomas
- Schwannomas
- Hemangiomas
- Leiomyomas
- Leiomyosarcomas and
  those that are uniquely found in the GI tract
- Gastrointestinal stromal tumor – GIST.

Gastrointestinal stromal tumor (GIST) is most commonly found in the stomach and duodenum, but may occur at any location in the GI tract. The annual incidence of GIST is about 10–20 cases per one million people, though these data are constantly being reevaluated as understanding of these tumors evolves [11].

Initially, GISTs were believed to be smooth muscle tumors based on their histologic appearance and as such were often grouped together with leiomyomas and leiomyosarcomas. However, as these were further studied, it became clear that not only did they rarely show histologic features of complete muscle differentiation, but they were also immunophenotypically different from smooth muscle tissues of other organs (including leiomyomas of the GI tract). Ultimately it was noted that these tumors universally expressed CD117 antigen, part of the c-kit membrane tyrosine kinase, a well known proto-oncogene. This soon led researchers to identify the cell of origin as the interstitial cell of Cajal, believed to be the so-called "GI pacemaker," which has both smooth muscle and neuronal characteristics and functions to regulate peristalsis throughout the GI tract [11].

Clinical behavior of GIST tumors lies on a spectrum between benign and malignant. This is largely dependent on macroscopic, histologic, and molecular features. Tumors greater than 5 cm and with more than 5 mitosis per 50 high powered fields are considered more likely to adopt malignant behavior.

The first line of treatment in GIST should always be surgical resection. Characteristically these tumors possess a so-called "pseudocapsule," and care must be taken not to violate this capsule during the operation (Fig. 16.3). Fortunately, these tumors rarely invade adjacent structures despite being often large in size and this feature makes them an ideal disease to address laparoscopically. Laparoscopic resection is feasible, but some centers recommend limiting this approach to lesions less than 2 cm in diameter. In our experience, however, tumor size is more a factor dictating the ultimate size of incision and not laparoscopic resectability [11–13].

Despite complete surgical excision with negative margins, the 5-year recurrence rate of GIST remains around 50%. Imatinib (Gleevec®) is a tyrosine kinase inhibitor that has shown promise in the management of these tumors. Trials are underway not only as an adjuvant mode of therapy, but also as a neoadjuvant agent to shrink tumors that are unresectable due to location as well as for treatment of metastatic disease.

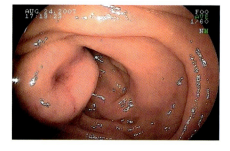

Fig. 16.3 Gastrointestinal stromal tumor (GIST): endoscopic view. Note the characteristic submucosal appearance

16.3.5 Metastatic Tumors

A metastasis from a distant primary tumor is by far the most common malignant neoplasm of the small bowel. Direct spread from a colonic or pancreatic primary is the most frequent origin of local invasion. Tumors may arise from any source via hematogenous spread, intraperitoneal seeding, or even swallowing of microscopic tumor fragments from a lung or oropharyngeal primary. The most common tumors metastazing to the small bowel are breast cancer and melanoma followed by renal cell cancer. Management of these tumors aims to only treat symptoms, and rarely has curative intent. Resection or bypass should be done as a palliative measure in patients with bleeding, pain, or especially obstructive symptoms. There are conflicting reports in the literature regarding prolonged survival of patients undergoing resection for solitary metastases, but without control of primary disease, further progression of metastatic disease is by far the most common course [14].

16.4 Benign Small Bowel Tumors

Benign small bowel tumors are slightly more common than malignancies of the small intestine, but are still overall an uncommon diagnosis. These tumors are usually asymptomatic, but may reach sufficient size to cause bowel obstruction or ischemia due to mass effect. In addition, they may be the cause of an occult GI bleed.

16.4.1 Leiomyoma

This is the most common benign small bowel tumor. The cell of origin is the smooth muscle cell of the small bowel muscularis and as such, the tumors are almost exclusively extralumenal. These tumors are often hypervascular and, if they do protrude intralumenally, are prone to ulceration and bleeding. Treatment of these lesions should always be resection, even if asymptomatic, as it is difficult to distinguish these lesions from leiomyosarcomas even on histologic examination [15].

16.4.2 Small Bowel Adenoma

Small bowel adenoma follow the same classification as colonic polyps and are divided into tubular, villous, or tubulo-villous (Fig. 16.4). Once diagnosed, they should be resected. The area of origin in the duodenum is believed to be the Brunner's gland, a submucosal duodenal cell responsible for the secretion of bicarbonate and mucus to neutralize gastric acid. Not surprisingly, these tumors have a in higher incidence in patients with concomitant *H. pylori* infection, and Brunner's gland hyperplasia in response to increased acid production is thought to universally precede adenoma formation. The majority of these lesions are located in the duodenum, particularly in the periampullary region; rare reports of proximal jejunal tumors exist. Up to 25% of adenomas have been found to harbor adenocarcinoma on histologic examination. Additionally, the literature suggests up to a 40% 10-year recurrence rate of duodenal adenomas, with 25% of these recurrences showing malignancy. Because of this pattern, some centers advocate pancreatico-duodenectomy in selected cases. Regardless, because of the high risk of recurrence, close endoscopic surveillance is mandatory in all patients [16].

16.4.3 Hamartoma

Harmatoma are frequent found in patients with Peutz-Jeghers syndrome and occur predominantly in the jejunum or ileum. These lesions have an extremely low potential for malignant transformation and should be resected only if they cause obstruction or

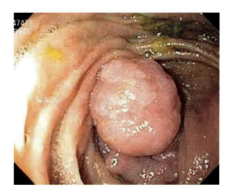

Fig. 16.4 Small bowel adenoma: polypoid variant

intussusception. Complete removal of all hamartomas is not only unnecessary, but impractical due to the diffuse nature of the condition. Synchronous adenocarcinoma of the colon and small bowel does occur with higher incidence in this population, and patient with Peutz-Jeghers should undergo routine surveillance with endoscopy [17, 18].

16.4.4 Hemangioma

Hemangiomas are usually solitary, congenitally acquired, and located in the jejunum and ileum. They follow an indolent course, growing slowly over a period of decades and are usually discovered as the source in the workup of an acute or chronic GI bleed. Peak incidence is in the third decade of life. They may be classified as cavernous, capillary, or mixed. Treatment options include endoscopic ablation, radiographic embolization, or surgical resection.

16.4.5 Lipoma

Lipomas are adipose tumors that may occur in any fat-containing tissue of the body, including the small bowel. Usually asymptomatic, they are most often found incidentally on abdominal CT scans done for other reasons. The most common symptom is obstruction or abdominal pain due to intussusception. Treatment of a solitary lipoma is observation only unless symptomatic, though surgical excision may be performed if the tumor is noted during laparotomy or laparoscopy. Lipomas that are larger than 2 cm or are rapidly growing should be excised to rule out liposarcoma.

16.5 Diagnostic Work-up

16.5.1 Endoscopic Evaluation

Using standard endoscopic equipment, visualizing the small intestine is limited to the duodenum during an upper endoscopy or to the ileum at the time of colonoscopy.

16.5.1.1 Push Enteroscopy and Overtubes

This technique allows for a pediatric colonoscope or a dedicated enteroscope, which is usually 250 cm in length, to be passed orally and advanced as far as possible. With or without the aid of an overtube, rarely does it advance more than 80 cm past the ligament of Treitz. Overtubes have been used to prevent gastric looping of the endoscope and try and maintain a more direct transfer of force into the small intestine. A new overtube, the Endosease Discovery SB®, with a spiral distal appendage, has shown that it can pleat the small intestine by spiraling the coupled endoscope and overtube deeper, while accordioning the small bowel past the ligament of Treitz onto the proximal portion of the overtube. This novel product and the technique for its use show great promise in the preliminary data [19].

16.5.1.2 Capsule Endoscopy

In 2001, the FDA approved the use of a wireless capsule endoscope which has since become the gold standard for visualizing the small intestine in a noninvasive fashion. This procedure uses the advantages of image acquisition and wireless transmission of data, as the capsule passes naturally through the gastrointestinal tract with the use of physiologic peristalsis. It captures 2 frames/s and stores the information on a data-recorder which is essentially a hard drive and battery supply. This is later downloaded and viewed as a video using proprietary software. This technique has allowed for a noninvasive view of the entire small intestine. Additional specialized capsules have been manufactured to specifically visualize the esophagus and colon. While this has revolutionized small bowel mucosal imaging, this is only a diagnostic tool, as currently no therapeutics can be applied using the device. It may create additional questions as the physician can only review the images acquired, without the usual ability to wash, use any standard accessory instruments, or close in on the spot in question. These are just some of the shortcomings compared to traditional endoscopy. As a result, other modalities are needed for potential therapeutic intervention and there are currently two systems, Given Imaging® and Olympus®, being sold in the USA to address some of these. The future of such technology will be aided by the current work on propulsive mechanism such as "legs," wireless steering, and potential interventions such as biopsies or tattooing [20].

16.5.1.3 Balloon-assisted Endoscopy

Pan-endoscopy for both, diagnostic and therapeutic purposes, is now possible in the ambulatory setting using balloon assisted endoscopy. The first such system was the double balloon endoscope (Fujinon®), whereby separate balloons can be insufflated and deflated on the endoscope and its specific overtube. The endoscope itself is 200 cm and the overtube 135 cm in length. Once the coupled device passed the ligament of Treitz, the balloons are inflated and deflated in a sequence to achieve greater depth of insertion. First, the endoscope is advanced – the push component of the procedure – to then be anchored at its distal depth by insufflating the endoscope balloon. This is followed by advancement of the overtube and its balloon insufflation. The pull part of the procedure will be used when the combination is shortened and will accordion the traversed small intestine onto the overtube. With the overtube balloon remaining inflated, it will hold the pleated bowel in place and allow for the endoscope, with the balloon deflated, to be advanced further. While reaching the cecum from the oral approach has been successful, this is not always the case. Should a pan-endoscopy be desired, then tattooing the depth of insertion from above should be done and subsequently a retrograde double balloon endoscopy performed in order to visualize the complete length of the small intestine. Recently, a single balloon system with similar lengths has been released by Olympus® whereby the overtube has the only balloon with which to facilitate the anchoring and pleating of the traversed small intestine [19].

16.5.1.4 Intraoperative Enteroscopy

Given the major advancements in small bowel imaging with new endoscopic equipment, the number of intraoperative enteroscopies has decreased, especially as a diagnostic modality. However, there are times when these procedures are still needed as other modalities cannot answer the question at hand. Different routes of insertion include the mouth, an enterotomy, or the anus. All attempts should be made to occlude the terminal ileum at the time of endoscopy to decrease the distention of the colon with air, which may increase the risk for complications and prolong hospital stay.

A major paradigm shift has occurred such that we no longer think of the small intestine as a black box. An increased ability to access this area endoscopically in the ambulatory setting allows for greater diagnostic yield. Noninvasive capsule endoscopy, that can take images wirelessly as it traverses the small intestine, balloon-assisted endoscopy whereby one can tattoo a lesion to mark for future surgical resection, sample or perform a polypectomy, dilate a stricture, place a stent or perform any other therapeutic intervention are only a few of the advancements in recent years. Using these new modalities we are as well able to reach areas such as the excluded stomach or biliary tree after Roux-en-Y reconstruction.

16.6 Preoperative Management

16.6.1 Indications

Given the greater ability to diagnose small bowel tumors at an earlier stage the opportunity to offer a minimally invasive procedure to selected patients has increased. Although no studies have shown a particular tumor size limiting laparoscopic resection, it is more difficult to manage tumors that are too small to visualize. However, when tumor size begins to dictate the size of the incision required to remove the specimen, an open approach might be more appropriate in managing that particular patient. Additionally, larger tumors invading adjacent structures may require en bloc resection, which is potentially a difficult task to accomplish laparoscopically, even in the most experienced hands. Despite suffering from bulky disease, it may be reasonable to perform a diagnostic laparoscopy to exclude metastatic disease, take biopsies or mobilize certain structures to facilitate a following open procedure. Initial laparoscopic exploration can allow for a more accurate placement of the actual incision and thus improve open performance as well limit the incision size necessary to perform the open procedure. It is known, that minimizing incision size results in early recovery due to decreased inflammatory response [21]. In addition, exposure of the peritoneum to CO_2 insufflation has also been associated with less inflammatory response [22].

16.6.2 Contraindications

There are currently, unlike in the past, only a few absolute contraindications to laparoscopic exploration. Hemodynamic instability due to significant hemorrhage or profound dehydration is perhaps the clearest contraindication. The deleterious effects of pneumoperitoneum on central venous return and thus cardiac output have been well documented, as have the effects on increasing afterload.

A history of multiple previous abdominal operations can be considered a relative contraindication and is dependent on the level of experience of the particular surgeon.

16.6.3 Preoperative Localization of Small Bowel Tumors

CT enterography, capsule endoscopy and double balloon endoscopy are three modalities, which led to more accurate preoperative tumor localization. Despite recent advancements all the above technologies have specific limitations. CT enterography is best suited to localize smaller tumors in the proximal or distal small bowel. Tumors in the mid-portion of the small bowel can often be mistaken as being located more distally or even more proximally towards the ligament of Treitz due to lack of permanent peritoneal attachments. Localization by capsule endoscopy is based on a local triangulation system that maps out the course of the capsule. This method is highly unreliable for accurate localization given the length of the small bowel, its peristaltic motion, and changes of a patient's position. The most reliable method for preoperative localization using a capsule is by having a close look at the time tracking feature. This feature documents in minutes the time the capsule enters the duodenal bulb and passes through the ileocecal valve into the colon. This can give some estimation of proximal, middle, or distal location of tumors based on the time the capsule took to traverse the small bowel.

Perhaps the most reliable preoperative tool for localization of small bowel tumors is double balloon endoscopy. Using this technique, it has recently become possible to map the entire length of the small bowel. The endoscopist can mark tumors with ink or at least the farthest point the scope was capable of reaching to aid in a surgeon's preoperative and/or intraoperative decision. Despite its diagnostic accuracy it is still capable of missing lesions and doesn't substitute a careful intraoperative inspection of the small bowel.

16.6.4 Relevance of Tumor Size

Tumor size matters in surgical decision making – should laparoscopy be attempted or not. Small tumors are difficult to localize intraoperatively, given the limitation of current instrumentation. We limit a laparoscopic resection to those small bowel tumors that are greater than 1 cm. All other tumors still undergo laparoscopic exploration, but if the tumor, documented by preoperative imaging, cannot be visualized, then we switch to a hand port to facilitate palpation. Patients who require significant lysis of adhesions after previous abdominal surgeries present usually with bowel wall thickening and scarring which can make it difficult to identify tumors larger than 1cm.

16.6.5 Preoperative Considerations

An extensive history and physical examination is completed to identify any comorbidity, which could be a contraindication for a laparoscopic approach. The anesthesia team evaluates patients with complicated medical problems preoperatively.

On physical examination, special attention is paid to previous abdominal incisions, which may influence surgical decision making. Every patient is consented for intraoperative push enteroscopy and hand port, should the tumor not be identifiable laparoscopically. The intraoperative push enteroscopy is performed by a gastroenterologist.

Patients are instructed to avoid aspirin and NSADS for 7 days prior to operation. Patients are put on a liquid diet the day prior to operation. A bowel preparation is not necessary. All patients are given 5,000 units of subcutaneous Heparin and have bilateral pneumatic compression stockings placed in the preoperative staging area. A first generation cephalosporin is given and occasionally we add Metronidazole in patients with significant tumor obstruction. A naso-gastric tube and Foley catheter is inserted, once the patient is asleep.

16.7 Surgical Technique

16.7.1 Patient Positioning

Patients should be placed on an operating table that is capable of assuming Trendelenburg, reverse Trendelenburg, as well as steep left and right tilted positions. Patients are placed supine position with the both arms tucked. The primary surgeon and camera assistant are positioned on the patient's left side. The patient is secured well to the table with straps across the lower body. Once the patient has been positioned, we place the operating table in all positions – a "tilt test" – to ensure ventilator tubing and intravenous lines are of appropriate length.

16.7.2 Trocar Placement

Appropriate port placement is paramount to ensure the surgical task at hand can be accomplished laparoscopically. The small bowel with its mesenteric root is located in the central compartment of the abdominal cavity. The length of the mesentery is dictated by patient factors like obesity, previous abdominal surgeries, history of inflammatory bowel disease etc. Tumor factors like desmoplastic reactions and invasion of neighboring structures play an important role as well. A shortened mesentery increases the difficulty of a complete small bowel examination and obtaining an adequate lymph node harvest and less commonly, can contribute to anastomotic tension. These are some very important considerations before placing the first port.

Our commonly used port configuration includes four ports, one 10-mm port for the camera, two 12-mm ports to allow the introduction of stapling devices and

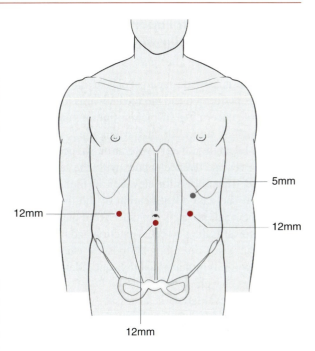

Fig. 16.5 Trocar placement. (Drawing by Hippmann GbR, Schwarzenbruck, Germany)

one 5-mm trocar (Fig. 16.5). Choice of peritoneal access is dictated by surgeon experience and the patient's past surgical history. We establish pneumoperitoneum using a Veress needle inserting it in the left upper quadrant of the abdomen. This has proven to be reliable and safe, even in patients who are morbidly obese. The only contraindication to this technique is patients with previous incisions close to the left upper quadrant. In these cases we perform an open entry in the left upper quadrant and subsequent lysis of adhesion using 5-mm ports. If access to the left upper quadrant is impossible we switch to the right upper quadrant. Access above the liver is usually associated with fewer complications, and adhesions in this location are not very common.

Following establishment of a pneumoperitoneum up to 15 mmHg, a 10-mm bladeless optical trocar is introduced, approximately two finger breaths below the umbilicus. This allows for full visualization of the small bowel. Three additional trocars will be used, two 12-mm trocars and one 5-mm trocar. It is possible to perform a small bowel resection using only three trocars, however, obtaining a large enough mesenteric resection with adequate lymph node harvest can be somewhat compromised by this approach.

16.7.3 Diagnostic Laparoscopy and Small Bowel Exploration

A complete diagnostic laparoscopy of all abdominal contents is performed and targeted towards identifying any area of concern. All suspicious findings are marked with a long silk suture for later evaluation.

At the beginning of our exploration we position the patient in reverse Trendelenburg with the table right side down. This allows for elevation of the transverse mesocolon and easy identification of the ligament of Treitz. The small bowel is run twice from the ligament of Treitz towards the ileo-cecal junction and back. This ensures that gross disease is not missed, evaluates the mesentery for lymphadenopathy, and identifies the tattoed sites as well.

A second evaluation is necessary to palpate the small bowel to identify intraluminal lesions. For this part of the procedure we slide two large, low-pressure bowel graspers along the small bowel. This allows for the identification of lesions within the lumen; however, small lesions can be missed entirely or mucosal folds be mistaken as real lesions.

We pay close attention not to create any serosal tears and in the event it happens, they are oversewn immediately.

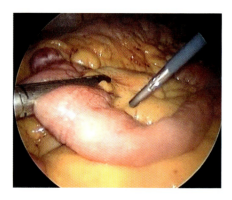

Fig. 16.6 Transection: a 45-mm EndoGIA, white load is usually sufficient. Strict perpendicular application is key!

mesentery. We examine the proximal and distal small bowel, the ends we intend to use to create our anastomosis, for pulsatile blood flow prior to firing of any stapler along the small bowel mesentery. If the mesentery is very short and the resection lines located in the proximal small bowel, we have to be very careful not to staple across the SMA.

An alternative approach to transect the mesentery is the use of a harmonic scalpel rather than using multiple firings of a stapler. This technique is quick and less expensive but has the disadvantage that we are not able to test the bowel segment for pulsatile blood flow.

The specimen will now be placed in a thick, tear resistant retrieval bag and the bag dropped into the pelvis for later retrieval.

16.7.4 Dissection and Transection of the Small Bowel

After identifying the pathology and the necessary extent of lymphadenectomy, we begin our dissection maintaining a safe margin towards the tumor. The small bowel is grasped close to the lesion and elevated by the surgeon. "No touch technique" is key! The first assistant inserts a 45-mm EndoGIA® from the opposite side (Fig. 16.6). Most of the small bowel is safely transected using a white load with a closed staple height of 1 mm. In the event of much thickened bowel wall, a blue cartridge should be used. This is often the case in patients suffering from longstanding partial small bowel obstruction. The stapler should be fired perpendicular to the small bowel. After transecting proximally and distally, we turn our attention to the mesentery. Typically, at least two 45-mm stapler loads are needed to create a wedge shaped excision along the

16.7.5 Creation of Anastomosis

We perform an intra-corporeal anastomosis. The two staple lines from the previous resection are aligned and we ensure that there is no torsion. We place a stay suture about 1 cm proximal to the cut edge to facilitate the insertion of the stapler (Fig. 16.7). The stay suture is placed on the anti-mesenteric side of the small bowel using a 3/0 silk. This will as well provide traction during creation of the side-to-side anastomosis. The first assistant holds the target small bowel segment in place by grabbing this suture and the surgeon performs the two mirror eneterotomies by using the harmonic scalpel. An Endo GIA®, 60-mm blue load, is inserted and fired assuring its antimesenteric position (Fig. 16.8). The staple line is routinely inspected for any bleeding and if present, this can be controlled by applying clips.

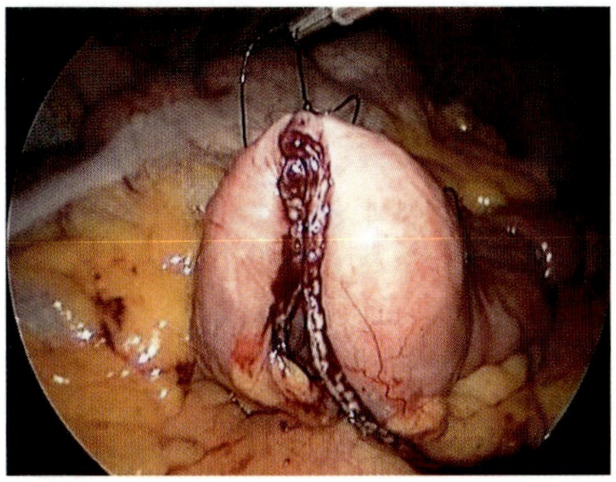

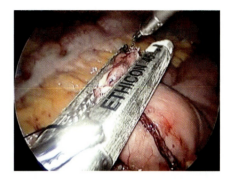

Fig. 16.7 Small bowel anastomosis: alignment of the two stapled limbs and placement of a stay suture on the anti-mesenteric side

Fig. 16.9 Small bowel anastomosis: closure of the common enterotomy with an EndoGIA 60-mm, blue load

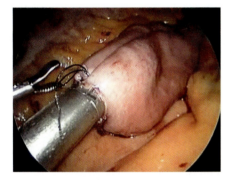

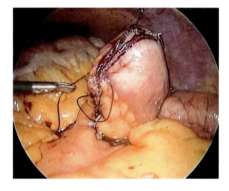

Fig. 16.8 Small bowel anastomosis: creation of two mirror enterotomies with the harmonic scalpel and firing of an EndoGIA, 60-mm blue load

Fig. 16.10 Small bowel anastomosis: closure of the mesenteric defect with a running 2/0 silk suture

Another tacking stitch is then placed exactly opposite to the previously placed stitch. These two stitches will oppose the small bowel edges and allow for placement of another 60-mm EndoGIA® blue load to close the common enterotomy (Fig. 16.9). The mesenteric defect is closed by a running 2-0 silk suture to prevent internal herniation. Only the two peritoneal edges should be incorporated into this suture line and deep stitches should be avoided in order not to compromise the blood flow towards the anastomosis (Fig. 16.10).

Intracorporeal anastomosis can be created using a double staple technique as described above or a triple staple technique by firing a second blue load to create a wider opening. In the event of using the triple staple technique, we recommend using two firings of a 45-mm blue load rather than two firings of a 60-mm blue load. The benefit of the triple staple technique is a decreased incidence of anastomotic stricture by creating a large side-to-side anastomosis. In our experience, the incidence of anastomotic strictures, using a single firing of a 60-mm blue load, is extremely low as long as we close the common enterotomy very carefully. In the event of shortened mesentery and short gut syndrome, we recommend closing the common enterotomy using a hand-sewn technique with two layers to preserve bowel length [8].

16.7.6 Hand-assisted Approach

In the event of a nonidentifiable lesion during diagnostic laparoscopy, it might become necessary to insert a hand port. The hand port is placed in the midline and the camera switched to the left lower quadrant. Using this configuration it will be possible to perform a push enteroscopy as well if necessary. In this event, the small bowel should be gently clamped, just proximal to the ileocecal valve, using a locking bowel grasper. The hand is used to prevent the distal small bowel from filling with air as well as to guide the enteroscope into the bowel.

16.7.7 Retrieval of Specimen and Wound Closure

As last step of the procedure we retrieve the Endo-bag with the specimen either through a hand port, if previously placed, or by enlarging one of the 12-mm port sites. Be patient in removing the specimen and do not rupture the bag in order to prevent port site recurrence.

All trocar sites greater than 10 mm are closed using an endo stitch device. Skin incisions are closed with a 4/0 subcuticular suture.

16.8 Postoperative Management and Outcome

The naso-gastric tube and Foley catheter are removed in the operating room unless further resuscitation is required. This would be necessary in patients with longstanding or acute partial small bowel obstruction where we expect a certain delay in return of bowel function. In all other patients, we begin a clear liquid diet on postoperative day 1. They are advanced as tolerated. If no complications occur, patients are discharged on postoperative day 2.

16.9 Conclusion

Given the recent advances in imaging and endoscopy and the use of these modalities as screening tools, small bowel tumors are being identified at a much earlier stage than in previous years. This translates into direct patient benefits in terms of long term outcome, and allows application of minimally invasive procedures in absence of advanced disease. Short-term complications such as wound infections, pneumonia and ileus are significantly decreased. Long-term complications like ventral hernias, formation of intra abdominal adhesions resulting in more difficult reoperations, if necessary, are less frequent. These tumors recur frequently and often require reoperation; therefore the benefits of a minimal invasive approach during the first surgery cannot be underestimated.

Quick Reference Guide

1. Reliable preoperative tumor localization is key to successful completion of the surgical procedure
2. Always perform a full diagnostic laparoscopy and address any area of concern prior to making a decision to proceed with resection
3. In the event of advanced disease involving nearby structures, have a low threshold to convert to open or at least to a hand assisted approach
4. If localization by laparoscopy is not possible, use a hand port
5. Resect the tumor segment with an appropriate margin each side using a white load EndoGIA®, applied perpendicular to the small bowel
6. Assure adequate lymphadenectomy down to the mesenteric root without compromising the vascular supply to the distal bowel
7. Create a side-to-side anastomosis in double staple technique by firing a single load of a 60-mm EndoGIA®, blue load
8. Always check your newly created anastomosis for internal bleeding. If necessary, control it with single clips
9. Close the mesenteric defect with a running suture by only approximating the peritoneal edges
10. Retrieve the specimen by strictly using a retrieval bag to prevent port site metastasis. All port sites larger than 10 mm should be closed

References

1. Matsuo, S., Eto, T., Tsunoda, T., et al.: Small bowel tumors: an analysis of tumor-like lesions, benign and malignant neoplasms. Eur. J. Surg. Oncol. **20**, 47–51 (1994)
2. Howe, J.R., Karnell, L.H., Menck, H.R., et al.: Adenocarcinoma of the small bowel: review of the National Cancer Data Base, 1985–1995. Cancer **86**, 2693–2706 (1999)
3. Memon, M.A., Nelson, H.: Gastrointestinal carcinoid tumors; current management strategies. Dis. Colon Rectum **40**, 1101–1118 (1997)

4. Clinical Outcomes of Surgical Therapy (COST) Study Group: A comparison of laparoscopically assisted and open colectomy for colon cancer. N. Engl. J. Med. **350**, 2050–2059 (2004)
5. Jayne, D.G., Guillou, P.J., Thorpe, H., et al.: Randomized trial of laparoscopic-assisted resection of colorectal carcinoma: 3-year results of the UK MRC CLASICC Trial Group. J. Clin. Oncol. **25**, 3061–3068 (2007)
6. Bertucci, W., Yadegar, J., Takahashi, A., et al.: Antecolic laparoscopic Roux-en-Y gastric bypass is not associated with higher complication rates. Am. Surg. **71**, 735–737 (2005)
7. Weller, W.E., Rosati, C.: Comparing outcomes of laparoscopic versus open bariatric surgery. Ann. Surg. **248**, 10–15 (2008)
8. Koppman, J.S., Li, C., Gandsas, A.: Small bowel obstruction after laparoscopic Roux-en-Y gastric bypass: a review of 9, 527 patients. J. Am. Coll. Surg. **206**, 571–584 (2008)
9. Soreide, J.A., van Heerden, J.A., Thompson, G.B., et al.: Gastrointestinal carcinoid tumors: long-term prognosis for surgically treated patients. World J. Surg. **24**, 1431–1436 (2000)
10. O'Boyle, C.J., Kerin, M.J., Feeley, K., et al.: Primary small intestinal tumours: increased incidence of lymphoma and improved survival. Ann. R. Coll. Surg. Engl. **20**, 332–334 (1998)
11. Miettinen, M., Lasota, J.: Gastrointestinal stromal tumors – definition, clinical, histological, immunohistochemical, and molecular genetic features and differential diagnosis. Virchows Arch. **438**, 1–12 (2001)
12. Fletcher, C.D., Berman, J.J., Corless, C., et al.: Diagnosis of gastrointestinal stromal tumors: a consensus approach. Hum. Pathol. **33**, 459–465 (2002)
13. Emory, T.S., Sobin, L.H., Lukes, L., et al.: Prognosis of gastrointestinal smooth muscle (stromal) tumors: dependence on anatomic site. Am. J. Surg. Pathol. **23**(1), 82–87 (1999)
14. Cunningham, J.D., Aleali, R., Aleali, M., et al.: Malignant small bowel neoplasms; histopathologic determinants of recurrence and survival. Ann. Surg. **225**, 300–306 (1997)
15. von Mehren, M.: New therapeutic strategies for soft tissue sarcomas. Curr. Treat. Options Oncol. **4**, 441–451 (2003)
16. Adeonigbagbe, O., Lee, C., Karowe, M., et al.: A Brunner's gland adenoma as a cause of anemia. J. Clin. Gastroenterol. **29**, 193–196 (1999)
17. Zangara, J., Kushner, H., Drachenberg, C., et al.: Iron deficiency anemia due to a Brunner's gland hamartoma. J. Clin. Gastroenterol. **27**, 353–356 (1998)
18. Dong, K., Li, B.: Peutz-Jeghers syndrome: case reports and update on diagnosis and treatment. Chin. J. Dig. Dis. **5**, 160–164 (2004)
19. Disario, J.A., Petersen, B.T., Tierney, W.M., et al.: Enteroscopes. Gastrointest. Endosc. **66**, 872–880 (2007)
20. Mishkin, D.S., Chuttani, R., Croffie, J., et al.: Wireless capsule endoscopy. Gastrointest. Endosc. **63**, 539–545 (2006)
21. Jesch, N.K., Vieten, G., Tschernig, T., et al.: Minilaparotomy and full laparotomy, but not laparoscopy, alter hepatic macrophage populations in a rat model. Surg. Endosc. **19**, 804–810 (2005)
22. Hanly, E.J., Aurora, A.A., Shih, S.P., et al.: Peritoneal acidosis mediates immunoprotection in laparoscopic surgery. Surgery **142**, 357–364 (2007)

Part V

Special Topics: Cancer of the Colon and Rectum

Right Hemicolectomy and Appendix

Antonio M. Lacy

17.1 Introduction

Colorectal Cancer (CRC) is the second most common cause of cancer death in the USA. The lifetime risk for colon cancer in America is 1 in 17. Surveillance Epidemiology and End Results (SEER) program data estimates that the incidence of colon cancer has decreased by 20%, whereas the mortality has also decreased by approximately 30% in the last 25 years. Nevertheless, SEER data estimate that CRC constitutes approximately 10.6% of all new cancer cases and is responsible for approximately 10% of all cancer deaths in the USA [1]. In Europe, CRC is the third most common type of cancer in men (12.8%) and ranks second in women (13.2%). Moreover, CRC is the second leading cause of cancer mortality with an estimated annual deaths of 103,300 (10.7%) in men and 100,400 (13.4%) in women.

The increased incidence of colon cancer is attributed to an accumulation of random somatic mutations over time. Population projections for the European Union have estimated a 22% increase in the age group >65 years and a 50% increase in the number of persons aged >80 years by 2015. Given the strong association between cancer risk and age, this will lead to a major increase in the cancer burden [2]. In addition to this finding, there is recently an increasing incidence of CRC in patients under the age of 40 [3].

The relative frequency of right-sided colon cancer has increased gradually during the past several decades. These days, approximately one half of colon cancers are located on the right side [4]. This effect is attributed in part to a decreased frequency of left-sided cancers resulting from polypectomies of pre-malignant left-sided polyps during flexible endoscopy [5]. The National Polyp Study is a multicenter, prospective, and randomized trial, designed to evaluate the effectiveness of routine surveillance of patients discovered to have colorectal adenomas. This study identified a change in the distribution and characteristics of adenomatous polyps in association with advanced age. According to this national-based study, patients older than 60 years were associated with an increased risk for high-grade dysplasia [6]. Furthermore, a population-based study of Medicare beneficiaries in patients 65 years and older found that the proportion of proximal tumors increases with age [7]. The fact that older patients are more likely to present with right-sided colon cancers has important implications regarding the use of screening programs in the elderly if there is only a flexible sigmoidoscopy and not a full colonoscopy performed [1]. In a Spanish study of 1,522 patients with CRC, the presence of a proximal tumor was found to be, among others, a risk factor for the development of synchronous adenomas and carcinomas. Other risk factors include TNM stage, male gender, personal history of colorectal adenoma, and mucinous pathology [8].

17.2 Factors Associated with Colorectal Cancer

17.2.1 Colorectal Cancer After Cholecystectomy

The relationship between cholecystectomy and the incidence of CRC is conflicting. Cholecystectomy is known to alter the enterohepatic circulation of bile

A.M. Lacy
Department of Gastrointestinal Surgery, Hospital Clínic,
University of Barcelona, Villarroel 170,
08036 Barcelona, Spain
e-mail: alacy@clinic.ub.es

acids exposing the colonic mucosa to continuous bile flow. This allows fecal bacteria to metabolize primary bile acids into secondary, potentially carcinogenic bile acids [1]. A first meta-analysis of over 30 studies demonstrated a positive association with a pooled relative risk of 1.34. This risk increased to 1.88 when lesions in the proximal colon were considered [9]. In 1993, the Netherlands Prospective Cohort study investigated this association in over 120,000 patients. After a 3-year follow-up, 478 CRC cases were identified, representing a relative risk of 1.78 in men and 1.51 in women [10]. The most recent meta-analysis of 35 studies reveals a less remarkable risk association between cholecystectomy and CRC, but once again, it increases to 1.86 for right-sided cancers [11, 12].

17.2.2 Hyperplastic Polyps

Hyperplastic polyps are better described as a precursor lesion [13]. Risk factors for malignancy in hyperplastic polyps include large polyp size (>1 cm in diameter), location in the right colon, a focus of adenoma within the polyp (mixed hyperplastic-adenomatous polyp), more than 20 hyperplastic polyps in the colon, a family history of hyperplastic polyposis, and a family history of colon cancer [14]. Hyperplastic polyps seem to be linked to colon cancer via the recently reclassified (sessile) serrated adenoma, previously classified as a hyperplastic polyp.

17.2.3 The Serrated Adenoma

A serrated adenoma arises within a hyperplastic polyp, but differs from an ordinary hyperplastic polyp by abnormal proliferation of crypt epithelium and by nuclear atypia [15]. The serrated adenoma is a precursor lesion for CRC with high microsatellite instability (MSI-H), which constitutes approximately 15% of sporadic colon cancers [16]. In a retrospective study by Goldstein et al, 91 MSI-H colorectal cancers developed in the same area of the proximal colon where hyperplastic polyps had been identified previously by colonoscopy. The polyps were examined by a pathologist. On re-review, all previously removed polyps were re-classified as serrated adenomas [17]. Patients who have hyperplastic polyposis and who have 30 or more hyperplastic polyps distributed throughout the colon (or at least five hyperplastic polyps proximal to the sigmoid colon, of which two at least are > 1 cm in diameter) frequently have serrated adenomas and frequently develop colon cancer [18]. If separating the high-risk serrated adenomas from hyperplastic polyps by applying the new nomenclature, the remaining conventional hyperplastic polyps are believed to harbor a negligible risk for developing colon cancer.

17.3 Appendiceal Malignancies

17.3.1 Histological Subtypes

An estimated 1% (0.9–1.4%) of all appendectomy specimens contain a neoplasm of some sort. These rare tumors are seldom suspected prior to surgery and less than one half of all the cases are diagnosed during the intervention. Epithelial tumors of the appendix have been classified into four distinct types:

- Carcinoid tumors
- Mucinous adenocarcinoma (often called mucinous cystadenocarcinoma or malignant mucocele)
- Colonic-type adenocarcinoma
- Adenocarcinoids with a dual cell origin

Carcinoid tumors account for 85% of the epithelial appendiceal tumors, followed by mucinous adenocarcinoma (8%), colonic-type adenocarcinoma (4%), and the unusual adenocarcinoid type (2%). The adenocarcinoid type contains goblet cells as pathognomonic feature [19]. A population-based study using the SEER Program (1,645 cases, 1973–1998) on primary malignant neoplasms of the appendix found an age-adjusted incidence of appendix cancer of 0.12 cases per 1,000,000 people per year [20]. The SEER study included carcinoid tumors only if they were labeled "malignant." In the SEER review, mucinous adenocarcinoma was the most frequent diagnosed, with 613 cases (37% of total). The mean age at diagnosis varied significantly among the different tumor types. Patients diagnosed with a malignant carcinoid were significantly younger (mean age of 38 years) than those diagnosed with any of the other tumor types. The mean age at diagnosis for goblet cell carcinoid was 52 years, for mucinous adenocarcinoma 60 years, and for colonic-type adenocarcinoma 62 years. Malignant carcinoid showed a sex preference and was significantly more common in women (ratio of 2.6 women to 1 man) when compared to other tumor types [20]. Tumor extension beyond the colon and/or metastases at the time of diagnosis differed according to histology and was significantly more likely in the presence of a mucinous adenocarcinoma or a signet ring cell carcinoma. Furthermore, 64% of the patients with signet ring cell carcinoma presented with lymph node involvement. Survival for patients with this type of tumor is significantly worse than for patients with other tumor histologies. Patients with malignant carcinoid had a better overall survival and this was the only other histology that had an impact on survival independent of age and extent of disease at the time of diagnosis [20].

The majority of the published literature on appendiceal malignancies is case series. Nitecki et al. reviewed their institutional experience from 1976 to 1992 in treating 94 consecutive patients with primary adenocarcinoma of the appendix. The authors found acute appendicitis to be the most common form of presentation (50%). Additionally, 46% of the patients had an appendiceal perforation (56% with the colonic type). The crude 5-year survival rate was 55%, but it varied with stage (Stage A 100%, Stage B 67%, Stage C 50%, Stage D 6%, $P < 0.01$) and with grade (Grade I 68% Grade III 7%, $P < 0.01$). Patients diagnosed with the mucinous type had a better prognosis than those with the colonic type ($P < 0.01$) [19]. Ito et al. from Brigham and Women's Hospital (Boston, Massachusetts) published a retrospective case series of 36 patients with appendiceal adenocarcinoma treated between 1981 through 2001. The mean age of the patient cohort was 52 years. Eighty eight percent of patients presented with symptoms of acute appendicitis. Eighteen (50%) patients underwent a curative resection (seven primary right hemicolectomies, ten appendectomies + subsequent right hemicolectomy, and one appendectomy alone). Mean length of follow-up was 55 months. Overall 5-year survival rate was 46%. The 5-year survival rate after curative resection was 61% and after palliative surgery was 32% ($P < 0.05$) [21].

alone for patients with primary invasive, non-mucinous adenocarcinoma of the appendix, undergoing resection with curative intent [19, 22, 23]. It is to be emphasized that in the SEER review, 64% of patients with signet ring cell carcinoma of the appendix had lymph node involvement [20] and in Nitecki's series, 17 of 42 patients with the colonic or adenocarcinoid type had nodal metastases (40%). Even though this is only a descriptive review, it is worth mentioning that the survival rate was superior after right hemicolectomy compared to appendectomy alone (68% vs 20%, $P < 0.001$) [19]. Ito et al. found that 27% of patients who underwent right hemicolectomy after initial appendectomy had residual cancer in the cecum or regional lymph node metastasis. All of these patients had T2 or T3 primaries [21]. It is clear that existing evidence supports to perform a right hemicolectomy in patients diagnosed with T2 or higher stage appendiceal cancers, who have been initially treated with appendectomy alone. The lack of information regarding the incidence of regional lymph node metastasis in the presence of T1 appendiceal cancer obliges us to apply the available knowledge on the natural history of colon cancer to treat this subgroup of patients. The incidence of associated regional lymph node metastasis in T1 colorectal cancers has been reported to be as high as 13% [24]. Assuming that the adenocarcinoma of the appendix and colorectal cancer has similar biological behavior, the best treatment option for T1 appendiceal cancers should be a formal hemicolectomy. Because in this disease the preoperative diagnosis is rarely evident, in many patients, the histology and invasiveness can only be defined a few days after the specimen of a simple appendectomy has been reviewed. In this common scenario, patients are best managed by reoperation and completion right hemicolectomy because of the risk of missed nodal metastases. Interestingly, in the study by Nitecki et al., a right hemicolectomy performed as a secondary procedure resulted in the upstaging of 38% of the patient's tumor [19]. It is important to point out that an adequate staging will identify those subjects who may benefit from adjuvant chemotherapy.

17.3.2 Non-mucinous Tumor

Although limited to retrospective data, the available evidence suggests that a right hemicolectomy is associated with improved survival compared with appendectomy

17.3.3 Mucinous Neoplasm

A mucocele of the appendix is an obstructive dilation of the appendix by intraluminal accumulation of mucoid material. They may be associated with a benign condition, such as retention cyst, mucosal hyperplasia, mucinous cystadenoma, or be the result of a malignant process termed as mucinous cystadenocarcinoma. Mucoceles are seen in 0.2–0.3% of all appendix specimens and, if perforated, may be associated with mucoid material in the peritoneal cavity. This mucoid material may be acellular or can contain cells either with low-grade dysplasia or high-grade dysplasia. Clinical presentation of a mucocele is usually nonspecific. Up to 50% are found incidentally at the time of operation and 51% of patients will be asymptomatic [25]. Stocchi et al. reported that the presence of clinical symptoms such as abdominal pain, abdominal mass, weight loss, and vomiting was associated with a higher incidence of cystadenocarcinoma. Mucoceles of benign origin are rarely larger than 2 cm. Mucoceles caused by cystadenoma or cystadenocarcinoma are usually larger, measuring up to 6 cm, and are associated with a 20% incidence of perforation [26].

17.3.4 Pseudomyxoma Peritonei

Pseudomyxoma peritonei (PMP) is the condition characterized by the presence of mucinous ascites and mucinous implants diffusely involving the peritoneal surfaces. Ronnett et al. analyzed the clinical and pathologic features of 109 cases of multifocal peritoneal mucinous tumors to develop a pathologic definition of cases characterized by the clinical condition PMP [27].

The authors defined two distinct entities:

17.3.4.1 Peritoneal Mucinous Carcinomatosis (PMCA)

Cases classified as PMCA consistent with origin from an appendiceal or intestinal mucinous adenocarcinoma were characterized by peritoneal lesions composed of more abundant mucinous epithelium with architectural and cytological features of carcinoma. There was a statistically significant difference in 5-year survival between cases classified as DPAM, cases classified as PMCA with intermediate (hybrid) or discordant features, and those classified as PMCA (84%, 37.6%, and 6.7%, respectively). The authors conclude that the term DPAM should be used to classify histologically benign peritoneal lesions associated with ruptured appendiceal mucinous adenomas. Additionally, cases with pathologic features of adenocarcinoma should be classified as PMCA because they have recognizably different pathologic features and a significantly worse prognosis [27].

17.3.4.2 Disseminated Peritoneal Adenomucinosis (DPAM)

Cases classified as DPAM consistent with origin from an appendiceal mucinous adenoma were characterized by peritoneal lesions composed of abundant extracellular mucin containing focally proliferative mucinous epithelium with little cytologic atypia or mitotic activity.

17.3.5 Therapy of Peritoneal Carcinomatosis and the Role of Laparoscopy

Traditionally, surgical treatment consisted of debulking that was repeated until no further benefit for the patient could be achieved. A new treatment option for mucinous appendiceal tumors with peritoneal seeding has emerged as a result of multiple phase II studies [28–31]. Nowadays, visible disease tends to be removed through peritonectomy and multiple visceral resections if necessary. Cytoreductive surgery is combined with intraperitoneal chemotherapy (IPC) using Mitomycin at 42°C in order to avoid entrapment of tumor cells at operative sites and to destroy small residual mucinous tumor nodules. Complementary systemic postoperative therapy is then given using Fluorouracil for 5 days. Applying this technique, Sugarbaker et al. have reported a 70% survival rate at 20 years in patients with minimally invasive mucinous tumors if complete cytoreductive surgery was performed. In the absence of phase III studies, the new combined treatments should be regarded as the standard of care for epithelial appendiceal neoplasms and pseudomyxoma peritonei syndrome and should replace serial debulkings [32]. Experienced surgeons recommend conversion to laparotomy for safe excision when a mucocele is visualized at the time of initial laparoscopy [25]. Open laparotomy is necessary to prevent rupture of the mucocele and seeding of trocar sites, ensuring that a benign process will not be changed to a malignant one. Additionally, laparotomy allows palpation and direct inspection of all sites that are at high risk for progression of mucinous carcinomatosis and mucoid fluid accumulation. If a cytological examination of the mucinous fluid confirms the presence of epithelial cells outside the appendix, then a diagnosis of pseudomyxoma peritonei syndrome or mucinous peritoneal carcinomatosis of appendiceal origin is established. Some surgeons may disagree with the recommendation that a mucocele requires laparotomy. If laparoscopy is performed, grasping of the mucocele should be avoided and an endo-bag must be used [33, 34]. The respect for an intact peritoneum as the first line of defense against carcinomatosis and limiting resection to avoid tumor cell entrapment are both new and key concepts in the management of dysplastic mucoceles. Accordingly, when a surgeon finds himself/herself facing appendiceal mucinous carcinomatosis or pseudomyxoma peritonei, a full cytoreductive procedure should be avoided in the general setting unless proper combined treatment with IPC is available. A cytoreductive procedure would include resection of greater and lesser omentum, often a splenectomy, and possibly resection of the recto-sigmoid colon to remove pelvic peritoneum. Under most circumstances, the goal of surgery should be to establish the diagnosis with generous sampling of mucinous fluid, completing appendectomy with clear margins at the base and lymphadenectomy of the meso-appendix. Limiting the extent of surgery must be emphasized and a thorough irrigation of the abdominal cavity and abdominal incision to minimize tumor cell entrapment should always be performed. After the pathology and cytology reports are reviewed and a diagnosis of mucinous carcinomatosis or pseudomyxoma peritonei is confirmed, the patient is referred to a peritoneal carcinomatosis treatment center for definitive and potentially curative treatment [25]. The indication for a formal right hemicolectomy in patients with the mucinous variant of appendiceal adenocarcinoma is more controversial. Traditionally, epithelial malignancies of the appendix, with or without carcinomatosis, have been treated with right hemicolectomy. Moreno-Gonzalez and Sugarbaker prospectively analyzed the clinical data on 501 patients with epithelial malignancy of the appendix with peritoneal dissemination, who were treated by cytoreductive surgery and perioperative, intraperitoneal chemotherapy [35]. With a median follow-up of 4 years, only the surgical procedure (appendectomy alone vs right hemicolectomy) demonstrated to have an influence on patient survival by univariate analysis ($P < 0.001$). Right hemicolectomy did not contribute to a survival advantage in patients with mucinous appendiceal tumors already having peritoneal seeding. With the data obtained, the authors proposed the following recommendations for limited use of right hemicolectomy in patients with appendiceal cancer having peritoneal seeding: A right hemicolectomy should be performed

- To clear the primary tumor or to achieve complete cytoreduction
- If lymph node involvement is demonstrated by histopathological examination of the appendiceal or ileocolic lymph nodes
- If a non-mucinous histological type is identified by histopathological examination

These recommendations imply a specifically targeted intraoperative management of patients with peritoneal seeding from a perforated epithelial appendiceal malignancy. The appendix is removed en bloc with mesoappendix and lymph nodes, and a gross pathological exam in the operating room is performed. If gross examination suggests cancerous involvement, a frozen-section examination should be obtained. If positive, a radical right hemicolectomy with lymph node dissection would be the next step. However, if a clear margin can be obtained and no lymph nodes are shown to be involved, a right hemicolectomy should not be performed.

17.3.6 Carcinoid Tumors

17.3.6.1 Indications for Right Hemicolectomy

It is a neoplasm derived from neuroendocrine tissue. The appendix is the most common single site, followed by the ileum. Goblet cell carcinoid is a rare histological variant of appendiceal carcinoid, also known as adenocarcinoid. These adenocarcinoids arise from a pluripotent cell that differentiates into both mucinous and neuroendocrine cells, and typically have an aggressive and unpredictable behavior. The prevalence of appendiceal carcinoid is 0·3–0·9% in patients undergoing appendectomy. Epidemiological studies show a slight predominance in females. The peak for women is reported between 15 and 19 years of age and between 20 and 29 years for men [36]. In the 2002 SEER review, Goblet cell carcinoids were found to present at a later age (mean of 52 years) [20]. The majority of carcinoid tumors (62–78%) are located at the tip of the appendix as an incidental finding associated with acute appendicitis in 54% of the cases [37, 38]. Tumor characteristics that predict aggressive behavior include histological subtype, presence of meso-appendiceal involvement, and size of the primary lesion as the most important factor. When reviewing the current literature, evidence regarding size as a determinant of tumor biology has been consistent. Moertel et al. described a cohort of 150 patients with appendiceal carcinoids, of which 127 had lesions less than 2 cm in diameter and none developed metastasis during follow-up [39]. Additionally, three of 14 patients with lesions larger than 2 cm but smaller than 3 cm had metastatic disease, and four of nine patients with lesions greater than 4 cm had metastatic disease. Based on these observations, the authors concluded that the risk of metastatic disease in tumors smaller than 2 cm was sufficiently low to treat them by appendectomy alone. Anderson and Wilson, in their series of 147 patients, found metastatic disease in two patients with lesions larger than 1.5 cm but smaller than 2 cm. These authors recommended subsequent right hemicolectomy for patients with lesions greater than 1.5 cm [40]. Syracuse et al. proved that meso-appendiceal extension correlated well with nodal metastases and also with tumor size. Positive regional lymph nodes were reported after prophylactic right hemicolectomy in two patients with meso-appendiceal involvement [41]. Goblet cell carcinoids are more aggressive tumors with a tendency for early, intra abdominal metastases. In the SEER review by McCusker et al., only 17% of the 227 patients with goblet cell carcinoids after a right hemicolectomy had positive lymph nodes, but surprisingly 65% of the patients showed spread through the serosa, invasion of the meso-appendix, and extension to adjacent organs or peritoneum. Based on this data, it is clear that in the presence of an adenocarcinoid lesion, serosal involvement and meso-appendiceal extension are more important predictors of outcome than lymph node status. In this series, 51% of goblet cell tumors had meso-appendiceal involvement [20]. Patients with tumors of 1–2 cm toward the tip of the appendix, with typical carcinoid histology, no angiolymphatic or meso-appendiceal invasion, and a low proliferative index, a right hemicolectomy does not appear to be justified. Although there is limited evidence for right hemicolectomy, in general, acceptable indications would be:

- Carcinoids larger than 2 cm in size
- Any high-grade malignant carcinoid with a high mitotic index (more than 2 cells/mm^2)
- High Ki67 index (more than 2% of positive cells/mm^2) may be indicative of more aggressive biological behavior
- Angioinvasion should be regarded as a feature of malignant behavior
- Presence of meso-appendiceal invasion
- Lesions at the base of the appendix with positive margins
- Goblet cell adenocarcinoid tumors

However, in the presence of advanced metastatic disease, there is no evidence that right hemicolectomy prevents additional distant metastases. In cases of advanced disease, there is again no clear evidence that a right hemicolectomy improves symptom control or survival [36]. Patients with tumors between 1 and 2 cm or larger than 2 cm should have plasma chromogranin levels measured, a blood marker elevated in 80–100% of neuroendocrine tumors. Chromogranin levels correlate well with tumor load and levels greater than 5,000 μg/L are generally associated with a poor outcome [42]. Patients with raised levels require further imaging with computed tomography and octreotide scintigraphy to rule out metastatic disease.

Appendiceal carcinoids usually metastasize to regional lymph nodes rather than to the liver. Patients with local disease are reported to have a 5-year survival rate of 92%, those with regional metastases 81%, and drops to 31% when distant metastases is present [43]. Patients with goblet cell carcinoid have a worse prognosis in general, as they tend to be widely invasive. Patients with appendiceal carcinoids have a high incidence of metachronous and synchronous gastrointestinal neoplasms, and consideration should be given to additional screening of this particular group of individuals. Appendiceal carcinoid series, such as Connor's, reported a 33% synchronous or metachronous incidence of mainly colorectal cancer [37]. Modlin et al. identified 18% of patients with coexisting neoplasms [43]. In patients undergoing re-exploration for right hemicolectomy after an initial appendectomy, preoperative colonoscopy is indicated to detect the 12% prevalence of a synchronous colonic or rectal carcinoma. Colonoscopic examination would also be indicated in patients with incidentally discovered appendiceal tumors, especially in patients in their 6th–8th decades [44].

17.3.7 Conclusions

While evidence of the benefits associated with laparoscopic approach continues to accumulate, an increasing number of appendiceal resections are being performed via laparoscopy. Appendiceal tumors are very rare entities. As previously mentioned, application of Minimally Invasive Surgery (MIS) for the treatment of appendiceal, epithelial neoplasms has not been generally assessed. Nevertheless, en bloc appendectomy, appendiceal lymphadenectomy, and right hemicolectomy are feasible, low-complex procedures that theoretically could be performed. Curative treatment of carcinoids and primary non-mucinous or colonic-type adenocarcinomas of appendiceal origin, without compromising on oncologic outcomes, has been attempted. Multi-institutional studies would be needed to validate the application of MIS in this setting. On the other hand, the specific biologic behavior and natural history of appendix mucinous neoplasms limit the application of laparoscopic approach for diagnosis and definitive curative treatment. Cytoreductive surgery and peritonectomy are long lasting, highly complex procedures that seem not to be designed for a minimally invasive approach. In experienced hands, laparoscopic resection of a mucocele with sampling of free intraperitoneal fluid for cytology could be considered.

17.4 Cancer of the Right Colon — Treatment

17.4.1 Non Surgical Therapies

Despite significant improvements in multimodality treatment over the last several decades, surgical resection of solid tumors continues to be the primary method for treating right-sided colon cancers. Fifty percent of patients with a diagnosed colon cancer are cured with surgery alone, most of them being stage I or stage II. Prognosis for patients with advanced CRC has substantially improved with the introduction of new chemotherapy agents. Median survival rates for patients with metastatic tumor have almost doubled over the past 10 years as a result of better chemotherapy strategy [45–48]. Nevertheless, the rate of success of adjuvant or neo-adjuvant therapies remains dependent on the ability to control the primary tumor with a complete R0 oncologic resection. Moreover, the low cure rate for surgical and medical treatment in recurrent colon cancer dictates that there is a very small margin for errors when surgically removing a potentially curable tumor. The quality of surgery is the main determinant for a good clinical outcome and the limiting factor when performing complex intra-abdominal resections.

17.4.2 Surgical Treatement

17.4.2.1 Laparoscopic Approach

Surgical R0 resection is the cornerstone for treatment of right-sided colon cancer and was first described in 1888 by Lubarsh. Maybe one of the most important advances in the last 2 decades was the development of laparoscopic surgery. In fact, laparoscopy is emerging as the preferred approach for different types of colectomies in benign and malignant disease processes.

The evidence-based support for oncologic equivalency of laparoscopic-assisted colectomy (LAC) when compared to open colectomy (OC) is now available. Oncologic concerns raised from high wound recurrence rates [49] prompted a series of multi-institutional randomized trials to test the hypothesis that disease-free and overall survival are equivalent, regardless of whether patients receive LAC or OC. Our single-institution randomized controlled trial (RCT) of LAC versus OC with a median follow-up of 43 months and 219 patients (111 LAC group, 108 OC group), identified a cancer-related survival advantage in patients with stage III CRC treated with laparoscopy. The patients experienced lower tumor recurrence and longer overall and cancer-related survival. LAC was also associated with lower perioperative morbidity and a shorter hospital stay [50]. Recently, we published long-term results of this trial with a median follow-up of 95 months confirming the initial findings. There was a tendency of higher cancer-related survival for the LAC group ($P = 0.02$) when compared to the OC group. The regression analysis showed that LAC was independently associated with reduced tumor relapse (hazard ratio 0.47, 95% CI 0.23–0.94), reduced death from a cancer-related cause (0.44, 0.21–0.92), and reduced death from any cause (0.59, 0.35–0.98). In this study, LAC proved to be more effective than OC for colon cancer treatment [51]. Our specific findings for the subset of patients with stage III disease have not been confirmed by other RCT.

The Three Major Multi Institutional Trials

COST, 2004
Clinical Outcome of Surgical Therapy, 2004

CLASSIC, 2005
The UK, Medical Research Council Trial of Conventional versus Laparoscopic-Assisted Surgery in Colorectal Cancer, 2005

COLOR, 2005
Colon Cancer Laparoscopic or Open Resection, 2005.

A recent pooled analysis, all consistently confirm these outcomes for early tumors [52–55]. Another meta-analysis of oncologic outcomes published by Jackson et al. found no significant differences in CRC-related mortality, CRC recurrence, or number of lymph nodes harvested between patients undergoing resection of CRC with laparoscopic surgery, when compared with those having traditional OC. For both cancer-related survival and recurrence, there was a trend toward improved survival and fewer recurrences in the laparoscopic group, although these differences were not statistically significant [56]. Also recently, the COST Study group published their long-term results with a median follow-up of 7 years. They found a 5-year survival rate of 90% of patients, disease-free 5-year survival (open 68.4%, laparoscopic 69.2%, $P = 0.94$), and overall 5-year survival (open 74.6%, laparoscopic 76.4%, $P = 0.93$) to be similar for the two groups. Overall recurrence rates were similar in both groups as well (open 21.8%, laparoscopic 19.4%, $P = 0.25$). According to the design of this study, LAC for curable colon cancer is not inferior to open surgery based on long-term oncologic endpoints [57].

Quality of Life and Postoperative Recovery

Quality of life and recovery data have been well analyzed in different trials performed, identifying low but measurable differences in postoperative pain, return of bowel function, and length of stay. The benefits of LAC in the early postoperative period described by our single institution trial were confirmed by the COST study group [50, 52]. On average, bowel function after laparoscopy returns 1 day earlier than in open surgery. Oral intake, either liquids or solid food, also occurs, on average, 1 day earlier [50, 58, 59]. In terms of postoperative pain control, the COLOR trial observed that LAC patients had a lower need for analgesia in the first 3 days after surgery [55]. In the COST trial, patients undergoing open colectomy required 4 days of intravenous narcotics, whereas patients in the laparoscopic group required parenteral narcotics for 3.2 days ($P = 0.001$). Shorter duration of parenteral narcotics and earlier return of bowel function most likely contributed to the decreased length of stay observed in patients undergoing laparoscopic colectomy. In the COST study, the median length of stay was 5 days for patients undergoing laparoscopic resection, 1 day shorter than that in the open group [57]. Reports of intraoperative blood loss have not been consistent. The COLOR and Barcelona trial showed that although the duration of surgery for LAC was longer than that of OC, patients who underwent laparoscopy had less blood loss during surgery. On the other hand, Milsom and Hasegawa did not find any difference in their comparative studies [59, 60]. Based on the current data available, there is no difference in operative mortality between patients undergoing OC or LAC. The short-term outcomes of different international multicenter trials are consistent with the findings of a meta-analysis for short-term outcomes of laparoscopic colorectal surgery published by Abraham et al. [61]. There is now substantial evidence to support early recovery benefits and modest quality of life improvements for patients treated with LAC [62].

Economical Considerations

Delaney et al. analyzed the clinical and economic outcomes of a patient cohort of 32,733 individuals (Premier Inc.'s Perspective Rx Comparative Database), having elective colectomies ($n = 11,044$ for laparoscopic and $n = 21,689$ for open) across 402 hospitals. Laparoscopic colectomy had a longer mean operative time and higher total hospital costs ($8076 vs $7678; $P = 0.0002$), but shorter mean length of stay and fewer mean intensive care unit days. The laparoscopic cohort also had lower rates of transfusions, in-hospital complications, and readmissions within 30 days. Reoperation rates were slightly, but significantly, increased in the LAC group. Laparoscopic colectomy patients were more likely to be discharged home without nursing care. This is the first national-level study describing short-term resource utilization of LAC and OC. The authors conclude that the benefits of LAC (including a reduction in post hospital nursing support) may outweigh its slightly higher in-hospital cost. The investigators are convinced that the routine use of enhanced recovery postoperative care pathways in conjunction with improved laparoscopic surgical techniques and reduced variability in resource use is the definite path to optimize the benefits of this surgical approach [63].

Miscellaneous Considerations

The Elderly Patient

Elderly patients, as expected, are more likely to have comorbidities that increase their risk for surgery. Yamamoto showed that surgical outcome after LAC for patients 80–90 years old were much the same as for those 60 years or younger [64]. Furthermore, Sklow et al. reported faster recovery after laparoscopic colectomy than after OC in patients older than 75 years, despite a longer operating time compared with open surgery [65].

Morbid Obesity

At the initial phase of laparoscopic colon surgery, obesity was regarded as a factor of technical challenge that could influence perioperative morbidity. In recent years, various publications have evaluated the effect of obesity in LAC. Leroy et al. assessed the outcome of LAC in obese and non-obese patients who had diverticular disease or CRC, and found that the two groups did not differ in operating times, radicality of resection, and morbidity. Moreover, none of the 23 patients with a BMI of more than 30 kg/m^2 needed conversion to open surgery [66]. Delaney et al. studied patients with a BMI higher than 30 kg/m^2 who had either LAC or OC, and the authors reported that operating times and morbidity did not differ between the groups, and hospital stay was 2 days shorter after LAC than after OC. However, the conversion rate from laparoscopic surgery to open surgery was 30% [67]. Thus, patients who are obese can benefit from laparoscopic surgery and obesity should not be regarded as a contraindication to laparoscopic colectomy. Nevertheless, this observation is valid for high-volume referral LAC centers, where expertise can compensate for the technical difficulties that a surgeon can encounter when operating on such patients.

Conversion from Laparoscopic Colectomy (LAC) to Open Colectomy (OC)

Conversion during LAC has been studied by several groups, and it varies in frequency according to surgeon's experience and case selection (14–20%). In LAC, the learning curve is longer than that in OC. A caseload of 50 LAC is thought to be sufficient to reach a level of proficiency to perform an LAC safely and with acceptable oncological outcome. In general, there is a concern that conversion could be associated with increased morbidity and higher hospital costs. In the MRC CLASIC trial, patients who underwent conversion had a higher death rate than those who completed a straight open or laparoscopic procedure (9% vs 5% and 1%, respectively). This difference, however, was not significant after adjustment for stratification factors. Complication rates were also higher in converted than in non-converted patients. The conversion rate for right-sided colectomies was 20% (28 out of 94 patients) [53]. The rate of intraoperative conversions fell in every year of the study, from 34 of 89 (38%) laparoscopic operations attempted in year 1–18 of 111 (16%) in year 6. Others have also reported a worse outcome if a conversion deemed to be necessary [68, 69]. Law et al. found that patients undergoing conversion had a higher incidence of complications (43.5% vs 12.9%, $P = 0.001$) and the hospital stay was significantly longer (8.5 days vs 6.0 days, $P = 0.001$) [70]. Casillas et al. compared 51 converted cases from a cohort of 430 LAC (12% conversion rate) with a matched series of 51 OC, and concluded that conversion did not result in inappropriately prolonged operative times, increased morbidity or length of stay, increased direct costs, or unexpected readmissions when compared with similarly complex OC. They support a policy of commencing most cases suitable for a laparoscopic approach offering patients the benefits of LAC without adversely affecting perioperative risks [71]. An early conversion in case of technical difficulties is generally recommended to save operating time and increased costs of the instruments used, as well as to avoid complications due to difficult dissection. The reality of this event is that patients with conversion cannot experience the benefits of laparoscopic surgery and the result will only be comparable to that of an open resection. A better selection of patients to avoid conversion is definitively necessary to improve operative outcome. The COST trial did not identify the differences in oncologic outcomes between patients converted to an open procedure and those completed laparoscopically [52].

Contraindications to LAC

The finding of a perforated neoplasia or infiltration of nearby structures has been historically considered an absolute contraindication for a laparoscopic approach. Tumor size greater than 8 cm and effects of pneumoperitoneum with CO_2 are thought to increase the risk for tumor dissemination. Nowadays, a relative contraindication for laparoscopy is tumor-related complications, such as hemorrhage, perforation, and bowel obstruction without septic shock. These factors combined with tumor location require great skills and experience when laparoscopy will be deployed. However, with surgical techniques being refined and increased training levels of surgeons, there are no absolute contraindications for laparoscopic colonic resections in centers where expertise and excellence in advanced laparoscopic surgery are combined.

Summary

Current available evidence suggests that laparoscopic approach for CRC achieves oncologic outcomes comparable to those in conventional open resection. Given the demonstrated short-term benefits, a laparoscopic approach has emerged as the new standard of care in appropriately selected patients. There is now a consensus that oncologic results are not compromised by laparoscopic surgery. With this perspective in mind, credentialing of surgeons, standardization of technique, and monitoring of outcomes become more important. Our challenge as surgeons is to balance the potential for improvement in the quality of life for patients performing less invasive procedures, with the risk of poor cancer outcomes as a result of a new technique.

17.5 Laparoscopic Right Hemicolectomy — the Technique

17.5.1 The Surgical Steps

Basic oncologic principles are the same as those in open surgery and are maintained at all times.

1. The first step of the operation is a complete diagnostic laparoscopy identifying local tumor characteristics and to rule out systemic dissemination that could change the operative strategy. Some authors perform a liver ultrasonography in every case (US) to look for liver metastases that could not be detected by preoperative imaging.
2. Proximal mesenteric vascular ligation at the base.
3. Avoid surgical maneuvers handling the tumor: A "*no touch technique*" is a must!
4. En bloc resection is mandatory.
5. Adequate proximal and distal margins of 4 cm should be obtained and are determined by the intestinal vascularization.
6. Lymph node count of 12 lymph nodes is a predictor of oncological quality and necessary for correct staging of the disease.
7. Restoring intestinal tract anatomy with either a hand-sewn or stapled anastomosis.

17.5.2 Tumor Localization: Pre-operative and Intra-operative

One of the few drawbacks of a laparoscopic approach is the lack of tactile feedback. When planning to treat right-sided lesions, a colonoscopy is sufficient and useful if the tumor is located close to a reliable landmark, such as the ileocecal valve or the cecum. However, if the lesion is endoscopically described to be in the ascending or proximal transverse colon and has a small size, we consider a barium enema or CT scan in combination with endoscopic tattooing as the most reliable localization procedure (0.2 cc of India ink is injected into the submucosa). If preoperative localization is unsuccessful, an intraoperative colonoscopy using CO_2 insufflation can be used to identify the exact location of the tumor. CO_2 is absorbed more rapidly than air, thus can decrease persistent bowel distension.

17.5.3 Preoperative Preparation of the Patient

A right hemicolectomy does not require bowel preparation and patients are usually admitted 12 h before surgery after being NPO, starting the night before. Antithrombotic and antibiotic prophylaxis are routinely administered prior to making incision and an oro-gastric tube and Foley catheter are placed in the operation room (OR).

17.5.4 Patient Positioning and Operating Room Setup

The patient is placed in supine position with both arms tucked. An alternative position would be to place the patient in a modified lithotomy position using Allen stirrups. In our clinic, the surgeon stands on the patient's left side and the second assistant holding the camera on the right side. The first assistant positions himself on the patient's right side next to the surgeon. The scrub nurse stands near the patient's right knee. The main monitor is placed over the patient's right shoulder to give the surgeon and second assistant an optimal view of the operative field. We use another monitor over the patient's left shoulder for the first assistant and the scrub nurse. If a third screen is available, it is placed at the patient's feet. The patient is placed in Trendelenburg position with a left lateral oblique rotation (minimum of 30° elevation) (Fig. 17.1).

17.5.5 Trocar Placement

Four trocars are generally required; an additional one is used if necessary. We use a set of two 10-/12-mm trocars and two 5-mm trocars. The first 10-/12-mm trocar is placed close to the umbilicus and used for the camera. We use a 30° scope for this procedure because it greatly helps in mobilizing the hepatic flexure; another option would be to use a flexible tip. As an initial step, we perform a diagnostic laparoscopy to rule out contraindications before we further proceed with the

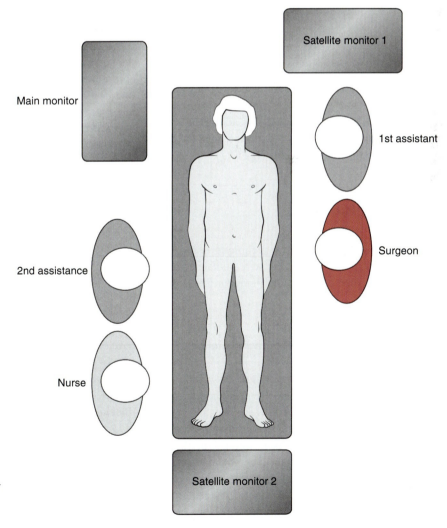

Fig. 17.1 Patient positioning and operation room setup. Copyright by Springer. (Drawing by Hippmann GbR, Schwarzenbruck, Germany)

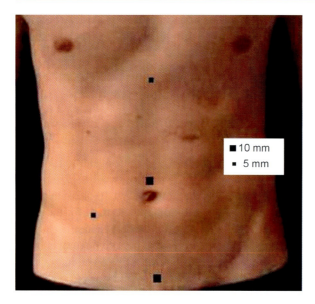

Fig. 17.2 Trocar placement

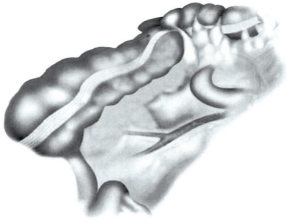

Fig. 17.3 The operative field

placement of the remainder of the trocars. The following trocars are placed under direct vision. The second 10-/12-mm trocar is inserted at the xyphoid, two fingerbreadths below the costal margin and to the left of the midline. The two 5-mm trocars are placed suprapubic and above the right iliacal crest. For additional exposure, we would insert another 5-mm trocar in the right upper quadrant of the abdomen (Fig. 17.2).

17.5.6 Surgical Steps

An efficient and safe operative technique is essential for good clinical outcomes. We use a medial approach for right hemicolectomy and apply standardized operative steps.

17.5.6.1 Exposure of the Operative Field

The surgical field is exposed with three easy steps. As a first step, we bring the table into Trendelenburg position with the left side down. Next, we move the greater omentum and transverse colon toward the upper abdomen. Last, the small bowel is positioned in the left abdominal cavity. With this maneuver, obtain great visualization of the right colon, right half of transverse colon, and ventral side of the right mesocolon. Graspers should never be used to grasp the colon directly, but can be applied to the mesentery or omental folds (Fig. 17.3).

17.5.6.2 Control of Vascular Pedicles

The blood supply for the right colon derives from the superior mesenteric vessels. The ileocolic and the right colic artery are the two main branches off the superior mesenteric artery (SMA). These arteries communicate with each other to form the often fragile marginal artery network. This branch originates at the right side of the SMA. The superior mesenteric vein (SMV) runs to the right of the SMA (Fig. 17.4). In a standard right hemicolectomy, the following vessels have to be transected: ileocolic vessels, right colic vessels, and right and marginal branch of the middle colic vessels. If an extended right hemicolectomy is performed, the surgeon has to take the middle colic artery as well. In any case, the vessels have to be clearly identified and transected at their base, coming off the SMA/SMV to ensure a complete nodal excision. The ileocolic vessels are easily exposed by grasping the right mesocolon and lifting it up close to the ileocecal junction (Fig. 17.5). The surgeon opens the peritoneum overlying the ileocolic vessels at the base of the superior mesenteric vessels using hot scissors or hook cautery (Fig. 17.6). After that, we proceed with dissecting beneath the vessels creating a tunnel until we reach the duodenum (Fig. 17.7). Special care must be taken to make sure that the plane of dissection is anterior to the layer of peritoneum covering the retroperitoneal structures, such as Gerota's fascia, duodenum, and right ureter. As long as this layer of peritoneum is preserved and the dissection is anterior to the duodenum, we do not routinely display the right ureter. The transection of the vessels can be performed in many different ways.

The surgeon can divide those using scissors after placing a proximal clip, use a sealing device such as harmonic scalpel or Ligasure, or fire a stapler across the base (Endo GIA®, grey cartridge). The dissection of the mesocolon continues cephalad along the right side of the SMA and the anterior surface of the SMV. This exposes the right colonic vessels and the right branch of the middle colic artery. The left branch of the middle colic artery has to be preserved in order to have sufficient vascular supply to the left transverse colon. With an adequate traction on the mesocolon and the ileocolic pedicle, lifting it toward the right upper quadrant, the posterior avascular plane is exposed. A careful dissection anterior to the duodenum is carried out to adequately mobilize the right side of the transverse colon. The right mesocolon is dissected away from the retroperitoneal structures using a medial to lateral approach. The pneumoperitoneum, laparoscopic instruments, and gauze are used at this step of the procedure. Exposing of the right gonadal vessels and right ureter is not necessary. A complete medial dissection along this plane is important to facilitate the next step of the procedure.

17.5.6.3 Mobilization of the Ascending Colon

The assistant grasps the ascending mesocolon and pulls it anteriorly. The surgeon grasps the proximal transverse colon and applies traction on the ascending colon by gently pulling it medially and inferiorly. By this combined maneuver, we put the hepatic flexure under tension and expose it nicely for further dissection. The gallbladder is retracted and lifted above the anterior edge of the liver. Now the right flexure is easily taken down by dividing the hepatocolic ligament and by

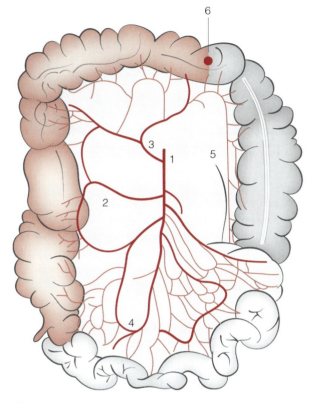

Fig. 17.4 Superior Mesenteric Artery (SMA) branches involved in right hemicolectomy (*1*) SMA, (*2*) Right colic Artery, (*3*) Middle Colic Artery, (*4*) Ileocolic Artery, (*5*) Marginal Artery), (*6*) Cannon-Boehm point-Border between Superior Mesenteric Artery (SMA and Inferior Mesenteric Artery (IMA). (Drawing by Hippmann GbR, Schwarzenbruck, Germany)

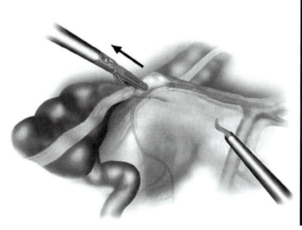

Fig. 17.5 Exposure of the ileocolic vascular pedicle

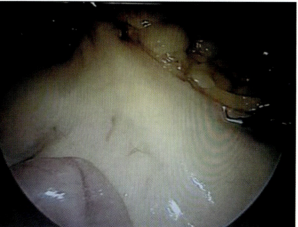

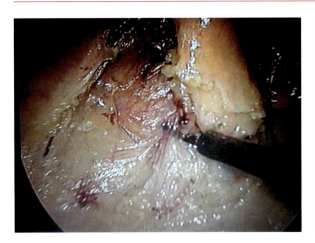

Fig. 17.6 Opening of the peritoneum and access to the ileocolic vascular pedicle at the base

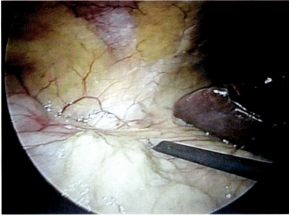

Fig. 17.8 Take down of the hepatic flexure

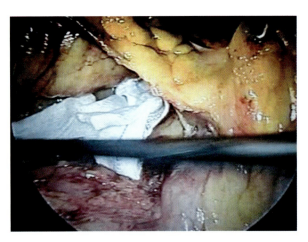

Fig. 17.7 Creation of a tunnel beneath the ileocolic vessels toward the duodenum

freeing the proximal transverse colon by dividing the gastrocolic ligament (Fig. 17.8). Mobilization of the right colon continues laterally along the white line of Told fascia heading down to the base of the cecum. The appendix and the base of the cecum are mobilized toward the midline. At that point of the procedure you have to be very cautious not to injure the underlying ureter. Now we identify the base of the attachment between small bowel, mesentery of the terminal ileum, and retro peritoneum. Usually, there is only a thin layer of peritoneum that remains intact and needs to be divided. The ileocecal region and ileal mesentery is mobilized lateral to the medial at this phase of the procedure. The entire right colon is now completely mobilized and free from peritoneal attachments. Before we

proceed with specimen extraction, we grasp the right colon and pull it to the left side of the abdomen to make sure that it is well mobilized. It is important that the root of the ileal mesentery is as mobile as possible to allow easy extraction of the small bowel through the chosen incision.

17.5.6.4 Transection and Extraction of the Surgical Specimen

The division of the right colon and performance of the anastomosis is accomplished extra corporeally. There are various options to choose the extraction site. It can be transverse in the right upper quadrant (RUQ) or vertical in the midline near the umbilicus. We prefer the transverse incision in the RUQ because of improved cosmetics, requiring a smaller incision for extraction. However, if the patient had previous abdominal surgery, then we try to remove the specimen through one of the old skin incisions. After performing the incision and gaining access to the peritoneal cavity, we routinely insert a wound protector (3M®) and carefully exteriorize the right colon. Extraction through the wound protector prevents parietal and peritoneal contamination. The distal small bowel mesentery is divided extra corporeally using Ligasure™. The terminal ileum is divided with a linear stapler device (Endo GIA™ 45 mm, blue load) about 20 cm from the ileocecal valve. A stitch is placed on the proximal end of the small bowel for easier identification. Mesocolon and greater omentum are divided using Ligasure® as well to allow vessels to be sealed without applying excessive heat.

After this, the transverse colon is divided with a linear stapler (Endo GIA™ 60 mm, blue load). The specimen is now removed from the operative field and carefully examined to verify that we have adequate proximal and distal margins.

17.5.6.5 Creation of the Anastomosis

We perform an extracorporeal side-to-side, isoperistaltical anastomosis applying a linear stapler (Endo GIA™ 60 mm, blue load). The resulting opening after firing of the Endo GIA™ stapler is closed with either a TEA stapler or a running suture (Fig. 17.9).

The anastomosis is then checked for hemostasis and returned to the abdominal cavity. The mesenteric defect does not require to be closed. The risk of internal hernias resulting in intestinal obstruction seems to be low. The extraction site is closed with non-interrupted sutures in two layers using absorbable suture material.

17.5.6.6 The Final Look

This is the last step of the operation, but not less important. Pneumoperitoneum is re-established and the abdominal cavity explored again. The small bowel loops are repositioned and checked for injuries due excessive manipulation. The anastomosis is then examined for bleeding or torsion. The greater omentum is placed over the anastomosis. At the end of the operation, we routinely explore the trocar sites to assure hemostasis. The routine use of an intra-abdominal drain is not necessary.

17.6 Postoperative Care

At the end of the procedure, the gastric tube is removed. Depending on intestinal peristalsis, patients start oral intake 12 h after the operation. No more antibiotic treatment during the postoperative phase is necessary after an elective right laparoscopic colectomy.

17.7 Complications

Despite being a procedure with a low complication rate, the surgeon must be aware of eventual complications. In our experience (289 cases until 2006), we had an intraoperative complication rate of 2.25%: two small bowel injuries, one trocar hemorrhage, one duodenal injury, one common bile duct injury, and two significant bleedings with hemodynamic stability. There were significant major complications in 44 patients (14.1%): anastomotic leaks were identified in 11 patients (3.5%), intraluminal hemorrhage in 6 cases (1.92%), intra-abdominal abscess formation in 5 cases (1.6%), intestinal obstruction was documented in 1 case (0.3%), intra-abdominal bleeding appeared in 2 cases (0.64), and one colo-cutaneous fistula was observed (0.3%). Re-interventions were necessary in nine patients (2.8%), 8 due to an anastomotic leak and one for diffuse abdominal sepsis. Mostly, we observed minor complications in which wound infection was the most frequent (13 cases – 4.1%) (Table 17.1).

17.8 Future Trends

Nowadays, the benefits of a laparoscopic approach are well known and universally accepted being the "gold standard" in right-sided colon lesions. Current efforts aim toward reducing the physiological injury and wound complications, to improve outcomes, psychological aspects, and patient's cosmetics.

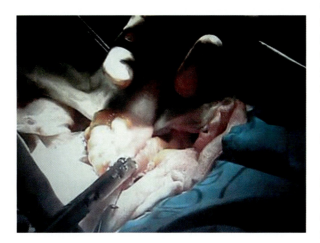

Fig. 17.9 Extracorporeal creation of a side-to-side anastomosis using an Endo GIA™

Table 17.1 Complications after laparoscopic right hemicolectomy: Personal experience

	Patients (*n*)	Patients (%)
Major Complications		
Anastomotic leaks	11	3.5
Ileus	16	5.14
Intraluminal hemorrhage	6	1.92
Intra-abdominal infection	5	1.6
Intestinal obstruction	1	0.32
Intra-abdominal bleeding	2	0.64
Pulmonary complication	4	1.28
Colo-cutaneous fistula	1	0.32
Minor Complications		
Wound infection	13	4.18
Urinary tract infection	4	1.28
Diarrhea	1	0.32
Surgical wound hematoma	1	0.32
Febrile syndrome	3	0.96

17.8.1 Reducing the Number of Ports

In the last few years, some procedures, such as cholecystectomy and appendectomy, have been performed through a transumbilical approach using single-port technology. Many definitions for this "new wave" have subsequently been crafted: Natural Orifice Trans Umbilical Surgery (NOTUS), Trans Umbilical Endoscopic Surgery (TUES), Trans Umbilical Laparoscopic Assisted (TULA), Laparo Endoscopic Single port Surgery (LESS), and Single Incision Laparoscopic Surgery (SILS). Results and benefits associated with single-port endoscopic surgery require long-term follow-up. However, benefits related to minimally invasive surgery could be increased in this new endoscopic single-site surgery.

17.8.2 Decreasing the Size of Ports or Mini Laparoscopy

Generally, 2-mm trocars are used. The disadvantages of mini-laparoscopy tools are reduced power and reduced performance.

17.8.3 Eliminating Skin Incisions or Surgery with No Scars

It is the greatest surgical revolution after the introduction of laparoscopy almost 2 decades ago. Known as Natural Orifice Transluminal Endoscopic Surgery (NOTES), it involves breaking dogmas established in general surgery during the past decades. A hollow viscus is intentionally perforated to gain access to the abdominal cavity using natural orifices. The transgastric, transanal, transrectal, transcolonic, or transvaginal route are described in the literature. Potential advantages of NOTES over standard laparoscopy should be: better cosmetics (scar-less surgery), less postoperative pain, easier access to the retroperitoneum, and decreased incidence of wound complications, such as infections or incisional hernias. More cases could be performed as outpatient surgery, and potentially, the operating room will be replaced by the endoscopy suite. However, barriers to NOTES surgery were highlighted by the NOSCAR group [72] and involved the access to the peritoneal cavity, lack of secure enterotomy closure, and prevention of infection by transluminal contamination. A big drawback as well is the necessary development of suture and anastomotic devices, difficult spatial orientation, and development of multi-tasking platforms incorporating robotics. Management of intraperitoneal complications remains challenging. In April 2007, at the University Hospital of Strasbourg (France), Professor J. Marescaux successfully performed the first no-scar surgery, a transvaginal cholecystectomy, using a flexible endoscope. It was called "operation Anubis" [73]. The development of NOTES surgery requires RCT and improvement in endoscopic devices, as well as development of safe instrumentation to adequately establish if this new technology will have a future.

> **Quick Reference Guide**
>
> 1. Expose the right colon and mesocolon to facilitate identification of vessels.
> 2. Meticulous dissection of the ileocolic pedicle is a must and it should be divided at the base.
> 3. The duodenum and its adhesions must be dissected before any vascular dissection is carried out.

4. The dissection plane you have to stay in is medial avascular plane, above the duodenum and right ureter.
5. Opening the right line of Told from lateral completes the mobilization of the right colon.
6. Choose the extraction site wisely, so that your specimen reaches easily.
7. It is important to assure that the colon reaches the anterior abdominal wall without tension.
8. Exteriorize the right hemicolon, transect, and perform a side-to-side isoperistaltic anastomosis.
9. Routinely re-establish the pneumoperitoneum and check all trocar sites for hemostasis. Check the anastomosis for torsion and hemostasis.
10. Placement of an intra-abdominal drain is not necessary after a routine procedure.

References

1. Bridges, L., O'Connell, J.B., Ko, C.Y.: Colorectal cancer: epidemiology and health services research. Surg. Oncol. Clin. N. Am. **15**, 21–37 (2006)
2. Boyle, P., Ferlay, J.: Cancer incidence and mortality in Europe, 2004. Ann. Oncol. **16**, 481–488 (2005)
3. O'Connell, J.B., Maggard, M.A., Liu, J.H., et al.: Rates of colon and rectal cancers are increasing in young adults. Am. Surg. **69**, 866–872 (2003)
4. Jessup, J.M., McGinnis, L.S., Steele Jr., G.D., Menck, H.R., Winchester, D.P.: The National Cancer DataBase: report on colon cancer. Cancer **78**, 918–926 (1996)
5. Cress, R.D., Morris, C.R., Bm, W.: Cancer of the colon and rectum in California: trends in incidence by race/ethnicity, stage, and subsite. Prev. Med. **31**, 447–453 (2000)
6. O'Brien, M.J., Winawer, S.J., Zauber, A.G., et al.: The national polyp study: patient and polyp characteristics associated with high grade dysplasia in colorectal adenomas. Gastroenterology **98**(2), 371–379 (1990)
7. Cooper, G.S., Yuan, Z., Landefeld, C.S., et al.: A national population-based study of incidence of colorectal cancer and age: implications for screening older Americans. Cancer **75**(3), 775–781 (1995)
8. Pinol, V., Andreu, M., Jover, R.: Synchronous colorectal neoplasms in patients with colorectal cancer: predisposing individual and familial factors. Dis. Colon Rectum **47**, 1192–200 (2004)
9. Giovannucci, E., Colditz, G.A., Stampfer, M.J.: A meta-analysis of cholecystectomy and risk for colorectal cancer. Gastroenterology **105**(1), 130–141 (1993)
10. Goldbohm, R.A., Van den Brandt, P.A., Van't Veer, P., et al.: Cholecystectomy and colorectal cancer: evidence from a cohort study on diet and cancer. Int. J. Cancer **53**(5), 753–759 (1993)
11. Reid, F.D., Mercer, P.M., Harrison, M.: Cholecystectomy as a risk factor for colorectal cancer: a meta-analysis. Scand. J. Gastroenterol. **31**(2), 160–169 (1996)
12. Todoroki, I., Friedman, G.D., Slattery, M.L., et al.: Cholecystectomy and the risk of colon cancer. Am. J. Gastroenterol. **94**(1), 41–46 (1999)
13. Cappell, M.S.: Pathophysiology, clinical presentation, and management of colon cancer. Gastroenterol. Clin. N. Am. **37**, 1–24 (2008)
14. Jass, J.R.: Hyperplastic polyps and colorectal cancer: is there a link? Clin. Gastroenterol. Hepatol. **2**, 1–8 (2004)
15. Higuchi, T., Jass, J.R.: My approach to serrated polyps of the colorectum. J. Clin. Pathol. **57**, 682–686 (2004)
16. Thibodeau, S.N., Bren, G., Schaid, D.: Microsatellite instability in cancer of the proximal colon. Science **260**, 816–819 (1993)
17. Goldstein, N.S., Bhanot, P., Odish, E., et al.: Hyperplastic-like colon polyps that preceded microsatellite-unstable adenocarcinomas. Am. J. Clin. Pathol. **119**, 778–796 (2003)
18. Jeevaratnam, P., Cottier, D.S., Browett, P.J., et al.: Familial giant hyperplastic polyposis predisposing to colon cancer: a new hereditary bowel cancer syndrome. J. Pathol. **179**, 20–25 (1996)
19. Nitecki, S.S., Wolff, B.G., Schlinkert, R., Sarr, M.G.: The natural history of surgically treated primary adenocarcinoma of the appendix. Ann. Surg. **219**(1), 51–57 (1994)
20. McCusker, M.E., Cote, T.R., Clegg, L.X., Sobin, L.H.: Primary malignant neoplasms of the appendix: a population-based study from the surveillance, epidemiology and end-results program, 1973–1998. Cancer **94**(12), 3307–3312 (2002)
21. Ito, H., Osteen, R.T., Bleday, R., Zinner, M.J., Ashley, S.W., Whang, E.E.: Appendiceal adenocarcinoma: long-term outcomes after surgical therapy. Dis. Colon Rectum **47**(4), 474–480 (2004)
22. Cortina, R., McCormick, J., Kolm, P., Perry, R.R.: Management and prognosis of adenocarcinoma of the appendix. Dis. Colon Rectum **38**, 848–852 (1995)
23. Lenriot, J.P., Huguier, M.: Adenocarcinoma of the appendix. Am. J. Surg. **155**, 470–475 (1988)
24. Nascimbeni, R., Burgart, L.J., Nivatvongs, S., Larson, D.R.: Risk of lymph node metastasis in T1 carcinoma of the colon and rectum. Dis. Colon Rectum **45**, 200–206 (2002)
25. Dhage-Ivatury, S., Sugarbaker, P.H.: Update on the surgical approach to mucocele of the appendix. J. Am. Coll. Surg. **202**(4), 680–684 (2006)
26. Stocchi, L., Wolff, B.G., Larson, D.R., Harrington, J.R.: Surgical treatment of appendiceal mucocele. Arch. Surg. **138**, 585–590 (2003)
27. Ronnett, B.M., Zahn, C.M., Kurman, R.J., Kass, M.E., Sugarbaker, P.H., Shmookler, B.M.: Disseminated peritoneal adenomucinosis and peritoneal mucinous carcinomatosis. A clinicopathologic analysis of 109 cases with emphasis on distinguishing pathologic features, site of origin, prognosis, and relationship to "pseudomyxoma peritonei. Am. J. Surg. Pathol. **19**(12), 1390–1408 (1995)
28. Deraco, M., Baratti, D., Inglese, M.G., Allaria, B., Andreola, S., Gavazzi, C., Kusamura, S.: Peritonectomy and intraperitoneal hyperthermic perfusion: a strategy that has confirmed its efficacy in patients with pseudomyxoma peritonei. Ann. Surg. Oncol. **11**, 393–398 (2004)
29. Loungnarath, R., Causeret, S., Bossard, N., Faheez, M., Sayaq-Beaujard, A.C., Brigand, C., Gilly, F., Glehen, O.:

Cytoreductive surgery with intraperitoneal chemohyperthermia for the treatment of pseudomyxoma peritonei: a prospective study. Dis. Colon Rectum **48**, 1372–1379 (2005)
30. Sugarbaker, P.H., Chang, D.: Results of treatment of 385 patients with peritoneal surface spread of appendiceal malignancy. Ann. Surg. Oncol. **6**, 727–731 (1999)
31. Witkamp, A.J., de Bree, E., Kaag, M.M., van Slooten, G.W., van Coevorden, F., Zoetmulder, F.A.: Extensive surgical cytoreduction and intraoperative hyperthermic intraperitoneal chemotherapy in patients with pseudomyxoma peritonei. Br. J. Surg. **88**, 458–463 (2001)
32. Sugarbaker, P.H.: New standard of care for appendiceal epithelial neoplasms and pseudomyxoma peritonei syndrome? Lancet Oncol. **7**, 69–76 (2006)
33. Lau, H., Yuen, W.K., Loong, F., Lee, F.: Laparoscopic resection of an appendiceal mucocele. Surg. Laparosc. Endosc. Percutan. Tech. **12**, 367–370 (2002)
34. Miraliakbari, R., Chapman, W.H.: Laparoscopic treatment of an appendiceal mucocele. J. Laparoendosc. Adv. Surg. Tech. **9**, 159–163 (1999)
35. Gonzalez-Moreno, S., Sugarbaker, P.H.: Right hemicolectomy does not confer a survival advantage in patients with mucinous carcinoma of the appendix and peritoneal seeding. Br. J. Surg. **91**, 304–311 (2004)
36. Goedel, A.C., Caplin, M.E., Winslet, M.C.: Carcinoid tumor of the appendix. Br. J. Surg. **90**, 1317–1322 (2003)
37. Connor, S.J., Hanna, G.B., Frizelle, F.A.: Appendiceal tumors: retrospective clinicopathologic analysis of appendiceal tumors from 7970 appendectomies. Dis. Colon Rectum **41**, 75–80 (1998)
38. Roggo, A., Wood, W.C., Ottinger, L.W.: Carcinoid tumors of the appendix. Ann. Surg. 217, 385–390 (1993)
39. Moertel, C.G., Weiland, L.H., Nagorney, D.M., Dockerty, M.B.: Carcinoid tumor of the appendix: treatment and prognosis. N Engl J. Med. **317**, 1699–1701 (1987)
40. Anderson, J.R., Wilson, B.G.: Carcinoid tumours of the appendix. Br. J. Surg. **72**, 545–546 (1985)
41. Syracuse, D.C., Perzin, K.H., Price, J.B., Wiedel, P.D., Mesa-Tejada, R.: Carcinoid tumors of the appendix. Mesoappendiceal extension and nodal metastases. Ann. Surg. **190**, 58–63 (1979)
42. Janson, E.T., Holmberg, L., Stridsberg, M., Eriksson, B., Theodorsson, E., Wilander, E.: Carcinoid tumors: analysis of prognostic factors and survival in 301 patients from a referral center. Ann. Oncol. **8**, 685–690 (1997)
43. Modlin, I.M., Lye, K.D., Kidd, M.: A 5-decade analysis of 13 715 carcinoid tumors. Cancer **97**, 934–959 (2003)
44. Bucher, P., Mathe, Z., Demirag, A., Morel, Ph: Appendix tumors in the era of laparoscopic appendectomy. Surg. Endosc. **18**, 1063–1066 (2004)
45. Cunningham, D., Glimelius, B.: A phase III study of irinotecan (CPT-11) versus best supportive care in patients with metastatic colorectal cancer who have failed 5-fluorouracil therapy. V301 Study Group. Semin. Oncol. **26**, 6–12 (1999)
46. De Gramont, A., Figer, A., Seymour, M., Homerin, M., Hmissi, A., Cassidy, J., et al.: Leucovorin and fluorouracil with or without oxaliplatin as first-line treatment in advanced colorectal cancer. J. Clin. Oncol. **8**, 2938–2947 (2000)
47. De Gramont, A., Tournigand, C., Andre, T., Larsen, A.K., Louvet, C.: Targeted agents for adjuvant therapy of colon cancer. Semin. Oncol. **33**(Suppl 11), S42–S45 (2006)
48. Saltz, L.B., Cox, J.V., Blanke, C., Rosen, L.S., Fehrenbacher, L., Moore, M.J., et al.: Irinotecan plus fluorouracil and leucovorin for metastatic colorectal cancer. Irinotecan Study Group. N. Engl. J. Med **343**, 905–914 (2000)
49. Alexander, R., Jaques, B., Mitchell, K.: Laparoscopic assisted colectomy and wound recurrence. Lancet **341**, 249–250 (1993)
50. Lacy, A.M., García-Valdecasas, J.C., Delgado, S., Castells, A., Taurá, P., Piqué, J.M., Visa, J.: Laparoscopic-assisted colectomy versus open colectomy for treatment of nonmetastatic colon cancer: a randomised trial. Lancet **9**, 2224–2229 (2002)
51. Lacy, A.M., Delgado, S., Castells, A., Prins, H.A., Arroyp, V., Ibarzabal, A., Piqué, J.M.: The long-term results of a randomised clinical trial of laparoscopy assisted versus open surgery for colon cancer. Ann. Surg. 248(**1**), 1–7 (2008)
52. Clinical Outcomes of Surgical Therapy (COST) Study Group: A comparison of laparoscopically assisted and open colectomy for colon cancer. N Engl J. Med. **0**, 2050–2059 (2004)
53. Guillou, P.J., Quirke, P., Thorpe, H., Walker, J., Jayne, D.G., Smith, A.M.H., Heath, R.M., Brown, J., for the MRC CLASICC trial group: Short-term endpoints of conventional versus laparoscopically assisted surgery in patients with colorectal cancer (MRC CLASSIC Trial): multicentre, randomized control trial. Lancet **365**, 1718–1726 (2005)
54. Fleshman, J., Sargent, D.J., Green, E., Anvari, M., Stryker, S.J., Beart, Jr R.W., Hellinger, M., Flanagan, Jr R., Peters, W., Nelson, H., for The Clinical Outcomes of Surgical Therapy Study Group.: Laparoscopic colectomy for cancer is not inferior to open surgery based on 5-year data from the COST Study Group Trial. Ann. Surg. 246 (**4**), 655–664 (2007)
55. Veldkamp, R., Kuhry, E., Hop, W.C., Jeekel, J., Kazemier, G., Bonjer, H.J., Haglind, E., Pahlman, L., Cuesta, M.A., Msika, S., Morina, M., Lacy, A.M., The COlon cancer Laparoscopic or Open Resection Study Group (COLOR): Laroscopic surgery versus open surgery for colon cancer: short-term outcomes of a randomised trial. Lancet Oncol. **6**, 477–484 (2005)
56. Jackson, T.D., Kaplan, G.G., Arena, G., et al.: Laparoscopic versus open resection for colorectal cancer: a meta-analysis of oncologic outcomes. JACS 204, 439–446 (2007).
57. Finlayson, E., Nelson, H.: Laparoscopic colectomy for cancer. Am. J. Clin. Oncol. **28**, 521–525 (2005)
58. Braga, M., Vignali, A., Gianotti, L., Zuliani, W., Radaelli, G., Gruarin, P., Dellabona, P., Di Carlo, V.: Laparoscopic versus open colorectal surgery: a randomized trial on shortterm outcome. Ann. Surg. **236**, 759–767 (2002)
59. Milsom, J., Bohm, B., Hammerhofer, K.A., Fazio, V., Steiger, E., Elson, P.: A prospective randomized trial comparing laparoscopic versus conventional techniques in colorectal cancer surgery: a preliminary report. J. Am. Coll. Surg. **187**, 46–57 (1998)
60. Hasegawa, H., Kabeshima, Y., Watanabe, M., Yamamoto, S., Kitayima, M.: R andomized controlledtrial of laparoscopic versus open colectomy for advanced colorectal cancer. Surg. Endosc. **17**, 636–640 (2003)
61. Abraham, M.S., Young, J.M., Solomon, M.J.: Meta-analysis of short term outcomes after laparoscopic resection for colorectal cancer. Br. J. Surg. **91**, 1111–1124 (2004)

62. Schwenk, W., Haase, O., Neudecker, J., Muller, J.M.: Short term benefits for laparoscopic colorectal resection. Cochrane Database Syst. Rev. **20**(3), 3145 (2005)
63. Delaney, C.P., Chang, E., Senagore, A.J.: Clinical outcomes and resource utilization associated with laparoscopic and open colectomy using a large national database. Ann. Surg. **247**, 819–824 (2008)
64. Yamamoto, S., Watanabe, M., Hasegawa, H., Baba, H., Kitayima, M.: Short-term surgical outcomes of laparoscopic colonic surgery in octogenarians: a matched case-control study. Surg. Laparosc. Endosc. Percutan. Tech. **13**, 95–100 (2003)
65. Sklow, B., Read, T., Birnbaum, E., Fry, R., Fleshman, J.: Age and type of procedure influence the choice of patients for laparoscopic colectomy. Surg. Endosc. **17**, 923–929 (2003)
66. Leroy, J., Ananian, P., Rubino, F., Claudon, B., Mutter, D., Marescaux, J.: The impact of obesity on technical feasibility and postoperative outcomes of laparoscopic left colectomy. Ann. Surg. **241**(1), 69–76 (2005)
67. Delaney, C.P., Pokala, N., Senagore, A.J., Casillas, S., Kirna, R.P., Km, B., VWl, F.: Is laparoscopic colectomy applicable to patients with body mass index > 30? A case-matched comparative study with open colectomy. Dis. Colon Rectum **48**(5), 975–981 (2005)
68. Gervaz, P., Pikarsky, A., Utech, M., et al.: Converted laparoscopic colorectal surgery. Surg. Endosc. 15, 827–832 (2001)
69. Marusch, F., Gastinger, I., Schneider, C., et al.: Importance of conversion for results obtained with laparoscopic colorectal surgery. Dis. Colon Rectum **44**, 207–214 (2001)
70. Law, W., Lee, Y.M., Choi, H.K., Seto, C.L., Ho, J.: Impact of laparoscopic resection for colorectal cancer on operative outcomes and survival. Ann. Surg. 245(**1**), 1–7 (2007)
71. Casillas, S., Delaney, C.P., Senagore, A.J., Brady, K., Fazio, V.W.: Does conversion of a laparoscopic colectomy adversely affect patient outcome? Dis. Colon Rectum **47**, 1680–1685 (2004)
72. Hawes, R.: ASGE/SAGES working group on natural orifice translumenal endoscopic surgery. Gastrointest. Endosc. **63**, 199e–203 (2006). [34] Varadarajulu S, Tamhane A, Drelichman ER. Patient perception
73. Marescaux, J., Dallemagne, B., Perreta, S., Wattiez, A.: Surgery without scars. Arch. Surg. **142**(9), 823–826 (2007)

Left Hemicolectomy and Sigmoid Colon

Joel Leroy, Ronan Cahill, and Jacques Marescaux

18.1 Introduction

While laparoscopic cholecystectomy, adrenalectomy, and selected other procedures rapidly gained wide acceptance among the surgical community after their introduction in the early 1990s, the development and integration of laparoscopic colectomy has taken a slower course. Questions arose about the oncological quality of laparoscopy for the treatment of colorectal cancer following initial reports of a high incidence of port-site metastases. However this has been dispelled now and increasing evidence supports great advantages for the patient without oncological compromise [1]. Indeed, the laparoscopic approach for left sided colonic cancers respects all the governing principles of its open counterpart and, with expanding acceptance, seems likely to become the access route of preference in leading surgical departments worldwide, even in obese patients [2].

18.2 Current Literature

After more than a decade of controversies [3], recent reports have now provided considerable evidence indicating that laparoscopic colectomy is safe, effective, and offers some definite advantages over conventional surgery [4]. High quality trials have documented decreased morbidity, decreased pain, shorter hospital stay, quicker return to work activities, and better immunologic status after laparoscopic colectomy compared to open colonic resection [5–13]. One randomized controlled study on colectomy for cancer has even favored the laparoscopic approach over open operation for stage III patients as it resulted in improved 5-year survival rates [14]. The results of other multicenter trials at least confirm both the oncological propriety [15, 16] and overall safety of the use of laparoscopy for colonic cancer when performed by an experienced team [17]. Therefore the laparoscopic approach for sigmoid cancer has been confirmed as an apposite oncological procedure and, even though, it has yet to become "gold standard" for sigmoid cancer, it is likely to play an increasingly important role in the surgical management of malignant colonic diseases [18–20]. Furthermore, the recognition conferred by consensus conference of experts' bodies such as SAGES and the ASCRS is likely to progress its acceptance and adoption (Tables 18.1 and 18.2).

18.3 Surgical Approach

The smooth performance of laparoscopic left hemicolectomy and sigmoidectomy depends on each of the following cornerstones:

- Appropriate patient selection
- High quality equipment
- Perfect knowledge of surgical anatomy
- Respect of operative strategic principles (e.g. "vessel first approach")
- Experience and expertise of the surgical team

J. Leroy, R. Cahill, and J. Marescaux (✉)
Department of Digestive and Endocrine Surgery, IRCAD-EITS Institute, University Hospital, 1 Place de L'Hopital, 67091 Strasbourg, France
e-mail: joel.leroy@ircad.fr; cahillra@gmail.com; jacques.marescaux@ircad.fr

Table 18.1 CLASSIC trial

Randomized trial of laparoscopic-assisted resection of colorectal carcinoma: 3-year results UK MRC CLASICC Trial Group *Journal of Clinical Oncology 2007; 25(21): 3061–3068*				
	Laparoscopic-assisted group	Open group	Difference (95% confidence interval)	p value
Randomization ratio	2	1	–	–
Number of patients (total = 749)	526	268	–	–
Overall survival	68.4%	66.7%	1.8% (−5.2% to 8.8%)	0.55
Disease free survival	66.3%	67.7%	−1.4% (−9.5% to 6.7%)	0.70
Local recurrence	8.6%	7.9%	−0.8% (−5.7% to 4.2%)	0.76
Wound/port-site recurrence	2.5%	0.6%	−2.0% (−4.0% to 0.02%)	
Quality of life	No significant difference between groups			>0.1

Table 18.2 Laparoscopic colectomy versus open colectomy: Survival

Survival after laparoscopic surgery versus open surgery for colon cancer: long-term outcome of a randomized clinical trial The Colon Cancer Laparoscopic or Open Resection Study Group *Lancet Oncology 2009; 10(1):44–52.*			
	Laparoscopic group	Open group	p value
N	258	252	0.66
OR Time (min) Median (range)	145 (102–230)	115 (70–180)	<0.001
Blood Loss (mL)	100 (19–410)	175 (40–500)	0.003
Size of tumor (cm) Median (range)	4.0 (2.0–7.5)	4.5 (2.1–8.0)	0.07
Positive resection margins (n/%)	10 (2%)	10 (2%)	0.96
Lymph nodes in resected specimen Median (range)	10 (3–20)	10 (3–20)	0.32
Early morbidity (<28 days) (n/%)	111 (21%)	110 (20%)	0.90
Early mortality (<28 days) (n/%)	6 (1%)	10 (2%)	0.47
Chemotherapy within 28 days (n/%)	55 (105)	57 (11%)	0.99
Overall survival at 3 and 5 years	81.8% and 73.8%	76.2% and 67.9%	ns
Disease free survival at 3 and 5 years	74.2% and 66.5%	76.2% and 67.9%	ns

ns nonsignificant

18.3.1 Indications and Contraindications to Laparoscopic Colectomy

Laparoscopy for cancer is safe as long as oncological principles are respected [3]. The presence of a large palpable malignancy suggesting local advanced disease, or the suspicion of perforation though still represent absolute contraindications to a laparoscopic approach. These cases should therefore still be routinely managed by conventional open surgery.

18.4 Operative Technique

A comprehensive demonstration of our preferred technique is available in the associated video as well as online through Websurg [21].

18.4.1 Instruments and Equipment

In order to facilitate exposure of the pelvic space and of the splenic flexure, it is advisable to use an operating table that can be easily tilted laterally and placed into both steep Trendelenburg and reverse Trendelenburg position. The laparoscopic unit with the monitor is located on the left side of the table.

18.4.2 Patient Positioning

A proper patient position is key to both facilitating operative maneuvers and preventing complications such as nerve and vein compression and traction injuries to the brachial plexus. The patient is placed supine in modified Lloyd-Davis position, with legs abducted and slightly flexed at the knees. The patient's right arm is tucked alongside the body. The left arm is placed at a 90° angle. Adequate padding is used to avoid compression on bony prominences (Fig. 18.1).

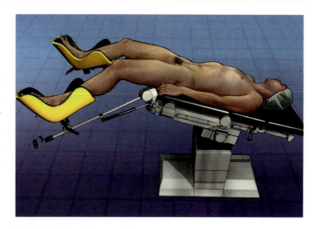

Fig. 18.1 Patient positioning: The patient legs are placed in stirrups and the table is tilted into a steep Trendelenburg position at the beginning of the operation (courtesy of WeBSurg© IRCAD®)

18.4.3 Preoperative Considerations

A nasogastric tube to decompress the stomach and a urinary catheter are routinely placed prior to commencing the surgery. We routinely use a heating device to prevent patient hypothermia. Adequate thrombo-embolism prophylaxis should be employed, as preferred by the surgeon, and intermittent leg compression can be used as well. Patients should receive peri-operative single-shot antibiotic prophylaxis as well.

18.4.4 Team Positioning

The procedure is usually performed with two assistants and a scrub nurse. The surgeon stands on the right side of the patient with the first assistant laterally to the right shoulder of the patient. The second assistant stands between the patients' legs and the scrub nurse at the lower right side of the table. The team usually remains in this position through the entire procedure (Fig. 18.2).

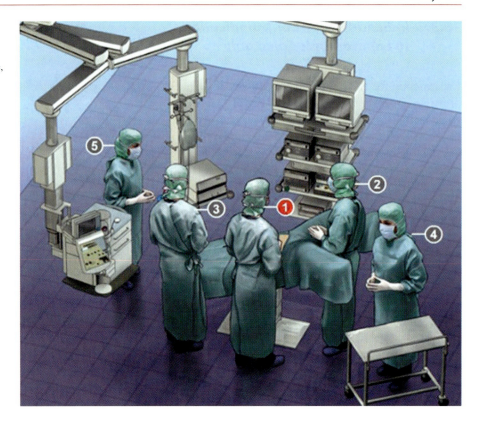

Fig. 18.2 Positioning of the surgical team: *1* main surgeon, *2* second ssistant, *3* first assistant, *4* scrub nurse, *5* anesthesiologist (courtesy of WeBSurg© IRCAD®)

18.4.5 Placement of Trocars

The number of trocars, unlike their size and the length of the wound incision, has very little impact, if any, on postoperative outcomes. Although as few as three trocars can be sufficient in uncomplicated cases, and is preferred by some surgeons, we choose to standardize trocar placement and routinely use five or six trocars for operations on the left-sided colon. This allows us to achieve perfect exposure in every case, which may be particularly valuable at the beginning of a surgeon's learning curve. Trocar fixation to the abdominal wall is also important, to avoid CO_2 leaks, and in cases of malignancy, to minimize the passage of tumor cells and therefore to help reduce the incidence of port site metastases.

We usually perform an "open" technique for the insertion of the first trocar (12 mm) which is used for the optical 0° laparoscope and is positioned in the midline 3–4 cm above the umbilicus (*Trocar A*). The two operating trocars are then introduced under endoscopic vision, one at the junction of the umbilical line and the right midclavicular line (*Trocar B*), and the other, 8–10 cm inferiorly to this along the same line (*Trocar C*). The latter should also be 12 mm in diameter to allow the introduction of a linear stapler at the time of bowel resection. During the course of the operation, this trocar will also accommodate:

- Scissors (monopolar, bipolar or ultrasonic hemostasis devices)
- Clips and staplers
- A suction-irrigation device
- Atraumatic graspers

The fourth trocar (*Trocar D*) is placed in the left midclavicular line, at the level of the umbilicus. A 5-mm trocar suffices in this position and is used to accommodate an atraumatic grasper for retraction and exposure during the medial approach for the dissection of the left mesocolon. When mobilizing the splenic flexure, this trocar may become an "operating" trocar rather than an "assisting" trocar. The fifth 5-mm trocar (*Trocar E*) is placed 8–10 cm above the pubic bone, in the midline and is also used for retraction. For most of the procedure, it accommodates a grasper used to expose the sigmoid and descending mesocolon. At the end of the case, the incision at this trocar's site is

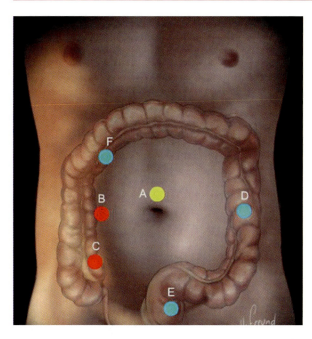

Fig. 18.3 Standardized port placements: The letters correspond to the positions described in the main text (courtesy of WeBSurg© IRCAD®)

effective as it ensures an empty digestive tract and decompressed small bowel, both of which facilitate the layering of intestinal loops, a crucial point for achieving adequate exposure. Alternatively, orthograde bowel lavage with polyethylene glycol can be used. In this case, administration 2 full days prior to surgery is preferable to avoid distension of small bowel loops that would be difficult to handle during the operation. In addition, creation of the working space is aided by

- Ensuring adequate pneumoperitoneum with a pressure of 12 mmHg
- Complete relaxation of the abdominal wall
- Sequential optimal patient positioning during the different operative steps

To then obtain exposure intra-operatively, the greater omentum and the transverse colon are placed in the left subphrenic region and maintained there by putting the operating table into Trendelenburg position (Figs. 18.4 and 18.5). An atraumatic retractor, introduced through trocar D, may also be helpful. Subsequently, the proximal small bowel loops are placed in the right upper quadrant by gently grasping them with atraumatic laparoscopic instruments. The distal small bowel loops are placed in the right lower quadrant with the cecum and maintained there with the help of gravity. If gravity is not sufficient, as it occurs especially in the presence of abundant intra-abdominal fat or dilated bowel loops, an additional maneuver is used. This involves passing an instrument through *Trocar F* to the root of the mesentery which then grasps the parietal peritoneum of the right

lengthened to allow extraction of the surgical specimen and so optimizes cosmetics for the patient. Finally, we sometimes use an additional trocar (*Trocar F*), which is 5 mm in diameter and is situated in the right mid-clavicular line in the subcostal area. This port accommodates an atraumatic grasper that is used to retract the terminal portion of the small intestine laterally, at the beginning of the dissection, and to retract the transverse colon or the greater omentum during the mobilization of the splenic flexure (Fig. 18.3).

18.4.6 Exposure of the Operative Field

Very often, conversion to open surgery is caused by difficulty in exposure, not only at the beginning but also throughout the procedure. Because we choose a medial to lateral approach, time is dedicated to perfect achievement of this exposure. This serves not only for the initial vascular approach, but also for about half of the remaining operative time.

Good preoperative bowel preparation is essential to facilitate exposure of the operative field. For this, we ask the patients to follow a strict fiber-free diet 8 days prior to admission and then take a phosphodisodic oral solution the day before surgery. This method is very

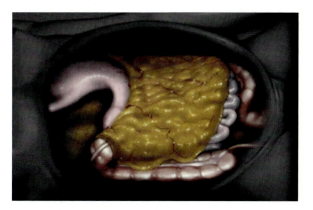

Fig. 18.4 Obtaining exposure by patient positioning: Initially the omentum and small bowel loops obstruct the view of the sigmoid colon and its mesentery (courtesy of WeBSurg© IRCAD®)

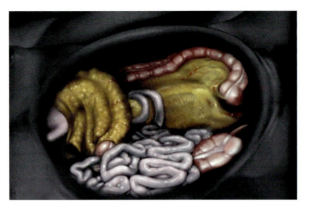

Fig. 18.5 Obtaining exposure by patient positioning: The patient is first tilted into Trendelenburg position and the omentum is retracted cephalad. Then the patient is tilted with right side down and the small bowel is placed in the right upper quadrant (courtesy of WeBSurg© IRCAD®)

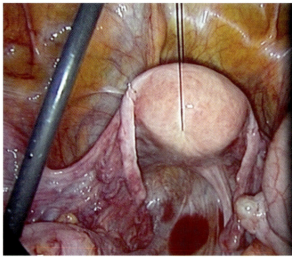

Fig. 18.6 Exposure of the operative field in a female patient: Suture suspension to retract the uterus and therefore to optimize the visualization in the pelvis (courtesy of WeBSurg© IRCAD®)

iliac fossa. Thus, the shaft of the grasper provides an "autostatic" retraction of the bowel loops, keeping them away from both the midline and the pelvic space. This technique of exposure provides an excellent view of the sacral promontory and the aorto–iliac axis. This particular view of the operative field is essential for the medio to lateral vascular approach that we perform routinely.

The uterus may be an additional obstacle to obtain adequate exposure in the pelvis. In postmenopausal female patients, it can be suspended to the abdominal wall by a suture (Fig. 18.6). This suture is introduced halfway between the umbilicus and the pubis, and ensures fully display of the rectovaginal space. In younger women, the uterus can be retracted using a similar suspension technique by inserting a suture around the round ligaments or by using a 5-mm retractor passed through the suprapubic port (*Trocar E*).

After adequate exposure has been obtained, the following operative steps follow in sequence:

- Approach to the vascular pedicle
- Medio-lateral mobilization of the sigmoid colon
- Resection of the target bowel segment
- Extraction of the surgical specimen
- Creation of the anastomosis

Additional steps could include the mobilization of the splenic flexure, performed when further lengthening of the colon is needed to perform a tension-free anastomosis.

18.4.7 Vascular Approach (Medio-lateral)

In approaching a patient with cancer, the vascular approach represents the first step of the dissection. We feel, that it allows us to avoid unnecessary manipulation of the colon and tumor, which may otherwise cause malignant cell exfoliation. Strictly following the vascular anatomy we are able to perform a good lymphadenectomy. We have to preserve the vascular supply of the nonresected left colon and rectum (Fig. 18.7). The vessels are gradually exposed, once the peritoneum at the base of the sigmoid mesocolon is incised. The medio-to-lateral approach allows us to see the trunks of the sympathetic nerve plexus and the left ureter. This is essential to avoid injuries to the ureter and to preserve urogenital function. Before approaching the vessels we visualize the tumor when possible and confirm its location.

We standardized the following three steps to achieve vascular control.

18.4.7.1 Identification of the Inferior Mesenteric Artery (IMA)

We begin the actual operation by making a peritoneal incision that facilitates the identification of the Inferior Mesenteric Artery (IMA) at its origin. To achieve that, we retract the sigmoid mesocolon anteriorly using a grasper introduced through *Trocar E*. This maneuver exposes the base of the sigmoid mesocolon (Fig. 18.8).

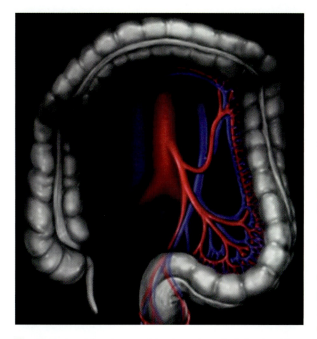

Fig. 18.7 Arterial and venous blood supply to the left colon: Note how the main venous tributaries mirror their arterial counterparts except for the main inferior mesenteric vessel. The inferior mesenteric artery is a direct branch of the aorta while the inferior mesenteric vein proceeds cephalad where it joins the splenic vein (courtesy of WeBSurg© IRCAD®)

The visceral peritoneum is incised at the level of the sacral promontory and this incision is carried on upwards along the right anterior border of the aorta up to the ligament of Treitz (Fig. 18.9). The pressure of the pneumoperitoneum, in combination with anterior traction of the mesosigmoid, facilitates the dissection, as the diffusion of CO_2 opens the avascular plane.

18.4.7.2 Division of Sigmoid Branches and IMA

The dissection is continued upwards by gradually dividing the sigmoid branches and the right sympathetic trunk to expose the origin of the IMA. To ensure an adequate lymphadenectomy, the first 2 cm of the IMA are dissected free and the artery is skeletonized before its division (Fig. 18.10). This dissection, at the origin of the IMA, involves a risk of injury to the body of the left sympathetic trunk located on the left border of the IMA. A meticulous dissection of the artery helps to prevent this, as only the vessel will then be divided rather than the surrounding tissue. Dissecting close to the artery also minimizes the risk of ureteral injury during the division of the IMA, indeed, the ureter should be routinely exposed and its position confirmed. Once fully isolated, the IMA can be divided between clips, by using a linear stapler (vascular 2.5 or 2.0 mm cartridges) or by using a sealing device like the Ligasure™ (Covidien).

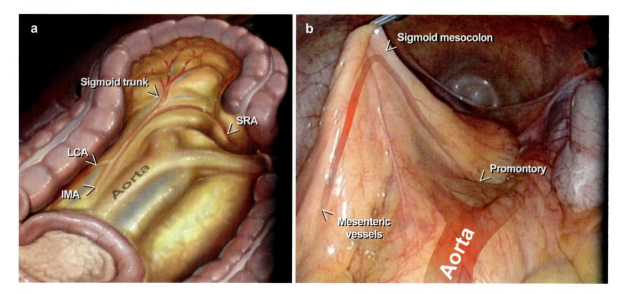

Fig. 18.8 Exposure of the sigmoid colon and its mesentery: Combination of retraction and patient positioning. (**a**) Schematic view (**b**) Real view (courtesy of WeBSurg© IRCAD®)

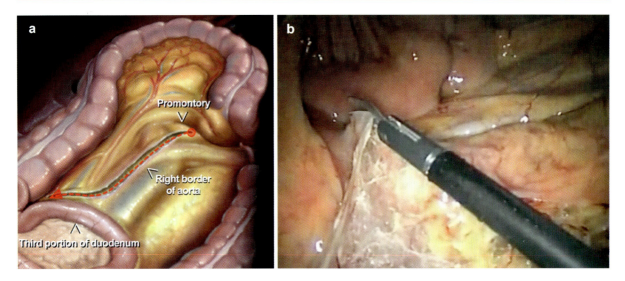

Fig. 18.9 Dissection of the IMA: Opening of the retroperitoneum to gain access to the root of the inferior mesenteric artery (IMA) (**a**) Schematic view (**b**) Real view (courtesy of WeBSurg© IRCAD®)

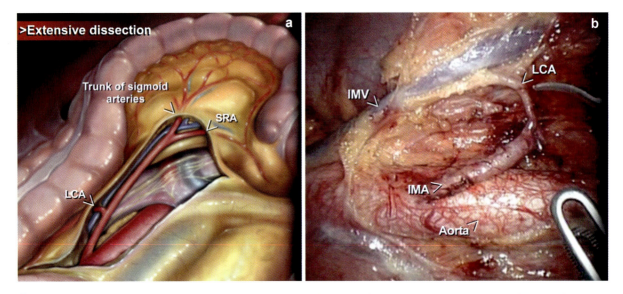

Fig. 18.10 Dissection of the IMA: Operative view of the skeletonized root of the inferior mesenteric artery (IMA). (**a**) Schematic view (**b**) Real view (courtesy of WeBSurg© IRCAD®)

18.4.7.3 Identification and Division of Inferior Mesenteric Vein (IMV)

The IMV is then identified to the left of the IMA or, in cases of difficult exposure higher up, on the left side of the ligament of Treitz. The vein is divided below the inferior border of the pancreas or above the left colic vein. Once again, clips or the Ligasure Atlas™ are both safe options for ligation and division of this structure.

18.4.8 Mobilization of the Sigmoid and Descending Colon

The mobilization of the sigmoid colon is performed after the division of the vessels. This step includes dissection of the posterior and lateral attachments of the sigmoid colon and mesocolon as well as the division of the rectal and sigmoid mesenteries. This step can be performed from medial or lateral. We, however, routinely perform the entire dissection from the medial side. The medial approach is well adapted for laparoscopy as it preserves the working space and demands the least handling of the sigmoid colon.

In a randomized trial comparing the medio-to-lateral laparoscopic dissection to the classical lateral-to-medial approach for resection of rectosigmoid cancer, Liang et al. demonstrated that the medial approach reduces the operative time and the postoperative pro-inflammatory response [22]. In addition, besides the potential oncological advantages of early vessel division and "no-touch" dissection [23, 24], we also feel that, the longer the lateral abdominal wall attachments of the colon are preserved the easier is the exposure and dissection (Table 18.3).

We standardized the following two steps to mobilize the sigmoid and descending colon.

18.4.8.1 Exposure of the Posterior Space

The sigmoid mesocolon is retracted anteriorly (*Trocar E*) in order to expose the posterior space. The plane between the line of Toldt and the sigmoid mesocolon can then be identified. This plane is avascular and easy to dissect. The dissection continues posterior to the sigmoid mesocolon heading laterally towards the line of Toldt.

18.4.8.2 Lateral Dissection

The sigmoid colon is now completely free, and the lateral attachments can now be divided. For this, the sigmoid loop is pulled towards the right upper quadrant by using a grasper inserted through *Trocar F* to apply traction on the line of Toldt. The peritoneal fold is opened cephalad and caudal, and the dissection joins the one previously performed, coming from the medial side. During this step, care must be taken to avoid injury to the gonadal vessels and the left ureter, as they can be tented up by traction exerted on the mesentery. Ureteral stenting using infrared stents can be useful in cases where inflammation, tumor tissue, adhesions, and/or endometriosis has made the anatomic planes difficult to recognize.

Table 18.3 Laparoscopic colectomy: Medial-to-lateral versus lateral-to-medial dissection

Comparison of medial-to-lateral versus traditional lateral-to-medial laparoscopic dissection sequences for resection of recto-sigmoid cancers: Randomized controlled clinical trial National Taiwan University Goup *World Journal of Surgery* 2003 27(2):190–6.			
	Medial to lateral group ($n=36$)	Lateral to medial group ($n=36$)	p value
Intra-operative parameters			
Operating Time (min)	198.0 ± 26.0	260 ± 32.0	<0.05
Intra-operative complications	2 (5.6%)	2 (6.5%)	ns
Conversion rate (n/%)	2 (5.6%)	2 (6.5%)	ns
Postoperative ileus (h)	50.0 ± 10.5	56.0 ± 18.4	ns
Postoperative pain (visual analog scale)	4.2 ± 1.0	4.8 ± 1.2	
Length of wound (cm)	5.0 ± 0.5	6.2 ± 1.0	ns
Rise in Inflammatory markers in first 24 h (CRP/ESR)	4.90 ± 1.3/1.6 ± 0.43	9.30 ± 1.50/2.46 ± 0.40	<0.05
Postoperative parameters			
Hospital stay (days)	8.5 ± 1.5	9.0 ± 2.0	ns
Overall cost (US $)	5,429 ± 121	5,657 ± 155	<0.05
Postoperative complications	6 (17%)	7 (19%)	ns
Return to work (weeks)	4.3 ± 0.4	4.6 ± 1.5	ns
2 year recurrence rate	5.6%	6.5%	ns

ns nonsignificant

18.4.9 Dissection of the Proximal Mesorectum

This area of dissection should be approached with caution, especially on the left side, as the mesorectum is closely attached to the parietal fascia, where the superior hypogastric nerve and the left ureter run. The upper portion of the rectum is mobilized posteriorly following the avascular plane, described above, and then laterally until an adequate distal margin is achieved.

18.4.10 Distal Division of the Rectum

Once the proximal rectum is freed up, the level of distal transection is determined to ensure a margin beyond the tumor of at least 5 cm. At this level, the colon is cleared from its surrounding fat using monopolar cautery, ultrasonic dissection, or the Ligasure™ device. After doing so, the superior haemorrhoidal artery is divided in the posterior upper mesorectum. Although we do not routinely perform it, the colon may now be closed using an umbilical tape before a rectal washout is performed. This should reduce tumor cell implantation at the staple line.

The distal division is performed using a linear stapler. The stapler is introduced through *Trocar C*. We use stapler loads (3.5-mm, 45-mm blue cartridges), which are applied perpendicular to the bowel. Articulated staplers can also be useful, although they are usually unnecessary at the level of the upper rectum.

18.4.11 Proximal Division of the Colon

The proximal division site should be chosen at least 10 cm proximal to the tumor. It is performed by first dividing the mesocolon and subsequently, the bowel. The division of the mesocolon is performed using the harmonic scalpel, Ligasure™, or linear staplers. The distal portion of the divided IMA is identified, and the division of the mesocolon starts at this level and continues towards the chosen proximal transection level at a 90° angle. The proximal end of the colon, which will be anastomosed later, is grasped with an atraumatic grasper through *Trocar B* or *Trocar D*. A linear stapler, best introduced through *Trocar C*, is then fired across the bowel.

18.4.12 Mobilization of the Splenic Flexure

In the frequent event where a long segment of sigmoid colon has been resected, mobilization of the splenic flexure is required. This can be achieved in different ways, and it is important for the surgeon to be familiar with all approaches, in order to select the one most suitable for the particular setting.

Mobilization of the entire splenic flexure may not be necessary when sufficient lengthening is obtained by simply freeing the posterior and lateral attachments of the descending colon. If the mobilized colon reaches the right lower quadrant easily, it may be safely assumed the anastomosis will be tension-free. When necessary, a full mobilization of the splenic flexure can be achieved, by first mobilizing the posterior attachments of the descending and distal transverse colon from the medial side, followed by taking down the lateral attachments. This step can be performed in reverse order. The medial mobilization is perfectly suited to our laparoscopic approach as the surgeon, standing at the patient's right side, has an excellent view of the anterior surface of the pancreas and the base of the left transverse mesocolon. This is especially true in obese patients. A lateral mobilization alone is sometimes sufficient. In addition, division of colo-colic adhesions or sometimes transection of additional vascular structures must be performed in order to achieve adequate bowel length for a tension-free anastomosis.

18.4.12.1 Medial Mobilization of the Splenic Flexure

This approach allows freeing the posterior attachments of the transverse and descending colon first. The dissection plane follows the plane of the previous mobilization of the sigmoid colon cephalad, anterior to the line of Toldt. The transverse colon is retracted anteriorly to expose the inferior border of the pancreas. We enter the lesser sac in order to divide the root of the transverse mesocolon anterior to the pancreas. The dissection then follows towards the base of the descending colon and distal transverse colon, dividing the posterior attachments of these structures. The division of the lateral attachments, as described above, then follows the full mobilization of the splenic flexure.

18.4.12.2 Lateral Mobilization of the Splenic Flexure

This approach is commonly used in open surgery and can be also used in straightforward laparoscopic colectomies. The first step is the division of the lateral attachments of the descending colon. An ascending incision is made along the line of Toldt using scissors inserted via *Trocar D*. The phreno-colic ligament is then divided. Retraction of the descending colon and the splenic flexure towards the right lower quadrant, using graspers introduced through *Trocar C* and *Trocar E*, helps in exposing the right plane. The attachments between the transverse colon and the omentum are divided close to the colon until the lesser sac is opened. Division of these attachments is continued, as needed, to reach adequate length.

18.4.13 Extraction of the Surgical Specimen

The size of the incision, its location, and the extraction technique are determined by

- Volume of the specimen
- Patient's body shape
- Cosmetic concerns
- Type of disease

The incision is generally placed in the suprapubic region. The proximal division of the colon is performed intra-corporeally, as described above. The specimen will be placed into a solid retrieval bag before being extracted through the suprapubic incision (Fig. 18.11).

The extraction of the specimen is performed using double protection: a plastic wound protector and a retrieval plastic bag. The wound protector is also helpful to ensure that there is no CO_2 leak during the intra-corporeally performed colorectal anastomosis. It also allows a smaller size incision and minimizes the risk of tumor cell seeding.

18.4.14 Creation of the Anastomosis

We always use a mechanical circular stapling device to transfix the rectal stump. Performing the anastomosis includes two steps:

- Extra-abdominal step
- Intra-abdominal step performed laparoscopically

The extra-abdominal step takes place after the extraction of the specimen. The laparoscopic instrument

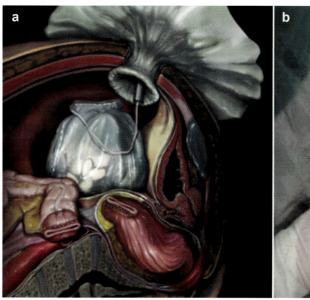
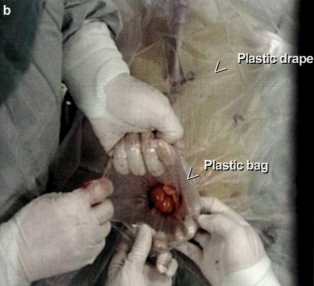

Fig. 18.11 Specimen extraction: use of a double wound protection to extract the resected specimen. (**a**) Schematic view (**b**) real view (courtesy of WeBSurg© IRCAD®)

holding the proximal bowel presents the colon at the incision site where it can easily be grasped with a Babcock forceps. The proximal colon is now inspected for viability and, if necessary, divided again. The anvil, at least 28 mm in diameter, is then introduced into the bowel lumen and the transected end is closed with a purse string suture. The colon is now reintroduced into the abdominal cavity.

The abdominal incision is temporarily closed to reestablish the pneumoperitoneum. For an airtight closure, it is sufficient to twist the previously placed wound protector and hold it in place applying a large clamp.

The well lubed circular stapler is introduced into the rectum after gently dilating the anus. The rectal stump is then held in place with the tip of the head of the circular stapler. In women, the posterior vaginal wall should be retracted anteriorly.

Once the anvil is engaged we check for twisting of the colon. The stapler is then fired, after ensuring that the neighboring organs are away from the stapling line. The device is opened and withdrawn through the anus.

Finally, the anastomosis is checked for leaks by

- Verifying the integrity of the proximal and distal donuts
- Performing an air test

Some authors complete the evaluation of the anastomosis with a rectoscopy. We do not routinely place a drain.

18.4.15 Wound Closure

The trocar sites are each checked laparoscopically for possible hemorrhage. With hemostasis ensured, the pneomoperitoneum is desufflated through the trocars, and the trocars are removed under direct visualization. The suprapubic incision is closed in layers using running absorbable sutures and all fascial defects greater than 10 mm are closed. The skin is closed using staplers or with a subcuticular running suture.

18.5 Complications and Pitfalls and How to Avoid Them

Laparoscopic sigmoid resection and open sigmoidectomy share a number of complications that include

- Anastomotic leak
- Abscess formation
- Wound infection
- Wound dehiscence
- Bleeding

The laparoscopic approach is also associated with some general complications such as thrombo-embolism, pneumonia, cardiovascular problems, as like any other operation of similar extent and duration. Some complications are however specific to the laparoscopic technique and mostly derive from the use of trocars. These include

- Trocar site hemorrhage
- Trocar site hernias
- Port site metastasis
- Veress needle or trocar-related puncture injuries of abdominal organs

18.5.1 Bleeding from the Abdominal Wall

Prevention of hemorrhage from the abdominal wall starts with careful evaluation of the site of the skin incision for trocar insertion. Transillumination may help to recognize the course of epigastric vessels. Small vessels may also be injured during trocar insertion, but the damage can be concealed by both the tamponading effect of the trocar and the pressure of the pneumoperitoneum. Because of this we check the trocar site for bleeding by removing the trocar over the shaft of a grasper.

18.5.2 Trocar Site Hernias

All trocar sites ≥10 mm are at risk of herniation and closure of the fascia at these sites is recommended. This can be done either open or laparoscopically using an endoclosure device. The endoclosure device is particularly helpful in closing the fascial defect in obese patients.

18.5.3 Port Site Metastasis

The use of laparoscopy to treat cancer has been very controversial largely due to fear of port site metastases and inadequate oncologic resections [25, 26]. Recently published large multicenter series show that recurrence of cancer at the trocar site is no longer to be considered a complication attributable to laparoscopy as a technique [22, 1], but, rather, a consequence of inexperience and improper tumor handling during the operation [27]. Indeed, with appropriate technique, the incidence of this phenomenon is about 1% in most recent series and in many cases, it seems to approach 0% [3].

18.5.4 Puncture Injuries of Abdominal Organs

To minimize the risk of trocar injuries, we use an open technique for the insertion of the first trocar.

18.5.5 Ureteral Injuries

The inability to use direct palpation to help identify important anatomic structures and the lack of tactile feedback during difficult dissections may also cause problems during laparoscopy especially where the ureter is of concern. The most important step to avoid injuries to the ureter is to achieve perfect exposure and to stay in the correct plane for further dissection. If the dissection is performed above the Toldt's fascia, the ureter will not be exposed and accidental injuries will be avoided. Major inflammatory or desmoplastic reactions, cancer invasion into surrounding structures, or adhesions may alter the anatomy and make it difficult to identify the ureter in its course. In these special cases, insertion of infrared ureteral stents is very helpful. The infrared light is a cold source, safe for use in close contact with ureteral tissue and can be easily visualized using a laparoscope.

18.6 Future Trends

The ease with which a colonic resection is performed laparoscopically is likely to be further enhanced in the future by increasingly sophisticated technology. Developments such as high definition (HD) screens have greatly improved the visual acuity of the surgeon, while instrument technology allows more precise dissection and results in less blood loss. In addition, evolutions in trocar technology may alleviate the requirement for a physical seal at the entry site. This will allow the passage of multiple instruments simultaneously through a single port. Reduction in the caliber of standard instruments for ensuring haemostatic dissection and even stapling is likely to allow reduced trocar size. With increasing numbers of patients suffering from cancer being detected at an early stage by improved screening, laparoscopy [28] may also have a role in augmenting endoscopic techniques such as endoscopic submucosal dissection [29]. Sentinel node mapping might be routinely applied [30]. Robotic devices improved clinical colorectal practice substantially and will be added to innovations such as Natural Orifice Transluminal Endoscopic Surgery (N.O.T.E.S.). This will greatly advance this nascent subspecialty without any doubt. Alteration of a surgeon's mindset and approach even in conventional situations will be the logical consequence [30]. Thus, an era of truly minimally *invasive* surgery, as opposed to mere minimal *access* surgery, may be on the horizon.

18.7 Conclusions

Laparoscopic sigmoid resection is a well standardized technique in this day and age. Whereas the open surgical approach is most commonly performed by using a standard lateral-to-medial dissection, with or without primary vascular approach, the medial-to-lateral approach seems to be more suitable to laparoscopy and is our favored operative strategy. Indeed, the medial-to-lateral approach permits a safe primary dissection and avoids manipulation of the colon. Surgeons learning the technique should ideally train with a skilled and experienced team. A good learning strategy may be to reproduce the steps of the laparoscopic technique during an open procedure.

Quick Reference Guide

1. Good equipment is key:
   - Laparoscopic unit with 3chip camera or preferably a HD video camera
   - Sealing devices like Ligasure or harmonic scalpel are essential
2. Obtain optimal exposure by:
   - Correct patient setup
   - Preoperative bowel preparation
   - Sufficient trocars of appropriate size
   - Ensure good anchoring of the trocars

3. Respect correct indications for a laparoscopic colectomy:
   - T1 and T2 cancers
   - T3, if indicated
4. Perform a primary vascular approach with extensive lymphadenectomy
5. No touch technique is mandatory!
   Limit manipulation of the colon and if necessary do it in an atraumatic way
   Don't manipulate the tumor!
6. Mobilize the entire left colon and splenic flexure to assure a tension-free anastomosis. If the mobilized left colon reaches the left lower abdominal quadrant, it can be safely assumed that the following anastomosis will be tension-free
7. Avoid a too small incision at the extraction site in order to extract the specimen appropriately
8. Use a retrieval bag in combination with a wound protector to avoid contamination. Abdominal wall and abdominal cavity protection is necessary
9. Perform a mechanical, tension-free anastomosis. Leak test with air insufflation or rectoscopy should always be performed
10. We recommend cleaning the instruments in use with a Betadine solution throughout the procedure

References

1. Martel, G., Boushey, R.P.: Laparoscopic colon surgery: past, present and future. Surg. Clin. North Am. **86**, 867–897 (2006)
2. Leroy, J., Ananian, P., Rubino, F., Claudon, B., Mutter, D., Marescaux, J.: The impact of obesity on technical feasibility and postoperative outcomes of laparoscopic left colectomy. Ann. Surg. **241**, 69–76 (2005)
3. Kohler, L., Eypash, E., Troidl, H.: Myths in management of colorectal malignancy. Br. J. Surg. **84**, 248–251 (1997)
4. Liang, Y., Li, G., Chen, P., Yu, J.: Laparoscopic versus open colorectal resection for cancer: a meta-analysis of results of randomized controlled trials on recurrence. Eur. J. Surg. Oncol. **34**, 1217–1224 (2008)
5. Franklin, M.E., Rosenthal, D., Abrego-Medina, D., Dorman, J.P., Glass, J.L., Norem, R., Diaz, A.: Prospective comparison of open vs. laparoscopic colon surgery for carcinoma. Five-year results. Dis. Colon Rectum **39**, S35–S46 (1996)
6. Hewitt, P.M., Kwok, S.P., Somers, S.S., Li, K., Leung, K.L., Lau, W.Y., Li, A.K.C.: Laparoscopic-assisted vs. open surgery for colorectal cancer: comparative study of immune effects. Dis. Colon Rectum **41**, 901–909 (1998)
7. Kockerling, F., Reymond, M.A., Schneider, C., Wittekind, C., Scheidbach, H., Konradt, J., Kohler, L., Barlehner, E., Kuthe, A., Bruch, H.P., Hohenberger, W.: Prospective multicenter study of the quality of oncologic resections in patients undergoing laparoscopic colorectal surgery for cancer. The Laparoscopic Colorectal Surgery Study Group. Dis. Colon Rectum **41**, 963–970 (1998)
8. Kwok, S.P., Lau, W.Y., Carey, P.D., Kelly, S.B., Leung, K.L., Li, A.K.: Prospective evaluation of laparoscopic-assisted large bowel excision for cancer. Ann. Surg. **223**, 170–176 (1996)
9. Milsom, J.W., Bohm, B., Hammerhofer, K.A., Fazio, V., Steiger, E., Elson, P.: A prospective, randomized trial comparing laparoscopic versus conventional techniques in colorectal cancer surgery: a preliminary report. J. Am. Coll. Surg. **187**, 46–54 (1998)
10. Nishiguchi, K., Okuda, J., Toyoda, M., Tanaka, K., Nobuhiko Tanigawa, N.: Comparative evaluation of surgical stress of laparoscopic and open surgeries for colorectal carcinoma. Dis. Colon Rectum **44**, 223–230 (2001)
11. Read, T.E., Mutch, M.G., Chang, B.W., McNevin, M.S., Fleshman, J.W., Birnbaum, E.H., Fry, R.D., Caushaj, P.F., Kodner, I.J.: Locoregional recurrence and survival after curative resection of adenocarcinoma of the colon. J. Am. Coll. Surg. **195**, 33–40 (2002)
12. Tang, C.L., Eu, K.W., Tai, B.C., Soh, J.G., MacHin, D., Seow-Choen, F.: Randomized clinical trial of effect of open versus laparoscopically assisted colectomy on systemic immunity in patients with colorectal cancer. Br. J. Surg. **88**, 801–807 (2001)
13. Weeks, J.C., Nelson, H., Gelber, S., Sargent, D., Schroeder, G., Clinical Outcomes of Surgical Therapy (COST) Study Group: Short-term quality-of-life outcomes following laparoscopic-assisted colectomy vs open colectomy for colon cancer: a randomized trial. J. Am. Med. Assoc. **287**, 321–328 (2002)
14. Lacy, A.M., Garcia-Valdecasas, J.C., Delgado, S., Castells, A., Taura, P., Pique, J.M., Visa, J.: Laparoscopy-assisted colectomy versus open colectomy for treatment of non-metastatic colon cancer: a randomised trial. Lancet **359**, 2224–2229 (2002)
15. Lacy, A.M., Delgado, S., Garcia-Valdecasas, J.C., Castells, A., Piqué, J.M., Grande, L., Fuster, J., Targarona, E.M., Pera, M., Visa, J.: Port site metastases and recurrence after laparoscopic colectomy. A randomised trial. Surg. Endosc. **12**, 1039–1042 (1998)
16. Zmora, O., Gervaz, P., Wexner, S.D.: Trocar site recurrence in laparoscopic surgery for colorectal cancer. Myth or real concern? Surg. Endosc. **15**, 788–793 (2001)
17. Marusch, F., Gastinger, I., Schneider, C., Scheidbach, H., Konradt, J., Bruch, H.P., Köhler, L., Bärlehner, E., Köckerling, F., Laparoscopic Colorectal Surgery Study Group (LCSSG): Experience as a factor influencing the indications for laparoscopic colorectal surgery and the results. Surg. Endosc. **15**, 116–120 (2001)
18. Franklin, M.E., Kazantsev, G.B., Abrego, D., Diaz-E, J.A., Balli, J., Glass, J.L.: Laparoscopic surgery for stage III colon cancer: long-term follow-up. Surg. Endosc. **14**, 612–616 (2000)
19. Poulin, E.C., Mamazza, J., Schlachta, C.M., Gregoire, R., Roy, N.: Laparoscopic resection does not adversely affect

early survival curves in patients undergoing surgery for colorectal adenocarcinoma. Ann. Surg. **229**, 487–492 (1999)
20. Veldkamp, R., Gholghesaei, M., Brunen, M., Meijer, D.W., Bonjer, H.J., Lezoche, E., Himpens, J., Jacobi, C.A., Whelan, R.L., Lacy, A.M., Morino, M., Haglind, E., Jakimowicz, J.J., Cuesta, M.A., Neugebauer, E., Anderberg, B., Guillou, P.J., Monson, J.W., Jeekel, J., Fingerhut, A., Cuschieri, A., Koeckerling, F., Fleshman, J.W., Wexner, S.D.: Laparoscopic Resection of Colonic Carcinoma EAES consensus conference Lisbon. Online publication http://www.eaes-eur.org/rescolframe.html (2002)
21. Leroy, J., Milsom, J.W., Okuda, J.: Laparoscopic sigmoidectomy for cancer. http://www.websurg.com
22. Liang, J.T., Lai, H.S., Huang, K.C., Chang, K.J., Shieh, M.J., Jeng, Y.M., Wang, S.M.: Comparison of medial-to-lateral versus traditional lateral-to-medial laparoscopic dissection sequences for resection of rectosigmoid cancers: randomized controlled clinical trial. World J. Surg. **27**(2), 190–196 (2003)
23. Turnbull, R.B., Kyle, K., Watson, F.R., Spratt, J.: Cancer of the colon: the influence of the no-touch technique on survival rates. Ann. Surg. **166**, 420–427 (1967)
24. Wiggers, T., Jeekel, J., Arends, J.W., Brinkhorst, A.P., Kluck, H.M., Luyk, C.I., Munting, J.D., Povel, J.A., Rutten, A.P., Volovics, A.: No-touch isolation technique in colon cancer: a controlled prospective trial. Br. J. Surg. **75**, 409–415 (1988)
25. Allardyce, R., Morreau, P., Bagshaw, P.: Tumor cell distribution following laparoscopic colectomy in a porcine model. Dis. Colon Rectum **39**, S47–S52 (1996)
26. Balli, J.E., Franklin, M.E., Almeida, J.A., Glass, J.L., Diaz, J.A., Reymond, M.: How to prevent port-site metastases in laparoscopic colorectal surgery. Surg. Endosc. **14**, 1034–1036 (2000)
27. Yamamoto, H.: Technology insight: endoscopic submucosal dissection of gastrointestinal neoplasms. Nat. Clin. Pract. Gastroenterol. Hepatol. **4**, 511–520 (2007)
28. Cahill, R.A., Perretta, S., Leroy, J., Dallemagne, B., Marescaux, J.: Lymphatic mapping and sentinel node biopsy in the colonic mesentery by Natural Orifice Transluminal Endoscopic Surgery. Ann. Surg. Oncol. **15**(10), 2677–2683 (2008)
29. Franklin Jr., M.E., Leyva-Alvizo, A., Abrego-Medina, D., Glass, J.L., Treviño, J., Arellano, P.P., Portillo, G.: Laparoscopically monitored colonoscopic polypectomy: an established form of endoluminal therapy for colorectal polyps. Surg. Endosc. **21**, 1650–1653 (2007)
30. Wexner, S.D., Cohen, S.M.: Port site metastases after laparoscopic colorectal surgery for cure of malignancy. Br. J. Surg. **82**, 295–298 (1995)

Laparoscopic Rectal Procedures

19

Rolv-Ole Lindsetmo and Conor P. Delaney

19.1 Introduction

Until recently, surgery for rectal cancer was associated with unacceptable high local recurrence rates up to 30% or higher. Published rates of local recurrence have changed dramatically since the popularization and more widespread acceptance of total mesorectal excision (TME) as the standard approach for radical surgery for rectal cancer. This change in practice has reduced local recurrencem, rates to less than 10% in many centers, and has been associated with improved survival in rectal cancer patients [1–3].

Along with improvements in surgical technique, data are available showing a beneficial relationship between specialization, case volume, and clinical outcome [4–6]. In some European countries, this has led to a centralization of rectal cancer surgery to institutions with a multidisciplinary approach to the disease. Involvement of trained colorectal surgeons that decide individual treatment plans based on evidence-based guidelines, in cooperation with dedicated radiologists and oncologists, is becoming more widely accepted in ensuring optimal treatment and prognosis for rectal cancer patients.

In parallel with this standardization of rectal cancer treatment, laparoscopic approaches to the colon and rectum have been rapidly gaining in acceptance. This chapter outlines the place of laparoscopy in the current range of treatment options for rectal cancer. Issues relating to training and the integration of this technically challenging procedure are discussed.

R.-O. Lindsetmo
University Hospital of North Norway, 9038 Tromso, Norway

C.P. Delaney (✉)
University Hospitals Case Medical Center and Case Western Reserve University, 11100 Euclid Avenue, Cleveland, OH 44106-5047, USA
e-mail: conor.delaney@UHhospitals.org

19.2 Current Literature

Once a diagnosis of rectal cancer has been confirmed, several decisions need to be made. First, whether this lesion is suitable for transanal excision, either because of stage, location, or patient comorbidities. For lesions that are not suitable for local therapy, a decision must be made whether preoperative therapy will be required. Lastly, a decision is made as to whether a restorative procedure can be performed.

19.3 Preoperative Staging and Workup

A thorough history and physical examination, in conjunction with preoperative staging, are the pieces of information used to make these decisions. Other diagnoses and comorbidities, a continence history, and history of prior surgery are important considerations. Physical examination is extremely important, especially for low rectal tumors. Sphincter tone can be assessed and site, size, and degree of fixity of the tumor can be determined. The preoperative fecal and urinary continence as well as sexual function should also be ascertained. Rigid proctoscopy is used to define the distance between the tumor and the dentate line.

In our practice, patients undergo endoanal ultrasound at the initial office visit, giving immediate information about T and N staging, though limited to approximately 70–90% accuracy [7]. Patients with stricturing tumors that are not suitable for ultrasound, and more recently almost all patients with rectal cancer undergo MRI evaluation to determine expected resection margins, invasion of surrounding structures, and lymph node status. CT scan of the abdomen and chest is performed to evaluate the liver, lungs, and rule out the presence of metastatic disease. Although there have been some discussions of PET scan in the literature, we have not made this part of our routine practice, except for preoperative evaluation of patients referred with recurrent rectal cancer [8]. All patients planned for rectal cancer surgery should undergo preoperative colonoscopy to detect synchronous colonic cancer. The abdominal wall should be inspected, and possible stoma sites should be planned. The patient should be informed about the planned operative strategies, possible complications, and the expected postoperative course.

The decisions on a treatment plan should be taken by a multidisciplinary team dedicated to colorectal cancer treatment and based on standardized clinical and radiological investigations and in accordance to national guidelines.

19.4 Selecting Preoperative Treatment for Patients

There is significant international debate about which patients should be offered preoperative therapy. In Sweden and The Netherlands, most patients with a rectal cancer tend to be considered for radiation [1, 9] and the US National Comprehensive Cancer Network guidelines recommend chemoradiation for all patients with stage 2 or 3 disease [10]. Others [11–14] suggest that radiation should be performed more selectively, either for T3 and node positive tumors in the lower two third of the rectum [14], or perhaps only for those with preoperative imaging suggesting that there will be a close postoperative circumferential margin, less than 3 mm [13].

There is increasing evidence that in patients who have tumors in the upper rectum, or stage I disease, and undergo optimal surgery, there is no need for radiation [11]. The long-term follow-up from the Dutch TME trial confirms that stage I and even stage II rectal cancers do not differ in 5-year local recurrence rates comparing preoperative radiation therapy and TME to TME alone [15]. Sauer and colleagues provided important data suggesting that if radiation is to be given, this should be given preoperatively to minimize local recurrence rates and to reduce complications seen [16]. More recently, Bosset et al. for EORTC evaluated 1011 T3 and T4 rectal cancer, and showed that timing of chemotherapy did not affect survival, but when given pre- or postoperatively, local recurrence rates could be reduced [17]. Thus, our practice has been to offer preoperative chemoradiation to patients with T3 tumors within the lower two third of the rectum, particularly for those with threatened margins on preoperative MRI.

19.5 Selecting the Best Surgical Option for Patients

19.5.1 Transanal Excision and Transanal Endoscopic Microsurgery

These less invasive surgical options are considered for patients with early-stage disease, patients with tumors that will require a permanent end colostomy, and those with severe comorbidities that would be at risk from an abdominal surgical approach. Local excision procedures give little or no functional disturbances in genitourinary and rectal functions, but recent reports have raised concerns with high local recurrence rates [18–20]. In several recent studies, local recurrence rates of 18% were reported for T1 cancers and 30% for T2 cancers [19–21]. Results from histological studies of the mesorectum in rectal cancer show that about 10% of T1 cancers and 17–18% of T2 cancers have lymph node metastasis [22, 23]. As long as micrometastasis in lymph nodes are left behind in the mesorectum, local recurrence rates are likely to be higher after local excision than after resectional surgery.

Generally, local excision should be reserved for carefully selected patients. Recent data from Italy [24] suggest that combination with radiation might be useful for selected cases. RCT are underway and will hopefully clarify the position of local excision in combination with adjuvant chemoradiotherapy. Other recent data with TEM suggest that this may be an option to reduce local recurrence rates [25], although randomized trials comparing this with standard transanal excision have not been performed. Performing local excision after preoperative radiation is currently being studied in ACOSOG trial z6041, but is not yet standard of care.

19.5.2 Low Anterior Resection (LAR) Versus Abdominoperineal Resection (APR)

Perhaps the most concerning question for many patients is whether or not they will require a permanent colostomy. Although data comparing quality of life suggest that patients have similar QOL whether with an end colostomy or a low colo-anal anastomosis, naturally most patients would rather defecate as normally as possible after surgery.

Patients with poor continence or with tumors within 1–2 cm of the dentate line, or with local invasion of the sphincters or levator ani muscles will require an abdominoperineal excision with permanent end colostomy. Many studies have suggested that local recurrence rates may be higher with this operation than with colo-anal anastomosis. This is probably related to the more advanced tumors chosen for this procedure, but may also be related to inadequacy of obtaining clear lateral margins in the perianal region. Thus, similar to the popularization of adequate circumferential resection margins with TME, there is now increasing awareness that adequate circumferential margins are necessary for patients having an APR, and an effort must be made not to "cone-down" on the specimen at the level of the division of the levators.

19.5.3 Resection Margins: Mesorectal, Mucosal, Circumferential, and Proximal

Current guidelines suggest that upper rectal cancers should have 5-cm distal mesorectal resection margin when a partial mesorectal resection (PME) is performed because of potential distal spread of invasive cancer cells [26, 27]. Cancers located in the distal half of the rectum should be removed within a total mesorectal excision [28]. As long as the complete mesorectum is removed, the distal mucosal resection margin can be 2 cm [29]. In selected motivated patients who wish to preserve continence with ultralow rectal cancers, and with favorable pathology (well or moderately well differentiated, no lymphovascular invasion), a 1-cm margin appears to be adequate. In patients with a long anal canal, or with tumors very close to the anal canal, there may not be enough distance to place a stapler across the distal rectum to perform a double-stapled anastomosis. In these cases, an intersphincteric dissection may be performed from below, removing part or all of the internal sphincter, and performing a hand-sewn anastomosis, with or without a neo-rectal reservoir. Preoperative chemoradiation treatment should probably be given when a sphincter-saving procedure is chosen for the lowest rectal cancers [30, 31].

The importance of an adequate circumferential resection margin (CRM) is documented in several studies [13, 32–34]. Failure to achieve more than 2-mm CRM worsens the prognosis of local recurrence and survival.

A proximal resection margin of 5–10 cm above the rectosigmoid junction is oncologically safe. Above this level, the proximal resection site is chosen to secure a tension-free anastomosis with adequate blood supply.

19.5.4 Surgery for Locally Advanced Tumors

Patients who present with locally advanced tumors may need extended resections involving *en bloc* resections of the bladder, uterus, sacrum, or other surrounding structures. These patients obviously should receive preoperative CRT, but also need appropriate counseling about their surgery, and adequate planning to have other surgical specialists available if necessary. In our practice, we have the facilities for use of intraoperative radiotherapy, and have used this selectively, particularly for patients with local invasion into unresectable structures in pelvic sidewall, or to avoid the morbidity of sacrectomy in older patients. Results have been excellent with recurrence rates of less than 5 % for these most advanced tumors [35].

19.5.5 Minimally Invasive Approaches to Surgery

Initial concerns about poor oncological outcomes for colon cancer have been put to rest by major clinical trials [36–42]. Substantial data show that using a laparoscopic approach for colon cancer surgery is associated with shorter hospital stay, earlier recovery, and reduction in complications [39–43]. The situation for laparoscopic rectal cancer surgery is less clear, as fewer reports are available and there are few randomized data showing oncological equivalence with open surgery. The Hong Kong study has shown similar survival for patients with rectosigmoid cancers, but low rectal cancers were not included [44]. The CLASICC trial included low cancers, but conversion rates were high, and circumferential margin positivity rates were higher for patients having laparoscopic anterior resection. However, 3-year local recurrence and survival rates were similar to patients undergoing conventional rectal cancer surgery [36].

Having said this, several series have been published showing excellent results with a laparoscopic approach [45–48]. Extremely low local recurrence rates can be achieved in highly skilled hands. These surgeons are all far past their learning curves, and the generalizability of these results is unclear, particularly knowing how difficult it has been to standardize open surgery, a much less technically demanding venture.

19.6 Surgical Approach

19.6.1 Preoperative Planning and Strategy

A precise knowledge of the patient's general conditions including previous and actual comorbidities and medication is important in order to estimate the risk of the operation and in preventing cardiopulmonary, cerebrovascular, or musculoskeletal complications due to the general anesthesia or the planned positioning of the patient on the operating table. Severe obesity will with certainty make the laparoscopic approach more difficult, especially in males, and if also a large tumor and a narrow deep pelvis, a primary open approach might be advisable.

Before entering the operating room, the surgeon must be updated with all available information regarding the patient's condition, tumor location within the rectum, and the preoperative tumor stage. Tumor response to preoperative CRT, possible resection margins, and distance of tumor from the dentate line must be verified. With this information in mind, the surgeon has to decide the surgical procedure that will give the best chance for cure, minimize the risk for local recurrence, and gives best functional results. At the same time, the surgeon must also take into consideration strategies for optimal recovery for the patients in order to reduce morbidity, hospital stay, and total costs.

19.6.2 Laparoscopic Surgery for Rectal Cancer: The Different Procedures

Laparoscopic resection of the cancer-bearing rectum with an intact surrounding mesorectum is the main minimally invasive procedure for laparoscopic rectal cancer surgery. However, there are four different laparoscopic procedures that are performed in patients with rectal cancer. These procedures are:

- Diverting loop ileostomy
- Low anterior resection
- Abdominoperineal resection
- Hartman's procedure

The chosen procedure depends on the site of the tumor in the rectum and on individual considerations regarding the patients general condition, cancer stage, anastomotic safety, anal function, and patients preference.

19.6.3 Laparoscopic Loop Ileostomy

A diverting loop ileostomy will be very helpful for patients with obstructive symptoms and pain needing chemoradiotherapy for downstaging of the cancer. The loop ileostomy is kept after the laparoscopic rectal resection to protect the patients from pelvic sepsis if they develop leakage from the colorectal or coloanal anastomosis. The loop ileostomy is favored over colostomy because a sigmoid colostomy uses the section of colon that will be required for a tension-free anastomosis.

A laparoscopic loop ileostomy is easily performed with two 5-mm trocars in the left lower quadrant in addition to the camera port in the umbilicus. Alternatively, the stoma site is used as one of the trocar positions. The ileostomy limbs are oriented carefully, and any intra-abdominal lesion should be biopsied.

19.6.4 Laparoscopic Rectal Resections

The main laparoscopic surgical procedure in rectal cancer patients is the low anterior resection. Depending on how distal the tumor growth is, various anastomotic techniques can be applied, or abdominoperineal resection might be indicated. Sometimes a Hartmans' procedure is preferred. Independent of the performed procedure, laparoscopic rectal cancer surgery follows the same oncological principles as open rectal cancer surgery.

The laparoscopic surgical approach should follow a standardized operative procedure. The operative key steps, as outlined in the Quick Reference Guides, can serve as a practical guideline on how to perform laparoscopic rectal cancer surgery. The key steps should be familiar to all members of the operating team.

In the following section, the stepwise details of laparoscopic low anterior resection, laparoscopic abdominoperineal resection, and the laparoscopic Hartman procedure are outlined [49, 50]. The operating room setup is similar for all laparoscopic rectal procedures (Fig. 19.1).

19.7 Low Anterior Resection

19.7.1 Positioning of Patient and Equipment

The patient is positioned on a beanbag and secured to the table to allow steep Trendelenburg position during the

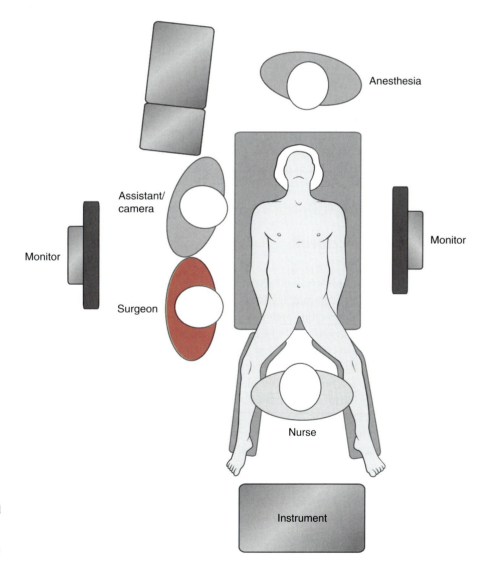

Fig. 19.1 Operating room setup for laparoscopic rectal surgery. (Drawing by Hippmann GbR, Schwarzenbruck, Germany)

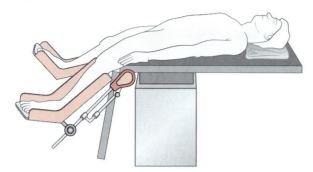

Fig. 19.2 Patient positioning on the table. (Drawing by Hippmann GbR, Schwarzenbruck, Germany)

operation. The legs are placed in stirrups, and the perineum should be at or below the break of the table (Fig. 19.2). An orogastric tube and Foley catheter are inserted. We favor the use of atraumatic 5-mm bowel graspers which can also be used as pelvic retractors. Dissection is performed with scissors cautery, but hook cautery may be required, especially at the right lower pelvic sidewall to avoid electrical short-circuiting into the sidewall. Energy-based devices are not usually required as the dissection plane in the pelvis is avascular.

Pitfalls to avoid: Prolonged Trendelenburg position might cause nerve injury to the brachial plexus if the patient's shoulders are not adequately protected from the shoulder support equipment at the head end of the table. For this reason, we do not use shoulder or chest strapping, but a beanbag alone.

19.7.2 Trocar Placement

Correct placement of the trocars will give optimal ergonomic position for surgeon and facilitate anatomical dissection of the mesorectum and mobilization of the splenic colonic flexure (Fig. 19.3). A 10-mm open cut down is made for the camera trocar in the umbilicus. In the right lower quadrant, a 12-mm port is inserted. For sigmoid colectomy, this is usually placed 2–3 cm medial and superior to anterior superior iliac spine, but when performing a low pelvic dissection, the right side of the pelvic brim limits access to the low pelvis, particularly in tall males. For this reason, the right lower quadrant trocar is moved medially in those patients where a low pelvic dissection is expected. In those marked for a temporary ileostomy, this site is often suitable. Further 5-mm trocars are placed in the right upper,

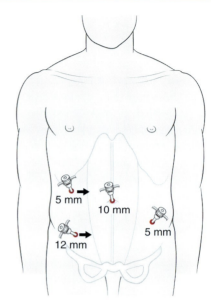

Fig. 19.3 Trocar positions. The right quadrant trocars should be inserted more medially compared to laparoscopic left-sided colectomies. (Drawing by Hippmann GbR, Schwarzenbruck, Germany)

left lower, and sometimes in the left upper quadrant for assistance with the splenic flexure. In some patients with narrow pelvis, a suprapubic trocar may be needed to insert the stapler for rectal transection, if it cannot be applied through the right lower quadrant trocar. The abdominal cavity is inspected in order to detect metastatic disease or other concomitant pathology.

Pitfalls to avoid: The trocar in the lower right quadrant placed too laterally.

19.7.3 Exposure of the Operating Field

The patient is placed in Trendelenburg position and rotated to the right. The colonic omentum is placed in the upper abdominal cavity and the loops of the small intestine carefully moved upward to expose the retroperitoneum from the pelvic cavity up to the ligament of Treitz. In obese patients, a 5-mm grasper may be required through an additional left upper quadrant trocar to help keeping the small bowel out of the operating field. A medial to lateral or lateral to medial approach is chosen according to the preference of the surgeon. However, both approaches should be mastered. The correct dissection plane in Toldt's fascia is most easily found with the medial to lateral approach as described below.

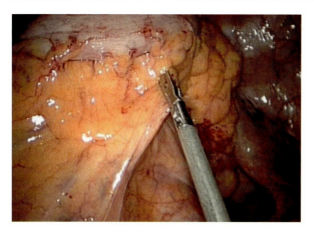

Fig. 19.4 The sigmoid mesocolon is lifted toward the abdominal wall exposing the inferior mesenteric groove at the level of the promontory

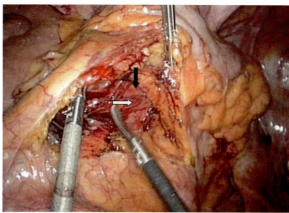

Fig. 19.5 The hypogastric nerves (*white arrow*) and left ureter (*black arrow*) are identified and kept away from the dissection plane

Pitfalls to avoid: Unintentional injury or contact with electrocautery on a small bowel loop not adequately put away from the operating field or injury during port or instrument insertion.

Pitfalls to avoid: With the patient tipped to the right, the horizontal plane will also be lifted. While dissecting medial to lateral, care must be taken to avoid going too deeply or posteriorly into the left pelvic sidewall in the search for the left ureter. This might cause damage to the left branches of the hypogastric nerve plexus or bleeding.

19.7.4 Identification of the Inferior Mesenteric Vessels and of the Left Ureter

The sigmoid colon should be put on stretch toward the abdominal wall in order to visualize the contours of the inferior mesenteric artery (IMA) pedicle at the level of the pelvic inlet (Fig. 19.4). The peritoneum is incised beneath the IMA groove. Care must be taken to preserve the hypogastric nerve plexus. The dissection plane should display the posterior surface of the capsule of the IMA, entering into the pelvis in the avascular presacral space. This keeps the hypogastric nerves posteriorly and ureter posterolaterally and safe from injury (Fig. 19.5).

If the left ureter cannot be found, the dissection may be too deep in the retroperitoneum. If there is any uncertainty about plane of dissection, a lateral to medial approach can be performed. Starting slightly distal to the sacral promontory is usually an easy way to find the correct plane. If the left ureter cannot be identified, conversion to open surgery should be done at this stage of the operation.

19.7.5 Division of the Inferior Mesenteric Artery (IMA)

The dissection continues on the posterior surface of the "mesorectal package," up toward the origin of the IMA. A high ligation (division above the left colic artery) is performed as this removes the apical lymphatic nodes within the resected surgical specimen. This also preserves the bifurcation of the ascending and descending branches of the left colic artery, maintaining collateral supply to the left colon [47]. A high ligation of the IMA will also assist in getting a tension-free colorectal or colo-anal anastomosis. The vascular division may be done with endovascular stapler, clips or with a laparoscopic electromechanical device.

Pitfalls to avoid: Traction on the sigmoid mesentery in an inferior or caudal direction and not toward the anterior abdominal wall will make the dissection of the IMA more difficult and increase the risk of injury to the hypogastric nerve plexus because of narrowing the operating space between the mesorectal package and the retroperitoneum posteriorly.

19.7.6 Division of the Inferior Mesenteric Vein (IMV) and Mobilization of the Left Colon and Splenic Flexure

The peritoneum is incised along the lower border of the inferior mesenteric vein (IMV) from the IMA up to the ligament of Treitz. The inferior mesenteric vein is divided at this level to ensure optimal mobilization of the left colon (Fig. 19.6). With gentle dissection, the left mesocolon can easily be lifted off the retroperitoneum from a medial approach. This dissection continues laterally until the lateral attachments are reached. The lateral side of the colon is then visualized, and the remaining peritoneal attachment is divided with cautery scissors. The splenocolic and gastrocolic ligaments are divided in the same way, bringing the splenic flexure as far medially as needed to avoid tension on the anastomosis.

Pitfalls to avoid: It is important to keep the left mesocolon intact to avoid damage to the arterial arcades including an intact left colonic artery and thereby minimize the chance for anastomotic leaks or colonic stoma dehiscence or necrosis because of ischemia.

19.7.7 Mobilization and Division of the Rectum

The 5-mm graspers are useful in elevating the uterus or bladder to optimize the access to the pelvic cavity, or a suture may be passed through the uterus on a Keith needle and suspended from the anterior abdominal wall.

The lateral mesorectal peritoneum is incised by cautery and opens into the avascular loose connective tissue behind the mesorectal fascia which is then dissected down to the pelvic floor. By dissection close to the mesorectal fascia just posterior to the inferior mesenteric artery, bleeding from the presacral veins and damage to the hypogastric nerves can be avoided. In this part of the dissection, traction and counter traction is especially important to stay in the avascular areolar tissues around the mesorectum. This helps avoid coning into the mesorectum and avoid going to laterally and thereby damaging the pelvic parasympathetic nerve ganglia close to the anterolateral surface of the mesorectum. The posterior and lateral mobilization is completed before an incision close to the peritoneal reflection is made and the dissection continues anteriorly to Denonvillier's fascia (Fig. 19.7). Care must be taken to avoid bleeding from the posterior vaginal venous system in females or vessels close to the seminal vesicles and prostate in men by staying in the correct anatomical plane. Complete hemostasis must be maintained during the whole dissection to reduce the risk of unintended damage to the nerve structures located posterolaterally and anterolaterally outside the mesorectum and avoid breaking of the mesorectal envelope.

The exact distal margin of the tumor must be verified before the distal resection site is determined. Digital examination and rigid proctoscopy may be performed intraoperatively. At the verified correct distal resection site, a tunnel is dissected between the posterior rectal wall and the mesorectum. A 5-mm dissector

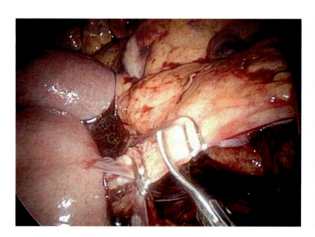

Fig. 19.6 Division of the inferior mesenteric vein at the level of ligament of Treitz

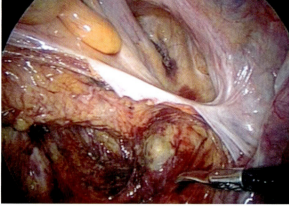

Fig. 19.7 Posterior and lateral mobilization is completed before the anterior dissection is performed

or an atraumatic grasper can be used for this dissection. A laparoscopic linear stapler is inserted through the 12-mm port in the lower right quadrant. One of the arms of the stapler is inserted through the tunnel behind the rectal wall. Low in the pelvis, the mesorectum tapers into the anal canal, and there is no separate mesorectum to divide and the bowel can be divided initially (Fig. 19.8).

Before the rectum is transected, the stapler instrument is closed to clamp the rectal lumen just above the planned resection line. Frequently, two cartridges have to be fired to get the rectum transected. Care must be taken to make sure the division is perpendicular to the plane of the rectum. Any mesorectum present is divided with an electromechanical device or electrocautery. In cases where it is difficult to get the stapler across the rectum, the rectum may be drawn to the left, opening the angle to insert the stapler low on the right side. If this is not enough, pressure can be applied to the perineum to elevate the anal canal. Finally, an additional suprapubic port may permit rectal transection. If all these options fail, a short open Pfannenstiel's incision can be made to permit a transverse stapler to be used. Another option is to complete the dissection from below, resulting in the possibility of removing the specimen through the anal canal. A hand-sewn anastomosis is then fashioned.

Pitfalls to avoid: The assistant must be able to perform traction and counter traction to facilitate the dissection while minimizing the risk of breakage of the mesorectal fascia, or dissection outside the correct plane.

19.7.8 Exteriorization of the Surgical Specimen

A 4–6-cm left lower quadrant incision is made. The exteriorization of the specimen should always be done through a wound protector to reduce the risk of implantation metastasis. The specimen is removed to a nearby table and opened to inspect the distal resection line. If not adequate, an additional resection of the rectal remnant/mesorectum must be performed.

Pitfalls to avoid: The opening must be wide enough to avoid squeezing, trauma, or perforation to the tumor-bearing intestine.

19.7.9 Creation of the Anastomosis

When performing a colo-anal or low colorectal anastomosis, a 6-cm colonic J-pouch is made with a linear stapler. Creation of a J-pouch will improve the functional results after rectal cancer surgery compared to coloplasty or straight anastomosis [51]. This option is preferred in patients in whom a J-pouch can fit into the pelvis, and in whom there is not too long an anal canal which might limit reach of the J-pouch. The colon end with the anvil is delivered into the abdominal cavity, the wound is closed, or the wound protector is twisted and clamped before the abdominal cavity is re-insufflated. The colonic mesentery must be oriented to avoid twisting. The circular stapler is inserted through the anal opening and carefully maneuvered up to the rectal remnant resection line. The anastomosis is made under direct vision.

The completeness of the anastomosis is confirmed with the finding of two intact, "all layers" tissue-doughnuts in the circular stapler and by insufflating air into the rectum with the pelvic cavity filled with water. If bubbling of air from the anastomosis, it should either be redone or strengthened with sutures until there is no leakage of air when tested.

Pitfalls to avoid: A large circular stapler head or not careful enough insertion and advancement of the stapler gun through the anus and rectal remnant might tear the sphincter muscles or perforate the rectal remnant.

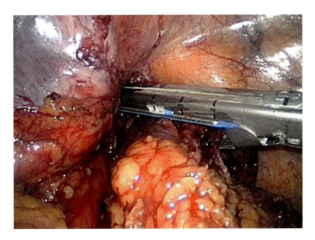

Fig. 19.8 Transection of the rectum with an endostapler

19.7.10 Desufflation of Pneumoperitoneum and Closure of Trocar Sites

The abdominal cavity should be desufflated through open trocars, before they are removed. The wound after the specimen extraction is closed in two layers. All trocar incisions larger than 5 mm are closed with fascial sutures. Placement of pelvic drains is as a rule not necessary.

Pitfalls to avoid: Failure or avoidance to close trocar incisions larger than 5 mm may increase the risk of Richter's or incisional hernia at the trocar sites.

19.8 Ultralow Anterior Resection with Transanal Intersphincteric Mobilization

As mentioned earlier, in selected patients with very low cancers with favorable histology and preoperative chemoradiotherapy, a distal resection margin of 1 cm can be oncologically safe. This permits the possibility of a transanal partial or total resection of the internal anal sphincter in order to avoid a permanent colostomy.

The intra-abdominal mobilization has been completed as described above in steps 3–7. Anal effacing sutures are placed to facilitate the intersphincteric dissection. Instrumental and digital contact with the cancer must be avoided. As soon as the transected internal sphincter is mobilized adequately to allow the lumen to be closed, this should be done to avoid spillage of tumor cells into the operative field. At the level of the dentate line, the dissection should continue perpendicularly to reach the levator muscle plane before continuing toward the pelvic cavity to meet the dissection from above. If a circumferential resection margin of 3 mm cannot be achieved, the risk of local recurrence will be increased [32, 33].

The specimen is pulled through the perineum and transected proximally at least 5 cm above the rectosigmoid junction. If a J-pouch or coloplasty cannot be performed from below and safely replaced through the anal channel for a hand-sewn anastomosis, a straight hand-sewn colo-anal anastomosis is fashioned.

If a decision has been made preoperatively to perform intersphincteric mobilization and partial or total internal sphincter resection, this step can be performed initially.

When making a colo-anal or a colorectal anastomosis in the lower third of the rectum or in cases with preoperative chemoradiation therapy, a diverting stoma is generally performed.

19.9 Abdominoperineal Resection

19.9.1 Closure of the Anal Opening

In cases with abdominoperineal resection, the first step of the operation is closure of the anus with a 2-0-nylon suture. Long thread ends are kept to help in traction during the perineal dissection.

19.9.2 Positioning of the Patient, Equipment, and Trocar Placement

The positioning of the patient on the operation table, the basic laparoscopic equipment, and trocar positions are identical to the laparoscopic low anterior resection procedure. Briefly, the patient is positioned on a beanbag and secured to the table to allow steep Trendelenburg position during the operation. The legs are placed in stirrups, and the perineum should be outside the break of the table. An orogastric tube and Foley catheter are inserted. A 10 mm open cut down is made for the camera trocar in the umbilicus. At the mark for the colostomy, a 5- or 10-mm trocar is placed for bowel graspers. As for low anterior resection, the right side of the pelvic brim limits access to the low pelvis. The right lower quadrant 12-mm trocar is therefore placed close to the lateral border of the abdominal rectus muscle, but without injury to the inferior epigastric vessels. This port is the main working port and must allow use of vascular clip equipment or an electromechanic device. A 5-mm trocar is placed in the right upper quadrant. The abdominal cavity is always inspected in order to detect metastatic disease or other concomitant pathology.

We favor the use of atraumatic 5-mm bowel graspers which can also be used as pelvic retractors. Dissection is performed with scissors cautery, but hook cautery is often required, especially at the right lower pelvic sidewall. Energy-based devices are not usually required as the dissection plane in the pelvis is avascular. Correct placement of the trocars will give optimal ergonomic position for surgeon and facilitate anatomical dissection of the mesorectum down to the pelvic floor.

19.9.3 Exposure of the Operating Field

The patient is placed in Trendelenburg position and rotated to the right. The colonic omentum is placed in the upper abdominal cavity and the loops of the small intestine carefully moved upward to expose the retroperitoneum from the pelvic cavity up to the ligament of Treitz. In obese patients, a 5-mm grasper may be required through the additional right upper quadrant trocar to help keeping the small bowel out of the operating field. A medial to lateral or lateral to medial approach is chosen according to the preference of the surgeon. The correct dissection plane is along the avascular Toldt's fascia which is most easily found with the medial to lateral approach.

19.9.4 Identification of the Inferior Mesenteric Vessels and of the Left Ureter

Identical to the laparoscopic low anterior resection procedure, the sigmoid colon is put on stretch toward the abdominal wall in order to visualize the contours of the inferior mesenteric artery (IMA) pedicle at the level of the pelvic inlet. The peritoneum is incised beneath the IMA groove. As always, when operating in this region, care must be taken to preserve the hypogastric nerve plexus. The dissection plane should display the posterior surface of the capsule of the IMA, entering into the pelvis in the avascular presacral space. This keeps the hypogastric nerves posteriorly. The left ureter can be identified posterolaterally as it crosses above the internal iliac artery and vein.

If the left ureter cannot be found, the dissection may be too deep in the retroperitoneum. If there is any uncertainty about plane of dissection, a lateral to medial approach can be performed. Starting slightly distal to the sacral promontory is usually an easy way to find the correct plane. If the left ureter cannot be identified, conversion to open surgery should be done at this stage of the operation.

19.9.5 Identification and Division of the Inferior Mesenteric Artery (IMA)

The dissection continues on the posterior surface of the "mesorectal package," up toward the origin of the IMA. A high ligation (division above the left colic artery) is favored as this removes the apical lymphatic nodes within the resected surgical specimen. The IMA is divided 1 cm distal to its origin from the abdominal aorta. A low tie (division after the branching of the left colonic artery) can be done without compromising long-term survival, and may help maintain optimal blood nutrition to a colostomy. This might be important in patients with concomitant severe atherosclerotic disease. The vascular division may be done with endovascular stapler, clips, or with a laparoscopic electromechanical device.

19.9.6 Mobilization of the Left Colon

The mesosigmoid and its lateral attachments are only mobilized enough to give adequate length to the colonic stoma. It is not necessary to take down the splenic flexure.

19.9.7 Mobilization of the Rectum

The initial mobilization of the rectum follows identical principles as during a low anterior resection. A sharp dissection with diathermy preserves the hypogastric nerves and keeps the mesorectal envelope intact in the avascular space between the presacral fascia and the fascia propria of the mesorectum. It is important to stop the dissection at the level of coccygus posteriorly and before the mesorectum cones in toward the pelvic floor muscles.

19.9.8 Proximal Division of the Left Colon

The level of division of the left colon is selected to secure a healthy and well-functioning stoma considering the risks of stoma complications as prolapse, parastomal hernia, ischemia, or necrosis. The mesocolon is divided at the preferred level, and the colon is divided with a laparoscopic linear stapler. The proximal division is done before the perineal dissection from below is completed because the pneumoperitoneum disappears at the time the perineal dissection reaches the abdominal cavity.

19.9.9 Perineal Dissection and Exteriorization of the Specimen

An oval incision around the closed anus is made with diathermy. The dissection plane should be outside the external anal sphincter and outside the levator ani muscle. If necessary, the puborectalis muscle or even the coccygus should be removed with the specimen to secure a safe resection margin. The most technically demanding dissection is in the anterior plane. The posterior vaginal wall in women and the urethra in men must not be injured. However, when involved by tumor, an anterior pelvic exenteration must be considered. Preferably, this should not be a surprise but is well planned and prepared for preoperatively. The direction of the dissection from below can be guided by using a grasper to push at the desired entry line into the abdominal side of the pelvic cavity. Once the perineal dissection is completed circumferentially, the specimen can be removed through the perineal opening.

19.9.10 Closure of Pelvic Wound and Trocar Sites; Creation of the Colostomy

The perineal opening is rinsed with warmed saline. Pelvic and perineal hemostases are secured before the wound is closed in layers. All trocar incisions larger than 5 mm undergo fascial closure. The lower left quadrant trocar incision is excised and a colostomy trephine fashioned. The colostomy is matured with absorbable sutures.

The decision for abdominoperineal resection with colostomy versus a low anterior resection with coloanal anastomosis after intersphincteric dissection and total or partial resection of the internal anal sphincter is based on oncological principles, in addition to the informed preference of the patient and the experience of the surgeon. Inexperience in radical perineal dissection and colo-anal anastomotic techniques should lead to referral of the patient to a surgeon and hospital with the necessary expertise.

19.10 Laparoscopic Hartman's Procedure

19.10.1 Indications

The main indications for performing a laparoscopic Hartman's procedure for rectal cancer include:

- A colorectal anastomosis cannot be safely performed
- The patient has anal incontinence making any colorectal or colonal anastomosis undesirable
- Concomitant anal or pelvic disease that will favor a colostomy
- Infirmity in patients in whom one wishes to avoid the morbidity of a perineal wound
- The wish of the patient

The initial procedural steps are identical to the laparoscopic low anterior resection, and the rectum is transected as described in low anterior resection, step 7, above. The exteriorization of the specimen after the distal resection is performed through the planned stoma site in the left lower quadrant, unless the bowel and mesentery are very bulky in which they may be brought out through a separate incision. The proximal division of the mesocolon and colon is performed extracorporeally with electrocautery. A colostomy is fashioned according to the surgeon's preferences.

19.11 Minimally Invasive Palliative Surgery

Surgeons taking care of patients with rectal cancer should be familiar with minimally invasive procedures for palliative reasons. When laparoscopic or open surgical resectional options are not recommended or contraindicated in a patient with unresectable rectal cancer, other palliative options might help the patient. Endoscopically placed rectal stents will avoid the need for a colostomy and maintain bowel function in cases with obstructive symptoms. These might also diminish symptoms of bleeding from the tumor. However, endoscopic stenting of unresectable cancers in the lower third of the rectum should be avoided because of the risk for increased pelvic pain and inducing fecal incontinence. Preoperative stenting should be avoided in cases with curative surgical intentions because of the potential detrimental effect of the stent expansion on dissemination of malignant cell into the circulation.

A laparoscopic colostomy with a distal mucocutaneous fistula will treat rectal obstructive symptoms when stent placement is not possible or contraindicated, or when a loop ileostomy is not indicated. Alternatively, fulguration can be performed on an obstructing or semi-obstructing rectal cancer. The risk of tumor perforation into the abdominal cavity must always be considered. Palliative laser ablation is also an option. In cases with disseminated disease, a laparoscopic intestinal anastomosis to bypass obstructing metastasis, or simply a diverting stoma, can help the patient in a difficult situation when survival may be short.

19.12 Future Trends

In order to improve rates of local recurrence and survival after treatment for rectal cancer and at the same time minimize the side effects of the treatment, several steps of care may be improved in the future:

1. Increased effort to reduce the impact of the surgeon on local recurrence rate is necessary to further improve the long-term results. Improved preoperative planning may reduce involuntary intraoperative contact with cancer cells during the pelvic or perineal dissection because of suboptimal technique or extensive local invasion.
2. Development of three-dimensional computer-guided programs might help direct operative dissection. Potentially, surgery may be performed by a computer-guided robot aided by three-dimensional imaging from intraoperative MRI or CT scans
3. Improved imaging, so we can better select candidates for chemoradiation or local resection.
4. Better understandings of biology (genetic chip analysis) so that we can predict which tumors are suitable for local excision, radical surgery, response to chemoradiation, or need chemoradiation alone.
5. Better understanding of which tumors need adjuvant therapy.
6. Continued development of new chemotherapy agents with improved effect.
7. One of the factors that have a significant negative impact on quality of life after rectal cancer treatment is the formation of a stoma. Improved experience and long-term results with total anorectal reconstruction using an artificial anal sphincter device would be a helpful solution for many patients that cannot adapt to a life with a traditional stoma. Reconstruction during the primary abdominoperineal resection might be advocated in selected cases.
8. Finally, many colo-anal anastomosis are complicated by development of anastomotic leak. Future techniques to reduce the frequency of this complication, or to standardize and improve our ability to treat this will undoubtedly improve clinical outcomes.

Quick Reference Guide

Laparoscopic Low Anterior Resection (LAR)

1. Positioning of the patient and equipment
2. Trocar placement
3. Exposure of the operating field
4. Identification of inferior mesenteric vessels and of the left ureter
5. Division of the inferior mesenteric artery (IMA)
6. Division of the inferior mesenteric vein (IMV) and mobilization of the left colon and splenic flexure
7. Mobilization and division of the rectum
8. Exteriorization of the surgical specimen
9. Creation of the anastomosis
10. Desufflation of pneumoperitoneum and closure of trocar sites

Laparoscopic Abdominoperineal Resection

1. Closure of the anal opening
2. Positioning of the patient, equipment, and trocar placement
3. Exposure of the operating field
4. Identification of inferior mesenteric vessels and of the left ureter
5. Identification and division of the inferior mesenteric artery (IMA)
6. Mobilization of the left colon
7. Mobilization of the rectum
8. Proximal division of the left colon
9. Perineal dissection and exteriorization of the specimen
10. Closure of pelvic wound and trocar sites; Creation of the colostomy

References

1. Kapiteijn, E., Matrijnen, C.A.M., Nagtegaal, I.D., et al.: Preoperative radiotherapy combined with total mesorectal excision for resectable rectal cancer. N. Engl. J. Med. **345**, 638–646 (2001)
2. Wibe, A., Moller, B., Norstein, J., et al.: A national strategic change in treatment policy for rectal cancer–implementation of total mesorectal excision as routine treatment in Norway: a national audit. Dis. Colon Rectum **45**, 857–866 (2002)
3. Cecil, T.D., Sexton, R., Moran, B.J., et al.: Total mesorectal excision results in low recurrence rates in lymph node-positive rectal cancer. Dis. Colon Rectum **47**(7), 1145–1149 (2004)
4. Borowski, D.W., Kelly, S.B., Bradburn, D.M., et al.: Impact of surgeon volume and specialization on short-term outcomes in colorectal cancer surgery. Br. J. Surg. **94**, 880–889 (2007)
5. Schrag, D., Panageas, K.S., Riedel, E., et al.: Hospital and surgeon procedure volume as predictors of outcome following rectal cancer resection. Ann. Surg. **236**(5), 583–592 (2002)
6. Rabeneck, L., Davila, J.A., Thompson, M., El-Seraq, H.B.: Surgical volume and long term survival following surgery for coorectal cancer in the Veterans Affairs Health-Care System. Am. J. Gastroenterol. **99**(4), 668–675 (2004)
7. Landmann, R.G., Wong, W.D., Hoepfl, J., et al.: limitations of early rectal cancer nodal staging may explain failure after local excision. Dis. Colon Rectum **50**(10), 1520–1525 (2007)
8. Hicks, R.J., Ware, R.E., Lau, E.W.: Cancer Imaging **6**, S52–S62 (2006)
9. Påhlman, L., Bohe, M., Cedermark, B., et al.: The Swedish rectal cancer registry. Br. J. Surg. **94**(10), 1285–1292 (2007)
10. Benson 3rd, A.B., Choti, M.A., Cohen, A.M., et al.: National Comprehensive Cancer Network NCCN Practice Guidelines for colorectal cancer. Oncology **14**(11A), 203–212 (2000)
11. Daniels, I.R., Fisher, S.E., Heald, R.J., Moran, B.J.: Accurate staging, selective therapy and optimal surgery improves outcome in rectal cancer: a review of the recent evidence. Colorectal Dis. **9**(4), 290–301 (2007)
12. Simunovic, M., Sexton, R., Rempel, E., Moran, B.J., Heald, R.J.: Optimal preoperative assessment and surgery for rectal cancer may greatly limit the need for radiotherapy. Br. J. Surg. **90**(8), 999–1003 (2003)
13. Eriksen, M.T., Wibe, A., Haffner, J., Wiig, J.N.: Norwegian Rectal Cancer Group prognostic groups in 1, 676 patients with T3 rectal cancer treated without preoperative radiotherapy. Dis. Colon Rectum **50**(2), 156–167 (2007)
14. Delaney, C.P., Brenner, A., Hammel, et al.: Pre-operative radiotherapy improves survival for patients undergoing total mesorectal excision for stage T3 low rectal cancers. Ann. Surg. **236**(2), 203–207 (2002)
15. Peeters, K., Marjinen, C.A., Nagtegaal, I.D., et al.: The TME trial after a median follow-up of 6 years. Increased local control but no survival benefit in irradiated patients with resectable rectal carcinoma. Ann. Surg. **246**, 693–701 (2007)
16. Sauer, R., Becker, H., Hohenberger, W., et al.: Preoperative versus postoperative chemoradiotherapy for rectal cancer. N. Engl. J. Med. **351**, 1731–1741 (2004)
17. Bosett, J.F., Colette, L., Calais, G., et al.: Chemotherapy with preoperative radiotherapy in rectal cancer. N. Engl. J. Med. **335**(11), 1114–1123 (2006)
18. Bentrem, D.J., Okabe, S., Wong, W.D., et al.: T1 adenocarcinoma of the rectum: transanal excision or radical surgery? Ann. Surg. **245**(2), 338–339 (2007)
19. Madbouly, K.M., Remzi, F.H., Erkek, B.A., et al.: Recurrence after transanal excision of T1 rectal cancer: should we be concerned? Dis. Colon Rectum **48**(4), 711–719 (2005)
20. Nascimbeni, R., Burgart, L.J., Nivatvongs, S., Larson, D.R.: Risk of lymph node metastasis in T1 carcinoma of the colon and rectum. Dis. Colon Rectum **45**(2), 200–206 (2002)
21. Endreseth, B.H., Myrvold, H.E., Romundstad, P., et al.: The Norwegian Rectal Cancer Group. Transanal excision vs. major surgery for T1 rectal cancer. Dis. Colon Rectum **48**(7), 1380–1388 (2005)
22. Ricciardi, R., Madoff, R.D., Rohtenberger, D.A., Baxter, N.N.: Population-based analyses of lymph node metastases in colorectal cancer. Clin. Gastroenterol. Hepatol. **4**(12), 1522–1527 (2006)
23. Fang, W.L., Chang, S.C., Lin, J.K., et al.: Metastatic potential in T1 and T2 colorectal cancer. Hepatogastroenterology **52**(66), 1688–1691 (2005)
24. Lezoche, E., Guerrieri, M., Paganini, A.M., et al.: Transanal endoscopic versus total mesorectal laparoscopic resections of T2-N0 low rectal cancers after neoadjuvant treatment: a prospective randomized trial with a 3-years minimum follow-up period. Surg. Endosc. **19**(6), 751–756 (2005)

25. Lesotho, E., Baldarelli, M., de Sanctis, A., Lezoche, G., Guerrieri, M.: Early rectal cancer: definition and management. Dig. Dis. **25**(1), 76–79 (2007)
26. Scott, N., Jackson, P., al-Jaberi, T., Dixon, M.F., Quirke, P., Finan, P.J.: Total mesorectal excision and local recurrence: a study of tumour spread in the mesorectum distal to rectal cancer. Br. J. Surg. **82**, 1031–1033 (1995)
27. Zhou, Z.G., Lei, W.Z., Yu, Y.Y., et al.: Pathological study of distal mesorectal cancer spread to determine a proper distal resection margin. World J. Gastroenterol. **11**(3), 319–322 (2005)
28. Cecil, T.D., Sexton, R., Moran, B.J., et al.: Total mesorectal excision results in low recurrence rates in lymph node-positive rectal cancer. Dis. Colon Rectum **47**, 1145–1149 (2004)
29. Andreola, S., Leo, E., Belli, F., et al.: Distal intramural spread in adenocarcinoma of the lower third of the rectum treated with total rectal resection and colo-anal anastomosis. Dis. Colon Rectum **40**, 25–29 (1997)
30. Guillem, J.G., Chessin, D.B., Shia, J., Suriawinata, A., Riedel, E., et al.: A prospective pathologic analysis using whole-mount sections of rectal cancer following preoperative combined modality therapy. Implications for sphincter preservation. Ann. Surg. **245**, 88–93 (2007)
31. Moore, H.G., Riedel, E., Minsky, B.D., et al.: Adequacy of 1-cm distal margin after restorative rectal cancer resection with sharp mesorectal excision and preoperative combined-modality therapy. Ann. Surg. Oncol. **10**(1), 80–85 (2003)
32. Nagtegaal, I.D., Marjinen, C.A., Kranenbarg, E.K., et al.: Circumferential resection margin involvement is still an important predictor of local recurrence in rectal carcinoma: not one millimetre but two millimetres is the limit. Am. J. Surg. Pathol. **26**(3), 350–357 (2002)
33. Wibe, A., Rendedal, P.R., Svensson, E., et al.: Prognostic significance of the circumferential resection margin following total mesorectal excision for rectal cancer. Br. J. Surg. **89**, 327–334 (2002)
34. Quirke, P., Durdey, P., Dixon, M.F., Williams, N.S.: Local recurrence of rectal adenocarcinoma due to inadequate surgical resection. Histopathological study of lateral tumour spread and surgical excision. Lancet **2**, 996–999 (1986)
35. Williams, C.P., Reynolds, H.L., Delaney, C.P. et al.: Clinical results of intraoperative radiation therapy for locally recurrent and advanced tumors with colorectal involvement. Am. J. Surg. **195**(3), 405–409 (2008)
36. Jayne, D.G., Guillou, P.J., Thorpe, H., Quirke, P., Copeland, J., Smith, A.M.H., Heath, R.M., Brown, J.M.: Randomized trial of laparoscopic-assisted resection of colorectal carcinoma: 3-year results of the UK MRC CLASSICC trial group. J. Clin. Oncol. **25**, 3061–3068 (2007)
37. Transatlantic Laparoscopically Assisted Vs Open Colectomy Trials Study Group: Laparoscopically assisted vs open colectomy for colon cancer. A meta-analysis. Arch. Surg. **142**, 298–303 (2007)
38. Reza, M.M., Blasco, J.A., Andradas, E., Cantero, R., Mayol, J.: Systematic review of laparoscopic *versus* open surgery for colorectal cancer. Br. J. Surg. **93**(8), 921–928 (2006)
39. COST: A comparison of laparoscopically assisted and open colectomy for colon cancer. N Engl J. Med. **350**, 2050–2059 (2004)
40. Lacy, A.M., Gracia-Valdecasas, J.C., Delgado, S., et al.: Laparoscopyassisted colectomy versus open colectomy for treatment of nonmetastatic colon cancer: a randomised trial. Lancet **359**, 2224–2229 (2002)
41. Abraham, N.S., Young, J.M., Solomon, M.J.: Meta-analysis of short-term outcomes after laparoscopic resection for colorectal cancer. Br. J. Surg. **91**(9), 111–124 (2004)
42. Tjandra, J.J., Chan, M.K.: Systematic review on the short-term outcome of laparoscopic resection for colon and rectosigmoid cancer. Colorectal Dis. **8**(5), 375–388 (2006)
43. Delaney, C.P., Kiran, R.P., Senagore, A.J., Brady, K., Fazio, V.W.: Case matched comparison of clinical and financial outcome after laparoscopic or open colectomy. Ann. Surg. **238**, 67–72 (2003)
44. Leung, K.L., Kwok, S.P., Lam, S.C., et al.: Laparoscopic resection of rectosigmoid carcinoma: prospective randomised trial. Lancet **363**(9416), 1187–1192 (2004)
45. Duluq, J.L., Wintringer, P., Stabilini, C., Mahamja, A.: Laparoscopic rectal resection with anal sphincter preservation for rectal cancer: long-term outcome. Surg. Endosc. **19**(11), 1468–1474 (2005)
46. Morinio, M., Parini, U., Giraudo, G., et al.: Laparoscopic total mesorectal excision: a consecutive series of 100 patients. Ann. Surg. **237**(3), 335–342 (2003)
47. Kim, S.H., Park, I.J., Joh, Y.G., Hahn, K.Y.: Laparoscopic resection for rectal cancer: a prospective analysis of thirty-month follow-up outcomes in 312 patients. Surg. Endosc. **20**(8), 1197–1202 (2006)
48. Bianchi, P.P., Rosati, R., Bona, S. et al.: Laparoscopic surgery in rectal cancer: a prospective analysis of patient survival and outcome. Dis. Colon Rectum **50**(12), 2047–2053 (2007)
49. Delaney, C.P., Neary, P., Heriot, A.G., Senagore, A.J.: Operative Techniques in Laparoscopic Colorectal Surgery. Lippincott Williams & Wilkins, Philadelphia, (2006)
50. Delaney, C.P.: Low anterior resection. Operative techniques in general surgery. 2003; 5: 214–223 (eds: van Heerden, F., et al.). W. B. Saunders Co., Philadelphia
51. Fazio, V.W., Zutshi, M., Remzi, F.H., et al.: A randomized multicenter trial to compare long-term functional outcome, quality of life, and complications of surgical procedures for low rectal cancers. Ann. Surg. **246**(3), 481–488 (2007)

Recommended Literature
The Role of Adjuvant Treatment

Bosett, J.F., et al.: Chemotherapy with preoperative radiotherapy in rectal cancer. N. Engl. J. Med. **335**(11), 1114–1123 (2006)

Kapiteijn, E., et al.: Preoperative radiotherapy combined with total mesorectal excision for resectable rectal cancer. N. Engl. J. Med. **345**, 638–646 (2001)

Peeters, K., et al.: The TME trial after a median follow-up of 6 years. Increased local control but no survival benefit in irradiated patients with resectable rectal carcinoma. Ann. Surg. **246**, 693–701 (2007)

Sauer, R., et al.: Preoperative versus postoperative chemoradiotherapy for rectal cancer. N. Engl. J. Med. **351**, 1731–1741 (2004)

The Feasibility and Results of Laparoscopic Surgery in Rectal Cancer Patients

Abraham, N.S., et al.: Meta-analysis of short-term outcomes after laparoscopic resection for colorectal cancer. Br. J. Surg. **91**(9), 111–124 (2004)

Bianchi, P.P., et al.: Laparoscopic surgery in rectal cancer: a prospective analysis of patient survival and outcome. Dis. Colon Rectum **50**(12), 2047–2053 (2007)

Delaney, C.P.: Low Anterior Sesection. Operative Techniques in General Surgery, vol. 5, pp. 214–223 (eds.: van Heerden, F., et al.). W. B. Saunders Co., Philadelphia, (2003)

Duluq, J.L., et al.: Laparoscopic rectal resection with anal sphincter preservation for rectal cancer: long-term outcome. Surg. Endosc. **19**(11), 1468–1474 (2005)

Kim, S.H., et al.: Laparoscopic resection for rectal cancer: a prospective analysis of thirty-month follow-up outcomes in 312 patients. Surg. Endosc. **20**(8), 1197–1202 (2006)

Morinio, M., et al.: Laparoscopic total mesorectal excision: a consecutive series of 100 patients. Ann. Surg. **237**(3), 335–342 (2003)

Tjandra, J.J., et al.: Systematic review on the short-term outcome of laparoscopic resection for colon and rectosigmoid cancer. Colorectal Dis. **8**(5), 375–388 (2006)

The Importance of Circumferential (CRM), Mesorectal and Mucosal Resection Margins in Rectal Cancer Patients

Andreola, S., et al.: Distal intramural spread in adenocarcinoma of the lower third of the rectum treated with total rectal resection and colo-anal anastomosis. Dis. Colon Rectum **40**, 25–29 (1997)

Guillem, J.G., et al.: A prospective pathologic analysis using whole-mount sections of rectal cancer following preoperative combined modality therapy. Implications for sphincter preservation. Ann. Surg. **245**, 88–93 (2007)

Moore, H.G., et al.: Adequacy of 1-cm distal margin after restorative rectal cancer resection with sharp mesorectal excision and preoperative combined-modality therapy. Ann. Surg. Oncol. **10**(1), 80–85 (2003)

Nagtegaal, I.D., et al.: Circumferential resection margin involvement is still an important predictor of local recurrence in rectal carcinoma: not one millimetre but two millimetres is the limit. Am. J. Surg. Pathol. **26**(3), 350–357 (2002)

Quirke, P., et al.: Local recurrence of rectal adenocarcinoma due to inadequate surgical resection.Histopathological study of lateral tumour spread and surgical excision. Lancet **2**, 996–999 (1986)

Scott, N., et al.: Total mesorectal excision and local recurrence: a study of tumour spread in the mesorectum distal to rectal cancer. Br. J. Surg. **82**, 1031–1033 (1995)

Wibe, A., et al.: Prognostic significance of the circumferential resection margin following total mesorectal excision for rectal cancer. Br. J. Surg. **89**, 327–334 (2002)

Zhou, Z.G., et al.: Pathological study of distal mesorectal cancer spread to determine a proper distal resection margin. World J. Gastroenterol. **11**(3), 319–322 (2005)

Laparoscopic Versus Open Rectal Cancer Surgery

Breukink, S., et al.: Laparoscopic versus open total mesorectal exicion for rectal cancer (review). The Cochrane database of systematic reviews 2006, Issue 4 Art no.: CD005200. DOI:10.1002/14651858.CD005200.pub2

Jayne, D.G., et al.: Randomized trial of laparoscopic-assisted resection of colorectal carcinoma: 3-year results of the UK MRC CLASSICC trial group. J. Clin. Oncol. **25**, 3061–3068 (2007)

Leung, K.L., et al.: Laparoscopic resection of rectosigmoid carcinoma: prospective randomised trial. Lancet **363**(9416), 1187–1192 (2004)

Reza, M.M., et al.: Systematic review of laparoscopic *versus* open surgery for colorectal cancer. Br. J. Surg. **93**(8), 921–928 (2006)

Treatment of Early Rectal Cancer

Bentrem, D.J., et al.: T1 adenocarcinoma of the rectum: transanal excision or radical surgery? Ann. Surg. **245**(2), 338–339 (2007)

Endreseth, B.H., et al.: Transanal excision vs. major surgery for T1 rectal cancer. Dis. Colon Rectum **48**(7), 1380–1388 (2005)

Lesotho, E., et al.: Early rectal cancer: definition and management. Dig. Dis. **25**(1), 76–79 (2007)

Madbouly, K.M., et al.: Recurrence after transanal excision of T1 rectal cancer: should we be concerned? Dis. Colon Rectum **48**(4), 711–719 (2005)

Nascimbeni, R., et al.: Risk of lymph node metastasis in T1 carcinoma of the colon and rectum. Dis. Colon Rectum **45**(2), 200–206 (2002)

Part VI

Special Topics: Cancer of the Hepato-Biliary System

General Considerations

Jonathan P. Pearl and Jeffrey L. Ponsky

20.1 Introduction

Both gallbladder cancer and extrahepatic cholangiocarcinoma are rare cancers with poor prognoses. Five-year survival historically ranges from 5% to 20% [1–4]. In recent years, improved survival rates have resulted from more radical operations, namely, major liver resections and extended lymph node dissections [2, 3, 5–8]. Despite the trend favoring radical conventional operations, minimally invasive therapy retains a role in diagnosis and palliation of both gallbladder cancer and cholangiocarcinoma. A therapeutic approach using minimally invasive surgery remains controversial.

20.2 Gallbladder Carcinoma

20.2.1 Epidemiology of Gallbladder Cancer

Gallbladder cancer is the fifth most common cancer of the gastrointestinal tract. In the USA the incidence of gallbladder cancer is 1.7 per 100,000 females and 0.9 per 100,000 males [9]. Higher incidences are reported in regions of South America, Eastern Europe, and Japan [10–12].

20.2.2 Symptoms of Gallbladder Cancer

The symptoms of gallbladder cancer mimic those of symptomatic gallstones. Nearly all patients with gallbladder cancer have gallstones, although less than 1% of those with symptomatic gallstones harbor gallbladder carcinoma [13, 14]. Many patients do not present with symptoms until regional or diffuse metastasis has ensued, and surgical resection for cure is possible in only 25–50% of patients [15, 16].

20.2.3 Preoperative Workup

Standard imaging studies are used to diagnose gallbladder cancer. Ultrasound is often the initial testing modality. Findings that portend possible gallbladder cancer are large polyps (>10 mm), local thickening and irregularity of the gallbladder wall, calcification of the gallbladder (porcelain gallbladder), and regional adenopathy [17, 18]. None of these findings is pathognomonic for gallbladder cancer, and such individual radiologic findings are associated with gallbladder cancer in less than 10% of cases [19, 20].

Suspicion of gallbladder cancer on ultrasound often prompts a CT scan of the abdomen, which can better assess local invasion and regional lymphadenopathy. Despite heightened suspicion from imaging studies, a surgical specimen is the only means to make the definitive diagnosis of gallbladder cancer.

20.2.4 Staging of Gallbladder Cancer

The TNM system is used for staging of gallbladder cancer and was recently revised in its seventh edition.

J.P. Pearl and J.L. Ponsky (✉)
Department of Surgery, University Hospitals Case Medical Center and Case Western Reserve University, 11100 Euclid Avenue, Cleveland, OH 44106-5047, USA
e-mail: jonathan.pearl@med.navy.mil;
jeffrey.ponsky@UHhospitals.org

Survival is closely correlated with T stage [16, 21]. T1a tumors are confined to the mucosa, and T1b lesions invade the muscularis. These tumors have 5-year survivals of 99% and 95%, respectively. T2 lesions invade the subserosa, and T3 lesions invade the serosa. The survival for T2 lesions is 70%, and 20% of those with T3 lesions survive 5 years. When the tumor invades adjacent organs (T4) there are virtually no long-term survivors.

20.2.5 Surgical Therapy

Gallbladder cancer spreads by direct hepatic invasion or via regional lymph nodes. To afford patients the best chance for long-term survival, standard therapy for T1b-T3 lesions is an extended cholecystectomy [6, 22–25]. This includes a cholecystectomy with en bloc resection of liver segments IV and V, lymphadenectomy of the nodes of the porta hepatis and superior pancreatic region, and common bile duct resection when the cystic duct margin is involved with tumor. Extended cholecystectomy as described above may not be adequate for T3 lesions, and some groups advocate extended right hepatectomy in those cases [15, 26].

20.2.6 Special Situations in the Operating Room

20.2.6.1 Laparoscopy and Incidental Gallbladder Cancer

Although laparoscopic therapy is not advocated for most cases of gallbladder cancer, incidental gallbladder cancer occurs in 0.3–1% of all laparoscopic cholecystectomies [27, 28]. Approximately 10% of all gallbladder cancers are discovered incidentally at laparoscopic cholecystectomy [27, 28]. Laparoscopy provides adequate therapy for carcinoma in situ and T1a lesions, with 5-year survivals approaching 100% in these cases [29–31]. Any lesions which penetrate the muscularis require conventional operations. There is no survival disadvantage in cases when the initial procedure was a laparoscopic cholecystectomy, rather than a conventional cholecystectomy, provided that liver resection and lymphadenectomy are subsequently performed [32, 33]. These procedures are more commonly performed laparoscopically but the current literature is still sparse.

When suspected gallbladder cancer is encountered intraoperatively, the surgeon has two options: convert to laparotomy or complete the cholecystectomy laparoscopically and obtain a frozen section pathological examination of the specimen during the same anesthesic. In such cases, the laparoscopic cholecystectomy must be performed with meticulous technique without spillage of bile. The specimen should be removed in an impermeable bag without exposure to the abdominal wall, and leakage of the pneumoperitoneum around the trocars should be avoided out of concern for seeding the trocar sites with tumor cells.

20.2.6.2 Management of Intraoperative Positive Frozen Section

Frozen section confirmation of gallbladder cancer does not necessitate conversion to laparotomy during the same anesthesia. A recent study revealed that survival is not adversely affected when definitive resection for gallbladder cancer is performed at a later date [34]. In this study, optimizing survival depended on performing an extended cholecystectomy with liver resection and meticulous lymphadenectomy at a center with expertise in the field of hepatobiliary surgery.

20.2.6.3 The Problem of Intraoperative Bile Spillage

Bile spillage has been reported to occur in 20–40% of laparoscopic cholecystectomies [35, 36]. Spilled bile can disseminate tumor cells and increase recurrence rates. Some studies have shown lower survival rates in gallbladder cancer when bile spillage occurred during the initial laparoscopic cholecystectomy [37, 38]. Thus, routinely avoided bile spillage in laparoscopic cholecystectomy, especially in patients older than 50 years, is strongly advocated.

20.2.6.4 Port Site Metastasis

Management of trocar sites after laparoscopic cholecystectomy for gallbladder cancer remains controversial. Port site recurrences may occur in up to 17% of patients with gallbladder cancer [39, 40], although this parallels the rate of wound recurrences in conventional laparotomy [40]. Some groups advocate routine trocar site excision for all incidental gallbladder cancers [37], although there is little evidence that this provides a survival advantage for T1a lesions. For tumors which require a laparotomy the trocar sites should be routinely excised [40, 41].

20.2.7 Laparoscopy for Staging of Gallbladder Cancer

Incidental gallbladder cancer represents only a fraction of gallbladder cancer cases. Many patients present with radiological evidence of advanced loco-regional disease. These patients may be candidates for laparotomy for potential cure if there is no metastatic disease. In cases of advanced gallbladder cancer laparoscopy may accurately stage the disease and select those patients without metastatic disease, who might be candidates for an extended cholecystectomy.

Recent studies have confirmed the value of laparoscopy for selecting patients for laparotomy. In two series, one-third of patients with potentially curable gallbladder cancer were spared a laparotomy due to the findings on laparoscopy [42, 43]. The most common findings precluding radical resection for cure were peritoneal metastases and liver metastases. Of the two-thirds of patients operated by laparotomy, up to half were found to have incurable disease due to lymph node metastases and local invasion. The patients in the laparoscopy-only groups were discharged to home earlier and experienced less postoperative pain, thus substantiating the value of staging laparoscopy in locally advanced gallbladder cancer.

20.2.8 Adjuvant Therapy

At present there are little data to support the use of adjuvant therapy outside of investigational protocols [44, 45], and most palliative chemotherapy regimens are extrapolated from the management of pancreas cancer. In Chile, where the most common cause of cancer death in women is gallbladder cancer, some investigators report success with adjuvant chemotherapy [46, 47]. There may be up to a 30% response rate with Gemcitabine and possibly even better results with a triple regimen of Cisplatin, Capecitabine, and Gemcitabine [48]. Most groups report little value in the use of radiotherapy for gallbladder cancer [47, 49].

20.2.9 Future Trends

Conventional operations will likely prevail in the management of gallbladder cancer even though more and more case series of laparoscopic management for locally advanced disease are reported. Poor survival rates in patients with advanced disease merit attention directed toward improving adjuvant therapies. Since the disease is rare in the USA and Europe, large-scale chemotherapy trials will likely occur in South America and Asia. The results with Gemcitabine are encouraging, although future studies with Gemcitabine in combination with other agents will likely yield enhanced long-term survival.

20.3 Extrahepatic Cholangiocarcinoma

20.3.1 Epidemiology of Cholangiocarcinoma

Cholangiocarcinoma represents 3% of all gastrointestinal tumors [50]. In the USA the incidence is 1.0 per 100,000 women and 1.5 per 100,000 men [51, 52]. Approximately 5% of cholangiocarcinomas are intrahepatic and are managed as liver tumors. Over 25% of cholangiocarcinomas are located in the distal bile duct and are treated similar to cancer in the head of the pancreas. The remaining 70% of cholangiocarcinomas are in the hilar and perihilar regions, commonly referred to as Klatskin's tumors [53]. These tumors are staged according to the TNM classification.

20.3.2 Classification of Extrahepatic Cholangiocarcinomas

Hilar cholangiocarcinomas are categorized according to the Bismuth-Corlette system [54] (Fig. 20.1). Bismuth Type I lesions are located below the bifurcation of the common hepatic duct. Type II tumors involve the bifurcation but do not extend into the main right or left ducts. Type III lesions involve either the right or left hepatic ducts, and Type IV involve both the right and left hepatic ducts.

20.3.3 Risk Factors and Symptoms in Cholangiocarcinoma

Risk factors for contracting cholangiocarcinoma include primary sclerosing cholangitis [51], infection with the parasite Opisthorchis viverrini [55], and viral hepatitis [56, 57]. Most patients present with jaundice, which incites a radiologic investigation.

20.3.4 Preoperative Workup

The extent of ductal involvement can be assessed with a form of cholangiography, be it magnetic resonance cholangiography, endoscopic retrograde cholangiography, or percutaneous transhepatic cholangiography. Furthermore, a CT scan may be useful in the search for metastatic disease.

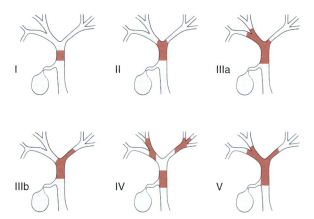

Fig. 20.1 The Bismuth-Corlette classification for hilar cholangiocarcinomas (The location of the tumor is shaded). (Drawing by Hippmann GbR, Schwarzenbruck, Germany)

20.3.5 Conventional Surgical Therapy

Cholangiocarcinoma is a slow growing tumor that spreads along the bile ducts with neural, perineural, and subepithelial extensions. Cholangiocarcinoma tends to recur locally after resection, thus an aggressive surgical approach may be warranted to improve long-term survival. Increasingly radical operations, often including liver resection, have led to improved survival over the last decade [58–60]. With current radical R0 resections (no evidence of residual disease) 5-year survival rates approach 30% [61–63].

The historical approach to cholangiocarcinoma included excision of the supraduodenal biliary tract, cholecystectomy, and biliary-enteric anastomosis [64, 65]. Recent innovations add a routine partial hepatectomy with caudate lobe resection and portal lymphadenectomy [4, 66–70]. Various degrees of liver resection are advocated ranging from routine resection of segments IV and V to major hepatic resection such as lobectomy or trisegmentectomy.

20.3.6 Laparoscopy for Staging of Cholangiocarcinoma

A priori contraindications to radical resection include evidence of involvement of the main hepatic artery or portal vein. Lymph node metastases, which is evident in up to 50% of patients at diagnosis [71, 72], also preclude resection for cure. Peritoneal implants and liver metastases contravene consideration for resection, although these typically elude conventional imaging. Laparoscopy has been shown to detect occult metastatic disease in approximately one-third of patients being considered for curative resection [42, 73–75].

In one series, 84 patients with suspected hilar cholangiocarcinoma underwent staging laparoscopy [73]. Nearly 25% were found to have metastatic disease by laparoscopy alone. The yield of detecting unresectable disease was improved with the addition of intraoperative ultrasound, and over 40% of patients were found to be unresectable through a combination of laparoscopy and intraoperative ultrasound.

Two other series found similar rates of unresectability [42, 75]. Approximately one-third of all patients considered for resection were found to have metastatic disease, and another one-third were found

20.3.7 Pathology of Cholangiocarcinoma

The pathologic diagnosis can be achieved by brush cytology or transpapillary biopsies in up to 50% of cases [76, 77]. The accuracy of cytologic diagnosis can be enhanced with the techniques of digital image analysis and fluorescent in situ hybridization [78]. Furthermore, both the sensitivity and specificity for diagnosing cholangiocarcinoma are improved with the addition of intraductal ultrasound, ultrasound-guided fine needle aspiration, or choledochoscopy [76, 79, 80]. Despite technological advances, the diagnosis of cholangiocarcinoma remains elusive in many patients.

20.3.8 Endoscopic Diagnosis and Palliation of Unresectable Disease

Endoscopy is useful for the diagnosis of cholangiocarcinoma (Fig. 20.2). Most patients without prior biliary surgery who present with jaundice and a stricture on cholangiogram will prove to have cholangiocarcinoma. The most characteristic finding on cholangiogram is a long, irregular, asymmetric stricture in the extrahepatic bile duct.

As the only chance for cure of cholangiocarcinoma relies on conventional surgery, endoscopic therapy is reserved for palliation. Stenting of strictures associated with cholangiocarcinoma relieves jaundice and pruritus, prevents cholangitis, avoids liver failure, and enhances patients' quality of life [80, 81]. Median survival of unresectable cholangiocarcinoma is 3 months without biliary drainage and 6 months with biliary drainage [82, 83], thus supporting broad application of endoscopic stenting in such cases.

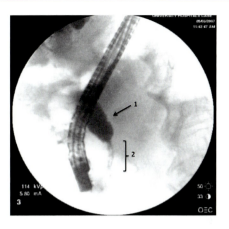

Fig. 20.2 ERCP with classical picture of proximal dilatation of the extrahepatic bile ducts (*1*) and distal malignant stricture (*2*) in cholangiocarcinoma

20.3.9 Advantages and Disadvantages of Different Stent Types

Both metal and plastic (polyethylene) biliary stents are available for transpapillary endoscopic deployment. Plastic endoprostheses require removal and replacement every 3 months due to accumulation of debris within the lumen of the stent. Self-expanding metal stents are generally considered permanent and offer a longer duration of patency (up to 1 year) before obstructing [84]. Metal stents have been shown to be efficacious in patients whose life expectancy exceeds 3 months [85, 86]. Recently, covered metal stents have been introduced which offer the patency rates of a conventional metal stent but can be removed and replaced should obstruction occur [87].

20.3.10 Endoscopic Photodynamic Therapy

This modality has been shown to prolong survival and enhance quality of life in patients with unresectable cholangiocarcinoma [88–90]. Patients are administered an intravenous photosensitizing agent, which accumulates in neoplastic tissue followed by intraductal exposure to laser light [91]. In the initial German trial investigating photodynamic therapy for unresectable cholangiocarcinoma, survival was prolonged to nearly 500 days compared to 100 days in an untreated cohort [92]. Further trials have shown photodynamic therapy to yield equivalent survival compared to R1 and R2 resections [93]. The prolonged survival from photodynamic therapy likely results from improved biliary drainage rather than reduction in tumor mass [94].

20.3.11 Adjuvant Therapy

There is currently no evidence to support radiotherapy in cholangiocarcinoma. Neither preoperative nor adjuvant radiotherapy in R0 resection has been shown to improve survival [48, 95]. Results of chemotherapy for cholangiocarcinoma have been generally disappointing, although some responses have been reported with single agent Gemcitabine or combination therapy using Gemcitabine and another agent [96, 97].

20.3.12 Future Trends

As with gallbladder cancer, conventional surgery will likely prevail in the management of cholangiocarcinoma. Enhanced survival in the future will likely depend on improving chemotherapy regimens and refinement of surgical technique.

The prospect of liver transplantation for unresectable cholangiocarcinoma depends on improved neoadjuvant therapy. While there is one study from the Mayo clinic showing encouraging results with chemotherapy and irradiation prior to liver transplantation in select patients [98], larger scale trials are imperative before transplantation should be routinely considered for unresectable cholangiocarcinoma.

Delineating benign from malignant strictures might be performed using endoscopic optical coherence tomography. Optical coherence uses backscatter from infrared light to create a two-dimensional image at high resolution. A choledochoscope can be outfitted to perform optical coherence. Using this technique, histologic features, such as ductal epithelium and supepithelium, can be imaged, thereby providing an "optical biopsy" of the bile duct.

Endoscopic palliative therapies will likely evolve. Techniques of endoscopic ablation are available for dysplasia within other areas of the gastrointestinal tract and might be applied to the biliary tree. Improved imaging and sampling will enhance the diagnostic capabilities of ERCP. Furthermore, covered metal stents which resist tumor ingrowth, and possibly even apply local chemotherapeutic agents, could further prolong survival in unresectable disease.

20.4 Conclusions

Gallbladder cancer and cholangiocarcinoma are rare tumors with poor prognoses. R0 resection offers the only chance for improved long-term survival. Recently, increasingly radical surgery, including anatomic liver resection and extended lymph node dissections, have improved survival somewhat.

On the whole, minimally invasive techniques play a limited role in gallbladder cancer and cholangiocarcinoma. Diagnostic laparoscopy can limit the number of patients who undergo nontherapeutic laparotomy. Furthermore, minimally invasive techniques, such as stenting and photodynamic therapy, can enhance survival and improve quality of life in unresectable cholangiocarcinoma patients.

Quick Reference Guide

1. Routinely avoid bile spillage in laparoscopic cholecystectomy to limit risk of disseminating gallbladder cancer.
2. T1a gallbladder cancer is adequately treated with laparoscopic cholecystectomy.
3. T1b-T4 gallbladder cancer requires extended cholecystectomy.
4. Trocar site excision for >T1a gallbladder cancer may be warranted.
5. Laparoscopic exploration reduces nontherapeutic laparotomy in 1/3 of patients with potentially resectable gallbladder cancer.
6. Laparoscopy combined with intraoperative ultrasound spares 40% of patients with cholangiocarcinoma a nontherapeutic laparotomy.
7. Routine hepatectomy improves survival in cholangiocarcinoma.
8. Endoscopic stenting improves survival and quality of life in unresectable cholangiocarcinoma.

9. Endoscopic photodynamic therapy prolongs survival in unresectable cholangiocarcinoma.
10. Self-expanding metal stents are suitable in patients with >3 months anticipated survival.

References

1. Piehler, J.M., Crichlow, R.W.: Primary carcinoma of the gallbladder. Arch. Surg. **112**(1k0), 26–30 (1977)
2. Wilkinson, D.S.: Carcinoma of the gall-bladder: an experience and review of the literature. Aust. N. Z. J. Surg. **65**(10), 724–727 (1995)
3. Hadjis, N.S., Blenkharn, J.I., Alexander, N., et al.: Outcome of radical surgery in hilar cholangiocarcinoma. Surgery **107**(6), 597–604 (1990)
4. Okuda, K., Kubo, Y., Okazaki, N., et al.: Clinical aspects of intrahepatic bile duct carcinoma including hilar carcinoma: a study of 57 autopsy-proven cases. Cancer **39**(1), 232–246 (1977)
5. Burke, E.C., Jarnagin, W.R., Hochwald, S.N., et al.: Hilar Cholangiocarcinoma: patterns of spread, the importance of hepatic resection for curative operation, and a presurgical clinical staging system. Ann. Surg. **228**(3), 385–394 (1998)
6. Cubertafond, P., Gainant, A., Cucchiaro, G.: Surgical treatment of 724 carcinomas of the gallbladder. Results of the French Surgical Association Survey. Ann. Surg. **219**(3), 275–280 (1994)
7. Lillemoe, K.D., Cameron, J.L.: Surgery for hilar cholangiocarcinoma: the Johns Hopkins approach. J. Hepatobiliary Pancreat. Surg. **7**(2), 115–121 (2000)
8. Madariaga, J.R., Iwatsuki, S., Todo, S., et al.: Liver resection for hilar and peripheral cholangiocarcinomas: a study of 62 cases. Ann. Surg. **227**(1), 70–79 (1998)
9. Sicklick, J.K., Choti, M.A.: Controversies in the surgical management of cholangiocarcinoma and gallbladder cancer. Semin. Oncol. **32**(6 Suppl 9), S112–S117 (2005)
10. Medina, E.: Digestive diseases in Chile: epidemiologic outlook. Rev. Med. Chil. **116**(3), 282–288 (1988)
11. Randi, G., Franceschi, S., La Vecchia, C.: Gallbladder cancer worldwide: geographical distribution and risk factors. Int. J. Cancer **118**(7), 1591–1602 (2006)
12. Levi, F., Lucchini, F., Negri, E., La Vecchia, C.: The recent decline in gallbladder cancer mortality in Europe. Eur. J. Cancer Prev. **12**(4), 265–267 (2003)
13. Hsing, A.W., Bai, Y., Andreotti, G., et al.: Family history of gallstones and the risk of biliary tract cancer and gallstones: a population-based study in Shanghai, China. Int. J. Cancer **121**(4), 832–838 (2007)
14. Kapoor, V.K.: Cholecystectomy in patients with asymptomatic gallstones to prevent gall bladder cancer – the case against. Indian J. Gastroenterol. **25**(3), 152–154 (2006)
15. Foster, J.M., Hoshi, H., Gibbs, J.F., et al.: Gallbladder cancer: defining the indications for primary radical resection and radical re-resection. Ann. Surg. Oncol. **14**(2), 833–840 (2007)
16. Balachandran, P., Agarwal, S., Krishnani, N., et al.: Predictors of long-term survival in patients with gallbladder cancer. J. Gastrointest. Surg. **10**(6), 848–854 (2006)
17. Rooholamini, S.A., Tehrani, N.S., Razavi, M.K., et al.: Imaging of gallbladder carcinoma. Radiographics **14**(2), 291–306 (1994)
18. Archer, A., Horton, K.: Radiologic evaluation and treatment of gallbladder and biliary tree carcinoma. Cancer Treat. Res. **69**, 157–183 (1994)
19. Polverosi, R., Zambelli, C., Sbeghen, R., et al.: Ultrasonography and computerized tomography in the diagnosis of gallbladder carcinoma. Radiol. Med. (Torino) **87**(5), 643–647 (1994)
20. Akatsu, T., Aiura, K., Shimazu, M., et al.: Can endoscopic ultrasonography differentiate nonneoplastic from neoplastic gallbladder polyps? Dig. Dis. Sci. **51**(2), 416–421 (2006)
21. Fong, Y., Wagman, L., Gonen, M., et al.: Evidence-based gallbladder cancer staging: changing cancer staging by analysis of data from the National Cancer Database. Ann. Surg. **243**(6), 767–771 (2006). discussion 771-4
22. Shirai, Y., Wakai, T., Hatakeyama, K.: Radical lymph node dissection for gallbladder cancer: indications and limitations. Surg. Oncol. Clin. N. Am. **16**(1), 221–232 (2007)
23. Rodriguez Otero, J.C., Proske, A., Vallilengua, C., et al.: Gallbladder cancer: surgical results after cholecystectomy in 25 patients with lamina propria invasion and 26 patients with muscular layer invasion. J. Hepatobiliary Pancreat. Surg. **13**(6), 562–566 (2006)
24. Misra, S., Chaturvedi, A., Misra, N.C.: Gallbladder cancer. Curr. Treat Options Gastroenterol. **9**(2), 95–106 (2006)
25. Aramaki, M., Matsumoto, T., Shibata, K., et al.: Factors influencing recurrence after surgical treatment for T2 gallbladder carcinoma. Hepatogastroenterology **51**(60), 1609–1611 (2004)
26. Principe, A., Del Gaudio, M., Ercolani, G., et al.: Radical surgery for gallbladder carcinoma: possibilities of survival. Hepatogastroenterology **53**(71), 660–664 (2006)
27. Misra, M.C., Guleria, S.: Management of cancer gallbladder found as a surprise on a resected gallbladder specimen. J. Surg. Oncol. **93**(8), 690–698 (2006)
28. Shimizu, T., Arima, Y., Yokomuro, S., et al.: Incidental gallbladder cancer diagnosed during and after laparoscopic cholecystectomy. J. Nippon Med. Sch. **73**(3), 136–140 (2006)
29. Sun, C.D., Zhang, B.Y., Wu, L.Q., Lee, W.J.: Laparoscopic cholecystectomy for treatment of unexpected early-stage gallbladder cancer. J. Surg. Oncol. **91**(4), 253–257 (2005)
30. Akyurek, N., Irkorucu, O., Salman, B., et al.: Unexpected gallbladder cancer during laparoscopic cholecystectomy. J. Hepatobiliary Pancreat. Surg. **11**(5), 357–361 (2004)
31. Yeh, C.N., Jan, Y.Y., Chen, M.F.: Management of unsuspected gallbladder carcinoma discovered during or following laparoscopic cholecystectomy. Am. Surg. **70**(3), 256–258 (2004)
32. Taner, C.B., Nagorney, D.M., Donohue, J.H.: Surgical treatment of gallbladder cancer. J. Gastrointest. Surg. **8**(1), 83–89 (2004). discussion 89
33. Antonakis, P., Alexakis, N., Mylonaki, D., et al.: Incidental finding of gallbladder carcinoma detected during or after laparoscopic cholecystectomy. Eur. J. Surg. Oncol. **29**(4), 358–360 (2003)
34. Shih, S.P., Schulick, R.D., Cameron, J.L., et al.: Gallbladder cancer: the role of laparoscopy and radical resection. Ann. Surg. **245**(6), 893–901 (2007)
35. Manukyan, M.N., Demirkalem, P., Gulluoglu, B.M., et al.: Retained abdominal gallstones during laparoscopic cholecystectomy. Am. J. Surg. **189**(4), 450–452 (2005)

36. Tumer, A.R., Yuksek, Y.N., Yasti, A.C., et al.: Dropped gallstones during laparoscopic cholecystectomy: the consequences. World J. Surg. **29**(4), 437–440 (2005)
37. Steinert, R., Nestler, G., Sagynaliev, E., et al.: Laparoscopic cholecystectomy and gallbladder cancer. J. Surg. Oncol. **93**(8), 682–689 (2006)
38. Ouchi, K., Mikuni, J., Kakugawa, Y.: Laparoscopic cholecystectomy for gallbladder carcinoma: results of a Japanese survey of 498 patients. J. Hepatobiliary Pancreat. Surg. **9**(2), 256–260 (2002)
39. Giuliante, F., Ardito, F., Vellone, M., et al.: Port-sites excision for gallbladder cancer incidentally found after laparoscopic cholecystectomy. Am. J. Surg. **191**(1), 114–116 (2006)
40. Lundberg, O., Kristoffersson, A.: Wound recurrence from gallbladder cancer after open cholecystectomy. Surgery **127**(3), 296–300 (2000)
41. Wakai, T., Shirai, Y., Hatakeyama, K.: Radical second resection provides survival benefit for patients with T2 gallbladder carcinoma first discovered after laparoscopic cholecystectomy. World J. Surg. **26**(7), 867–871 (2002)
42. Goere, D., Wagholikar, G.D., Pessaux, P., et al.: Utility of staging laparoscopy in subsets of biliary cancers: laparoscopy is a powerful diagnostic tool in patients with intrahepatic and gallbladder carcinoma. Surg. Endosc. **20**(5), 721–725 (2006)
43. Agrawal, S., Sonawane, R.N., Behari, A., et al.: Laparoscopic staging in gallbladder cancer. Dig. Surg. **22**(6), 440–445 (2005)
44. Feisthammel, J., Schoppmeyer, K., Mossner, J., et al.: Irinotecan with 5-FU/FA in advanced biliary tract adenocarcinomas: a multicenter phase II trial. Am. J. Clin. Oncol. **30**(3), 319–324 (2007)
45. Sato, K., Kitajima, Y., Kohya, N., et al.: CPT-11 (SN-38) chemotherapy may be selectively applicable to biliary tract cancer with low hMLH1 expression. Anticancer Res. **27**(2), 865–872 (2007)
46. Gallardo, J.O., Rubio, B., Fodor, M., et al.: A phase II study of gemcitabine in gallbladder carcinoma. Ann. Oncol. **12**(10), 1403–1406 (2001)
47. de Aretxabala, X., Roa, I., Berrios, M., et al.: Chemoradiotherapy in gallbladder cancer. J. Surg. Oncol. **93**(8), 699–704 (2006)
48. Hong, Y.S., Lee, J., Lee, S.C., et al.: Phase II study of capecitabine and cisplatin in previously untreated advanced biliary tract cancer. Cancer Chemother. Pharmacol. **60**(3), 321–328 (2007)
49. Fuller, C.D., Thomas Jr., C.R., Wong, A., et al.: Image-guided intensity-modulated radiation therapy for gallbladder carcinoma. Radiother. Oncol. **81**(1), 65–72 (2006)
50. Jepsen, P., Vilstrup, H., Tarone, R.E., et al.: Incidence rates of intra- and extrahepatic cholangiocarcinomas in Denmark from 1978 through 2002. J. Natl. Cancer Inst. **99**(11), 895–897 (2007)
51. Fevery, J., Verslype, C., Lai, G., et al.: Incidence, diagnosis, and therapy of cholangiocarcinoma in patients with primary sclerosing cholangitis. Dig. Dis. Sci. **52**(11), 3123–3135 (2007)
52. Welzel, T.M., McGlynn, K.A., Hsing, A.W., et al.: Impact of classification of hilar cholangiocarcinomas (Klatskin tumors) on the incidence of intra- and extrahepatic cholangiocarcinoma in the United States. J. Natl Cancer Inst. **98**(12), 873–875 (2006)
53. Nakeeb, A., Pitt, H.A., Sohn, T.A., et al.: Cholangiocarcinoma. A spectrum of intrahepatic, perihilar, and distal tumors. Ann. Surg. **224**(4), 463–473 (1996). discussion 473-5
54. Bismuth, H., Nakache, R., Diamond, T.: Management strategies in resection for hilar cholangiocarcinoma. Ann. Surg. **215**(1), 31–38 (1992)
55. Kurathong, S., Lerdverasirikul, P., Wongpaitoon, V., et al.: Opisthorchis viverrini infection and cholangiocarcinoma. A prospective, case-controlled study. Gastroenterology **89**(1), 151–156 (1985)
56. Gatselis, N.K., Tepetes, K., Loukopoulos, A., et al.: Hepatitis B virus and intrahepatic cholangiocarcinoma. Cancer Invest. **25**(1), 55–58 (2007)
57. Wiwanitkit, V.: Seroprevalence of hepatitis virus B seropositive in the patients with cholangiocarcinoma: a summary. Asian Pac. J. Cancer Prev. **6**(1), 27–28 (2005)
58. Seyama, Y., Makuuchi, M.: Current surgical treatment for bile duct cancer. World J. Gastroenterol. **13**(10), 1505–1515 (2007)
59. Uchiyama, K., Nakai, T., Tani, M., et al.: Indications for extended hepatectomy in the management of stage IV hilar cholangiocarcinoma. Arch. Surg. **138**(9), 1012–1016 (2003)
60. Neuhaus, P., Jonas, S., Settmacher, U., et al.: Surgical management of proximal bile duct cancer: extended right lobe resection increases resectability and radicality. Langenbecks Arch. Surg. **388**(3), 194–200 (2003)
61. Miyazaki, M., Kato, A., Ito, H., et al.: Combined vascular resection in operative resection for hilar cholangiocarcinoma: does it work or not? Surgery **141**(5), 581–588 (2007)
62. DeOliveira, M.L., Cunningham, S.C., Cameron, J.L., et al.: Cholangiocarcinoma: thirty-one-year experience with 564 patients at a single institution. Ann. Surg. **245**(5), 755–762 (2007)
63. Hasegawa, S., Ikai, I., Fujii, H., et al.: Surgical resection of hilar cholangiocarcinoma: analysis of survival and postoperative complications. World J. Surg. **31**(6), 1258–1265 (2007)
64. Chung, C., Bautista, N., O'Connell, T.X.: Prognosis and treatment of bile duct carcinoma. Am. Surg. **64**(10), 921–925 (1998)
65. Strasberg, S.M.: Resection of hilar cholangiocarcinoma. HPB Surg. **10**(6), 415–418 (1998)
66. Patel, T., Singh, P.: Cholangiocarcinoma: emerging approaches to a challenging cancer. Curr. Opin. Gastroenterol. **23**(3), 317–323 (2007)
67. Liu, C.L., Fan, S.T., Lo, C.M., et al.: Improved operative and survival outcomes of surgical treatment for hilar cholangiocarcinoma. Br. J. Surg. **93**(12), 1488–1494 (2006)
68. Nagino, M., Kamiya, J., Arai, T., et al.: "Anatomic" right hepatic trisectionectomy (extended right hepatectomy) with caudate lobectomy for hilar cholangiocarcinoma. Ann. Surg. **243**(1), 28–32 (2006)
69. Hawkins, W.G., DeMatteo, R.P., Cohen, M.S., et al.: Caudate hepatectomy for cancer: a single institution experience with 150 patients. J. Am. Coll. Surg. **200**(3), 345–352 (2005)
70. Nagino, M., Kamiya, J., Arai, T., et al.: One hundred consecutive hepatobiliary resections for biliary hilar malignancy: preoperative blood donation, blood loss, transfusion, and outcome. Surgery **137**(2), 148–155 (2005)

71. Murakami, Y., Uemura, K., Hayashidani, Y., et al.: Prognostic significance of lymph node metastasis and surgical margin status for distal cholangiocarcinoma. J. Surg. Oncol. **95**(3), 207–212 (2007)
72. Grobmyer, S.R., Wang, L., Gonen, M., et al.: Perihepatic lymph node assessment in patients undergoing partial hepatectomy for malignancy. Ann. Surg. **244**(2), 260–264 (2006)
73. Connor, S., Barron, E., Wigmore, S.J., et al.: The utility of laparoscopic assessment in the preoperative staging of suspected hilar cholangiocarcinoma. J. Gastrointest. Surg. **9**(4), 476–480 (2005)
74. White, R.R., Pappas, T.N.: Laparoscopic staging for hepatobiliary carcinoma. J. Gastrointest. Surg. **8**(8), 920–922 (2004)
75. Corvera, C.U., Weber, S.M., Jarnagin, W.R.: Role of laparoscopy in the evaluation of biliary tract cancer. Surg. Oncol. Clin. N. Am. **11**(4), 877–891 (2002)
76. DeWitt, J., Misra, V.L., Leblanc, J.K., et al.: EUS-guided FNA of proximal biliary strictures after negative ERCP brush cytology results. Gastrointest. Endosc. **64**(3), 325–333 (2006)
77. Boberg, K.M., Jebsen, P., Clausen, O.P., et al.: Diagnostic benefit of biliary brush cytology in cholangiocarcinoma in primary sclerosing cholangitis. J. Hepatol. **45**(4), 568–574 (2006)
78. Chahal, P., Baron, T.H.: Endoscopic palliation of cholangiocarcinoma. Curr. Opin. Gastroenterol. **22**(5), 551–560 (2006)
79. Fritscher-Ravens, A., Broering, D.C., Sriram, P.V., et al.: EUS-guided fine-needle aspiration cytodiagnosis of hilar cholangiocarcinoma: a case series. Gastrointest. Endosc. **52**(4), 534–540 (2000)
80. Savader, S.J., Prescott, C.A., Lund, G.B., Osterman, F.A.: Intraductal biliary biopsy: comparison of three techniques. J. Vasc. Interv. Radiol. **7**(5), 743–750 (1996)
81. Rumalla, A., Baron, T.H.: Evaluation and endoscopic palliation of cholangiocarcinoma. Management of cholangiocarcinoma. Dig. Dis. **17**(4), 194–200 (1999)
82. Chang, W.H., Kortan, P., Haber, G.B.: Outcome in patients with bifurcation tumors who undergo unilateral versus bilateral hepatic duct drainage. Gastrointest. Endosc. **47**(5), 354–362 (1998)
83. Farley, D.R., Weaver, A.L., Nagorney, D.M.: "Natural history" of unresected cholangiocarcinoma: patient outcome after noncurative intervention. Mayo Clin. Proc. **70**(5), 425–429 (1995)
84. Soderlund, C., Linder, S.: Covered metal versus plastic stents for malignant common bile duct stenosis: a prospective, randomized, controlled trial. Gastrointest. Endosc. **63**(7), 986–995 (2006)
85. De Palma, G.D., Pezzullo, A., Rega, M., et al.: Unilateral placement of metallic stents for malignant hilar obstruction: a prospective study. Gastrointest. Endosc. **58**(1), 50–53 (2003)
86. Cheng, J.L., Bruno, M.J., Bergman, J.J., et al.: Endoscopic palliation of patients with biliary obstruction caused by nonresectable hilar cholangiocarcinoma: efficacy of self-expandable metallic Wallstents. Gastrointest. Endosc. **56**(1), 33–39 (2002)
87. Yoon, W.J., Lee, J.K., Lee, K.H., et al.: A comparison of covered and uncovered Wallstents for the management of distal malignant biliary obstruction. Gastrointest. Endosc. **63**(7), 996–1000 (2006)
88. Prasad, G.A., Wang, K.K., Baron, T.H., et al.: Factors associated with increased survival after photodynamic therapy for cholangiocarcinoma. Clin. Gastroenterol. Hepatol. **5**(6), 743–748 (2007)
89. Ortner, M.A., Dorta, G.: Technology insight: Photodynamic therapy for cholangiocarcinoma. Nat. Clin. Pract. Gastroenterol. Hepatol. **3**(8), 459–467 (2006)
90. Zoepf, T., Jakobs, R., Arnold, J.C., et al.: Palliation of nonresectable bile duct cancer: improved survival after photodynamic therapy. Am. J. Gastroenterol. **100**(11), 2426–2430 (2005)
91. Wiedmann, M.W., Caca, K.: General principles of photodynamic therapy (PDT) and gastrointestinal applications. Curr. Pharm. Biotechnol. **5**(4), 397–408 (2004)
92. Wiedmann, M., Berr, F., Schiefke, I., et al.: Photodynamic therapy in patients with non-resectable hilar cholangiocarcinoma: 5-year follow-up of a prospective phase II study. Gastrointest. Endosc. **60**(1), 68–75 (2004)
93. Witzigmann, H., Berr, F., Ringel, U., et al.: Surgical and palliative management and outcome in 184 patients with hilar cholangiocarcinoma: palliative photodynamic therapy plus stenting is comparable to r1/r2 resection. Ann. Surg. **244**(2), 230–239 (2006)
94. Khan, S.A., Sharif, A.W., Taylor-Robinson, S.D.: Photodynamic therapy significantly improves survival outcomes in people with non-resectable cholangiocarcinoma. Cancer Treat. Rev. **30**(3), 315–318 (2004)
95. Mazhar, D., Stebbing, J., Bower, M.: Chemotherapy for advanced cholangiocarcinoma: what is standard treatment? Future Oncol. **2**(4), 509–514 (2006)
96. Charoentum, C., Thongprasert, S., Chewaskulyong, B., Munprakan, S.: Experience with gemcitabine and cisplatin in the therapy of inoperable and metastatic cholangiocarcinoma. World J. Gastroenterol. **13**(20), 2852–2854 (2007)
97. Lee, J., Kim, T.Y., Lee, M.A., et al.: Phase II trial of gemcitabine combined with cisplatin in patients with inoperable biliary tract carcinomas. Cancer Chemother. Pharmacol. **61**(1), 47–52 (2008)
98. Heimbach, J.K., Gores, G.J., Nagorney, D.M., Rosen, C.B.: Liver transplantation for perihilar cholangiocarcinoma after aggressive neoadjuvant therapy: a new paradigm for liver and biliary malignancies? Surgery **140**(3), 331–334 (2006)

Liver: Nonanatomical Resection

21

Fumihiko Fujita, Susumu Eguchi, Yoshitsugu Tajima, and Takashi Kanematsu

21.1 Introduction

The first laparoscopic procedure, a laparoscopic cholecystectomy (LC), was initially performed in Europe in the mid-1980s [1, 2]. More complex procedures, like laparoscopic liver surgery, have developed more slowly in the years thereafter. The first laparoscopic hepatectomy was initially performed for benign liver disease in 1991; however, this procedure has been slow to gain acceptance for malignant disease processes [3, 4]. Since 1995, several reports of laparoscopic hepatectomies for liver cancer have been published [5, 6]. Laparoscopic liver surgery had been limited initially to tumors located in peripheral segments of the liver [7]. Some authors report using this procedure for successful anatomical lobe resections or living donor hepatectomies for liver transplantation [8–11].

Hepatocellular carcinoma (HCC) and metastatic liver cancer, especially colorectal cancer, are the two most frequent liver malignancies. Both disease processes can be treated with laparoscopic partial hepatectomy depending on their location. Especially for HCC, anatomic resection techniques are recommended in order to prevent dissemination of cancer cells into the portal vein. These techniques should also be applied if laparoscopy is used to perform a hepatectomy [12, 13]. A Glissonean pedicle transection is recommended as well to prevent cancer cells from being disseminated during a hepatectomy. This technique is thought to improve the postoperative survival in patients with HCC [14]. On the other hand, patients with HCC commonly have a history of chronic hepatitis and liver cirrhosis with an incidence of 74.1% and 63.3%, respectively [15]. This contributes not seldom to severe liver cirrhosis or a poor liver reserve in that subset of patients; hence, a partial, nonanatomic hepatectomy may be more suitable for these patients than major liver resections. HCC can be a secondary cause of viral infections, including hepatitis B virus (HBV) or hepatitis C virus (HCV). Unfortunately, if present, these viral infections seem to increase the incidence of recurrence after surgical resection of the liver. Especially in such cases, laparoscopic procedures may be best suited in order to avoid an unnecessary exploratory laparotomy if only a biopsy or a nonanatomical liver resection is planned.

Metastatic disease to the liver from colorectal cancer is a well-accepted indication for liver resection and it has been demonstrated to improve overall patient survival [16]. Laparoscopic partial hepatectomies are accepted indications for the treatment of liver metastasis, but its successful completion very much depended on the location of the tumor. Mala et al. compared the short-term outcome of laparoscopic and conventional liver resections in patients with colorectal liver metastasis and concluded that the laparoscopic procedure was superior to the traditional open approach in terms of shorter hospital stay and reduced postoperative pain [17].

21.2 Non-surgical Therapies for Liver Malignancies

Optimal treatment strategies for patients with advanced and unresectable HCC are still under investigation [18, 19]. The prognosis of patients with

---

F. Fujita (✉), S. Eguchi, Y. Tajima, and T. Kanematsu
Department of Transplantation and Digestive Surgery,
Nagasaki University Graduate School of Biomedical Science,
1-7-1 Sakamoto, Nagasaki, 852-8501, Japan
e-mail: ffujita@net.nagasaki-u.ac.jp

unresectable disease, multiple intrahepatic metastases, and major portal vein thrombosis is much worse, and most of these patients die within several months [20, 21]. Given this dismal outcome, the development of effective chemotherapeutic agents or targeted molecular therapies is urgent and mandatory. Transarterial embolization (TAE) or transarterial chemoembolization (TACE) are the most used treatment options for patients with unresectable HCC. In addition, if cirrhotic patients have a poorly preserved liver function, hepatic arterial infusion chemotherapy (HAIC) is another modality used [19, 22, 23]. The chemotherapeutic agents used, either individually or in combination, are Cisplatin, 5-Fluorouracil (5-FU), Epirubicin, Doxorubicin, and Mitomycin-C [19]. Of these agents, 5-FU and Cisplatin are the most commonly applied to treat HCC [24]. Several molecular targeted therapies with drugs like Sorafenib are in trial and the results are awaited with much anticipation.

21.3 Minimally Invasive Approach to Liver Malignancies

21.3.1 Microwave Coagulation Therapy (MCT)

This technique has been widely applied for the treatment of malignant liver disease. A monopolar antenna is inserted into the area harboring cancer and induces tissue necrosis by coagulation [25]. Microwave coagulation therapy (MCT) is applicable for small HCC's with a maximum diameter of less than 2 cm. The big advantage of MCT is that it can be repeated several times over the course of the disease [26]. MCT is especially recommended for patients with poor hepatic reserve, and can be performed via either an open or laparoscopic approach [27, 28]. Sadamori et al. analyzed the serum levels of Interleukin-6, cytokine antagonists, and C-reactive protein, which reflect the severity of surgical stress, between patients following laparoscopic and open MCT, and they concluded that laparoscopic MCT could be recommended for patients with poor hepatic reserve when their indocyanine green retention rate at 15 min (ICG R15) is over 30% [26].

21.3.2 Radiofrequency Ablation (RFA)

Radiofrequency ablation (RFA) is often used percutaneously. As a guidance tool either ultrasound (US), computed tomography (CT), or magnetic resonance imaging (MRI) can be used [29]. RFA has specific characteristics which makes it suitable to treat liver malignancies. It is easy to apply, very effective, and can be repeated if necessary [30, 31]. In comparison to MCT, it coagulates the target point more widely. In general, RFA is indicated for tumors with a maximum diameter of less than 3 cm.

21.4 General Aspects in Laparoscopic Hepatectomies

21.4.1 Preoperative Considerations

The absence of coagulopathy and a sufficient hepatic reserve are important prerequisites. The amount of ascites, the serum level of total bilirubin, and the indocyanine green (ICG) clearance test results are important factors to determine the best surgical strategy. Portal vein pressure is also a useful measurement to evaluate the extent of liver cirrhosis and to determine the area of liver to be resected.

21.4.2 Indications for Laparoscopic Hepatectomy

Indications for laparoscopic hepatectomy should be the same as those for open hepatectomy. Tumor location is still one of the major drawbacks to successful completion of laparoscopic hepatectomy. In general, tumors located in lateral segments (Couinaud segments 2 and 3 and 6) and on the surface of the liver are more suitable for a laparoscopic partial hepatectomy because of their easy access [6, 11, 32]. On the other hand, tumors located in the posterior or superior portion of the right lobe are associated with poor visualization and control of bleeding might be difficult. For those tumors, Huang et al. recommended a hand-assisted laparoscopic approach [33].

21.5 Complications in Laparoscopic Liver Surgery

21.5.1 Intraoperative Bleeding

Intraoperative bleeding is one of the major complications associated with laparoscopic major hepatectomies or even smaller wedge resections. Several authors have reported to intermittently apply the Pringle maneuver for vascular control to reduce blood loss especially during the parenchymal part of the transection [34–36]. In the event of a hemorrhage from the parenchyma of the liver, gauze can be placed over the bleeding site for temporary packing. This packing can usually be removed after 10–15 min. If hemostasis cannot be achieved, a suture or clip can be applied, but the surgeon should consider converting to open surgery under those conditions.

21.5.2 Gas Embolism

In order to obtain good visualization, establishing a pneumoperitoneum using carbon dioxide (CO_2) is recommended especially because of the solubility of CO_2. However, laparoscopic liver surgery using CO_2 carries a high risk of inducing gas embolism [37–39]. Although an accidental gas embolism is rare [40, 41], some authors recommend a gasless laparoscopic technique while resecting the hepatic parenchyma [5, 6, 42]. In addition, the elevated intra-abdominal pressure caused by CO_2 insufflation bears not only the risk of air embolism but also significantly decreases portal blood velocity [39]. Careful monitoring for a gas embolism and meticulous dissection of the liver are crucial preventive measures.

21.5.3 Trocar Site Metastasis

The possibility of port-site recurrence remains one of the main controversies in the use of laparoscopic surgery for malignancies [43–46]. Clinical evidence demonstrated the incidence of wound recurrences to be similar between laparoscopic and conventional procedures [35, 44, 47]. Lang et al. also concluded that laparoscopy does not increase the risk of either port-site or peritoneal metastases in patients with HCC [48]. Vittimberga et al. reported that the immune response is better preserved after laparoscopic surgery than compared with an open procedure. This would result in less port site recurrences [49].

21.6 Surgical Technique

21.6.1 Operating Room Setup and Patient Positioning

The patient is placed in supine position, with split-leg technique. The surgeon positions himself between the legs with one assistant on each side of the patient. Two monitors are placed at the head of the table and as close as possible to the surgeon (Fig. 21.1). For lesions in segment 6, the patient is placed in the left lateral decubitus position in order to expose the lateral aspect of the right lobe of the liver.

21.6.2 Trocar Placement

Four, sometimes five trocars are generally used. A set of two 5-mm and three 12-mm trocars, placing the camera trocar slightly supraumbilical, is used for our preferred setup (Fig. 21.2). Pneumoperitoneum using CO_2 is established and abdominal pressure monitored and maintained below 8 mmHg at all times to reduce the risk of gas embolism. An abdominal wall lift technique is sometimes used in order to reduce the risk of gas embolism (Fig. 21.3). We prefer a laparoscope with a flexible tip.

21.6.3 Diagnostic Laparoscopy and Determination of the Dissection Line

The liver is examined under direct visualization in conjunction with intraoperative ultrasound to confirm the number and size of the lesions to resect. It is important

Fig. 21.1 Patient positioning and operating room setup. *Su* surgeon, *As* assistant, *Ns* nurse, *Anes* anesthesiologist. (Drawing by Hippmann GbR, Schwarzenbruck, Germany)

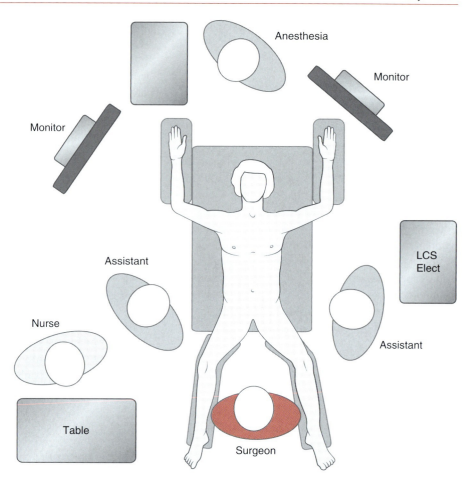

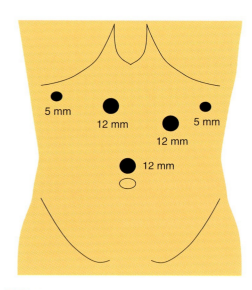

Fig. 21.2 Trocar placement

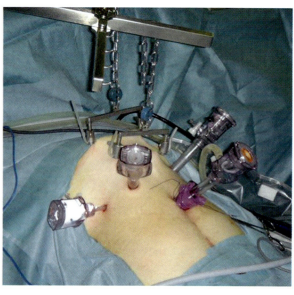

Fig. 21.3 Abdominal wall-lift technique is an alternative to pneumoperitoneum when dissecting the parenchyma of the liver. It is thought to reduce the risk of CO_2 gas embolism

to define their relationship to the intrahepatic vascular structures. In cases where a left lateral segmentectomy or wedge resection is planned, we determine and mark the transecting line on the surface of the liver using intraoperative ultrasound prior to starting the dissection (Fig. 21.4).

21.6.4 Dissection – The Operative Steps

As an initial step, we divide the falciform ligament, and the dissection is then carried on, down to the level of the inferior vena cava. After that, a small hole is made in the coronary ligament, which is located on the extended transecting line. The left triangular ligaments are usually preserved (Fig. 21.5). A penrose drain is inserted into the abdominal cavity and one side of it fixed to the abdominal wall. The other side is passed through the hole in the coronary ligament and positioned behind the posterior surface of the lateral segment of the liver (Fig. 21.6). During the hepatic parenchymal dissection, this penrose drain plays an important role in lifting up the liver and exposing the dissection plane (Figs. 21.7 and 21.8). The preserved

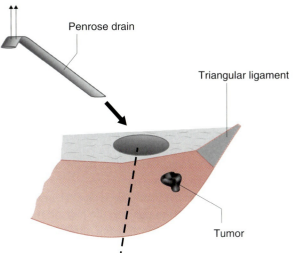

Fig. 21.6 A penrose drain is passed through the divided coronary ligament. One side is fixed to the abdominal wall. The triangular ligament is usually preserved, and helps to prevent the penrose drain from slipping out. (Drawing by Hippmann GbR, Schwarzenbruck, Germany)

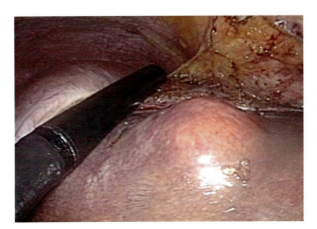

Fig. 21.4 Laparoscopic ultrasound is the key imaging modality to locate the target lesions and to define the dissection line

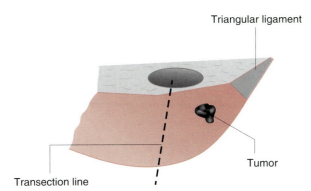

Fig. 21.5 The transection line is determined using intraoperative ultrasound. A hole is made in the coronary ligament that is located on the extended transecting line. This will help for further exposure. (Drawing by Hippmann GbR, Schwarzenbruck, Germany)

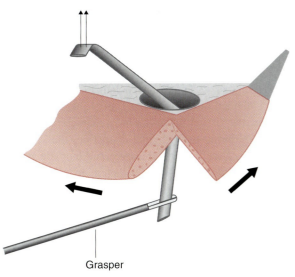

Fig. 21.7 The penrose drain is controled with a grasper. The transecting plane opens up nicely and we obtain great exposure. (Drawing by Hippmann GbR, Schwarzenbruck, Germany)

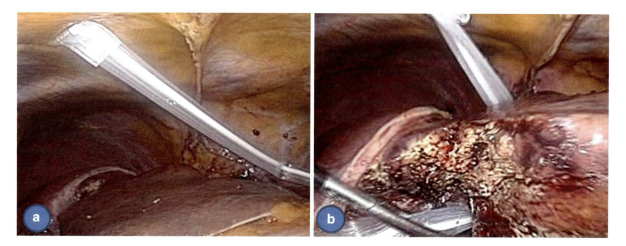

Fig. 21.8 (**a**) One side of the penrose drain is fixed to the abdominal wall. (**b**) The penrose drain allows good exposure of the transection plane, contributing to less intraoperative blood loss and safe dissection

left triangular ligaments are useful in preventing the penrose drain from slipping out.

We regularly use the harmonic scalpel (Ultracision; Ethicon Endo-Surgery) to perform the hepatic transection. This is a surgical device utilizing ultrasonic energy to cut and coagulate tissues. This device is sufficient to seal and divide vascular and biliary structures up to 3 mm in diameter. Other larger structures should only be divided after initial clipping. The TissueLink® device, an instrument using monopolar energy, is also used to dissect the parenchyma of the liver. This device provides excellent coagulation and limits bleeding to a great extent [40]. The surface of this radiofrequency device is covered by a continuous flow of saline, to keep the tissue temperature at or below 100°C without producing any char [50]. An important step at this point of the operation is to maintain constant contact with the liver tissue while dissecting the parenchyma. Smaller vessels can be divided safely using the TissueLink device only. Because the TissueLink device has a characteristic mode of action during parenchymal dissection, the vascular and biliary structures are preserved and they are sealed by shrinking the natural collagen in tissue [51] (Fig. 21.9). This sealing is effective for structures up to 3 mm in diameter. Larger structures should be secured with clips before division as we would do when using the harmonic scalpel. Portal pedicles and major hepatic veins are divided by applying a linear stapler using a vascular white load. When dividing the major hepatic veins, make sure that these structures are circumferentially freed off parenchyma in order to safely apply the stapler (Fig. 21.10).

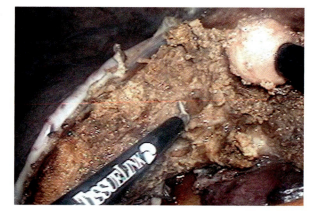

Fig. 21.9 TissueLink™ is used to dissect the parenchyma of the liver. The blunt force applied greatly reduces intraoperative blood loss

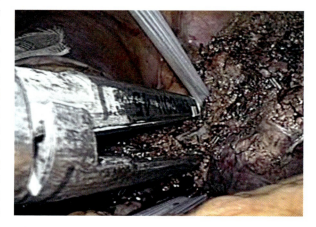

Fig. 21.10 The left hepatic vein is divided with a linear stapler. Make sure that the entire vein is freed off the parenchyma. Blind stapler application may cause major bleeding

21.6.5 Retrieval of the Specimen

The resected specimen is placed in an impermeable retrieval bag and externalized without fragmentation through a separate incision made in the suprapubic region. After retrieval of the specimen, we close this incision immediately and reestablish the pneumoperitoneum. The surgical field is now irrigated and checked for any bleeding or bile leakage. Residual fluid is removed by suction.

21.7 Hand-assisted Technique (HALS)

Hand-assisted laparoscopic surgery (HALS) can overcome some disadvantages associated with a total laparoscopic approach. In 2000, Fong et al. reported preliminary results using HALS for liver resections [36]. Recently, more authors reported the advantages of a HALS approach to the liver [10, 33, 34, 52, 53]. The benefits of HALS are mainly in facilitating manual retraction, in assessing safe resection margins using tactile feedback, and safe parenchymal dissection [10, 34]. The assisting hand can be used for blunt dissection, and to place stapling devices more precisely [34]. Cushieri et al. reported shorter operative times using HALS [52]. The most important advantage seems to be superior control of bleeding, because the fingers can be used to grasp the bleeding vessels immediately. HALS may be converted to an open procedure more easily, whenever it becomes necessary. In this case, we are able to extend the incision for the hand port to a full laparotomy incision much faster. Although HALS usually requires a larger incision of 6–8 cm when compared to a totally laparoscopic procedure, this wide incision will be used to deliver the specimen.

21.8 Future Trends

Will laparoscopic liver surgery become the "gold standard" for all types of liver procedures?

Laparoscopic techniques will probably take the place of open techniques with regard to wedge resections and segmentectomies for focal lesions. Most hepatobiliary surgeons already accept laparoscopic partial hepatectomies for benign liver tumors in various locations. However, for malignant disorders, many surgeons may choose a laparoscopic approach only for tumors located in peripheral segments. In cases, where the extent of the resection is bigger than just a wedge or one segment, an open approach may be chosen in many surgical departments because of safety concerns or out of technical reasons. Recent advancements in technology have made laparoscopic liver surgery safer. New instruments such as TissueLink™ or harmonic scalpel can reduce the amount of intraoperative blood loss. Laparoscopic liver surgery for major hepatectomies may be easily accepted by many surgeons in the near future as technology evolves and surgeons acquire advanced skills through specialized training. Laparoscopic procedures for malignant lesions should only be performed by surgical experts and the same oncological rules should apply when compared to an open resection.

Quick Reference Guide

1. Patient positioning and port placement are dependend on tumor location.
2. Maintain intra-abdominal pressure as low as possible while still achieving adequate visualization. A pressure of less than 8 mmHg should be used to reduce the risk of gas embolism.
3. Laparoscopic ultrasonography is useful to confirm the location of the tumor and to determine the dissection line.
4. Stitches placed on both sides of the dissection line can help to provide good counter traction while dissecting the parenchyma of the liver.
5. Appropriate devices should be selected to dissect the parenchyma of the liver. This can greatly reduce intraoperative blood loss.
6. The harmonic scalpel is used to incise the capsule of the liver and to seal vessels or intrahepatic bile ducts up to 3 mm in diameter. The TissueLink® device is used to dissect the parenchyma of the liver
7. Vessels or intrahepatic bile ducts more than 3 mm in diameter should be clipped before they are divided.
8. If bleeding occurs from the cut edge of the liver, immediate packing with gauze should be the

first choice. Thereafter, clips or stitches should be applied.
9. It is necessary to obtain great visualization when approaching the hepatic vein. If a linear cutting stapler is used to divide the hepatic vein, the surrounding parenchyma should be dissected carefully before firing the device.
10. Upon completion of the operation, confirm that there is no bleeding or bile leakage at the cut surface.

References

1. Dubois, F., Icard, P., Berthelot, G., et al.: Coelioscopic cholecystectomy. Preliminary report of 36 cases. Ann. Surg. **211**(1), 60–62 (1990)
2. Perissat, J., Collet, D., Belliard, R., et al.: Laparoscopic treatment for gallbladder stones and the place of intracorporeal lithotripsy. Surg. Endosc. **4**(3), 135–136 (1990)
3. Gagner, M., Rheault, M., Dubuc, J.: Laparoscopic partial hepatectomy for liver tumor. Surg. Endosc. **6**, 99 (1992)
4. Reich, H., McGlynn, F., DeCaprio, J., et al.: Laparoscopic excision of benign liver lesions. Obstet. Gynecol. **78**(5 Pt 2), 956–958 (1991)
5. Hashizume, M., Takenaka, K., Yanaga, K., et al.: Laparoscopic hepatic resection for hepatocellular carcinoma. Surg. Endosc. **9**(12), 1289–1291 (1995)
6. Kaneko, H., Takagi, S., Shiba, T.: Laparoscopic partial hepatectomy and left lateral segmentectomy: technique and results of a clinical series. Surgery **120**(3), 468–475 (1996)
7. Cherqui, D.: Laparoscopic liver resection. Br. J. Surg. **90**(6), 644–646 (2003)
8. Azagra, J.S., Goergen, M., Gilbart, E., et al.: Laparoscopic anatomical (hepatic) left lateral segmentectomy-technical aspects. Surg. Endosc. **10**(7), 758–761 (1996)
9. Cherqui, D., Soubrane, O., Husson, E., et al.: Laparoscopic living donor hepatectomy for liver transplantation in children. Lancet **359**(9304), 392–396 (2002)
10. Kurokawa, T., Inagaki, H., Sakamoto, J., et al.: Hand-assisted laparoscopic anatomical left lobectomy using hemihepatic vascular control technique. Surg. Endosc. **16**(11), 1637–1638 (2002)
11. Samama, G., Chiche, L., Brefort, J.L., et al.: Laparoscopic anatomical hepatic resection. Report of four left lobectomies for solid tumors. Surg. Endosc. **12**(1), 76–78 (1998)
12. Matsumata, T., Kanematsu, T., Takenaka, K., et al.: Lack of intrahepatic recurrence of hepatocellular carcinoma by temporary portal venous embolization with starch microspheres. Surgery **105**(2 Pt 1), 188–191 (1989)
13. Mizoe, A., Tomioka, T., Inoue, K., et al.: Systematic laparoscopic left lateral segmentectomy of the liver for hepatocellular carcinoma. J. Hepatobiliary Pancreat. Surg. **5**(2), 173–178 (1998)
14. Tsuruta, K., Okamoto, A., Toi, M., et al.: Impact of selective Glisson transection on survival of hepatocellular carcinoma. Hepatogastroenterology **49**(48), 1607–1610 (2002)
15. Ikai, I., Itai, Y., Okita, K., et al.: Report of the 15th follow-up survey of primary liver cancer. Hepatol. Res. **28**(1), 21–29 (2004)
16. Geoghegan, J.G., Scheele, J.: Treatment of colorectal liver metastases. Br. J. Surg. **86**(2), 158–169 (1999)
17. Mala, T., Edwin, B., Gladhaug, I., et al.: A comparative study of the short-term outcome following open and laparoscopic liver resection of colorectal metastases. Surg. Endosc. **16**(7), 1059–1063 (2002)
18. Han, K.H., Lee, J.T., Seong, J.: Treatment of non-resectable hepatocellular carcinoma. J. Gastroenterol. Hepatol. **17**(Suppl 3), S424–S427 (2002)
19. Park, J.Y., Ahn, S.H., Yoon, Y.J., et al.: Repetitive short-course hepatic arterial infusion chemotherapy with high-dose 5-fluorouracil and cisplatin in patients with advanced hepatocellular carcinoma. Cancer **110**(1), 129–137 (2007)
20. Fan, J., Wu, Z.Q., Tang, Z.Y., et al.: Multimodality treatment in hepatocellular carcinoma patients with tumor thrombi in portal vein. World J. Gastroenterol. **7**(1), 28–32 (2001)
21. Poon, R.T., Fan, S.T., Ng, I.O., et al.: Prognosis after hepatic resection for stage IVA hepatocellular carcinoma: a need for reclassification. Ann. Surg. **237**(3), 376–383 (2003)
22. Ueno, K., Miyazono, N., Inoue, H., et al.: Transcatheter arterial chemoembolization therapy using iodized oil for patients with unresectable hepatocellular carcinoma: evaluation of three kinds of regimens and analysis of prognostic factors. Cancer **88**(7), 1574–1581 (2000)
23. Yamamoto, T., Nagano, H., Imai, Y., et al.: Successful treatment of multiple hepatocellular carcinoma with tumor thrombi in the major portal branches by intraarterial 5-fluorouracil perfusion chemotherapy combined with subcutaneous interferon-alpha and hepatectomy. Int. J. Clin. Oncol. **12**(2), 150–154 (2007)
24. Ando, E., Tanaka, M., Yamashita, F., et al.: Hepatic arterial infusion chemotherapy for advanced hepatocellular carcinoma with portal vein tumor thrombosis: analysis of 48 cases. Cancer **95**(3), 588–595 (2002)
25. Tabuse, K.: Basic knowledge of a microwave tissue coagulator and its clinical applications. J. Hepatobiliary Pancreat. Surg. **5**(2), 165–172 (1998)
26. Sadamori, H., Yagi, T., Kanaoka, Y., et al.: The analysis of the usefulness of laparoscopic microwave coagulation therapy for hepatocellular carcinoma in patients with poor hepatic reserve by serial measurements of IL-6, cytokine antagonists, and C-reactive protein. Surg. Endosc. **17**(3), 510–514 (2003)
27. Seki, S., Sakaguchi, H., Kadoya, H., et al.: Laparoscopic microwave coagulation therapy for hepatocellular carcinoma. Endoscopy **32**(8), 591–597 (2000)
28. Yamanaka, N., Okamoto, E., Tanaka, T., et al.: Laparoscopic microwave coagulonecrotic therapy for hepatocellular carcinoma. Surg. Laparosc. Endosc. **5**(6), 444–449 (1995)
29. Mahnken, A.H., Buecker, A., Spuentrup, E., et al.: MR-guided radiofrequency ablation of hepatic malignancies at 1.5 T: initial results. J. Magn. Reson. Imaging **19**(3), 342–348 (2004)
30. Allgaier, H.P., Deibert, P., Zuber, I., et al.: Percutaneous radiofrequency interstitial thermal ablation of small hepatocellular carcinoma. Lancet **353**(9165), 1676–1677 (1999)
31. Livraghi, T., Goldberg, S.N., Lazzaroni, S., et al.: Small hepatocellular carcinoma: treatment with radio-frequency

ablation versus ethanol injection. Radiology **210**(3), 655–661 (1999)
32. Gugenheim, J., Mazza, D., Katkhouda, N., et al.: Laparoscopic resection of solid liver tumours. Br. J. Surg. **83**(3), 334–335 (1996)
33. Huang, M.T., Lee, W.J., Wang, W., et al.: Hand-assisted laparoscopic hepatectomy for solid tumor in the posterior portion of the right lobe: initial experience. Ann. Surg. **238**(5), 674–679 (2003)
34. Antonetti, M.C., Killelea, B., Orlando 3rd, R.: Hand-assisted laparoscopic liver surgery. Arch. Surg. **137**(4), 407–411 (2002)
35. Cherqui, D., Husson, E., Hammoud, R., et al.: Laparoscopic liver resections: a feasibility study in 30 patients. Ann. Surg. **232**(6), 753–762 (2000)
36. Fong, Y., Jarnagin, W., Conlon, K.C., et al.: Hand-assisted laparoscopic liver resection: lessons from an initial experience. Arch. Surg. **135**(7), 854–859 (2000)
37. Moskop Jr., R.J., Lubarsky, D.A.: Carbon dioxide embolism during laparoscopic cholecystectomy. South Med. J. **87**(3), 414–415 (1994)
38. Schmandra, T.C., Mierdl, S., Bauer, H., et al.: Transoesophageal echocardiography shows high risk of gas embolism during laparoscopic hepatic resection under carbon dioxide pneumoperitoneum. Br. J. Surg. **89**(7), 870–876 (2002)
39. Takagi, S.: Hepatic and portal vein blood flow during carbon dioxide pneumoperitoneum for laparoscopic hepatectomy. Surg. Endosc. **12**(5), 427–431 (1998)
40. Di Carlo, I., Barbagallo, F., Toro, A., et al.: Hepatic resections using a water-cooled, high-density, monopolar device: a new technology for safer surgery. J. Gastrointest. Surg. **8**(5), 596–600 (2004)
41. Yacoub, O.F., Cardona Jr., I., Coveler, L.A., et al.: Carbon dioxide embolism during laparoscopy. Anesthesiology **57**(6), 533–535 (1982)
42. Watanabe, Y., Sato, M., Ueda, S., et al.: Laparoscopic hepatic resection: a new and safe procedure by abdominal wall lifting method. Hepatogastroenterology **44**(13), 143–147 (1997)
43. Paolucci, V., Schaeff, B., Schneider, M., et al.: Tumor seeding following laparoscopy: international survey. World J. Surg. **23**(10), 989–995 (1999)
44. Pearlstone, D.B., Feig, B.W., Mansfield, P.F.: Port site recurrences after laparoscopy for malignant disease. Semin. Surg. Oncol. **16**(4), 307–312 (1999)
45. Schaeff, B., Paolucci, V., Thomopoulos, J.: Port site recurrences after laparoscopic surgery. A review. Dig. Surg. **15**(2), 124–134 (1998)
46. Shoup, M., Brennan, M.F., Karpeh, M.S., et al.: Port site metastasis after diagnostic laparoscopy for upper gastrointestinal tract malignancies: an uncommon entity. Ann. Surg. Oncol. **9**(7), 632–636 (2002)
47. Whelan, R.L.: Laparotomy, laparoscopy, cancer, and beyond. Surg. Endosc. **15**(2), 110–115 (2001)
48. Lang, B.H., Poon, R.T., Fan, S.T., et al.: Influence of laparoscopy on postoperative recurrence and survival in patients with ruptured hepatocellular carcinoma undergoing hepatic resection. Br. J. Surg. **91**(4), 444–449 (2004)
49. Vittimberga Jr., F.J., Foley, D.P., Meyers, W.C., et al.: Laparoscopic surgery and the systemic immune response. Ann. Surg. **227**(3), 326–334 (1998)
50. Topp, S.A., McClurken, M., Lipson, D., et al.: Saline-linked surface radiofrequency ablation: factors affecting steam popping and depth of injury in the pig liver. Ann. Surg. **239**(4), 518–527 (2004)
51. Sundaram, C.P., Rehman, J., Venkatesh, R., et al.: Hemostatic laparoscopic partial nephrectomy assisted by a water-cooled, high-density, monopolar device without renal vascular control. Urology **61**(5), 906–909 (2003)
52. Cuschieri, A.: Laparoscopic hand-assisted surgery for hepatic and pancreatic disease. Surg. Endosc. **14**(11), 991–996 (2000)
53. Inagaki, H., Kurokawa, T., Nonami, T., et al.: Hand-assisted laparoscopic left lateral segmentectomy of the liver for hepatocellular carcinoma with cirrhosis. J. Hepatobiliary Pancreat. Surg. **10**(4), 295–298 (2003)

Liver – Anatomical Liver Resections

Bruto Randone, Ronald Matteotti, and Brice Gayet

22.1 Introduction

The first footsteps in the field of laparoscopic liver surgery were marked by wedge resections limited to the marginal and anterior regions of the organ [1–3].

Since then, more technically demanding procedures have been performed with efficacy and safety equaling outcomes in open surgery when performed in highly specialized centers [4–6] (Table 22.1).

To propose laparoscopy as a valid and definitive alternative to open access in liver surgery, though, the feasibility of anatomical resections had to be established.

This has been now accomplished in centers with a solid expertise in hepato-biliary surgery and laparoscopic techniques [7–13].

This exciting evolution in minimally invasive liver surgery is the result of technological advances and modifications in laparoscopic equipment coupled with progression in surgical skills. Routine use of preoperative imaging like computed tomography (CT) scans, magnetic resonance imaging (MRI) or intra-operative ultrasound (US) contributed greatly to diagnostic accuracy and planning of the resection. Improved anesthesia and critical care was essential in having good outcomes.

22.2 Indications for Laparoscopic Liver Resection

Indications for laparoscopic resections in malignancies are nowadays practically comparable to the ones applied to open resections. In cases of benign tumors, indications should not be overstretched because of laparoscopic feasibility. According to the *Louisville Statement on Laparoscopic Liver Surgery*, the best indication for a laparoscopic approach is a solitary lesion, 5 cm or less in size, located on the anterior segments II–VI [14].

Although the laparoscopic approach to the posterior segments I, IVa, VII and VIII is not universally accepted as a good indication, our group has a solid experience in this type of resections (Fig. 22.1). In our department tumors larger than 5 cm in size, tumors centrally located or in contiguity with major hepatic veins or the inferior vena cava (IVC), as well multifocality are no longer contraindications to surgical therapy. We assure that there is enough hepatic reserve and use selective portal vein embolization if necessary. In cirrhotic patients 40% of remaining liver parenchyma is considered to be a sufficient hepatic reserve. In non-cirrhotic patients or patients with small livers, 25–30% of liver parenchyma is considered to be enough functional tissue. Attention should be paid, when considering remnant liver volume, to parenchyma alterations following chemotherapy as *steatofibrosis* or sinusoidal obstructive syndrome, the so-called yellow and blue liver, could develop.

22.2.1 Main Indications for Anatomical Liver Resection

- Primary malignant tumors
- Isolated metastases or multiple metastases confined to one lobe

---

B. Randone and B. Gayet (✉)
Department of Digestive Pathology, Institut Mutualiste Montsouris, Université Paris Descartes, 42 Bd Jourdan, 75014 Paris, France
e-mail: bruto.randone@imm.fr; brice.gayet@imm.fr

R. Matteotti
Surgical Oncologist/Minimally Invasive Surgeon,
263 Osborn Street, Philadelphia, PA 19128, USA
e-mail: ronald.matteotti@gmail.com

Table 22.1 Laparoscopic versus Open approach for liver resection: Major hepatectomies

	Year	n	Malignancies (%)	Major hepatectomies (n/%)
Sasaki et al. [48]	2009	82	93	0
Buell et al. [12]	2008	253	42	62/24
Cho et al. [45]	2008	128	61	36/28
Chen et al. [13]	2008	116	100	4/3.5
Topal et al. [49]	2008	109	71	21/19
Koffron et al. [17]	2007	273	37	96/35
Dagher et al. [11]	2007	70	54	19/27
Cai et al. [44]	2006	62	32	2/3
Vibert et al. [8]	2006	89	73	38/43
Mala et al. [47]	2005	53	89	0
Descottes et al. [46]	2003	87	0	3/3.5

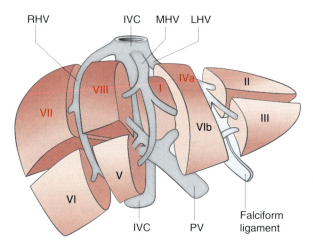

Fig. 22.1 The liver segments are the basis of anatomical resections and are classified (According to Couinaud). Posterior segments are displayed in *red*. RHV right hepatic vein; IVC inferior vena cava; MHV middle hepatic vein; LHV left hepatic vein; PV portal vein. (Drawing by Hippmann GbR, Schwarzenbruck, Germany)

- Benign lesions
- Living-donor resection for transplant

Reduced intra-operative bleeding, higher rates of negative margins in the surgical specimen and better visualization are only a few observed benefits due to which surgeons adopted a laparoscopic approach to the liver.

22.2.2 Primary Liver Tumors and Hepatocellular Carcinoma (HCC)

Surgical resection is considered the primary treatment for hepatocellular carcinoma (HCC) in compensated cirrhotic patients because of the shortage of liver allografts. Anatomic resections are demonstrated to assure lower recurrence rates and longer survival when compared to wedge resections [15]. Moreover, in cirrhotic patients, laparoscopic resection is associated with lower morbidity because of reduced postoperative ascites production and lower rates of liver failure. This is in part explained by preservation of portosystemic venous collaterals running along the abdominal wall and reduced liver trauma from less manipulation of the organ using laparoscopy only [16].

22.2.3 Role of Laparoscopy in Liver Transplants

Laparoscopic resection can also be performed to bridge a patient before a transplantable organ becomes available. Transplantation is often seen as a salvage procedure in case of recurrence and might be possible in 50% of the cases. A laparoscopic approach to resect a liver tumor prior to transplantation is particularly of interest because of fewer postoperative adhesions and lesser morbidity compared to an open procedure.

22.2.4 Radiofrequency Ablation (RFA) Versus Resection in HCC

Radiofrequency ablation (RFA) may be a valid alternative to resection for solitary HCC smaller than 3 cm in diameter. At our institution we prefer a resection over an RFA because of the possibility to assess histology and identify markers of aggressiveness, such as microvascular invasion, satellite nodules and grade of differentiation. These histological findings, if present, will greatly affect outcome and possibly result in tumor recurrence.

Laparoscopic major liver resections offer the same benefits over open surgery as other minimally invasive surgical procedures: less pain, better cosmetics, shorter length of hospital stay and faster return to everyday activities.

Gas embolism during laparoscopic liver resections has been the greatest fear in the recent past. This is thought to be less dramatic because CO_2 has a greater solubility when compared to nitrogen. If suspected, an intra-operative trans-esophageal echocardiography can be obtained and the insufflation should be stopped immediately because of the risk of resulting arrhythmias and hemodynamic instability.

22.3 Different Approaches to Minimally Invasive Liver Surgery

Laparoscopic procedures in liver surgery can be divided into three main categories [17]:

- Total laparoscopic approach
- Hand-assisted approach
- Hybrid technique

In applying a total laparoscopic approach, the entire resection of the liver is completed through ports. One port site is enlarged for specimen extraction at the end of the procedure. Hand-assisted technique utilizes a hand-port device to perform the resection, for easier manipulation of anatomical structures and to retrieve the specimen at the end of the procedure. The pneumoperitoneum stays established at all times. If the procedure is started laparoscopically but the actual resection performed through a mini-laparotomy, then we call it a hybrid procedure.

We perform almost exclusively a total laparoscopic approach even for major hepatectomies. If the preoperative work-up demonstrates extensive disease with suspected vena cava invasion, then we place a hand-port device proximal to the umbilicus at the beginning of the operation. This allows us to control major bleeding by applying manual compression and for a fast conversion to an open procedure in the event this becomes necessary. We believe that every attempt should be made to control major bleeding laparoscopically prior to a conversion in order to avoid excessive blood loss exaggerated by the laparotomy itself. If the hand-port is not utilized during resection, it will be adopted for specimen extraction at the end of the procedure.

Laparoscopic liver resections can be divided into three levels according to technical difficulty:

- Biopsies and small-wedge resections
- Left lateral segment and the anterior segments II, III, IVb, V, VI
- Hemihepatectomies, trisegmentectomies and the posterior segments I, IVa, VII, VIII

The mainstay of anatomical liver resections consists of the delineation of a proper dissection plane which starts with critical appraisal of the preoperative contrast CT scan to define the relationship between the tumor and the major intra-hepatic vessels or bile duct pedicles and is further evaluated intra-operatively by US.

22.4 The Role of Intra-operative Ultrasound in Liver Surgery

Without knowledge of the relationship between the tumor and the major intra-hepatic structures, unexpected damage can occur during resection, leading to massive bleeding, bile duct injury or tumor exposure at the dissection plane.

Intra-operative US of the liver should be considered as an integral part of any liver surgery, since it provides vital information to the surgeon during the procedure which may affect surgical decision making. It permits detection of accessory tumors not visualized on routine preoperative cross-sectional imaging, and helps to clarify the relationship between tumor and vascular structures. US is crucial in defining the anatomical limits of a planned resection based on the relationship between portal pedicles and hepatic veins according to Coineaud's segments. It is a great tool to establish the proper dissection plane. When an intravascular thrombus is identified, it permits the surgeon to distinguish between a tumor-associated thrombus that is avascular and a tumor thrombus that has an arterial waveform upon pulsed Doppler evaluation. Intra-operative US also allows distinguishing between vessel invasion and vessel occlusion. Tumor invasion into a major vessel is usually a contraindication to resection. Intra-operative US has been shown to supply additional information in up to 38% of surgical procedures [18]. Intra-operative ultrasound compared to preoperative contrast-enhanced MRI has a much higher tumor detection rate for liver lesion, 94% versus 86% respectively [19]. Furthermore, different studies concluded that intra-operative US will change clinical management in up to 50% of patients undergoing hepatic resection for malignancy [20, 21].

22.5 Laparoscopic Liver Surgery in Malignancy

During the last decade, laparoscopic liver surgery has proven itself to be a valid alternative to open surgery [7, 22].

One of the first studies, a retrospective, multicenter study conducted in 2003 in 11 European surgical centers, looked at the role of laparoscopic liver resections for malignant tumors [23]. Limitations of that study were the small sample number of only 37 patients, the type of resections performed and tumor location. Only two major hepatectomies were included and 89% of all the tumors were located in the left or anterior right lobe of the liver. Conversion from laparoscopy to laparotomy was necessary in 10–20% of all reported cases.

In the last 5 years increasing literature on laparoscopic liver resections was published and especially more cases of anatomical and major liver resections were reported (Table 22.2).

Our group published in 2004 the first series of laparoscopic liver surgery reporting exclusively on anatomical resections in 46 patients [24]. Eighty percent of the patients suffered from a malignant lesion. We included 26 major hepatectomies (56%) and found that perioperative and postoperative results were comparable to previous series which included a lower rate of anatomical resections.

The most important single-center experience in laparoscopic liver resection was reported by Northwestern University in Chicago [17]: 300 anatomical resections, 110 segmentectomies, 63 bisegmentectomies, 47 left hepatectomies, 64 right hepatectomies including 20 living donor-related interventions, 8 extended right hepatectomies and 8 caudate lobe resections. A total laparoscopic approach was used in 241 cases, a hand-assisted approach in 32 cases and a hybrid approach in 27 patients. Only one third of these resections were performed for malignancy. A matched-pair analysis was done adding 100 open liver resections. Minimally invasive resections compared favorably with the open group in terms of operative time (99 vs. 182 min), blood loss (102 vs. 325 mL), transfusion requirement (2 out of 300 vs. 8 out of 100), length of stay (1.9 vs. 5.4 days) and overall operative complications (9.3% vs. 22%). Complications in the laparoscopic group were mainly biliary leaks. There was no ascites, liver failure or port-site recurrence in the laparoscopic group. Conversions from a total laparoscopic to a hand-assisted approach occurred in 6% of cases. In the hybrid group 7% of the patients required a conversion to a laparotomy. There was no difference between the two groups when looking at recurrence rates, supporting the equality of the two techniques from an oncological point of view.

In the largest series of minimally invasive hepatic procedures published, Buell et al. described 590 procedures in 489 interventions [12]. Of these interventions, 253 were anatomical resections: there were 72 segmentectomies, 64 resections of two or more segments, 42 left lateral lobectomies and 69 major hepatectomies. Resections for malignant lesions accounted for 42% of the patients and cirrhosis was present in 12% of the liver specimens. The rest of the hepatic procedures were laparoscopic RFAs and explorations with

Table 22.2 Largest series of laparoscopic liver resections: Comparison with open resections

	Year	Patients Lap/open	OR time (min)	Blood loss (ml)	Length of stay (d)	Morbidity (%)
Gayet and Castaing [29] ccs	2009	60 vs. 60	278 vs. 294	NA	10 vs. 11	27 vs. 28
Cai et al. [51] ccs	2008	31 vs. 31	140 vs. 152	503 vs. 588	7.5 vs. 7.2	0 vs.16
Lee et al. [52] ccs	2007	25 vs. 25	220 vs. 195	100 vs. 250 s	4 vs. 7 s	4 vs. 4
Troisi et al [53] ccs	2008	20 vs. 20	220 vs. 242	NA	7.1 vs. 10.4 s	20 vs. 45
Polignano et al. [54] ccs	2008	25 vs. 25	362 vs. 366	135 vs. 420 s	7.4 vs. 13.1 s	12 vs. 40 s
Aldrighetti et al.[55] ccs	2008	20 vs. 20	260 vs. 220	165 vs. 214 s	4.5 vs. 5.8 s	10 vs. 25
Topal et al. [49] ccs	2008	76 vs. 76	NA	150 vs. 300 s	6 vs. 8 s	8 vs. 32 s
Koffron et al. [17]	2007	273 vs. 100	99 vs. 182	102 vs. 325	1.9 vs. 5.4	9 vs. 22
Belli et al. [56] ccs	2007	23 vs. 23	148 vs. 125 s	260 vs. 377	8.2 vs. 12	13 vs. 48 s
Simillis et al. [30] ma	2007	165 vs. 244	NS	−123 s	−2.6 s	12 vs. 17
Laurent et al. [16] ccs	2003	13 vs. 14	267 vs. 182 s	620 vs. 720	15.3 vs. 17.3	36 vs. 50
Morino et al. [28] ccs	2003	30 vs. 30	148 vs. 142	320 vs. 479	6.4 vs. 8.7 s	7 vs. 7
Lesurtel et al. [25] ccs	2003	18 vs. 20	202 vs. 145 s	236 vs. 429 s	8 vs. 10	11 vs. 15
Farges et al. [26] ccs	2002	21 vs. 21	177 vs. 156	218 vs. 285	5.1 vs. 6.5	10 vs. 10
Rau et al. [50] ccs	1998	17 vs. 17	184 vs. 128 s	458 vs. 556	7.8 vs. 11.6 s	6 vs. 6

ccs Case control study, ma Meta analysis, s Significant difference ($p < 0.05$), *NA* not available, *NS* not significant biopsies to establish a diagnosis. Results were compared to modern cohorts of open liver resections. In comparison with other case series, laparoscopic liver resections were associated with reduced operative time, reduced blood loss, less complications, lower transfusion rate and shorter hospital stay. The rate of bile leaks and local tumor recurrence were comparable with the open groups.

There is, in fact, no prospective comparison between open and laparoscopic hepatectomies but different case control series have been reported [16, 25–29]. Advantages of a laparoscopic approach over open surgery are uniformly reported in these different studies and included mainly less blood loss, less narcotic usage and shorter hospital stay. Morbidity and the rate of close tumor margins (<1 cm) are comparable between the two groups.

Only one meta-analysis comparing the two approaches has been published so far and is based on eight series including 409 resections [30]. Forty percent of the procedures were completed laparoscopically. No significant difference between the two groups was identified in terms of transfusion requirement, operative time, length of Pringle maneuver and obtaining of adequate margins. There was no significant difference in complication rates. Intra-operative blood loss, length of hospital stay and time to oral intake were decreased with laparoscopy. Three of these studies included a long-term follow-up and overall and disease-free survival at 5 years was comparable in the two groups.

These findings support the initial hypothesis of a laparoscopic procedure to be oncologically equivalent, if not superior, to an open procedure, when taking into account all the added benefits of a minimally invasive procedure itself.

22.6 Surgical Approach

22.6.1 Preoperative Evaluation

Resectability is assessed preoperatively by either US, CT scan or MRI. If metastatic disease is suspected, we add a positron emission tomography (PET) scan. Any imaging obtained will be carefully analyzed to define the relationship between the target lesion, major intrahepatic vessels and bile ducts. Based on this evaluation we determine a surgical strategy. In patients with large tumors of the right or left lobe it is mandatory to identify the middle hepatic vein in order to decide whether an extended left or right hepatectomy will be necessary. The proximity of the target lesion to the right or left main hepatic vein may influence the decision to perform a hepatectomy instead of a segmentectomy.

We obtain a 3D reconstruction of the vascular supply for all lesions close to the hepatic or portal veins (Fig. 22.2). As a first step of every attempted hepatic resection we perform an intra-operative US to finally decide about the type of resection to be performed and especially to assess resectability once more.

22.6.2 Operating Room Setup and Equipment

We use a high-definition camera (EndoEye HD®, Olympus) and two monitors, placed at the head side of the table. The insufflation device and video system are located on a platform suspended from the ceiling for better ergonomics (Video system Exera II®, Olympus). All monitors and the devices on the platform are coordinated by a computerized system (Advanced Endo Alpha®). The camera is mounted to a voice-controlled robotic arm (AESOP 3000®; Intuitive Surgical Inc, CA; and Vicky®; Endocontrol-medical, France). A flexible laparoscopic US probe with color-flow Doppler capability is used routinely for the reasons mentioned above. The image of the intra-operative US (Super Focus®, BK medical) can be displayed directly on the surgeon's monitor using picture-in-picture (PIP) technology. Standard laparoscopic instruments and a self-retaining liver retractor are used. As a transaction or dissection tool we found it very useful to combine any type of ultrasonic dissector (Harmonic ACE®, Ethicon or Sonosurg®, Olympus) with bipolar cautery forceps. The bipolar cautery forceps is utilized for hemostasis but also for dissection and identification of vascular branches in a sort of "gentle clamp and crush" technique. Laparoscopic vascular linear staplers (Endo-GIA®, Covidien) are useful to divide hepatic veins and

22 Liver – Anatomical Liver Resections

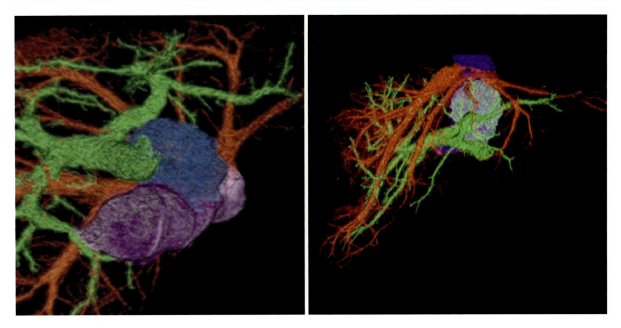

Fig. 22.2 CT scan with 3D vascular reconstructions. The tumor (*blue*) is located in segment I, in close contact with the anterior aspect of the IVC (*red*: hepatic veins; *green*: portal triad; *violet*: IVC)

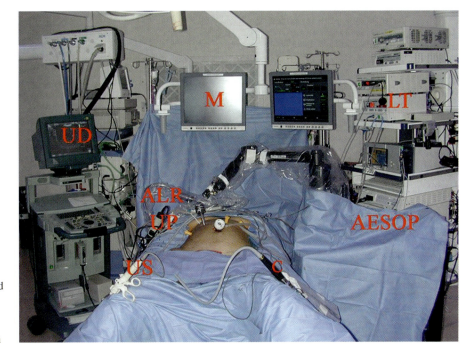

Fig. 22.3 Operating room setup and equipment. *M* high-definition monitor, *UD* ultrasound cart, *ALR* autostatic liver retractor, *AESOP* robotically controlled camera holder, *LT* laparoscopic tower, *UP* laparoscopic ultrasound probe, *USS* ultrasonic shears system

occasionally portal structures. A hand-port device (Gel port, Applied Medical®, CA, USA) is readily available in the operating room. A wound protector (Vi-Drape, Medical Concepts Development®, MN, USA) is routinely used to protect the abdominal wall during the specimen extraction (Fig. 22.3).

22.6.3 Patient Positioning

The patient is placed supine in a low lithotomy position (Fig. 22.4). The arms are placed along the sides of the patient and are tucked. The upper portion of the trunk is strapped securely to the table to permit reverse Trendelenburg position. The holder for the liver retractor is placed on the patient's right, and the robotic holder for the camera on the left side of the operating room table. The surgeon stands between the patient's legs, the assistant positions himself or herself at the patient's left side while the scrub nurse stands at the right side. Central venous pressure (CVP) is monitored during the intervention. For lesions localized in the right lobe of the liver, we prefer elevating the right upper portion of the abdomen with pads.

22.6.4 Trocar Placement

Trocar placement in laparoscopic liver surgery varies with type of resection and patient anatomy. We usually use a configuration of six trocars. Initially we establish pneumoperitoneum using a Veress needle and maintain it at 12 mmHg. The first trocar, a 12-mm port, is placed to the right of the umbilicus and slightly superior to it. This port will be used for the camera and is ideally located between the mid-clavicular line and the midline. To place this first trocar we elevate the pneumoperitoneum temporarily to 20 mmHg. Two 5-mm trocars are placed on the right and on the left of the camera port and used as primary working channels. Another 5-mm trocar is placed inferior to the left costal margin and is used by the first assistant. We place two additional ports inferior to the right costal margin, a 5-mm port for the liver retractor on the anterior axillary line and a 12-mm port on the mid-clavicular line. The two 12-mm ports will be used alternatively for stapling devices, US probe or camera placement (Fig. 22.5).

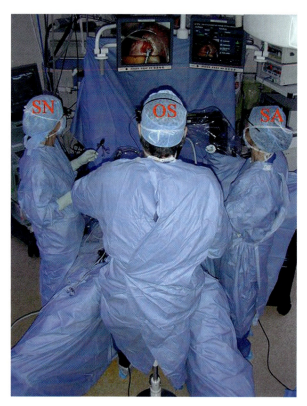

Fig. 22.4 Positioning of patient and operating room personnel. The patient is placed supine in split leg technique and reverse Trendelenburg. The operating surgeon (OS) stands between the legs of the patient, the surgical assistant (AS) stands to the left of the patient and the scrub nurse (SN) on the patient's right. The anesthesia team (A) is at the head of the table

22.6.5 Special Considerations for Anesthesia

One of the most important advances in liver surgery in recent years is the practice of low CVP anesthesia. This is achieved by a combination of fluid restriction, diuretics, vasodilatators, low-pressure and high-frequency ventilation, and anesthetic agents such as Isoflurane that produce vasodilatation. The CVP should ideally be lowered to <5 mmHg, provided that the patient remains hemodynamically stable. Low CVP anesthesia is usually well tolerated by patients. It is more effective in reducing intra-operative blood loss than total vascular occlusion. A recent randomized

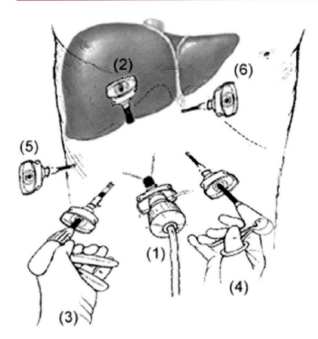

Fig. 22.5 Trocar placement. A combination of two 12-mm trocars and four 5-mm trocars is used

controlled trial involving 50 patients with either low (2–4 mmHg) or normal CVP showed that the use of low CVP during transection of the liver parenchyma led to a significant reduction in intra-operative blood loss and length of hospital stay [31]. The real factor influencing intra-operative blood loss is the actual volemic state of the patient. The CVP alone is not a reliable value to assess the intravascular volume of the patient because of its frequent changes due to alteration in intra-abdominal pressure induced by the pneumoperitoneum. In our opinion the best way to monitor a low volemic state remains direct visualization of the IVC, which should be half empty and "breathe" along with the cyclic variations of intra-thoracic pressure.

22.7 Intra-operative Ultrasound

22.7.1 General Remarks

As a first step, in all our cases, we perform a diagnostic laparoscopy to exclude carcinomatosis and hepatic or porto-caval lymph node involvement. If stage 4 disease can be excluded, we move ahead with an intra-operative US.

The objectives of intra-operative US are

- Defining the anatomy of the different segments in relationship to intra-hepatic vascular and biliary structures
- Localizing the target lesion
- Detecting additional lesions missed on preoperative imaging
- Finalizing surgical strategy and extent of resection

We think that this intra-operative imaging is the most crucial step in making any surgical decision in liver surgery, no matter how the surgery is performed, laparoscopically or open. Therefore any hepato-biliary surgeon has to master this technique in order to make sound intra-operative decisions.

22.7.2 Technique and Major Steps

To facilitate this step and to gain access especially to the dome of the liver we preferably excise the falciform ligament. If a decision is made to go ahead with resection, we recommend repeating the US after mobilizing the liver to identify artifacts due to air.

The surgical anatomy of the liver is defined by the intersection of hepatic veins and portal pedicles. Initially we place the probe on segment IV and angle the transducer toward the heart to identify the confluence of the major hepatic veins and the IVC. We follow these veins out to their terminal branches in both lobes. Do not put too much pressure on the probe, otherwise these veins will disappear. Any anomalous hepatic vein is noted as well as eventual vascular involvement by the tumor. By tilting the transducer inferiorly, the main portal vein is identified at the base of segment IV and its division in the right and left portal branches is found. The right portal branch is then followed distally until it divides into the anterior (segments V and VIII) and posterior (segments VI and VII) branches. Portal pedicles can easily be recognized by US. Once they enter the liver they are surrounded by the Glissonian capsule, which creates a hyper-echogenic zone around the pedicle. The anterior and posterior branches are followed to their superior or inferior segmental branches. The left portal branch is then visualized at the base of the umbilical fissure as it turns anteriorly toward the probe. As it ascends in the umbilical fissure, it has the appearance of a tree trunk with branches extending to the right and the left. The branches to the right of the falciform ligament supply segment IV, while vessels going to the left of the falciform ligament supply segment III and II [32]. Once the segmental anatomy is verified, we perform a systematic scanning of the entire parenchyma with multiple overlapping sagittal sweeps of the transducer. Known lesions are confirmed and localized in relationship to major vessels. Additional hepatic neoplasms will be noted. If a right hepatectomy is planned, particular attention is paid to the drainage of segment VIII. The outflow vein of segment VIII might end directly at the IVC or at the middle vein close to its confluence with a course adjacent to the IVC within the parenchyma.

22.8 Parenchyma Dissection – Different Techniques

Clamp crushing and ultrasonic dissection are the two most widely used dissection techniques in open surgery. In recent years, new instruments using different types of energy to coagulate or to seal vessels have become available. These include radiofrequency devices, Harmonic Scalpel®, Ligasure®, EnSeal® and TissueLink™® dissecting sealer. As with open surgery, no single method of parenchyma dissection has been shown to be superior to others, mostly because the result of each dissection technique fluctuates significantly with the individual surgeon's experience [33]. Other techniques of liver dissection, like water-jet or radiofrequency-assisted devices exist but are at the current stage reserved for open surgery.

When comparing different devices for liver resection, parameters to be considered should be

- Efficacy in sealing vascular structures with low blood loss
- Efficacy in sealing bile ducts with a low rate of bile leaks
- Relative speed of dissection
- Potential complications
- Costs

Currently the only available randomized controlled trials concern the open approach [34].

22.8.1 The CUSA® System

With ultrasonic dissection (CUSA®, Radionics, Burlington, MA), the liver parenchyma is fragmented and aspirated, thus exposing vascular and biliary structures that can be ligated or clipped. The preferred clip in our hands is a titanium hemoclip.

22.8.2 Harmonic Scalpel® and Sonosurg®

Ultrasonic shears (Harmonic Scalpel®, Ethicon Endosurgery, Cincinnati, USA; Sonosurg®, Olympus medical Systems, JA) use ultrasonically activated shears to seal small vessels between the vibrating blades. A frequency of 55.5 kHz permits to dissect liver parenchyma. The sealing effect on vessels is due to protein coagulation and is applicable to blood vessels up to 3 mm in diameter. This device is commonly used in laparoscopic liver resection. The Sonosurg® shears are equipped with an automatic aspiration device which considerably reduces "fog" during laparoscopic resections. There are still concerns about the efficacy of sealing bile ducts [35, 36]. In our experience, the harmonic scalpel is a great device to reduce bile leaks at the cut edge of the liver.

22.8.3 Ligasure®

Ligasure® (Valley Lab, Tyco Healthcare, Boulder, CO, USA) seals small vessels by a combination of mechanical compression and bipolar radiofrequency energy. It causes collagen and elastin shrinkage in the vessel wall. It is effective in sealing small vessels up to 7 mm in diameter. Similarly to Ultracision, there is still some concern regarding its capability of sealing bile ducts and the results in the literature are controversial [37, 38]. It is useful when dissecting cirrhotic livers, where the ultrasonic dissector (CUSA®) is usually less effective.

22.8.4 TissueLink™

The TissueLink™ device (Tissuelink Medical, Inc, Dover, NH, USA) uses saline solution which runs to the tip of the electrode to couple electric energy to the liver surface and achieve coagulation. The device has a pointed tip that allows dissection and sealing of vessels and bile ducts simultaneously. Currently there are only preliminary experiences reported in the literature [39].

22.8.5 EnSeal®

The EnSeal® vessel fusion system (SurgRx Inc, Redwood City, CA) is a bipolar instrument that combines a high-compression jaw with a tissue dynamic energy delivery mechanism. The tissue impedance feed-back is monitored, so each tissue type receives a different energy dose. In comparison with other sealing and cutting devices, EnSeal® showed less radial thermal damage to the adventitial collagen of the vessels, but the highest bursting pressure [40]. It is recommended for vessels up to 7 mm in diameter.

22.8.6 Stapling Devices

Vascular staplers are mostly applied to divide the major trunk of hepatic veins and less frequently to transect portal pedicles. Some surgeons, especially in the United States, utilize them to directly divide liver parenchyma. The use of staplers for this purpose loses its efficacy if the liver is fibrotic. Once again, a problem associated with the use of stapling devices for liver dissection is the increased risk of bile leaks, since the stapler is not very effective in sealing small bile ducts. This could potentially be overcome by using staple reinforcement material.

22.8.7 Personal Technique

In our institution, we have adopted the combined use of a bipolar forceps and ultrasonic shears for parenchyma dissection. The ultrasonic shears are controlled by the dominant hand and the bipolar forceps by the opposite hand. At the surface, near the capsule of the liver, we predominantly use ultrasonic shears. The bipolar forceps is used simultaneously in the event the harmonic scalpel fails to seal small vessels. While getting deeper into the liver parenchyma, the bipolar forceps takes more relevant action and leads the dissection with a gentle "clamp and crush" technique while coagulating. The ultrasonic shears are used to transect or can participate in dissection with the active blade in the open position. Keep in mind that the active blade of the Sonosurg® shears has a very low cutting effect when used alone.

We no longer use and would not recommend the ultrasonic dissector because the combination of irrigation and aspiration reduces visibility and deflates the pneumoperitoneum constantly.

Whatever device is used meticulous hemostasis should be obtained to maintain a good visualization and to recognize important vascular structures.

22.9 Specimen Removal

The specimen is placed into an impermeable endobag and removed from the abdomen through either a suprapubic incision or a previously performed abdominal incision. If a hand-port is used for the procedure, it will be utilized for specimen removal. In the case of dense adhesions in the pelvis we will use another site for extraction. We always use a wound protector to avoid tumor seeding. Once the specimen is extracted we will close the incision and reestablish the pneumoperitoneum.

22.10 Leak Test and Final Considerations

We control the cut surface of the liver for any bleeding or bile leak. A small catheter is then inserted into the cystic duct and air is injected to check for leaks from the biliary tree and to proof adequate bile drainage from the rest of the liver. A US probe is placed on the liver surface. The previously injected air results in a diffuse hyperechogenic signal in the entire remnant of the liver as an indirect proof that the essential bile ducts have not been violated. The cut surface is inspected for air bubbles that would demonstrate a bile leak. We prefer the air test over the use of Methylene blue to test for leaks because it can be repeated several times without staining the liver surface. As a final step fibrin glue is sprayed on the raw liver surface with the aim of reducing postoperative bile leaks or hemorrhage. Drains are not routinely placed. The pneumoperitoneum is evacuated and all ports are removed under direct vision. The fascial defects of all port sites larger than 5 mm will be closed. The skin is adapted with a subcuticular running suture using 4/0 absorbable suture material.

22.11 Hepatectomies-classification

Hepatectomies are classified according to the number of segments being removed and are divided generally into four categories.

1. Major hepatectomies
   a. Major hepatectomy right
      i. This involves resection of *four* segments
      ii. Segment V, VI, VII and VIII
   b. Major hepatectomy left
      i. This involves resection of *three* segments
      ii. Segments II, III and IV
   c. Trisegmentectomies
      i. Any combination of three segments, for example IV, V and VI
2. Limited hepatectomies
   This involves resection of up to *two* segments
   a. Left lobectomy
   b. Right posterior sectoriectomy
   c. Segmentectomy
   d. Subsegmentectomy
      i. Anterior segmnetectomy IV
      ii. Resection of the quadrate lobe
3. Extended hepatectomies
   a. Extended hepatectomy right
      i. Involves *five* segments
      ii. Extends into segment I or segment IV
   b. Extended hepatectomy left
      i. Involves *four* segments
      ii. Extends into segment I, V or VIII
4. Superextended hepatectomies
   a. Superextended hepatectomy right
      i. Involves *six* segments
      ii. Adds segment I and IV
   b. Superextended hepatectomy left
      i. Involves at least *five* segments, but no more than *six*
      ii. Adds segment V, VIII and possibly segment I

22.12 Hepatectomies-surgical Technique

22.12.1 Hemihepatectomies

22.12.1.1 Major Hepatectomy Right

The patient is placed in a supine position. Some surgeons place the patient in a left lateral decubitus position for this intervention, but, in our opinion, this changes the topographic anatomy of the porta hepatis. In addition, it would make it very difficult to treat a lesion in the left lobe of the liver. Therefore we prefer a supine position and rotate the patient to the left if necessary. After resectability is confirmed by diagnostic laparoscopy and intra-operative US, we divide the falciform ligament along with the umbilical ligament as a first step. The divided ligaments will be used to retract. The falciform ligament is divided next to the anterior abdominal wall to avoid a "curtain effect," which can jeopardize visualization during the entire procedure. Care must be taken to free all fibrous attachments between the umbilical ligament and the umbilical fissure in order to avoid capsule tears during retraction. The ligamentum teres is gently pulled cephalad and lateral to the left to expose the right portion of the porta hepatis. The hepato-duodenal ligament is opened and a small tape is passed through the foramen of Winslow to surround the hepatic pedicle twice to permit a Pringle maneuver if necessary. We advise adopting this safety step routinely, especially for surgeons at the beginning of their learning curve, even though improvement in surgical technique and development of new instruments have made portal clamping less necessary in recent years [41]. The triangle of Calot is dissected and the cystic duct and artery are divided. We ligate the cystic duct using an endoloop, while for the cystic artery bipolar coagulation is applied. The gallbladder is mobilized from its hepatic bed on the left side only. This gives us the possibility to use the gallbladder for retraction if necessary. Dissection is continued cephalad and lateral to the common bile duct in order to find the right hepatic artery, which usually passes posterior to the bile duct. Before approaching the right portion of the hepatic pedicle, the corresponding portion of the hilar plate is lowered by dissecting it free from the liver parenchyma. The artery should be ligated to the right of the common bile duct to avoid ischemic damage to the bile duct. Care must be taken to identify an accessory right hepatic artery originating from the superior mesenteric artery (SMA). The portal vein is dissected laterally and posteriorly until we identify and preserve the origin of the left portal branch. The right portal branch is now isolated enough to be divided by an Endo-GIA vascular stapler. We usually oversew the stump with a 5/0 Prolene suture. When passing a curved forceps around the right portal vein to isolate it, the first posterior branch, which supplies the caudate lobe, should be recognized and preserved if possible. If any difficulties are encountered we do not hesitate to ligate this branch. Sometimes the anterior and posterior branches of the right portal vein arise individually. This anatomical variant has to be known in order to obtain complete inflow control to the right lobe of the liver. Both branches will be divided separately. An ischemic demarcation should now be seen with the medial border corresponding to Cantlie's line. This line divides the liver in a functional left and right and runs from the middle of the gallbladder fossa anterior to the IVC posterior. We prefer to divide the right hepatic duct inside the parenchyma, to avoid leaving an ischemic stump, which may increase the risk of a biliary fistula. Then we mobilize the right portion of the liver by dissecting the right aspect of the coronary ligament, the right triangular ligament and taking down all the attachments to the posterior peritoneum until the right aspect of the IVC is exposed. The liver can now be retracted upward and medially to begin the dissection of the right portion of the anterior aspect of the IVC (Fig. 22.6). This is started distally and carried on cephalad. Spigelian veins are controlled with bipolar coagulation or by metallic clips of appropriate size

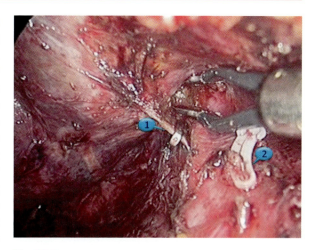

Fig. 22.6 Mobilization of the right liver. The right portion of the anterior aspect of the IVC is isolated from the liver: a venous branch from segment V has been clipped and divided (*2*). The retrocaval ligament is clipped (metallic clip) (*1*) and will be divided in order to expose the right aspect of the right hepatic vein

and then divided. For this part of the procedure, the laparoscopic approach poses a clear advantage when compared to open surgery, because it allows much better visualization. The right hepatic vein is reached and isolated. In order to do so, the hepato-caval ligament, which was first described by Gayet, has to be dissected. This fibrous ligament obscures the right aspect of the right hepatic vein and surrounds the posterior aspect of the IVC from the right to the left border of the liver. It can contain vessels, especially in cirrhotic livers, and should be ligated before transection. To facilitate control of the right hepatic vein we dissect all fibrous tissue anterior to the supra-hepatic IVC in order to expose the medial side of the IVC. This can be done either by an anterior approach during mobilization of the liver or by extending the dissection between the IVC and the posterior aspect of the liver toward the diaphragm passing between the right and middle hepatic veins. A tape can be placed between the right and middle hepatic veins should a hanging maneuver be done (Fig. 22.7). The liver is placed back in its original position over the IVC and we begin the parenchyma transection anteriorly. The ischemic demarcation line on the Glissonian capsule is incised using the harmonic scalpel. The dissection is deepened toward the IVC adding bipolar forceps to the harmonic scalpel. The fascia of the main portal pedicle is immediately encountered and the portion containing the bile duct is divided. The anterior and posterior branches are ligated and secured under

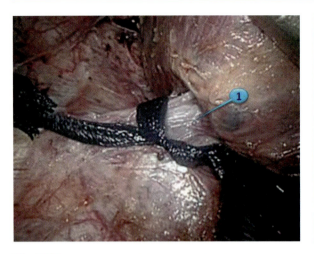

Fig. 22.7 Control of the right hepatic vein, lateral approach. The connective tissue between the right hepatic vein and the common trunk has been dissected and a tape is passed through to surround the right hepatic vein (*1*)

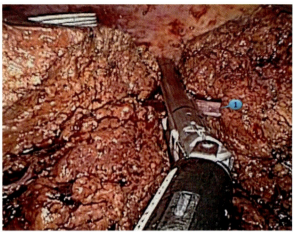

Fig. 22.8 Final step in right hepatic vein is ready to be divided using a vascular stapler, white load. The end of the middle hepatic vein is preserved (*1*)

direct vision with Prolene 5/0 stitches. The portal pedicles for segments V and VIII are then encountered and controlled by ligation, clips or stapler. The middle hepatic vein is kept medial to the dissection line and this can be verified by US while progressing through the parenchyma. If major bleeding occurs we tighten the tape, which we placed at the beginning of the procedure around the hepatic pedicle and fix it temporarily by double clipping. This allows us to perform a temporary Pringle maneuver. We remove the clips after 10–15 min to permit inflow for 5 min. After completion of the parenchyma transection the specimen remains attached to the right hepatic vein only. The right hepatic vein will now be divided using an Endo-GIA vascular stapler (Fig. 22.8). If you encounter a bulky liver which is difficult to handle, you can use a modified liver hanging maneuver, as first described by Belghiti, to facilitate the parenchyma dissection. A pediatric oro-gastric tube is passed in the plane between the posterior aspect of the liver and the IVC and between the middle and right hepatic veins and lifted upward and to the left.

22.12.1.2 Major Hepatectomy Left

The falciform ligament has been divided as described above to allow intra-operative US. The lesser omentum is now opened and an accessory left hepatic artery arising from the left gastric artery, if present, is identified and ligated. The hepatic pedicle is isolated and surrounded by a tape for reasons previously described. The triangle of Calot is dissected and the cystic duct and artery are divided. The inflow control is started by direct dissection at the base of the umbilical fissure. We prefer not to dissect the anterior aspect of the common hepatic duct, especially at the confluence of the cystic duct with the common hepatic duct to avoid ischemic lesions to the extra-hepatic biliary tree. To expose the umbilical fissure the round ligament is retracted cephalad and to the right. The left portion of the hilar plate is lowered by dissecting its superior border free from the parenchyma of the liver. The left hepatic artery is identified immediately after opening the peritoneum at the left border of the hepatic pedicle in its subhilar portion. The left hepatic artery is now excluded by double clipping. Dissection is continued posterior to the artery which exposes the left portal branch prior to its entry into the umbilical fissure. The left portal branch should be controlled at this point if the caudate lobe is not included in the resection. The main reason for this is because the portal branches for segment I arise to the right before the left portal branch. We ligate the vein before the takeoff of the caudate branches if the caudate lobe is going to be removed together with the left lobe. We divide the left portal branch either with an endoscopic vascular stapler or with a suture ligature (Fig. 22.9). The left hepatic duct is then identified and isolated superior and to the right of the left portal vein after limited lowering of the hilar plate. The left bile duct is divided with scissors along with the surrounding hilar plate and secured separately with a suture ligature. A demarcation line should now be visible on the Glissonian capsule extending from the gallbladder fossa to the left portion of the IVC delineating the resection plane. The left lobe is now mobilized by dividing the left triangular ligament and the left aspect of the coronary ligament and the liver will be retracted laterally and to the right. The ligamentum venosum is identified and divided (Fig. 22.10). This exposes the left hepatic vein before its confluence with the IVC. A US probe is positioned just laterally to it to identify the middle hepatic vein and its medial aspect is isolated by dissecting the parenchyma in a retrograde fashion (Fig. 22.11). The dissection plane is now perfectly delineated and is formed by a triangle with the gallbladder fossa at the base, the ischemic line on the Glissonian capsule anteriorly (Cantlie line) and the middle hepatic vein as a side border. The parenchyma dissection is then started posteriorly with the middle hepatic vein perfectly exposed and in vision at all times. After reaching midway through the

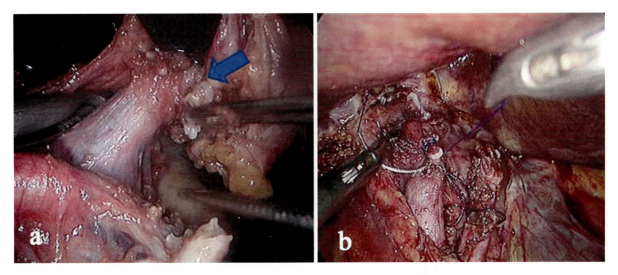

Fig. 22.9 The left portal branch is isolated and ready to be divided before starting the parenchyma dissection when performing a left hepatectomy. (**a**) After being clipped and divided (*arrow*) (**b**), the stump is secured with a nonabsorbable stitch

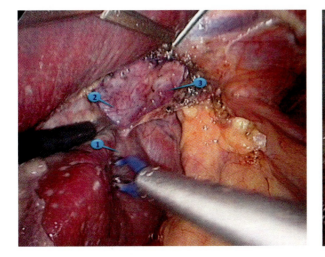

Fig. 22.10 The ligament of Arantius (*1*) is dissected to approach the confluence between the left hepatic vein (*2*) (common trunk) and the IVC (*3*)

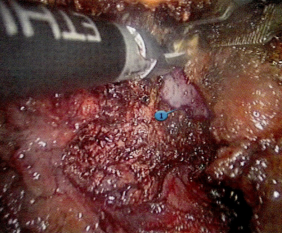

Fig. 22.11 Left hepatectomy can be performed with a posterior approach: the middle hepatic vein (*1*) is identified at its confluence and its left aspect will be isolated in cranio-caudal direction

parenchyma we put the left lobe of the liver back in its anatomical position and continue the transection of the parenchyma anteriorly until the left hepatic vein is encountered (Fig. 22.12). We divide the left hepatic vein proximal to its confluence with the middle hepatic vein using a laparoscopic Endo-GIA vascular load. The specimen is now free and will be placed in a non-permeable retrieval bag.

22.12.2 Central Hepatectomy

This procedure involves resection of segments IV, V and VIII. Mobilization of the liver is not necessary. Some surgeons leave the falciform ligament intact to take advantage of its suspensory function. A tape is passed around the hepatic pedicle as described above in the event a Pringle maneuver becomes necessary.

The hilum of the liver is now approached and we lower the hilar plate by dissecting its superior border off the parenchyma of segment IV. Dissection of the left portion of the hilum is easiest performed by retracting the umbilical ligament to the right. The left branch of the hepatic artery is isolated and followed distally until the paramedian branch is found. This branch supplies segment IV and is found directly medial to it. We divide it with scissors after careful placement of clips distally and proximally. The distal end of the left portal vein is approached at the base of the umbilical fossa, and the branches to the superior (IVa) and inferior (IVb) portion of the quadrate lobe are separated between clips. The bile ducts to segments IVa and IVb are divided to the right of the umbilical fissure during the dissection of the parenchyma to avoid any damage to the biliary drainage from the left lobe.

After the demarcation line is established we divide the parenchyma until the IVC is encountered. We follow the IVC cephalad to the right of the falciform ligament toward the confluence with the middle hepatic vein. Once the middle hepatic vein is we divide it with a vascular stapler. This step of the procedure becomes much easier if the right lobe is retracted upward and lateral to the right. The parenchyma is now dissected laterally to the right until the left lateral aspect of the right hepatic vein is encountered. The right portion of the hepatic pedicle is then approached. The bifurcation between the main right portal triad, the anterior pedicles of segments V–VIII and the postero-lateral pedicles of segments VI–VII is identified so that the anterior pedicle can be clearly identified and safely divided (Fig. 22.13). Anatomical variations sometimes allow an extra parenchymal dissection of the main right bifurcation, but most often a standard parenchyma dissection is necessary to approach this structure. This will be done under US guidance. The antero-lateral portal pedicle can be divided directly with a vascular stapler, but separate ligation of the vascular elements is preferred in order to correctly identify the bile ducts. The vascular stapler, if

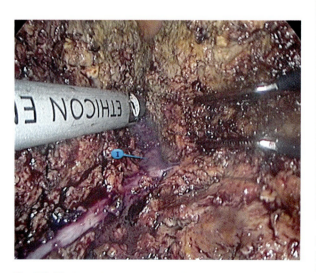

Fig. 22.12 Parenchyma transection in left hepatectomy. The middle hepatic vein (*1*) is preserved and kept laterally

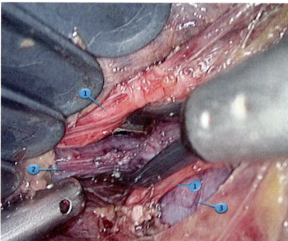

Fig. 22.13 Central or extended left hepatectomy. The anterior pedicle of the right portal triad is isolated and divided, while the posterior pedicle is preserved. *Red*: anterior and posterior segmental arteries (*1*); *blue*: anterior (*2*) and posterior (*3*) segmental portal veins

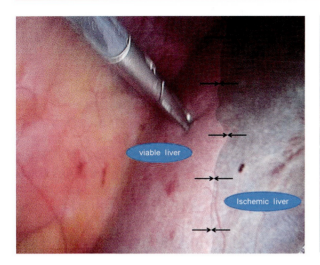

Fig. 22.14 Demarcation line. After complete inflow interruption, an ischemic demarcation line should be visible on the outside of the liver and will guide the parenchymal transection (*black arrows*)

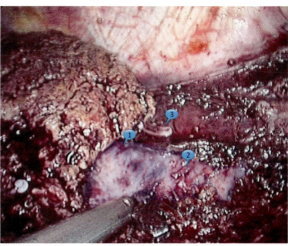

Fig. 22.15 Central hepatectomy. The right hepatic vein (*1*) is preserved and kept laterally, while the middle hepatic vein has been stapled (*2*) (veins are highlighted in blue). A plastic clip on the IVC corresponds to a variation of the vein of segment VIII draining directly into the IVC (*3*)

used, should be placed at least 5 mm from the origin of the pedicle, to avoid lesions to the bile duct of the posterior sector. An ischemic demarcation line between the postero-lateral and the anterior sectors should now appear (Fig. 22.14). The right dissection is started by separating the postero-lateral from the antero-lateral segments. The right hepatic vein is visualized on US and preserved, while segmental branches from segments V and VIII, draining into the right hepatic vein, are divided (Fig. 22.15). The central bloc, formed by segments IV, V and VIII is retracted upward and laterally to complete the resection approaching from the inferior plane. Great care must be taken to preserve the hilar plate in order to prevent an ischemic insult to the biliary tree. Ischemia of the bile ducts will result in postoperative bile leaks, which are not an uncommon complication after this type of resection. Bile leaks should be treated promptly by placing a stent.

22.12.3 Extended Hepatectomies

22.12.3.1 Extended Hepatectomy Left

A classical left hepatectomy will be extended into segments V and VIII.

The hepato-duodenal ligament is controlled by placing a small tape around it as previously described for other major hepatectomies. The falciform ligament, left triangular and left coronary ligaments are dissected to mobilize the liver. The hilar plate is lowered by dissecting its superior border off from the hepatic parenchyma. The left portion of the hilum is approached and the elements of the left main portal triad are resected as described for a left hepatectomy. The line of dissection is defined by US following the anterior side of the right hepatic vein, which of course will be preserved during the following dissection. As for central hepatectomy, the bifurcation between the postero-lateral and the antero-lateral pedicles is identified. The antero-lateral pedicle is then divided as described above. The fibrous tissue surrounding the supra-hepatic IVC is dissected and the common trunk of the left and middle hepatic veins isolated and controlled. During the dissection of the parenchyma we encounter veins from segments V and VIII draining directly into the right hepatic vein and divide them between clips. The right hepatic vein is followed toward its confluence with the IVC. At this point, the common trunk of hepatic veins, which has already been isolated, is transected with a laparoscopic vascular stapler to complete resection of the specimen.

22.12.3.2 Extended Hepatectomy Right

A classical right hepatectomy will be extended into segments IV, with or without segment I. Control of the hepatic pedicle, mobilization of the liver and division of the right portal triad are performed as already described for a right hepatectomy. The hilar plate is lowered prior to the division of the right portal triad. The line of dissection corresponds with the falciform ligament. The left branch of the porta hepatis is approached from the right side of the umbilical fossa and the elements of the portal triad of segment IVa and IVb are identified and divided as described above for a central hepatectomy. Dissection is carried on toward the IVC until the confluence of the middle and left hepatic vein is encountered. The middle hepatic vein is then resected using a vascular stapler, preserving the left hepatic vein. The right liver is completely split open after parenchyma dissection and positioned laterally. This maneuver exposes the right hepatic vein posterior to the middle vein. The right hepatic vein will be divided with a vascular stapler. The specimen is now completely detached and will be placed into an impermeable specimen retrieval bag.

22.12.4 Limited Hepatectomies Segmentectomies

Better understanding of the segmental anatomy of the liver has led to a wider practice of tissue-sparing procedures like segmental resections. Moreover, segmental resections reduce the risk of major bleeding and are more likely to result in a higher rate of negative microscopic margins when compared to wedge resections. Each segment is an autonomous unit, with its own biliary drainage and vascular inflow and outflow. We will therefore describe the surgical steps to perform single segmentectomies. The principles described will be applicable to any combination of segmental resections.

22.12.4.1 Resection of Segment I

Laparoscopy, when compared to the open approach, puts the caudate lobe into an anterior position. This provides a better exposure to perform the resection. The hepatic pedicle is isolated after opening the lesser sac and freeing up the hiatus of Winslow. We do not place a tape around the hepato-duodenal ligament. The hepato-duodenal ligament is retracted upward by the first assistant and the posterior aspect of the porta hepatis is dissected. The arterial and portal flow to the caudate lobe is divided. The right portion of the caudate lobe receives portal venous blood from the right portal vein and the bifurcation of the main portal trunk, while the left portion receives portal blood exclusively from the left portal branch. The arterial supply and biliary drainage of the right portion depends on the right posterior sectorial pedicle and on the left main pedicle [42]. The hepatic pedicle is lifted up and to the left to divide vessels to the right portion of segment I and to the right to disconnect the left portion. Segment I is unique from an anatomical point of view because it drains directly into the IVC through Spigelian veins. Usually one to nine Spigelian veins are found with a mean number of four reported in the literature [43]. The proximal aspect of the caudate lobe is lifted upward and the Spigelian veins are divided with scissors between clips or with the harmonic scalpel depending on their diameter. Further transection is carried on cephalad and follows the anterior aspect of the IVC (Fig. 22.16). Usually, the upper outflow vein drains directly into the left hepatic vein or into the IVC. In cases of caudate lobe hypertrophy the dissection may involve the lateral aspects of the IVC. Mobilization of segment I is completed by lifting up the left lateral segment and after dissection of the ligamentum venosum in a left to right direction. The bridge of

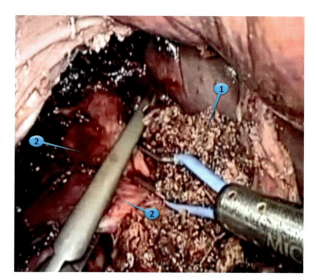

Fig. 22.16 Resection of segment I. In this patient a tumor (*1*) was invading the IVC. A laparoscopic vascular clamp is positioned laterally on the IVC (*2*), which is partially resected to completely remove the tumor. The vein is reconstructed with a 4/0 Polypropylene running suture

parenchymal tissue that connects the caudate lobe with segments VI and VII is divided and the specimen can be delivered. Great care must be taken when transecting the anterior border of segment I, to avoid any injury to the middle and left hepatic vein. In cases of large tumors, it may be wise to control the middle and left hepatic vein at the junction with the IVC before further dissection. In our most recent cases, we directly visualized the middle hepatic vein after lifting up the left lateral segment and dissecting the ligament of Arantius. This ligament is a fetal remnant of the ductus venosus, a thin fibrous cord, lying in the fissure of the ligamentum venosum. This was done prior to dissection of the anterior border of the caudate lobe, in order to avoid accidental injury to it.

22.12.4.2 Resection of Segment II and III

These two segments are usually resected together as a left lateral segmentectomy. In the event of a cirrhotic patient we use a tissue-sparing method and resect either segment II or segment III alone. The left triangular ligament is dissected. The falciform ligament is divided together with the round ligament which is pulled superiorly and laterally to the right by the first assistant. This exposes the proximal part of the dissection plane which runs on the left side of the umbilical fissure. The dissection line will follow the medial aspect of the falciform ligament. Sometimes a bridge of parenchyma is present between segments III and IV, anterior to the umbilical fissure, and this should be divided. Parenchyma dissection of the left portion of the umbilical fossa allows isolation of the pedicles of segments II and III, which will be divided with scissors between clips, right at their origin (Fig. 22.17). In cases of large tumors, isolation of the main left portal pedicle will be necessary. On further dissection cephalad we encounter the left hepatic vein, which is divided with an Endo-GIA stapler, vascular load. In fact, the entire dissection can be done with staplers alone and this method is preferred by many surgeons because it's easier and faster. The middle hepatic vein drains into the terminal end of the left hepatic vein. Therefore dissection and division of the left hepatic vein should be done right before the confluence in order to avoid any injury to the middle hepatic vein. After this final step the specimen will be totally freed up. Rarely, segments II and III are resected separately.

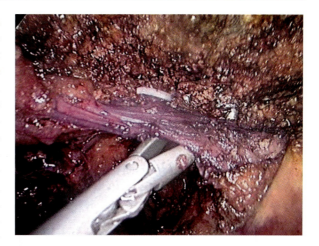

Fig. 22.17 Left lateral segmentectomy including segments II and III. The portal triad to segment III is isolated

The line of dissection between the two segments is oblique and antero-cranial. If you decide to resect segment II only, make sure to preserve the left hepatic vein to assure outflow of segment III.

22.12.4.3 Resection of Segment IV

Mobilization of the liver is not mandatory if addressing segment IV only. The hepato-duodenal ligament is surrounded by a tape in the event a Pringle maneuver will be needed. Like in central and extended right hepatectomies, we approach the left portion of the hilum from the umbilical fossa while the ligamentum teres is pulled laterally to the left. The left branch of the hepatic artery is identified at this level and followed to find, isolate and divide the left para-median branch at its takeoff. The superior aspect of the left portal branch is then dissected in its distal part to identify and divide the para-median branch that frequently originates alone or is separated into two branches, directed to sub-segments IVa (apical) and IVb (basal). At this point an ischemic demarcation line should be noted just lateral to the falciform ligament. The medial dissection is now carried out, starting from the umbilical fossa toward the IVC and continued cranially at the right border of the falciform ligament. Every bile duct recognized during the dissection will be ligated separately. The further the dissection progresses we identify the confluence between the middle and the left hepatic vein and preserve it. The lateral dissection starts with a cholecystectomy. The middle hepatic vein is identified on US and its projection on the Glissonian capsule marked with the harmonic scalpel. Dissection starts in the center of the gallbladder fossa and is continued cranially to the left side of the middle hepatic vein. Outflow branches, draining directly into the middle hepatic vein, are divided between clips or harmonic scalpel. As for all central hepatic resections, care must be taken not to injure the hilar plate in order to avoid ischemic lesions to the bile ducts.

Segment IV can be divided into two subunits with independent vasculature and biliary drainage: segment IVa superiorly and segment IVb inferiorly.

22.12.4.4 Resection of Segment *IVb*

The borders of the area to resect will be defined using intra-operative US. The inferior and lateral borders are the same as for segment IV. The superior extent is located between the portal pedicles for segments IVa and IVb. Their origin is found at the superior right aspect of the left portal branch just after the ligamentum teres enters the umbilical fossa. The portal pedicle should always be evaluated by US to make sure not to violate the inflow to sub-segment IVa.

22.12.4.5 Resection of Segment *IVa*

The anterior aspect of the liver is partially opened by dissecting the parenchyma immediately to the right of the falciform ligament, extending from the umbilical fossa to the right aspect of the left hepatic vein. This initial step helps to gain better exposure to carry out the planned resection. Depending on the localization of the tumor we control the common trunk of the left and middle hepatic veins before progressing further with the dissection. This is done from the lateral side after dissecting the anterior aspect of the supra-hepatic IVC and the left coronary ligament. US is used to define the inferior dissection plane. This allows localizing the portal pedicle to this sub-segment and makes it possible to preserve the portal pedicle to sub-segment IVb (Fig. 22.18). The pedicle is ligated and the parenchyma is dissected horizontally toward the middle hepatic vein. This part of the dissection is much easier after the previous opening of the parenchyma alongside a line corresponding with the falciform ligament. Once encountered, the middle hepatic vein is followed cranially toward the IVC and tributary branches are divided. Attention should be paid to the vein of segment VIII draining directly into the IVC

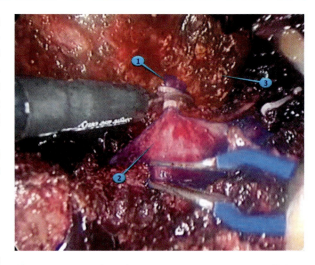

Fig. 22.18 Resection of segment IVa. (*1*) The portal pedicle to segment IVa is divided between clips. (*2*) Main left portal pedicle. (*3*) Inferior medial aspect of segment IVa

because of its proximity to the vein of segment IVa. The medial dissection line corresponds to the upper part of the dissection plane, next to the falciform ligament, that has already been performed to expose sub-segment IVa.

22.12.4.6 Resection of Segment *V*

Mobilization of the liver is not necessary for this type of resection. Only the falciform ligament is divided to facilitate intra-operative US. The triangle of Calot is dissected and the cystic duct and artery ligated. The gallbladder is dissected from its hepatic bed on the medial portion only. This will expose the further line of dissection and permits to use the gallbladder to expose the segment. The lateral border of the resection is defined by the right hepatic vein, while the superior border is presented by the bifurcation of the antero-lateral portal pedicle into the branches for segment VIII and V. These structures are identified with intra-operative US and their projection marked with ultrasonic shears on the capsule of the liver. As a next step we start the parenchyma dissection in the midline of the gallbladder fossa. The dissection is directed inferiorly toward the hilum and cephalad until the portal triad for this segment is encountered. We prefer to divide the portal structures separately in order to properly identify the segmental bile ducts. Outflow vessels to the middle and right hepatic vein will be divided between clips or using ultrasonic shears.

22.12.4.7 Resection of Segment *VI*

For this particular type of resection we position the patient supine with the right flank elevated by a pad. A left lateral decubitus position would be an alternative. The main portal pedicle is controlled by a tape as previously described. We mobilize the right lobe by dividing the ipsilateral triangular and coronary ligaments and by dividing the posterior attachments of the right liver. The borders of the resection are, once again, established by intra-operative US and are as follows: superior – the bifurcation of the postero-lateral portal pedicle into the branches for segment VII and segment VI; medially – the origin of the portal pedicle to the postero-lateral segment itself. The borders of the resection are marked on the liver surface and the dissection is started. The portal pedicle to segment VI is divided with vascular staplers and the proximal portion of the right hepatic vein is ligated at the level where it ends, between segments VI and VII.

22.12.4.8 Resection of Segment *VII* and *VIII*

The patient is brought into a left lateral decubitus position because of the posterior localization of these two segments in the right liver. A tape is passed around the hepatic ligament, as described above, to control inflow if necessary. The right lobe is fully mobilized by dividing the right triangular ligament and the right aspect of the coronary ligament. The dissection continues on the right lateral aspect of the IVC which is separated from the posterior aspect of the right liver This is accomplished by retracting the liver upward. The retro-caval ligament is encountered and divided with ultrasonic shears or between clips in the case of a cirrhotic liver. The surgeon, who was initially standing between the legs, moves on to the right side of the patient and two additional trocars are placed: one in the 11th intercostal space on the anterior axillary line for repositioning of the camera and one in the 9th intercostal space on the mid-axillary line. The mobilized right liver is pulled medially and inferiorly by the first assistant, who is now standing between the legs of the patient. With this positioning and exposure the surgeon obtains optimal control over the supra-hepatic IVC and the postero-superior portion of the right liver. The right aspect of the right hepatic vein is skeletonized and its medial border is dissected cranially until it reaches the space between the right hepatic vein and the common trunk and until the diaphragm is seen. A tape will now be passed around the isolated right hepatic vein to control outflow in the event massive bleeding occurs. The dissection of the supra-hepatic IVC is completed once the medial aspect of the common trunk is visualized. If it was not possible to pass a tape around the right hepatic vein during the posterior portion of the dissection, it will be easier to place it now. The borders of the resection are now defined by intra-operative US. For segment VII these will be: the right side of the right hepatic vein, which is preserved, and inferiorly the bifurcation of the portal triad into the segmentary pedicles for segments VII and VI. The borders are marked with ultrasonic shears on the outside of the liver and dissection is started and continued until the portal pedicle for segment VII is found. It will be divided between clips. All the efferent veins encountered during parenchyma dissection will be divided between clips. The borders of dissection for segment VIII are established as well by intra-operative US and are as follows: the right side of the common trunk and the middle hepatic vein, the left lateral aspect of the right hepatic vein and inferiorly the bifurcation between the portal pedicles for segments VIII and V. The inflow to the segment comes from the main portal pedicle and is divided between clips as well. The outflow is disconnected by dividing tributary veins to the right and middle hepatic vein. Care must be taken to strictly respect these two major veins. For tumors of segment VIII located near its medial border, we advise to isolate and control the middle hepatic vein prior to dissection (Fig. 22.19). At the end of the procedure, when removing the intercostal ports, we always aspirate first because they pass through the inferior portion of the pleural cavity. If a capnothorax is noted on a postoperative chest X-ray we usually only observe it and do not place a chest tube. The capnothorax is different from a pneumothorax in a sense that it should resolve rather quickly without intervention mainly due to the high solubility of carbon dioxide and lack of an injury to the visceral pleura.

22.13 Future Trends

Currently, a combination of preoperative imaging and intra-operative US provides the information to plan and perform liver surgery. To ameliorate and facilitate the

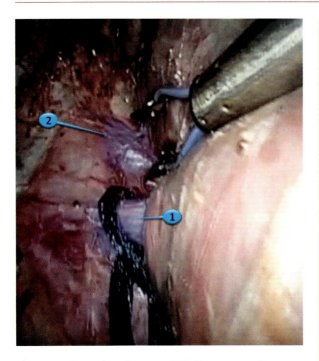

Fig. 22.19 Resection of segment VIII. For a tumor of segment VIII, close to the IVC, the supra-hepatic portion of the IVC must be dissected prior to parenchyma dissection, when using a lateral approach. *Blue*: Isolated right hepatic vein (*1*) and the common trunk (*2*)

performance of parenchyma dissection, an intra-operative, image-guided, 3D liver surgical system has been developed to furnish a real-time liver navigation device which would assist the surgeon in visualizing the tumor and its blood supply while still surrounded by parenchyma. This system will most probably gain acceptance and will be used routinely for liver resections.

Quick Reference Guide

1. Choose your patient wisely and base your operative strategy on appropriate preoperative imaging. 3D reconstructions should ideally be obtained to delineate all vascular structures and bile ducts.
2. A surgeon has to be familiar with intra-operative US if performing liver surgery. Intra-operative US is the key imaging modality to finally decide about:
   - To resect or not to resect
   - Extent of resection

   Intra-operative US is absolutely mandatory if an anatomical resection is planned.
3. Place the patient appropriately to gain optimal exposure. This will vary with the type of resection planned. Generally a supine, low lithotomy position is sufficient for major resections.
4. Trocar placement varies with the type of resection planned. Usually a configuration of six trocars should be sufficient.
5. Always surround the hepatic pedicle with a tape if a major hepatectomy will be performed. This precaution is very useful in the event a Pringle maneuver becomes necessary and avoids excessive intra-operative bleeding.
6. Liver mobilization should be done by dividing all the embryologic attachments and carefully dissecting the liver off the IVC.
7. Control and divide all tributary portal veins before starting the parenchyma dissection.
   The same should be done to control the outflow by dividing Spigelian veins draining into the IVC.
8. Keep the intravascular volume low during the course of the parenchyma dissection to reduce intra-operative bleeding. The intra-operative CVP is ideally kept <5 mmHg to achieve that goal. The volume state can be controlled as well by direct visualization of a flat, emptied IVC.
9. As a final step of the procedure control the cut edge and remnant of the liver for accurate hemostasis, bile leaks and integrity of the biliary tree by injection of air into the cystic duct. US, placed on the outside of the liver remnant, will produce a diffuse hyper-echogenic signal as a proof of the patency of the biliary tree.
10. Always extract the specimen from the abdominal cavity using an impermeable endobag in combination with a wound protector to avoid tumor seeding.

References

1. Samama, G., et al.: Laparoscopic anatomical hepatic resection: report of four left lobectomies for solid tumors. Surg. Endosc. **12**, 763–778 (1998)
2. Cherqui, D., Husson, E., Hammoud, R., et al.: Laparoscopic liver resections: a feseability study in 30 patients. Ann. Surg. **232**, 753–762 (2000)
3. Descottes, B., et al.: Early experience with laparoscopic approach for solid liver tumors: initial 16 cases. Ann. Surg. **232**, 641–645 (2000)
4. Huang, M., et al.: Hand-assisted laparoscopic hepatectomy for solitary tumor in the posterior portion of the right lobe: initial experience. Ann. Surg. **238**, 674–679 (2003)

5. O'Rourke, N., Shaw, I., Nathanson, L., et al.: Laparoscopic resction of hepatic colorectal metastases. HPB **6**, 230–235 (2004)
6. Laurence, J.M., Lam, V.W.T., Langcake, M.E., et al.: Laparoscopic hepatectomy, a systemic review. ANZJ Surg. **77**, 948–953 (2007)
7. Koffron, A., Geller, D.A., Gamblin, T.C., et al.: Laparoscopic liver surgery – shifting the management of liver tumors. Hepatology **44**, 1694–1700 (2006)
8. Vibert, E., Perniceni, T., Levard, H., et al.: Laparoscopic liver resection. Br. J. Surg. **93**, 67–72 (2006)
9. Soubrane, O., Cherqui, D., Scatton, O., et al.: Laparoscopic left lateral sectionectomy in living donors: safety and reproducibility of the technique in a single center. Ann. Surg. **244**, 815–820 (2006)
10. Gayet, B., Cavaliere, D., Vibert, E., et al.: Totally laparoscopic right hepatectomy. Am. J. Surg. **194**, 685–689 (2007)
11. Dagher, I., Proske, J.M., Carloni, A., et al.: Laparoscopic liver resection: results for 70 patients. Surg. Endosc. **21**, 619–624 (2007)
12. Buell, J.F., Thomas, M.T., Rudich, S., et al.: Experience with more than 500 minimally invasive hepatic procedures. Ann. Surg. **248**, 475–486 (2008)
13. Chen, H.Y., Juan, C.C., Ker, C.G.: Laparoscopic liver surgery for patients with hepatocellular carcinoma. Ann. Surg. Oncol. **15**, 800–806 (2008)
14. Buell, J.F., Cherqui, D., Geller, D. et al.: The international position on laparoscopic liver surgery: The Lousiville Statement. Ann Surg. **250**(5), 825–830 (2009)
15. Billingsley, K.G., Jarnagin, W.R., Fong, Y., et al.: Segment-oriented hepatic resection in the management of malignant neoplasms of the liver. J. Am. Coll. Surg. **187**, 471–481 (1998)
16. Laurent, A., Cherqui, D., Lesurtel, M., et al.: Laparoscopic liver resection for subcapsular hepatocellular carcinoma complicating chronic liver disease. Arch. Surg. **138**, 763–769 (2003)
17. Koffron, A.J., Auffenberg, G., Kung, R., et al.: Evaluation of 300 minimally invasive liver resections at a single institution. Less is more. Ann. Surg. **246**, 385–394 (2007)
18. Boutkan, H., Luth, W., Meyer, S., et al.: The impact of intraoperative ultrasonography of the liver on the surgical strategy of patients with gastrointestinal malignancies and hepatic metastases. Eur. J. Surg. Oncol. **18**, 342–346 (1992)
19. Sahani, D.V., Kalva, S.P., Tanabe, K.K., et al.: Intraoperative US in patients undergoing surgery for liver neoplasms: comparison with MR imaging. Radiology **232**, 810–814 (2004)
20. Cervone, A., Sardi, A., Conaway, G.L.: Intraoperative ultrasound is essential in the management of colorectal liver lesions. Am. Surg. **66**, 611–615 (2000)
21. Conlon, R., Jacobs, M., Dasgupta, D., et al.: The value of intraoperative ultrasound during hepatic resection compared with improved preoperative magnetic resonance imaging. Eur. J. Ultrasound **16**, 211–216 (2003)
22. Nguyen, K.T., Gamblin, T.C., Geller, D.A.: Laparoscopic liver resection for cancer. Future Oncol. **4**, 661–670 (2008)
23. Gigot, J.F., Glineur, D., Azagra, J.S., et al.: Laparoscopic liver resection for malignant liver tumors. Preliminary results of a multicenter European Study. Ann. Surg. **236**, 90–97 (2002)
24. Vibert, E., Kouider, A., Gayet, B.: Laparoscopic anatomic liver resection. HPB **6**, 222–229 (2004)
25. Lesurtel, M., Cherqui, D., Laurent, A., et al.: Laparoscopic versus open left lateral hepatic lobectomy: a case control study. J. Am. Coll. Surg. **196**, 236–242 (2003)
26. Farges, O., et al.: Prospective assessment of the safety and benefit of laparoscopic liver resection. J. Hepatobiliary Pancreat. Surg. **9**, 242–248 (2002)
27. Mala, T., Edwin, B., Gladhaug, I., et al.: A comparative study of the short term outcome following open and laparoscopic liver resection of colorectal liver metastases. Surg. Endosc. **16**, 1059–1063 (2002)
28. Morino, M., Morra, I., Rosso, E., et al.: Laparoscopic vs open hepatic resection: a comparative study. Surg. Endosc. **17**, 1914–1918 (2003)
29. Castaing, D., Vibert, E., Ricca, L., Azoulay, D., Adam, R., Gayet, B.: Oncologic results of laparoscopic versus open hepatectomy for colorectal liver metastases in two specialized centers. Ann. Surg. **250**(5), 849–855 (2009 Nov)
30. Simillis, C., Costantinides, V.A., Tekkis, P.P., et al.: Laparoscopic versus open hepatic resections for benign and malignant neoplasms – a meta-analysis. Surgery **14**, 203–211 (2007)
31. Wanhg, W.D., Liang, L.J., Huang, X.Q., et al.: Low central venous pressure reduces blood loss in hepatectomy. World J. Gastroenterol. **12**, 935–939 (2006)
32. Adams, R.B.: Intraoperative ultrasound of the liver: techniques for liver resection and transplantation. In: Blumgart, L.H. (ed.) Surgery of the Liver, Biliary Tract and Pancreas. Saunders Elsevier, Philadelphia, (2007)
33. Poon, R.T.: Current techniques of liver transection. HPB **9**, 166–173 (2007)
34. Lesurtel, M., Selzner, M., Petrowsky, S., et al.: How should transection of the liver be performed ? a prospective randomised study in 100 consecutive patients: comparing four different transection strategies. Ann. Surg. **242**, 814–822 (2005)
35. Schmidbauer, S., Hallfeldt, K.K., Sitzmann, G., et al.: Experience with ultrasonic scissors and blades (Ultracision) in open and laparoscopic liver resection. Ann. Surg. **235**, 27–30 (2002)
36. Kim, J., Ahmad, S.A., Lowy, A.M., et al.: Increased biliary fistulas after liver resection with the harmonic scalpel. Am. Surg. **69**, 815–819 (2003)
37. Romano, F., Franciosi, C., Caprotti, R., et al.: Hepatic surgery using the Ligasure vessel sealing system. World J. Surg. **29**, 110–112 (2005)
38. Saiura, A., Yamamoto, J., Koga, R., et al.: Usefulness of Ligasure for liver resection: analysis by randomised clinical trial. Am. J. Surg. **192**, 41–45 (2006)
39. Poon, R.T., Fan, S.T., Wong, J.: Liver resection using a saline-linked radiofrequency dissecting sealer fior transection of the liver. J. Am. Coll. Surg. **200**, 308–313 (2005)
40. Person, B., Vivas, D., Ruiz, D., et al.: Comparison of four energy-based vascular sealing and cutting instruments: a porcine model. Surg. Endosc. **22**, 534–538 (2007)
41. Scatton, O., Massault, P.P., Dousset, B., et al.: Major liver resections without clamping: a prospective reappraisal in the era of modern surgical tools. J. Am. Coll. Surg. **199**, 702–708 (2004)
42. Mizumoto, R., Suzuki, H.: Surgical anatomy of the hepatic hilum with special reference to the caudate lobe. World J. Surg. **12**, 2–10 (1988)

43. Heloury, Y., Leborgne, J., Rogez, J.M.: The caudate lobe of the liver. Surg. Radiol. **10**, 83–91 (1988)
44. Cai, X.J., et al.: Laparoscopic hepatectomy by curettage and aspiration. Experiences of 62 cases. Surg. Endosc. **20**(10), 1531–1535 (2006)
45. Cho, J.Y., et al.: Experiences of laparoscopic liver resection including lesions in the posterosuperior segments of the liver. Surg. Endosc. **22**(11), 2344–2349 (2008)
46. Descottes, B., et al.: Right hepatectomies without vascular clamping: report of 87 cases. J. Hepatobiliary Pancreat. Surg. **10**(1), 90–94 (2003)
47. Mala, T., et al.: Laparoscopic liver resection: experience of 53 procedures at a single center. J. Hepatobiliary Pancreat. Surg. **12**(4), 298–303 (2005)
48. Sasaki, A., et al.: Ten-year experience of totally laparoscopic liver resection in a single institution. Br. J. Surg. **96**(3), 274–279 (2009)
49. Topal, B., et al.: Laparoscopic versus open liver resection of hepatic neoplasms: comparative analysis of short-term results. Surg. Endosc. **22**(10), 2208–2213 (2008)
50. Rau, H.G., et al.: Laparoscopic liver resection compared with conventional partial hepatectomy – a prospective analysis. Hepatogastroenterology **45**(24), 2333–2338 (1998)
51. Cai, X.J., et al.: Clinical study of laparoscopic versus open hepatectomy for malignant liver tumors. Surg. Endosc. **22**(11), 2350–2356 (2008)
52. Lee, K.F., et al.: Laparoscopic versus open hepatectomy for liver tumours: a case control study. Hong Kong Med. J. **13**(6), 442–448 (2007)
53. Troisi, R., et al.: The value of laparoscopic liver surgery for solid benign hepatic tumors. Surg. Endosc. **22**(1), 38–44 (2008)
54. Polignano, F.M., et al.: Laparoscopic versus open liver segmentectomy: prospective, case-matched, intention-to-treat analysis of clinical outcomes and cost effectiveness. Surg. Endosc. **22**(12), 2564–2570 (2008)
55. Aldrighetti, L., et al.: A prospective evaluation of laparoscopic versus open left lateral hepatic sectionectomy. J. Gastrointest. Surg. **12**(3), 457–462 (2008)
56. Belli, G., et al.: Laparoscopic versus open liver resection for hepatocellular carcinoma in patients with histologically proven cirrhosis: short- and middle-term results. Surg. Endosc. **21**(11), 2004–2011 (2007)

Cancer of the Gallbladder and Extrahepatic Bile Ducts

Andrew A. Gumbs, Angel M. Rodriguez-Rivera, and John P. Hoffman

23.1 Introduction

Gallbladder cancer is the most common biliary tract carcinoma both worldwide and in the USA, being the sixth most common gastrointestinal malignancy in the USA. It is an uncommon malignancy with only 9,250 new cases of gallbladder and other extrahepatic biliary duct cancers occurring in the USA in 2008 [1]. The incidence in the USA is estimated to be approximately 1.2 cases per 100,000 per year [2]. Gallbladder (GB) cancer is associated with a poor prognosis, having a 5-year survival of 5–10% and a median survival of 3–6 months from the time of diagnosis [3–6]. In the USA, it is estimated that approximately 98% of patients with GB cancer receive inadequate surgical management [7].

Ironically, laparoscopic gallbladder removal was one of the first laparoscopic procedures to be performed and is nowadays the most widespread application of minimally invasive surgery. Despite the fact that laparoscopic liver resection has been done for more than a decade, most cancer centers consider laparoscopic treatment of gallbladder cancers greater than Stage 1, an absolute contraindication. Despite this, and because of our growing experience with laparoscopic liver and pancreatic surgery, we have begun to develop techniques for minimally invasive management of gallbladder cancer.

Specifically, we have performed laparoscopic radical cholecystectomy with and without common bile duct excision, choledocho-jejunostomy, and laparoscopic hepatoduodenal lymphadenectomy for any gallbladder cancers of Stage 1b or greater.

23.2 Risk Factors for Gallbladder Cancer

Current evidence suggests that the female to male ratio of GB cancer is 2:1 [8]. A higher rate of occurrence in women is seen among major geographic, ethnic, and racial variations [8–11]. Other risk factors for GB cancer include: cigarette smoking, postmenopausal status, and age. However, the most common risk factor for GB cancer is chronic inflammation of the gallbladder wall/mucosa [10].

Chronic inflammation can lead to mucosal dysplasia and consequent GB cancer [12]. Infection, congenital anomalies, and drugs can all cause gallbladder mucosal inflammation. Known factors include but are not limited to:

- Salmonella typhi or Salmonella paratyphi-related infections
- Cigarette smoking
- Chemical exposure – rubber, metal, and wood finishing fabricating industries
- Choledochal cysts
- Congenital cystic dilatation of the biliary tree
- Anomalous junction of the pancreatico-biliary ducts
- Primary sclerosing cholangitis

The most important risk factor for gallbladder cancer is cholelithiasis [13].

A.A. Gumbs (✉) and J.P. Hoffman
Department of Surgical Oncology, Fox Chase Cancer Center, 333 Cottman Ave, C-308, Philadelphia, PA 19111, USA
e-mail: andrew.gumbs@fccc.edu; jp_hoffman@fccc.edu

A.M. Rodriguez-Rivera
Department of Surgery Mercy Catholic Medicial Center, 1500 Lansdowne Avenue, Darby, PA 19023, USA
e-mail: angelmcmc@gmail.com

23.2.1 Porcelain Gallbladder

Porcelain gallbladder is a sequela of a chronically inflamed GB and hence a risk factor for developing GB cancer. But interestingly, not all the patients with porcelain gallbladder develop GB cancer. The incidence of GB cancer in porcelain GB has been reported to be approximately 10–20% [14]. Like other GI cancers, adenomatous polyps within the GB represent an increased risk for carcinoma. This risk correlates with polyp size, and most investigators recommend a cholecystectomy for pedunculated polyps that are more than 10 mm in size. In comparison, small polyps <5 mm are more consistent with pseudotumors and are unlikely to be malignant processes.

23.3 Incidental Gallbladder Cancer

More than 750,000 cholecystectomies are performed annually in the USA and an estimated 0.3–1% have an associated tumor discovered "incidentally" [10]. The term "incidental gallbladder cancer" was given to imply the surprise histologic discovery of GB cancer in patients who underwent a cholecystectomy for presumed benign disease. However, it is estimated that up to 50% of patients with an "incidental gallbladder cancer" diagnosis actually had radiological findings suspicious for gallbladder cancer preoperatively [15].

23.4 General Consideration in Managing Gallbladder Cancer

23.4.1 Historical Overview

Until the 1950s, a cholecystectomy, with or without wedge resection of the GB bed, had been the recommended treatment for GB cancer [16]. In 1954, Glenn and Hays first proposed a "radical cholecystectomy" for the treatment of GB cancer. In this procedure, the GB bed with a 1 cm or greater rim of adjacent liver tissue and the lymphatic tissue within the hepatoduodenal ligament are excised *en bloc* with the gallbladder [17, 18]. Lymph drainage from the GB flows in a hepatofugal direction within the hepatoduodenal ligament. The sentinel lymph nodes include the cystic duct and the peri-choledochal node groups. The second draining lymph nodes are located postero-superior to the head of the pancreas or posterior to the portal vein and anterior to the common hepatic artery [9, 19, 20].

23.4.2 Staging and Re-resection

The need to perform re-resection following an "incidental GB cancer" is dependent on the pathologic stage of the tumor. T1a tumors only invade the lamina propia of the gallbladder wall and a cholecystectomy with negative margins is considered curative. Re-resection of the GB fossa with and without lymphadenectomy does not provide any survival benefit [21]. In contrast, re-resection is recommended in patients with T1b, T2, or T3 tumors due to an overall improved survival [10, 21–25].

Patients with "incidental" GB carcinoma often have a good prognosis because the majorities are early T1 or T2 lesions [26] (Table 23.1). In fact, patients with "incidental" GB cancer who undergo re-resection may have a better survival rate than patients with "nonincidental" GB cancer [27]. T2 tumors make up the majority (67%) of "incidental" GB cancers with re-resection having a 5-year survival rate of 61% compared to only 19% for those treated with a cholecystectomy only [27, 28] (Table 23.2).

T3 disease is defined as a tumor that invades the serosa and/or the liver and/or one other adjacent organ. These patients are at a higher risk of peritoneal metastases. In patients without evidence of peritoneal disease, formal re-resection and lymphadenectomy may provide a survival benefit. If untreated, T3 disease has a 5-year survival rate of 0–15%, as compared to 25–65% for T3 patients that have undergone re-resection [10] (Table 23.3).

23.4.3 Preoperative Workup for Re-resection

There are no defined guidelines or data that exist on how to stage prior to re-resection. High-resolution cross-sectional imaging is the most common radiographic workup employed in the setting of "incidentally" discovered

Table 23.1 Survival outcomes in retrospective reviews after resection of AJCC 6th edition Stage 1 non-metastatic GB cancer

	Year	N	Procedure	Survival 3 years (%)	Survival 5 years (%)
Donohue [10]	1990	6	83% simple cholecystectomy	100	100
Shirai [24]	1992	39	Simple cholecystectomy	100	100
Matsumoto [21]	1992	4	Extended cholecystectomy	100	100
Cubertanfond [3]	1994	20	Simple cholecystectomy	28	NR
De Aratxabala [29]	1997	32	69% simple cholecystectomy	94	94
Takayuki [30]	2003	22	Simple cholecystectomy	100	100
Shih [31]	2007	8	Simple cholecystectomy	NR	63

N number of patients

Table 23.2 Survival outcomes in retrospective reviews after resection of AJCC 6th edition T2 non-metastatic GB cancer

	Year	N	Re-resection (n)	Stage	Procedure	Operative mortality (%)	Survival 5 years (%)
Matsumoto [21]	1992	9	0	T2N0	Extended resection	4	100
Shirai [24]	1992	35	NR	T2N0	Simple cholecystectomy	NR	41
Shirai [24]	1992	10	NR	T2N0	Extended resection	NR	90
Fong [28]	2000	37	32	T2N0	Extended resection	4	61
Dixon [32]	2005	7	NR	T2N0	Extended resection	2	80

N number of patients, NR not specifically reported

Table 23.3 Survival outcomes in retrospective reviews after resection of AJCC 6th edition T3 and/or N1 nonmetastatic GB cancer

	Y	N	Re-resection (n)	Stage	Operative mortality (%)	Survival 3 years (%)	Survival 5 years (%)	Comments
Donohue [22]	1990	17	NR	T3N0 or T1-3N1	0	50	29	Extended resections only
Shirai [24]	1992	20	NR	T3N0 or T1-3N1	NR	NR	45	All patients had lymph node metastasis
Fong [28]	2000	24	NR	T3N0 or T1-3N1	4	28	28	Extended resections only
Fong [28]	2000	34	NR	T3N0 or T3N1	4	25	25	Extended resections only
Dixon [32]	2005	57	NR	T3N0	2	NR	63	Two time period cohorts
Dixon [32]	2005	57	NR	T3N0 or T1-3N1	2	NR	24	Two time period cohorts
Shih [31]	2007	34	NR	T3N0 or T1-3N1	4	NR	34	85% Extended resection

N number of patients, NR not reported

GB cancer. As with other liver tumors, an abdominal MRI with gadolinium may be superior to CT scanning to delineate intraparenchymal disease.

23.4.4 FDG-PET and Its Limitations

Because of the high risk of metastatic disease associated with GB cancer, some investigators have suggested that FDG (fluorodeoxyglucose) PET (positron emission tomography) may also be useful in the preoperative evaluation. It has been reported in one study that FDG-PET changed the management of nearly 25% of patients with gallbladder cancer [33]. FDG-PET may be able to identify residual tumor in patients who have previously undergone a cholecystectomy. Be aware that these findings can be false-positive due to activity related to early postoperative changes rather than actual residual disease. In conclusion, FDG-PET may be helpful to identify unsuspected distant metastatic disease in patients being considered for re-resection.

23.5 Non-surgical Management of Gallbladder Cancer

23.5.1 General Remarks

The roles of chemotherapy and radiation therapy are not well established in treating GB cancer. Complete surgical resection is the only therapy to date with curative intent. Unfortunately there are no prospective, randomized studies available mainly due to the low incidence of the disease and dismal prognosis. Retrospective data are limited and biased by selection factors. However, survival data following chemotherapy and/or chemoradiation are encouraging and should be considered in select patients with a high risk of recurrence.

23.5.2 Radiation Therapy

En bloc resections of the gallbladder and portal lymph nodes with adequate surgical margins are often difficult to achieve. The role of adjuvant radiotherapy is to control residual carcinoma in the tumor bed and to control regional lymph nodes. Significant increase in survival has been reported after curative surgery if there is only microscopic residual disease. Survival in this group of patients after surgery alone ranges from 6 to 7 months and can be prolonged to >12 months adding external beam radiotherapy [34]. This excludes patients with T1 or Stage 1 disease confined to the mucosa of the gallbladder, since their survival rates are high and they are at low risk for lymph node metastases [34, 35]. Surgical clips, placed at the conclusion of the initial resection, greatly help the radiation therapist to target the right field.

23.5.3 Chemotherapy

No evidence-based Phase III clinical study exists to demonstrate the benefit of any form of adjuvant therapy in GB cancer. 5-FU chemoradiation has shown a response rate of 10–24% in advanced disease, and is usually considered in both the adjuvant and neo-adjuvant setting [34]. Recently, Gemcitabine combination therapy has shown an increased response rate when compared to 5-FU alone. Gemcitabine has been studied in combination with S-1 with promising efficacy and acceptable toxicity [36]. Also, it has been studied with Cis-platinum and Capecitabine [34]. NCCN guidelines currently state that in a patient status post resection, a fluoropyrimidine chemoradiation (except T1b, N0), or fluoropyrimidine or Gemcitabine chemotherapy regimen should be considered [37]. However, there are limited clinical trial data to define a standard regimen or definitive benefit.

We have used neo-adjuvant therapy in settings where larger cancers have been incompletely removed. While there has never been a trial of adjuvant vs. neo-adjuvant therapy, it makes sense to treat those patients with tumors that have been violated during surgery and in the setting of bile spillage with adjuvant chemoradiation prior to re-excision [38]. It provides time to observe the patient for development of distant disease and it also allows adjuvant therapy to be delivered at the earliest time possible.

23.6 Surgical Management of Gallbladder Cancer

The two main components comprising surgical management of GB cancer are

- Partial resection of the liver
- Clearance of the loco-regional lymph nodes

23.6.1 Extent of Liver Resection

An R0 surgical margin is a major determinant of outcome [39]. A nonanatomic resection with ≥2 cm of hepatic parenchyma in the GB fossa is recommended for patients with no gross evidence of residual disease. Major liver resections have been controversial. Extended resections have an indeterminate or marginal survival benefit. Clearly, increased morbidity does no longer justify their application in routine management of GB cancer.

23.6.2 Extent of Lymphadenectomy

Lymphadenectomy is usually confined to the portal, hepatoduodenal ligament, pericholedochal, and hilar areas. Extended "radical N2" lymphadenectomy

- Celiac nodes
- Peripancreatic nodes
- Periduodenal nodes
- Superior mesenteric nodes
  is not routinely recommended. At our institution, we routinely sample the common hepatic artery lymph node. We have also begun obtaining peritoneal washings with intraoperative frozen section analysis to determine the extent of the disease.

23.6.3 Common Bile Duct Resection: Yes or No?

The belief that routine bile duct resection facilitates the lymphadenectomy and increases the number of lymph nodes in the pathological specimen has not been supported in the literature. Lymphadenectomy plus routine common bile duct resection has been associated with increased morbidity and no improvement in survival [40]. The cystic duct can often be biopsied at the time of repeat surgery. Patients with a positive duct margin, based on the initial cholecystectomy pathology or the intraoperative biopsy of the cystic duct stump, have an incidence of residual disease of 42% compared to 4% for those with a negative cystic duct margin. Therefore, in order to obtain R0 resection in patients with a positive cystic duct margin, a common bile duct resection in conjunction with a lymphadenectomy should be performed.

23.6.4 Choosing the Right Surgical Procedure

GB tumors may be identified in three distinct ways: preoperatively, intraoperatively, or postoperatively. Preoperatively, advanced radiological diagnostic modalities can identify asymptomatic GB tumors. The tumor can be identified intraoperatively at the time of cholecystectomy. But most commonly, the GB tumor is discovered on final histopathological examination following a routine cholecystectomy [41].

As mentioned, patients with "nonincidental" GB cancer have a significantly worse survival rate when compared to patients with "incidental" disease. As a result, there are currently two approaches to the management of preoperatively suspected gallbladder cancer. The patient can undergo cholecystectomy with intraoperative frozen section. If malignancy is confirmed and the tumor exceeds the T1a classification, a radical cholecystectomy should be performed. Alternatively, a radical cholecystectomy consisting of removal of the gallbladder and resection of hepatic segments IVb and V can be performed initially. Due to the fact that flat appearing GB cancers are not always picked up on intraoperative histopathologic analysis, we also perform a hepatoduodenal lymphadenectomy in these patients. Because of this fact, we routinely use the second approach in all patients with preoperative suspicion of gallbladder cancer. In patients with clear intraparenchymal spread who are considered for extended hepatectomies, liver volumetric studies need to be obtained to ensure an adequate functional liver remnant.

23.6.5 Role of Laparoscopy in Gallbladder Cancer

Although it has been recommended that laparoscopy should be avoided in the setting of preoperatively diagnosed GB cancer, we did not find clear contra-indications and started to use minimally invasive techniques routinely. Some studies have reported bile spillage of 15–45% leading to a significantly reduced survival, attributed to diffuse intraperitoneal tumor spread. However, we have not had bile spillage in any of our laparoscopic radical cholecystectomy patients [42]. Historically, as with all intraabdominal malignancies, in patients with GB cancer, there is a concern that laparoscopy may be associated with port-site recurrence. Over the last decade, long-term studies have shown that laparoscopy does not confer any increased risk of port site or incisional recurrence when compared to open procedures. This is believed to be due to improvement in technology and surgical skills and

- Routine use of wound protectors
- Impermeable specimen retrieval bags
- Evacuation of pneumoperitoneum with the trocars in place

23.6.6 Immediate Versus Staged Re-resection

Frozen section may confirm or suggest a gallbladder cancer. If the gallbladder mass is identified in situ, intraoperative ultrasound can be helpful to assess tumor extent and stage. According to a group in New York, there is no difference in long-term survival in patients managed with immediate versus staged re-resection for GB cancers. Nonetheless, our group performs a one-stage procedure whenever possible [28, 43].

23.6.7 Involvement of the Common Bile Duct

As previously discussed, in patients with T1b, T2, and T3 "incidental" GB cancers, re-resection is recommended after workup has been completed to exclude distant disease [44]. Definitive oncologic management requires re-resection of the liver (gallbladder bed), lymphadenectomy, and attention to the common bile duct. The extent of resection should be dictated by the ability to achieve an R0 resection. Routine common bile duct resection is unnecessary but should be performed in the setting of a positive cystic duct margin. When the intrapancreatic common bile duct is positive for malignancy, a Whipple procedure is indicated. When the proximal common bile duct is involved extending into the left or the right bile ducts, a corresponding major hepatectomy is indicated. If both the left and right hepatic ducts are found to be positive, we perform resection of the bifurcation with left and right hepatico-jejunostomies and place bilateral external biliary stents for postoperative brachytherapy.

23.7 Surgical Procedures

23.7.1 Laparoscopic Radical Cholecystectomy and Hepatoduodenal Lymphadenectomy

23.7.1.1 Preoperative Evaluation

All patients undergo a full medical evaluation including CBC, chemistry profile, and liver function tests to assess the Child–Pugh status. All patients with preoperative suspicion of GB cancer are offered an open or laparoscopic radical cholecystectomy with added lymphadenectomy. This includes patients with

- Gallbladder masses >1 cm
- Gallbladder masses combined with elevated serum tumor markers (CEA and/or CA19-9)
- Evidence for hepatic parenchymal spread
- Blood flow in gallbladder masses or polyps

Although most patients are initially diagnosed on right upper quadrant ultrasound, all patients receive cross-sectional imaging. As for liver tumors, abdominal MRI with gadolinium is preferred due to the enhanced visualization of the hepatic parenchyma. For patients with concerns for hepatic metastases or bulky disease, we also obtain a PET-CT scan. The serum tumor markers CEA and CA 19-9 are obtained preoperatively and when elevated used postoperatively to monitor treatment response. Patients who come to our institution diagnosed after cholecystectomy undergo the same workup. If there is a concern for peritoneal metastases, a preliminary laparoscopic exploration with peritoneal washings is performed. In addition to venous compression boots, all patients receive preoperative subcutaneous heparin injection for deep venous thrombosis prophylaxis. In the rare circumstance of contraindications to heparin, we will place an inferior vena cava filter preoperatively.

23.7.1.2 Patient Positioning and Operating Room Setup

The patient is placed on a bean-bag and positioned in the low lithotomy or French position. A safety strap is placed over the lower abdomen and all bony-prominences are given extra padding. The patient is brought in reverse Trendelenburg position at the beginning of the procedure. The operating surgeon stands in-between the patient's legs and his first assistant to the left of the patient. A set of three monitors is placed in a semicircle at the proximal end of the operating table.

23.7.1.3 Trocar Placement

As with standard laparoscopic cholecystectomy, four trocars are used. The first trocar is placed approximately one hand-breadth below the right subcostal margin along the mid-clavicular line. This is the camera trocar. Two working trocars are placed to the left and the right of this trocar. A final trocar is placed in the subxiphoid region and is used for the assistant. All trocars placed are dilating trocars (VersaStep™ System, Covidien, Norwalk, CT, USA). Ideally, a robotically controlled camera holder is used to provide a steady image and to reduce the surgeon's visual fatigue (ViKY™, Endocontrol, Grenoble, France). This is particularly useful if a biliary reconstruction becomes necessary (Fig. 23.1).

23.7.1.4 Dissection for Preoperative Suspected Gallbladder Cancer

Any adhesions to the gallbladder are transected using ultrasonic shears (Ethicon, Cincinnatti, OH, USA). Care is taken not to violate any attachments to the tumor. The assistant retracts the liver superiorly using a standard laparoscopic liver retractor. As with routine laparoscopic cholecystectomy, the dissection begins by identifying the triangle of Calot. The cystic duct and artery are then dissected and triple clipped prior to transection. The vascular anatomy of the porta hepatis is controlled at all times and if in doubt intraoperative ultrasound will be used (Fig. 23.2). We transect the cystic duct right at its confluence with the common bile duct. This is done to prevent multiple positive frozen sections requiring re-resection of the cystic duct. If the distal margin is positive for malignancy on frozen section, the decision can be made expeditiously to perform a laparoscopic common bile duct excision. The common bile duct will be transected with the ultrasonic shears proximally and with the laparoscopic GIA stapling device distally. The CBD is then cannulated with a 5 Fr. pediatric feeding tube prior to reconstruction (Fig. 23.3).

Prior to the parenchymal transection, a full-staging laparoscopic hepatic ultrasound is performed to rule out synchronous metastases and to delineate the extent

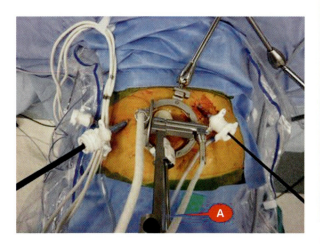

Fig. 23.1 Laparoscopic radical cholecystectomy: Trocar placement. A robotically controlled camera holder (ViKY, Endocontrol, Grenoble, France)

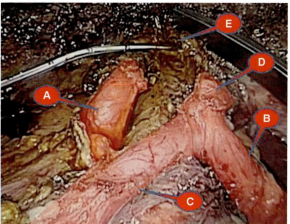

Fig. 23.2 Porta hepatis: Vascular anatomy. *A* replaced right hepatic artery, *B* common hepatic artery, *C* gastroduodenal artery, *D* left hepatic artery, *E* transected common bile duct with a 5 Fr. pediatric stent placed within it

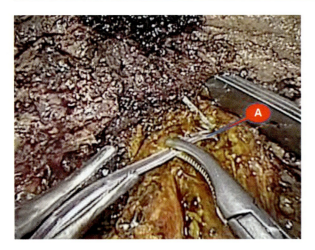

Fig. 23.3 Laparoscopic radical cholecystectomy: Common bile duct transection. *A* 5 Fr. pediatric feeding tube placed prior to construction of the laparoscopic choledocho-jejunostomy

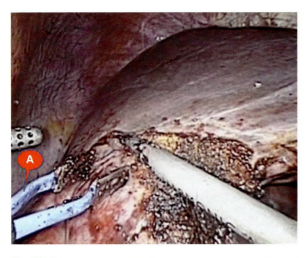

Fig. 23.4 Laparoscopic radical cholecystectomy: Parenchymal transection. *A* bipolar device

of disease. The parenchyma is then transected with the ultrasonic shears, trying to obtain a 3-cm margin of normal tissue. Hemostasis is reinforced with the laparoscopic bipolar forceps (Medtronic, Jacksonville, FL, USA). It is helpful to identify the middle hepatic vein using ultrasound so that this structure can be transected with minimal blood loss (Fig. 23.4). The specimen is then placed in a specimen retrieval bag and sent to pathology for further frozen section analysis. For large specimens, we use a trans-umbilical incision for specimen extraction, similar to the one used for single incision laparoscopic procedures [45].

23.7.1.5 Dissection for Postoperative Detected Gallbladder Cancer

For patients that present after laparoscopic cholecystectomy, a review of the pathology slides and operative reports is mandatory. This holds especially true if the cystic duct status was not analyzed. In the event the cystic duct margin cannot be determined, the cystic duct will be sought laparoscopically and sent for frozen section analysis [46]. If the cystic duct cannot be localized, a common bile duct excision may become necessary. Oftentimes, the operative report will specify whether or not a specimen retrieval bag was used and via what trocar site the specimen was removed. We routinely excise approximately 1 cm of skin and fascia from the extraction site due to concerns of bile spillage and possible development of port-site metastasis. If the extraction site is not clearly specified in the operative report, all trocar sites may have to be excised.

23.7.2 Laparoscopic Common Bile Duct Excision and Laparoscopic Roux-en-Y Choledocho-jejunostomy

If a common bile duct excision is required, this is done just below the confluence of the right and left hepatic duct and just above the intrapancreatic portion of the common bile duct using ultrasonic shears. If a Whipple procedure or left or right hepatectomy is required, this can be done open or laparoscopically [47–50]. To reconstruct the biliary system, we perform a Roux-en-Y choledocho-jejunostomy laparoscopically [51]. This is done with the patient initially in reverse Trendelenburg position. The transverse colon is elevated with laparoscopic graspers and the ligament of Treitz is identified. A 40 cm limb of jejunum is chosen and transected with a laparoscopic GIA stapling device. If the mesentery needs to be transected, this can be done with ultrasonic shears or with a firing of the laparoscopic GIA stapler device, white load. The Roux limb can be brought up either in an antecolic or retro-colic fashion, depending on the patient's anatomy. We create the choledocho-jejunostomy laparoscopically in a running fashion with absorbable sutures (Figs. 23.5 and 23.6). Bile ducts <5 mm are reconstructed with interrupted absorbable sutures. The jejuno-jejunostomy is then created after placement of two stay sutures at the edges. Mirror enterotomies for placement of the stapling device are created with ultrasonic shears. The jejuno-jejunostomy is then created with one firing of the laparoscopic GIA stapler device (blue load). The remaining enterotomy is closed with two layers of running 3/0 silk. The outer layer is fashioned with a horizontal Lembert stitch. Alternatively, the jejuno-jejunostomy can be created via the extraction site if a trans-umbilical site was used for specimen removal.

23.8 The FOX CHASE Data – Personal Experience

A total of seven patients have undergone laparoscopic radical cholecystectomy and hepatoduodenal lymphadenectomy at our institution. Four were found to have gallbladder cancer on final pathology. The other three patients with benign disease had cholelithiasis in the setting of a porcelain gallbladder. One of these patients underwent laparoscopic radical cholecystectomy via a single incision laparoscopic approach. The last patient had autoimmune cholecystitis in the setting of normal preoperative IgG4 levels. The autoimmune cholecystitis was diagnosed postoperatively when immunehistochemical analysis was positive for IgG4 [52]. Of the four patients with gallbladder cancer, two presented after routine laparoscopic cholecystectomies at outside institutions and two were suspected preoperatively. One patient who underwent primary resection was found to be Stage 1b and the second patient was Stage 2b. Of the two patients that underwent laparoscopic re-resection after an initial laparoscopic cholecystectomy elsewhere, one was Stage 1b and the other was found to be Stage 2a. The average operative time for minimally invasive radical cholecystectomies was 209 min (range = 95–360 min), average estimated blood loss of 133 cc (range = 50–300 cc), and the average length of stay was 3.7 days (range = 3–4 days). Average lymph node retrieval was three (range = 1–6). There have been no intraoperative complications nor postoperative morbidity or mortality at 30 days for all seven patients.

For the patients with cancer, the average operative time was 230 min (range = 120–360 min), average estimated blood loss of 115 cc (range = 50–200 cc), and the average length of stay was 4 days (range = 3–5 days). Average lymph node retrieval was three (range = 1–7). Currently all patients are alive and free of disease with an average follow-up of 7 months (range = 3–10 months). At 60 days, one patient developed a benign biliary stricture in the left ductal system that was stented endoscopically.

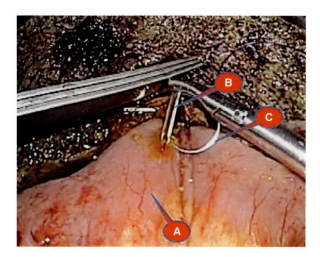

Fig. 23.5 Laparoscopic radical cholecystectomy: Choledocho-jejunostomy. *A* Jejunum, *B* distal limb of the 5 Fr. pediatric feeding tube used as stent, *C* start of the anterior layer of the choledocho-jejunostomy

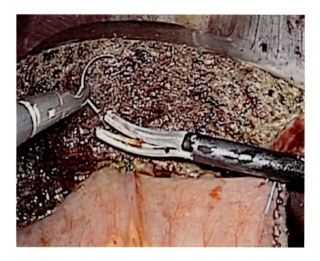

Fig. 23.6 Laparoscopic radical cholecystectomy: Completed choledocho- jejunostomy

23.9 Conclusion

Although laparoscopic gallbladder surgery is one of the most widespread minimally invasive procedures across the globe, laparoscopic management of gallbladder cancer > T1a has been slow to be adopted. As our laparoscopic experience with major hepatectomies and Whipple procedures has grown, we have begun adopting minimally invasive approaches for patients with T1b or greater tumors diagnosed postoperatively or suspected preoperatively. One of the main reasons why laparoscopy in treating gallbladder cancer has not been widely adopted is its low incidence. Traditionally, gallbladder cancers are referred to major cancer centers where the majority of surgeries are still performed open.

Historically cited reasons for not adopting laparoscopic approaches for cancer have been concerns for port site recurrences. We now know that laparoscopy does not have any increased incidence of port site or incisional metastasis when compared to traditional open surgery. This is due to the adoption of wound protectors and development of new techniques. A final concern has been the fear of air embolism during liver surgery. It is important to remember that carbon dioxide gas is used during laparoscopy. Although argon gas embolism has been reported, the risk of air embolism is probably decreased during laparoscopy [53]. To this end, it is interesting to recall that interventional radiologists often inject carbon dioxide gas during their procedures as a routine with no untoward events.

Many controversies exist as to the proper surgical resection for GB cancer. Although some centers advocate extended hepatectomies for GB cancer, at our center we perform radical cholecystectomies, either open or laparoscopic, depending on the surgeon's comfort level. It is important to note that even extended right hepatectomies for gallbladder cancer have been safely performed laparoscopically [48]. As common bile duct excision is often required, a mastery of laparoscopic suturing is needed prior to embarking on laparoscopic radical cholecystectomy so that biliary reconstruction can be performed intracorporally. During lymphadenectomy and hepatic parenchymal transection, the laparoscopic bipolar device is particularly useful to obtain hemostasis.

As an increasing number of surgical oncologists obtain minimally invasive surgical training, the minimally invasive approach to the surgical management of gallbladder cancers will most likely expand. Although we have a small series, this approach seems technically feasible and safe. When done for cancer, we have shown that an adequate lymph node retrieval of at least three nodes is possible and that hepatic parenchymal margins can be rendered negative. As our experience grows, we believe that our lymph node retrieval will continue to improve. Ultimately, it is important to remember that conversion to an open procedure should be done in a timely manner in the face of significant hemorrhage or if clear oncological margins or adequate lymph node retrieval cannot be obtained. Much larger trials are needed to fully answer open questions. Additionally, further follow-up is needed to see if the laparoscopic approach confers any advantage or disadvantage compared to traditional open techniques.

Quick Reference Guide

1. **T1a lesions:** Laparoscopic management is currently the standard of care if negative margins and no bile leak.
2. **T1b or greater lesions:** Laparoscopic management is still controversial.
3. **Required margin:** Although a minimum of 1 cm of normal hepatic parenchyma around the gallbladder cancer is required, ideally 3 cm of margin should be sought.
4. **Lymph node retrieval:** A minimum of three lymph nodes should be obtained during the hepatoduodenal lymphadenectomy.
5. Routine laparoscopic common bile duct excision is not required, but should be performed if

   - Cystic duct margin is positive
   - Lymph nodes are adherent to common bile duct

6. **Reason to convert:** When an adequate hepatic parenchymal or bile duct margin or a minimum of three lymph nodes cannot be obtained safely.
7. **Indications for radical cholecystectomy at FOX CHASE:**

   - All patients with gallbladder masses >1 cm
   - Gallbladder masses with elevated serum tumor markers (CEA and/or CA19-9)
   - Blood flow in the mass or polyp
   - Evidence for hepatic parenchymal spread

8. If the mass is on the peritoneal side of the gallbladder, a simple cholecystectomy with frozen section analysis should be considered.

9. Minimally invasive surgery for gallbladder cancer requires advanced laparoscopic skills.
10. The minimally invasive approach to GB cancers >T1a should be done in cancer centers with minimally invasive expertise and access to multidisciplinary treatment.

References

1. Jemal, A., Siegel, R., Ward, E., Hao, Y., Xu, J., Murray, T., et al.: Cancer statistics. CA Cancer J. Clin. **58**, 71–96 (2008)
2. Carriaga, M.T., Henson, D.E.: Liver, gallbladder, extrahepatic bile ducts, and pancreas. Cancer **75**, 171–190 (1995)
3. Cubertafond, P., Gainant, A., Cucchiaro, G.: Surgical treatment of 724 carcinomas of the gallbladder. Results of the French Surgical Association Survey. Ann. Surg. **219**, 275–280 (1994)
4. Lazcano-Ponce, E.C., Miguel, J.F., Munoz, N., Herrero, R., Ferrecio, C., Wistuba, I.I., et al.: Epidemiology and molecular pathology of gallbladder cancer. CA Cancer J. Clin. **51**, 349–364 (2001)
5. Levy, A.D., Murakata, L.A., Rohrmann, C.A.: Gallbladder carcinoma: radiologic-pathologic correlation. Radiographics **21**, 295–314 (2001)
6. Piehler, J.M., Crichlow, R.W.: Primary carcinoma of the gallbladder. Surg. Gynecol. Obstet. **147**, 929–942 (1978)
7. Jensen, E., et al.: A critical analysis of the surgical management of early-stage gallbladder cancer in the United States. J. Gastrointest. Surg. **13**, 722–727 (2008)
8. Goodman, M.T., Yamamoto, J.: Descriptive study of gallbladder, extrahepatic bile duct, and ampullary cancers in the United States, 1997–2002. Cancer Causes Control **18**, 415–422 (2007)
9. Fahim, R.B., McDonald, J.R., Richards, J.C., et al.: Carcinoma of the gallbladder: a study of its modes of spread. Ann. Surg. **156**, 114–124 (1962)
10. Hueman, T., et al.: Evolving treatment strategies for gallbladder cancer. Ann. Surg. Oncol. **16**, 2101–2115 (2009)
11. Randi, G., Malvezzi, M., Levi, F., Ferlay, J., Negri, E., Franceschi, S., et al.: Epidemiology of biliary tract cancers: an update. Ann. Oncol. **20**(1), 146–159 (2008)
12. Albores-Saavedra, J., Alcantara-Vazquez, A., Cruz-Ortiz, H., Her-rera-Goepfert, R.: The precursor lesions of invasive gallbladder carcinoma. Hyperplasia, atypical hyperplasia and carcinoma in situ. Cancer **45**, 919–927 (1980)
13. Lowenfels, A.B., Lindstrom, C.G., Conway, M.J., Hastings, P.R.: Gallstones and risk of gallbladder cancer. J. Natl. Cancer Inst. **75**, 77–80 (1985)
14. Kwon, A.H., Inui, H., Matsui, Y., Uchida, Y., Hukui, J., Kamiyama, Y.: Laparoscopic cholecystectomy in patients with porcelain gallbladder based on the preoperative ultrasound findings. Hepatogastroenterology **51**, 950–953 (2004)
15. Shukla, P.J., Barreto, G., Neve, R., et al.: Can we do better than incidental gallbladder cancer? Hepatogastroenterology **54**, 2184–2185 (2007)
16. Fahim, R.B., Ferris, D.O., McDonald, J.R.: Carcinoma of the gallbladder: an appraisal of its surgical treatment. Arch. Surg. **86**, 334–341 (1963)
17. Glenn, F.: Radical cholecystectomy for carcinoma of the gallbladder. In: Glenn, F. (ed.) Atlas of Biliary Tract Surgery. The Macmillan Company, New York (1963)
18. Glenn, F., Hays, D.M.: The scope of radical surgery in the treatment of malignant tumors of the extrahepatic biliary tract. Surg. Gynecol. Obstet. **99**, 529–541 (1954)
19. Japanese Society of Biliary Surgery: Classification of Biliary Tract Carcinoma. Kanehara & Co, Tokyo (2004)
20. Shirai, Y., Yoshida, K., Tsukada, K., et al.: Identification of the regional lymphatic system of the gallbladder by vital staining. Br. J. Surg. **79**, 659–662 (1992)
21. Matsumoto, Y., Fujii, H., Aoyama, H., Yamamoto, M., Sugahara, K., Suda, K.: Surgical treatment of primary carcinoma of the gallbladder based on the histologic analysis of 48 surgical specimens. Am. J. Surg. **163**, 239–245 (1992)
22. Donohue, J.H., Nagorney, D.M., Grant, C.S., Tsushima, K., Ilstrup, D.M., Adson, M.A.: Carcinoma of the gallbladder. Does radical resection improve outcome? Arch. Surg. **125**, 237–241 (1990)
23. Foster, J.M., Hoshi, H., Gibbs, J.F., et al.: Gallbladder cancer: defining the indications for primary radical resection and radical reresection. Ann. Surg. Oncol. **14**, 833–840 (2007)
24. Shirai, Y., Yoshida, K., Tsukada, K., Muto, T., Watanabe, H.: Radical surgery for gallbladder carcinoma. Long-term results. Ann. Surg. **216**, 565–568 (1992)
25. Shukla, P.J., Barreto, G., Kakade, A., Shrikhande, S.V.: Revision surgery for gallbladder cancer: factors influencing operability and further evidence for T1b tumours. HPB (Oxford) **10**, 43–47 (2008)
26. Shirai, Y., et al.: Radical lymph node dissection for gallbladder cancer: indications and limitations. Surg. Oncol. Clin. N. Am. **16**(1), 221–232 (2007)
27. Pawlik, T.M., Gleisner, A.L., Vigano, L., Kooby, D.A., Bauer, T.W., Frilling, A., et al.: Incidence of finding residual disease for incidental gallbladder carcinoma: implications for re-resection. J. Gastrointest. Surg. **11**, 1478–1487 (2007)
28. Fong, Y., Jarnagin, W., Blumgart, L.H.: Gallbladder cancer: comparison of patients presenting initially for definitive operation with those presenting after prior noncurative intervention. Ann. Surg. **232**, 557–569 (2000)
29. De Aretxabala, X., et al.: Curative resection in potentially resectable tumours of the gallbladder. Eur. J. Surg. **163**, 419–426 (1997)
30. Takayuki, T., et al.: Completion radical surgery after cholecystectomy for accidentally undiagnosed gallbladder carcinoma. World J. Surg. **27**, 266–271 (2003)
31. Shih, S., et al.: Gallbladder cancer: the role of laparoscopy and radical resection. Ann. Surg. **245**, 893–901 (2007)
32. Dixon, E., Vollmer Jr., C.M., Sahajpal, A., Cattral, M., Grant, D., Doig, C., et al.: An aggressive surgical approach leads to improved survival in patients with gallbladder cancer: a 12-year study at a North American Center. Ann. Surg. **241**, 385–394 (2005)
33. Corvera, C.U., Blumgart, L.H., Akhurst, T., DeMatteo, R.P., D'Angelica, M., Fong, Y., et al.: 18F-fluorodeoxyglucose positron emission tomography influences management decisions in patients with biliary cancer. J. Am. Coll. Surg. **206**, 57–65 (2008)

34. Denshaw-Burke, M. et al.: Gallbladder Cancer: eMedicine Specialties: Carcinomas of the Gastrointestinal Tract. Epub (2010)
35. Todoroki, T., Kawamoto, T., Otsuka, M., Koike, N., Yoshida, S., Takada, Y., Adachi, S., Kashiwagi, H., Fukao, K., Ohara, K.: Benefits of combining radiotherapy with aggressive resection for stage IV gallbladder cancer. Hepatogastroenterology **46**(27), 1585–1591 (1999)
36. Sasaki, T., Isayama, H., Nakai, Y., Ito, Y., Kogure, H., et al.: Multicenter, phase II study of gemcitabine and S-1 combination chemotherapy in patients with advanced biliary tract cancer. Cancer Chemother. Pharmacol. **62**, 849–855 (2009)
37. Macdonald, O.K., Crane, C.H.: Palliative and postoperative radiotherapy in biliary tract cancer. Surg. Oncol. Clin. N. Am. **11**(4), 941–954 (2002)
38. Sasson, A.R., Hoffman, J.P., Ross, E., Meropol, N.J., Szarka, C.E., Freedman, G., Pinover, W., Pingpank, J.F., Eisenberg, B.L.: Trimodality therapy for advanced gallbladder cancer. Am. Surg. **67**(3), 277–283 (2001). discussion 284
39. Pawlik, T.M., Choti, M.A.: Biology dictates prognosis following resection of gallbladder carcinoma: sometimes less is more. Ann. Surg. Oncol. **16**, 787–788 (2009)
40. D'Angelica, M., Dalal, K.M., DeMatteo, R.P., Fong, Y., Blumgart, L.H., Jarnagin, W.R.: Analysis of the extent of resection for adenocarcinoma of the gallbladder. Ann. Surg. Oncol. **16**, 806–816 (2009)
41. Steinert, R., Nestler, G., Sagynaliev, E., Muller, J., Lippert, H., Reymond, M.A.: Laparoscopic cholecystectomy and gallbladder cancer. J. Surg. Oncol. **93**, 682–689 (2006)
42. Blumgart, L.H.: Surgery of the Liver, Biliary Tract and Pancreas, vol. 1. WB Saunders, Philadelphia (2006)
43. Shih, S.P., Schulick, R.D., Cameron, J.L., Lillemoe, K.D., Pitt, H.A., Choti, M.A., Campbell, K.A., Yeo, C.J., Talamini, M.A.: Gallbladder cancer: the role of laparoscopy and radical resection. Ann. Surg. **245**(6), 893–901 (2007)
44. Shukla, P., et al.: Gallbladder cancer: we need to do better! Ann. Surg. Oncol. **16**, 2084–2085 (2009)
45. Gumbs, A.A., Milone, L., Sinha, P., Chabot, J.A., Bessler, M.: VIDEO: totally transumbilical laparoscopic cholecystectomy. J. Gastrointes. Surg. **13**(3), 533–534 (2009)
46. Gumbs, A.A., Hoffman, J.P.: Laparoscopic completion radical cholecystectomy for T2 gallbladder cancer. Surg. Endosc. Online First, Epub ahead of print (2010 May 25)
47. Gumbs, A.A., Gayet, B.: Laparoscopic Duodenopancreatectomy: the posterior approach. Surg. Endosc. **22**(2), 539–540 (2008 Feb)
48. Gumbs, A.A., Gayet, B.: Totally laparoscopic extended right hepatectomy. Surg. Endosc. **22**(9), 2076–2077 (2008 Sep)
49. Gumbs, A.A., Bouhanna, P., Bar-Zakai, B., Briennon, X., Gayet, B.: Laparoscopic partial splenectomy using radiofrequency ablation. J. Laparoendosc. Adv. Surg. Tech. **18**(4), 611–613 (2008 Aug)
50. Gumbs, A.A., Bar-Zakai, B., Gayet, B.: Totally laparoscopic extended left hepatectomy. J. Gastrointest. Surg. **12**(7), 1152 (2008 July)
51. Gumbs, A.A., Hoffman, J.P.: Laparoscopic completion radical cholecystectomy for T2 gallbladder cancer. Surg. Endosc. **24**(7), 1766–1768 (2010 May 25)
52. Gumbs, A.A., Milone, L., Geha, R., Delacroix, J., Chabot, J.A.: Laparoscopic radical cholecystectomy. J. Laparoendosc. Adv. Surg. Tech. **19**(4), 519–520 (2009)
53. Gumbs, A.A., Gayet, B., Gagner, M.: Laparoscopic liver resection: when to use the laparoscopic stapler device. HPB **10**(4), 296–303 (2008)

Part VII

Special Topics: Spleen

Spleen: Hematological Disorders

Eduardo M. Targarona, Carmen Balague, and Manuel Trias

24.1 Introduction

Hematological malignancies rarely require major surgical intervention. Major surgery in the management of hematological malignancy typically involves either splenectomy, removal of an intra-abdominal or retroperitoneal mass, or lymph node sampling for staging. Traditionally, these types of procedures require a large incision to access the abdominal cavity and the associated morbidity can be quite substantial.

The great advances in minimally invasive surgery (MIS) that have been made over the last two decades did also benefit patients suffering from hematological disease. The advantages of MIS for cancer treatment are widely accepted these days. It should be kept in mind that patients requiring splenectomy are usually elderly and frail, so a less invasive approach to their treatment may be an advantage.

Laparoscopic splenectomy (LS) is mainly indicated for hematological disorders that are not associated with splenomegaly, such as idiopathic thrombocytopenic purpura (ITP) [1–3]. Intra-abdominal manipulation of bulky organs during laparoscopic surgery is technically challenging, and retrieval of the specimen may be difficult. Splenomegaly was initially considered a contraindication for LS. Many hematological diseases associated with an enlarged spleen are malignant conditions and were traditionally a domain for open splenectomy with its associated increased morbidity. Improvements and refinement of LS techniques have resulted in the ability to remove an enlarged spleen using a laparoscopic approach and preserving all the advantages of a minimally invasive approach [4–12]. However, a large spleen is associated with considerable technical demands. In addition, operative time is longer and the conversion rate higher than in the case of a normal-sized spleen (Table 24.1).

24.2 Hematological Malignancies

24.2.1 Classification and Current Nonsurgical Therapies

Medical therapy has improved considerably in recent years, and only a few hematological malignancies require splenectomy as first-line treatment. Those, in which a splenectomy may be considered as part of the treatment strategy can be divided into six groups [13–16]:

- Hodgkin's lymphoma
- Non-Hodgkin's lymphoma
- Chronic lymphocytic leukemia
- Chronic myeloid leukemia
- Myelofibrosis
- Metastasis to the spleen

24.2.1.1 Hodgkin's Lymphoma (HL)

The incidence of Hodgkin's disease in European countries is about 2.2/100,000/year. Definitive diagnosis is

E.M. Targarona (✉)
Service of Surgery, Hospital de Sant Pau, Medical School of the Autonomous University of Barcelona, Barcelona, Spain
e-mail: etargarona@santpau.cat

C. Balague
Service of Surgery, Hospital de Sant Pau, Barcelona, Spain

M. Trias
Hospital de Sant Pau, Medical School of the University of Barcelona, Barcelona, Spain

Table 24.1 World Experience – Laparoscopic splenectomy in cases of splenomegaly

	Year	n	Spleen weight (g)	OR time (min)	Length of stay (day)	Conversion rate (%)	Morbidity (%)	Mortality (%)	Spleen weight mean (g)
Nicholson [5]	1998	12	>800	186*	5	0	0	0	1,500
Terrossu [6]	2001	20	>500	163	5.6	4	20	0	2,220
Todd [7]	2001	60	>500	172*	2.7	3.3	8.3	0	983
Kercher [8]	2001	41	>600	171*	2.3	0	9	0	–
Patel [9]	2003	27	>1,000	170	5	18	55	0	2,500
Mahon [10]	2003	10	>1,000	94	6	60	20	0	2,000
Kaban [11]	2004	39	>600	153*	5.3	3	24	5	1,285
Targarona [12]	2005	56	>700	150*	5	14	26	0	1,600

Includes series with >10 patients, *HALS technique

established by lymph node biopsy. Accurate staging (Stage I–IV) may be accomplished with different imaging techniques. The traditional surgical intra-abdominal staging has been replaced by imaging modalities like CT scan or PET. The choice of chemotherapeutic regimen combined with radiation therapy of 30–36 Gy depends on the clinical stage. ABVD, using a combination of four drugs (**A**driamycin, **B**leomycin, **V**inblastine, **D**acarbazine), or BEACOPP for advanced stage, (**B**leomycin, **E**toposide, **A**driamycin, **C**yclophosphamide, Vincristin=**O**ncovine, **P**rocarbazine, **P**rednisone), are the two most common applied regimens. Treatment for relapsing disease includes different drug combinations. Autologous stem cell transplantation after high-dose chemotherapy may be considered [17].

24.2.1.2 Non-Hodgkin's Lymphoma (NHL)

Non-Hodgkin's lymphoma is a group of lymphoid malignancies that rank fifth in cancer incidence and mortality in most countries. The incidence increased by 80% over the last 30 years. NHL presents as an indolent disease, mainly nodular or follicular variant or highly aggressive disease. B-cell lymphomas are more common than T-cell types.

The most common B-cell lymphoma types are:

- Diffuse large B-cell (31%)
- Follicular lymphomas (22%)

Less common variants are:

- Chronic Lymphatic Leukemia (5.5%)
- MALT lymphoma (8%)
- Peripheral T-cell (7%)
- Mantle cell lymphomas (6.9%)
- Other lymphoma types (3%)

Conventional treatment is based on the natural history of the disease, and ranges from a "watch-and-see policy," to radiation therapy alone, chemotherapy alone or chemoradiation therapy. Single-agent alkylation therapy and the CVP regimen (**C**yclophosphamide, **V**incristine, and **P**rednisone) are the mainstay treatments available for low-grade NHL. High-intensity therapy usually involves the CHOP regimen (Doxorubicin, Cyclophosphamide, Vincristine and Prednisone and Fludarabine). Treatment for relapsing disease after first-line therapy includes a number of drug combinations. In the setting of relapsing disease, the 5-year survival is reported to be below 50%. Monoclonal antibody treatment is currently in clinical trials and shows promising results as first-line and salvage therapy. Initial results with Rituximab, a chimeric anti CD-20 monoclonal antibody, and Alemtuzumab, a CDR-grafted human IgG monoclonal antibody, have led to the development of new medications and alteration of current therapies. Both medications are directed against the CD52 antigens expressed in leukemic T lymphocytes, macrophages, and monocytes [18–21].

24.2.1.3 Chronic Myeloid Leukemia (CML)

Chronic myeloid leukemia (CML) was one of the first hematological diseases to be linked to a chromosomal defect, the so-called Philadelphia chromosome. It is a rare disease with an incidence of 1–2/100,000/year. It is easily diagnosed by blood tests and confirmed by genetic analysis (Phi chromosome or BCR-ABL transcripts) of peripheral white blood cells or bone marrow. A number of hematological, cytogenetic and molecular markers can be used to predict a response to treatment or to identify a possible blast crisis. Treatment for CML has advanced considerably over the last 40 years due to improved understanding of the molecular and genetic basis of this disease. Treatment strategies evolved from using Hydroxyl Urea and Busulfan, to stem cell transplantation, alpha Interferon, and more recently to molecular targeted therapies like the tyrosine kinase inhibitor Imatinib. Current treatment protocols for chronic disease generally include Imatinib or allogenic stem cell transplantation. The selection of any of those therapies will depend on the existence of clinical predictors of blast crisis or the individual risk factors for stem cell transplantation. Novel therapies under development include additional tyrosine kinase inhibitors (Dasatinib or Nilotinib), immunotherapy with vaccines (BCR-ABL peptide vaccine), and immunochemotherapy combining Imatinib and interferon [22, 23].

24.2.1.4 Myelofibrosis

Myeloid metaplasia with myelofibrosis is a chronic myeloproliferative disorder characterized by

- Anemia
- Massive splenomegaly
- Extra-medullar hepatosplenic hematopoiesis
- Stromal bone marrow reactions including fibrosis
- Osteosclerosis and
- Angiogenesis.

Median survival is 5 years, ranging from 2 to 12 years, depending on the clinically defined prognostic factors. Clinical symptoms include portal hypertension, pulmonary hypertension, and leukemic changes and these patients often require blood transfusions. The only curative therapy is allogeneic bone marrow transplantation in younger, high-risk patients. Supportive therapy for clinically symptomatic anemia includes steroids, Danazol, EPO, Thalidomide, or a blood transfusion. In the event of splenomegaly Hydroxyl-urea, Busulfan, interferon, or surgery will be therapeutic options. Leukemic changes are associated with a grim prognosis. Evolving therapies include VEGF receptor inhibitors or a combination of therapies including Thalidomide or Etanercept [24, 25].

24.3 Malignancies Involving the Spleen Directly

24.3.1 Primary Tumors of the Spleen

Primary malignant tumors of the spleen are rare and include

- Splenic lymphoma
- Angiosarcoma
- Malignant fibrous histiocytoma

Local symptoms are very unspecific. Currently available imaging techniques demonstrate only indirect signs. Surgery is usually warranted to confirm the diagnosis and will be performed in curative intent.

24.3.2 Secondary Tumors of the Spleen

Secondary tumors of the spleen are also very rare. The most common primary cancers, metastasizing to the spleen are

- Breast cancer
- Lung cancer
- Colon cancer
- Ovarian cancer
- Melanoma

Splenectomy may be an option, if the spleen is the only site of disease. The primary tumor should already have been resected and be well controlled. Therefore, surgery is planned with curative intent [13–16, 26].

24.4 The Barcelona Data – Personal Experience

326 patients underwent LS over a period of 14 years. Malignancy was found in 94 of 326 (30%) patients. (Figs. 24.1–24.3)

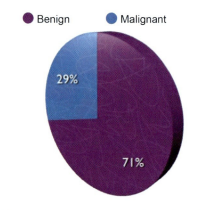

Fig. 24.1 The Barcelona data (1998–2007): Overall distribution of malignant and benign cases

24.4.1 Non-Hodgkin's Lymphoma (NHL)

The most frequent indication for LS was non-Hodgkin Lymphoma (NHL) (64/94, 60%). Diagnosis is usually made by biopsy of an enlarged peripheral lymph node. The spleen is rarely the primary site for NHL, but is involved in more than 70% of patients. Standard treatment is nonsurgical. LS is only indicated in cases where a diagnosis cannot be established by obtaining peripheral tissue and the clinical suspicion remains or when the patient experiences clinical symptoms related to massive splenomegaly or low platelet count. Laparoscopic splenectomy does not alter the natural history of the disease, but related thrombocytopenia may improve in up to 75% of patients. In our series, patients with NHL were older when compared with patients having a splenectomy for other indications. Enlargement of the spleen was moderate with a mean weight of 1,200 g (range 140–6,100 g) (Table 24.2).

24.4.2 Primary and Secondary Splenic Lymphoma

Therapeutic LS may also be beneficial to patients in cases of a primary spleen lymphoma or splenic marginal zone lymphoma. A splenic lymphoma is a rare disorder and seen in less than 1% of NHL.

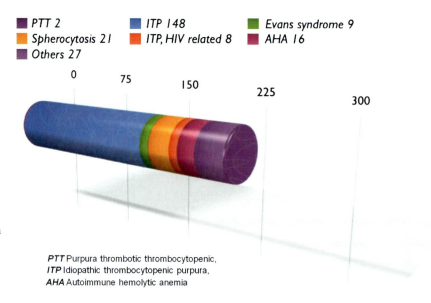

Fig. 24.2 The Barcelona data (1998–2007): Overall distribution of benign cases stratified by pathological diagnosis

PTT Purpura thrombotic thrombocytopenic, *ITP* Idiopathic thrombocytopenic purpura, *AHA* Autoimmune hemolytic anemia

24 Spleen: Hematological Disorders

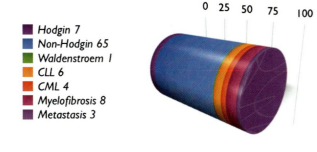

- Hodgin 7
- Non-Hodgin 65
- Waldenstroem 1
- CLL 6
- CML 4
- Myelofibrosis 8
- Metastasis 3

CLL Chronic lymphocytic leukemia, *CML* Chronic myeloid leukemia

Fig. 24.3 *The Barcelona data (1998–2007)*: Overall distribution of malignant cases stratified by pathological diagnosis

24.4.3 Myelofibrosis

The second most frequent indication in our series was myelofibrosis (8/94, 11%), a malignant condition without definitive cure. The spleen, in this particular subgroup, was greatly enlarged with a median weight of 2,700 g (range 300–3,300 g). It is characterized by bone marrow fibrosis, pancytopenia, extramedullar hematopoiesis and hepatosplenomegaly and associated with massive spleen enlargement, requiring repeat transfusions. Surgery is mainly performed to palliate symptoms but is also indicated in cases of massive enlargement and portal hypertension, and to reduce transfusion requirements. The completion rate, when performing a laparoscopic splenectomy, was 87%. HALS was necessary in 50% of the patients. A well-known potential risk of laparoscopic splenectomy, especially in this subgroup of patients, is development of postoperative portal vein thrombosis.

24.4.4 Hodgkin's Disease (HD)

LS was performed in seven patients suffering from Hodgkin's disease (HD) (7/94, 7.4%). These patients were younger, and the size of the spleen was generally normal.

Laparoscopy for staging purposes is currently indicated only in very few cases. Indications for LS in this subset are clinical suspicion of lymphoma without evidence of peripheral disease, or patients requiring re-staging after completion of chemotherapy due to suspicion of residual disease on conventional imaging or PET-CT.

24.4.5 Chronic Lymphocytic Leukemia (CLL)

Chronic lymphocytic leukemia (CLL), currently considered a NHL subtype, is an incurable disease. CLL was diagnosed in 6 of 94 cases (7%), and splenomegaly was moderate with a spleen weight of 1,094 g (range 440–2,952 g). LS is mainly indicated to treat cytopenia, massive spleen enlargement, or progressive splenomegaly refractory to medical treatment. Splenectomy did improve cytopenia in up to 90% of our patients. HALS was required in one patient and conversion in another.

Table 24.2 The Barcelona data: perioperative outcome after LS – Malignancy stratified by diagnosis

	Hodgkin	Non-Hodgkin	CLL	CML	Myelofibrosis	Metastasis
n	7	64	6	4	8	4
Age (year)	35 (27–55)	67 (34–84)	61 (40–72)	50 (22–50)	56 (48–72)	56 (25–81)
Spleen weight (g)	390 (248–1,158)	1,200 (140–6,100)	1,094 (440–2,952)	3,675 (3,200–4,500)	2,700 (300–3,300)	577 (373–640)
OR time (min)	105 (60–150)	130 (85–300)	150 (3,200–4,500)	165 (150–240)	200 (110–270)	132 (120–180)
HALS (*n*/%)	1 (14%)	28 (44%)	2 (33%)	3 (75%)	4 (50%)	0
Conversion (*n*/%)	0	9 (14%)	0	1 (25%)	1 (12%)	1 (25%)
Morbidity (*n*/%)	1 (14%)	15 (23%)	1 (16%)	4 (100%)	4 (50%)	1 (25%)
Mortality (*n*/%)	0	0	0	0	1 (12%)	0

CLL chronic lymphocytic leukemia, *CML* chronic myeloid leukemia

24.4.6 Waldenstrom's Macroglobulinemia

Waldenstrom's macroglobulinemia is a rare disorder, and 40% of these patients present with splenomegaly. LS is indicated in cases that are refractory to systemic therapy.

24.4.7 Chronic Myeloid Leukemia (CML)

Chronic myeloid leukemia (CML) is rarely an indication for LS. It is most common in males in their sixth decade of life. Splenomegaly develops in 55–70% of patients. The spleen is often massively enlarged with a median weight of 3,675 g (range 3,200–4,500 g) (Fig. 24.4). If splenomegaly develops rapidly, then it will be a predictor of a blast crisis. Splenectomy may be indicated in advanced disease and improves clinical symptoms in up to 15% of patients, but the risk to develop a blast crisis remains unchanged. Surgical risk in this subgroup is high because of associated coagulation disorders and platelet malfunction.

24.4.8 Secondary Tumors of the Spleen

Splenic metastases were found in 4/94 cases (4%). Metastases to the spleen are usually a sign of systemic disease and therefore rarely an indication for surgery [26]. Splenectomy may be performed, if it can be proven that the spleen is the sole site of cancer spread. The most frequent encountered primary sites are lung cancer, breast cancer, or melanoma. The four cases we treated included 4 patients with melanoma and one patient with a sarcoma metastatic to the spleen (Fig. 24.5). Spleen enlargement was not excessive, and all four patients had an uneventful perioperative and postoperative outcome (Table 24.3).

24.4.9 Diagnostic Laparoscopy for Hematological Malignancies

Diagnostic laparoscopy and biopsy for enlarged retroperitoneal masses may be indicated when CT-guided

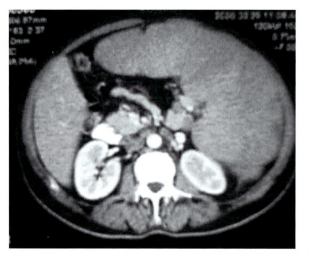

Fig. 24.4 CT scan of a patient with CML requiring splenectomy

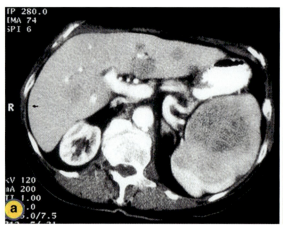
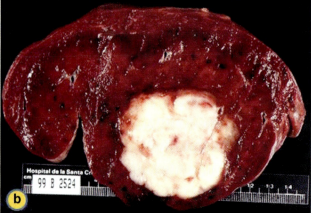

Fig. 24.5 Secondary splenic malignancy: Splenic metastasis of a sarcoma. (**a**) CT scan, (**b**) macroscopic appearance

Table 24.3 The Barcelona data: Perioperative outcome after LS: *Comparison between benign/malignant with ITP as reference*

	Overall	ITP	Benign	Malignant
n	326	148	230	94
Sex (m/f)	208/118	49/99	79/154	44/50
Age (year)	48 (3–85)	40 (12–85)	40 (3–85)	64 (22–84)
OR time (min)	120 (35–400)	100 (45–360)	120 (35–400)	150 (60–300)
Length of stay (day)	3 (1–29)	3 (2–16)	3 (1–23)	4 (2–29)
Spleen weight (g)	261 (40–6,100)	148 (40–602)	179 (40–3,420)	1,139 (140–6,100)
Conversion (*n/%*)	21/6.5	5/3.4	11/4.7	12/12.8
Morbidity (*n/%*)	63/19.3	19/12.7	34/14.6	2/2.1
Mortality (*n/%*)	2/0.6	1/0.7	1/0.4	1/1
Reoperation (*n/%*)	19/5.8	8/5.4	13/5.6	6/6.4
HALS (*n/%*)	44/13.5	1/0.7	8/3.5	36/38.2

ITP idiopathic thrombocytopenic purpura, *HALS* hand-assisted laparoscopic surgery

needle biopsy is not available, when percutaneous sampling is insufficient or when a large biopsy specimen is required for immunohistochemical studies [27, 28]. We performed a diagnostic laparoscopy and biopsy in 46 patients. Tissue sampling was adequate in 90% of the cases. Nine patients required a conversion to an open biopsy, and the morbidity in this short series was noted to be as low as 8% (Fig. 24.6).

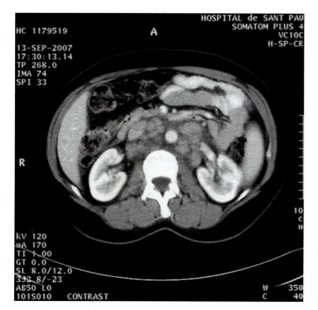

Fig. 24.6 Retropancreatic lymphoma: Indication for diagnostic laparoscopy and biopsy

24.5 Surgical Approach to the Spleen

24.5.1 Indications for Splenectomy

Splenectomy is indicated in a variety of clinical situations, and there are four main indications for laparoscopic splenectomy (LS) [13–16].

1. *Diagnostic splenectomy* for splenomegaly suggesting malignancy.
   This is especially true, if all other diagnostic studies, like biopsy of a peripheral lymph node or a bone marrow biopsy are negative. Radiological imaging does usually not allow narrowing the spectrum of possible differential diagnoses.
2. *Therapeutic splenectomy* is indicated in the following situations:
   - Primary splenic lymphoma; LS may be curative.
   - Thrombocytopenia secondary to splenomegaly; LS may reduce transfusion needs, thus increasing quality of life.
   - Autoimmune thrombocytopenia; LS is especially useful in the context of CLL
3. *Palliative splenectomy* to relieve from symptoms secondary to massive enlargement of the spleen.
4. *Staging splenectomy* to stage or re-stage Hodgkin's disease if noninvasive staging modalities are inconclusive.

24.5.2 Preoperative Workup and Special Considerations

Patients undergoing elective LS for malignancy require special attention. A thorough physical examination will allow the surgeon to determine the size of the spleen preoperatively. Normal-sized spleens are usually not felt below the costal margin. Moderate splenomegaly presents with a lower pole palpable in the left upper quadrant of the abdomen. Massive splenomegaly with a diameter ≥30 cm may occupy the entire abdominal cavity. The abdominal exam allows assessing mobility of the spleen, distensibility of the abdominal wall, which is important when planning a laparoscopic procedure and the projection of the lower pole of the spleen to the midline. All these preoperatively collected data will determine patient positioning on the operating table (supine, semi-supine or lateral), guide the placement of a hand-assisted device and finally will determine, if a laparoscopic approach is feasible or not. A preoperative blood transfusion should be considered depending on the result of the obtained blood work, taking in account, that an enlarged spleen pools a significant amount of blood. Coagulation profile should be obtained, and the patient typed and crossed in the event she/he requires fresh frozen plasma, platelets, or packed red blood cells perioperatively. All our patients get vaccinated preoperatively with a polyvalent pneumococcal, meningococcal, and hemophilus vaccine.

24.5.3 Preoperative Imaging

A preoperative computer tomogram (CT) or ultrasound (US) is recommended to evaluate the size and shape of the spleen. The shape of the spleen will influence operative planning and surgical strategy. Postoperative outcome is directly related to the shape of the spleen.

24.5.4 The Role of Preoperative Splenic Artery Embolization (SAE)

Preoperative splenic artery embolization (SAE) to facilitate any splenectomy, not only laparoscopic splenectomy and serves three major purposes:

- Occludes terminal vascular branches
- Diminishes the risk of intraoperative bleeding
- Reduces spleen size

In our series, patients who underwent SAE showed 10% less intraoperative blood loss and subsequently a lower rate of emergency blood transfusions. However, SAE is associated with other complications such as pain, hemorrhage, and hepatic or splenic abscesses. Preoperative SAE is not routinely recommended for LS but may play a role in spleens larger than 25 cm in maximum dimension [29, 30].

24.5.5 Essential Equipment for LS

Laparoscopic splenectomy does not require any special equipment. The use of two video monitors is recommended and improves surgeon's comfort and efficiency. We routinely use a set of three or four trocars. Our preference lies on an angled 30° laparoscope, which is often repositioned depending on the step of the procedure and visualization. Most grasping, dissecting, and cutting instruments used are 5 mm in diameter. It is not uncommon, particularly for large spleens, that 10-mm instruments are required to facilitate retraction.

To seal and divide vessels, a combination of clip appliers, endovascular stapling devices, monopolar, and bipolar cautery is used and readily available in the operating room. The harmonic scalpel is also a very useful tool to dissect the spleen. Clips should only be placed in areas where no stapler will be needed because they will prevent proper sealing and will lead to malfunctioning of the stapling device. Endovascular staplers are very useful, particularly in controlling the splenic hilum. A durable specimen retrieval bag is key equipment for LS. It has to withstand the final morcellation process prior to specimen extraction.

24.6 Surgical Technique

24.6.1 General Considerations

Antibiotic prophylaxis is given preoperatively as per national/international recommendations. LS is always performed under general anesthesia. An oral gastric tube (OGT) is inserted to decompress the stomach, which will greatly improve the visualization in the left upper quadrant. We remove the OGT upon completion of surgery. A Foley catheter should be placed due to the duration of the procedure.

24.6.2 Patient Positioning

Since LS was first described, several techniques and ways to position the patient have been reported; all geared toward controlling the hilar vessels. The most difficult part of the procedure is the mobilization of the spleen toward the midline. Some surgeons prefer to start the procedure in the French position, standing between the patient's legs and will move to the side, if the procedure warrants it. Patient positioning on the operating table will depend on surgeon's preference and on the size of the spleen. The patient can be placed in a low lithotomy position and further tilted laterally to elevate the left upper abdomen. The lateral tilt may be increased to 45°, if necessary. Currently the most accepted position is full lateral at 90°. We prefer the 90° full lateral approach in cases of a normal-sized spleen or moderate splenomegaly. A supine or semi-lateral position is more adequate in cases of massive splenomegaly or when the median border of the spleen crosses the midline when measured on the outer abdomen (Fig. 24.7).

24.6.3 Anterior Approach

The patient is placed supine or in Fowler position according to surgeon's preference. A sand bag is placed right below the left rib cage. After establishing the pneumoperitoneum, the first trocar is inserted at the umbilicus and an exploratory laparoscopy is performed. Three more trocars are inserted, one in the subxiphoid area, one in the midepigastrium, and a fourth in the left iliac fossa. The scope is introduced through the midepigastric trocar. The subxiphoid trocar and umbilical port are used for placement of grasping and dissecting instruments. The table is now placed in a right lateral tilt and brought into reverse Trendelenburg position. The lesser sac is opened, and the short gastric vessels are divided with the harmonic scalpel or bipolar cautery.

Several techniques are described in the literature to dissect the splenic hilum. The splenic vessels can either be controlled at their main trunk or a segmental devascularization near the splenic parenchyma will be performed. The remaining short gastric vessels are divided with the harmonic scalpel after division of the main splenic vessels. We pay close attention not to injure the pancreas by carefully dissecting off the main vessels. Takedown of the splenic flexure gives you access to the posterior attachments of the spleen which will be divided using harmonic scalpel.

24.6.4 Lateral Approach

The patient is positioned on the operating table in right lateral decubitus position. The table is flexed 20°–30° below level in both directions and brought into moderate reverse Trendelenburg position. This maximizes the window of access, which is between the patient's left iliac crest and the costal margin. Three or four trocars are then inserted in the patient's left upper abdominal quadrant. A 12-mm port is inserted in the anterior axillary line, superior to the patient's anterior superior iliac crest, and is used for the endovascular stapler and final specimen removal. In pediatric and non-obese patients, we place the camera port in the rim of the umbilicus. In obese patients, it is often necessary to move this site to the left upper abdominal quadrant. A subcostal and a subxiphoid trocar are used for

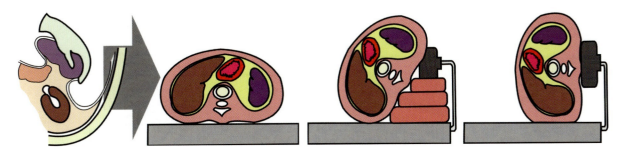

Fig. 24.7 Progressive lateral approach for LS: The spleen can be mobilized with lateral tilt taking advantage of gravity

retraction and dissection. Finally, a 2- or 5-mm trocar is placed under direct vision dorsally, below the 12th rib, in the mid- to post-axillary line. This trocar is used to retract and elevate the lower pole of the spleen.

Dissection starts with mobilization of the splenic flexure of the colon using a combination of sharp dissection and ultrasonic. The lateral peritoneal attachments of the spleen are incised as a second step. A cuff of peritoneum is left alongside the spleen for further safe mobilization. This maneuver avoids grabbing the spleen directly and greatly reduces the risk of splenic tears.

Dissection of the splenic hilum starts from the lower pole and progresses cephalad. An accessory splenic artery at the lower pole is often encountered and should be divided between clips or with the harmonic scalpel.

After mobilization of the lower pole of the spleen and division of the polar vessels, we obtain easy access to the lesser sac. With the spleen elevated, the short gastric vessels and main vascular pedicle are tented up. The short gastric vessels can be divided either with the harmonic scalpel, between clips or using an endovascular stapler. The tail of the pancreas is often visible at this point of the dissection. The vascular pedicle is now well exposed. Once the main artery and vein are dissected off the pancreas, they are divided with two separate firings of the endovascular stapler (Fig. 24.8).

24.6.5 Extraction of the Specimen

After the remaining splenic hilar and short gastric vessels are divided, a small cuff of avascular spleno-phrenic ligament is temporarily left in place. This serves to hold the spleen in its normal anatomic position and facilitates introduction into the retrieval bag. The specimen retrieval bag is introduced, opened, and placed over the relatively immobile spleen. The final spleno-phrenic attachments are now divided and the bag closed. The neck of the bag is withdrawn through the 12-mm trocar site. The spleen is morcellated within the bag and extracted in pieces. Great care is needed to insure not to rupture the bag and to avoid spillage and subsequent splenosis. Once the entire specimen and bag are removed, we perform a final laparoscopic inspection of the left upper abdomen and copious amounts of water are used for irrigation.

As placing a large spleen into a bag may be challenging, a retrieval bag with a wide opening which can be controlled from the exterior may be of great help (Endocatch II™, US Surgical).

An accessory incision is used in the event the spleen has to be removed as a whole. Widening of a trocar site, a Pfannenstiel incision, or the umbilicus are the most common used approaches.

24.6.6 Hand-Assisted Laparoscopic Splenectomy (HALS)

The main indication for a hand-assisted laparoscopic splenectomy (HALS) procedure is a patient with massive splenomegaly [31]. Position of choice is right lateral decubitus (Fig. 24.9). Pneumoperitoneum is created using a Veress needle inserted into the right

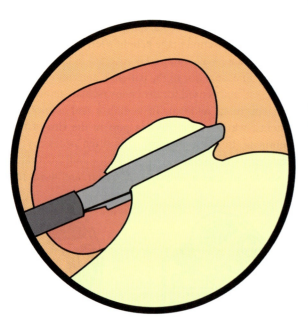

Fig. 24.8 Division of the vascular pedicle of the splenic hilum with the endostapler

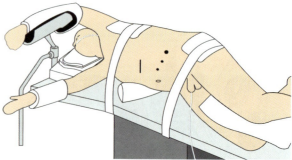

Fig. 24.9 HALS: Patient positioning in full lateral approach – 90°

iliac fossa, a good distance away from the spleen. A 12-mm. camera port is inserted in the periumbilical area to perform an exploratory laparoscopy and to select the best site for the hand-port, which usually requires an incision of 7–7.5 cm in length. The most common site is the right hypogastrium (Fig. 24.10), but in cases of massive splenomegaly, it will be placed in the right subcostal area or in the right iliac fossa. Several devices are commercially available (Lapdisc™, Ethicon, USA; Omniport™, Advanced Surgical Concepts Ltd, Dublin, Ireland; Handport™, Smith Nephew, Ma, USA).The left hand is inserted into the abdomen to examine the shape of the spleen and surrounding anatomy. A second 12-mm trocar is inserted lateral to the laparoscope under guidance of the intra-abdominal hand. All further instruments are introduced through this trocar (Fig. 24.11). For additional retraction, if needed, a 5-mm trocar is placed in the left flank and an endoretractor (Endoflex™, Genzyme, Tucker, GA, USA) is inserted to expose the anterior aspect of the spleen. As a first step in the procedure, we incise the gastro-splenic ligament to gain access to the retro-gastric plane. The opening of the lesser sac is widened, and the short gastric vessels are divided with the ultrasonic shears (Ultracision™, Ethicon, USA) or Ligasure™ (Valley lab, USA). The splenic artery is directly palpated at the upper border of the pancreas, and a ligature or clip is placed to interrupt the inflow to the spleen. With the hand in place, we mobilize the spleen medially to expose its posterior aspect and divide the retroperitoneal adhesions. The splenic hilum and pancreatic tail are bluntly dissected with the hand. Using this type of dissection, we are able to place the stapling device in the splenic hilum in

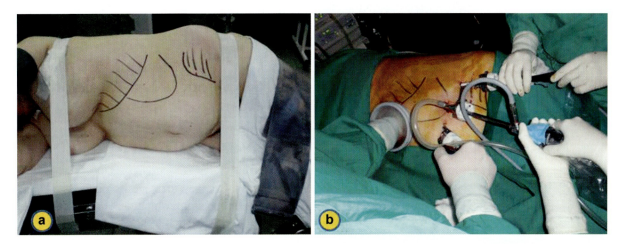

Fig. 24.10 HALS: full lateral approach, intermediate splenomegaly: (**a**) Patient positioning (**b**) trocar placement

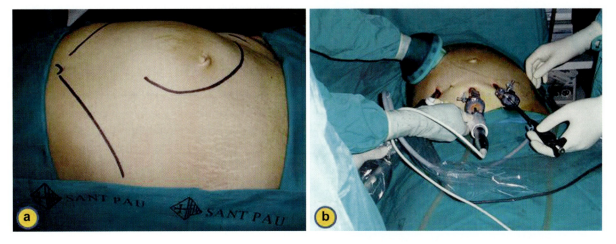

Fig. 24.11 *HALS*: supine approach, massive splenomegaly: (**a**) Patient positioning, (**b**) trocar placement

such a way that it can be fired without tension and the pancreatic tail is spared (Fig. 24.12). Once the hilar vessels are controlled, we dissect the upper pole from all posterior attachments which frees the spleen entirely. In most cases, the spleen is retrieved intact through the accessory incision. However, in cases of massive splenomegaly, a sterile plastic bag (Endocatch II™, Tyco, (Norwalk, USA)) is introduced and the spleen morcellated. The larger pieces are removed through the 7-cm incision (Fig. 24.13).

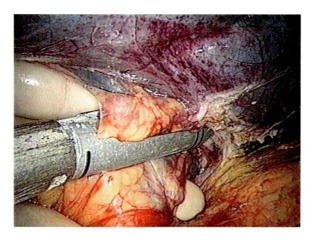

Fig. 24.12 HALS: Dissection of the splenic hilum; the inserted hand guides the endostapling device

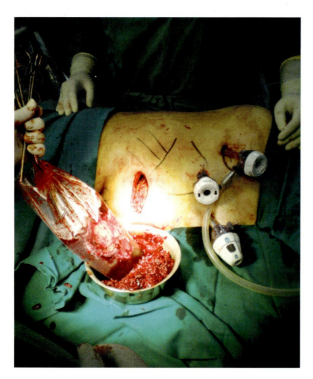

Fig. 24.13 HALS: Specimen extraction

24.6.7 Staging Laparoscopy and Lymph Node Biopsy

The French position, with the surgeon standing between the legs of the patient, is used. Trocar placement will depend on the location of the nodes to be sampled. Placement of a 30° scope in the midline, 3–4 cm above the umbilicus, is standard. Two or three additional trocars placed laterally will permit access to the peripancreatic and celiac artery regions. Place the patient differently to allow access to the pelvis if the nodes to be sampled are located in the iliac region. Efforts should be made to obtain a significant sample from one pathological area. Preoperative CT scan helps to localize the site of disease. Lymph node biopsy, partial resection of an entire lymph node station or tru-cut biopsy can be obtained and additional intra-abdominal fluid sampling or liver biopsy can be performed.

24.7 Complications Associated with Laparoscopic Splenectomy

24.7.1 Hemorrhage

In cases of malignancy, there are several potential perioperative complications which the surgeon should be aware of and able to treat [32]. The most likely problem is hemorrhage which is usually located at three distinct sites:

- Short gastric or polar vessels – small caliber vessels – constant ooze
- Hilar vessels – large caliber – life-threatening bleed
- Splenic parenchyma.

Though not life-threatening, the first may be a considerable hindrance as rapidly accumulating blood may impede visualization. In most of the cases, it can easily be stopped with clips, electrocautery, or ultrasonic dissector. Hemorrhage from a larger vessel may require immediate conversion to laparotomy. The best way to prevent this from happening is delicate dissection of the splenic artery and vein to prevent rupture of smaller splenic and pancreatic blood vessels. The dissected splenic artery and vein should then be clipped prior to any further mobilization of the spleen. Injury to these vessels can occur simply due to the rigidity of the clamping instruments. Hemorrhage from the parenchyma is less dangerous and can be managed either by clamping the artery, applying slight pressure with a gauze, or by using electrocautery.

24.7.2 Pancreatic Tail Injury

Another potential complication of LS is injury to the tail of the pancreas. This can be avoided by proper dissection and placement of the endostapler when dividing the hilar vessels. It may be more difficult in cases of malignancy due to extensive surrounding lymphadenopathy. The lateral approach to LS allows placing the stapling device more safely due to better exposure of the splenic hilum. In the event it happens and we realize it intraoperatively, we will place a drain in the left upper abdominal quadrant close to the pancreatic tail.

24.7.3 Perforation of the Diaphragm

This could happen during dissection of the superior pole of the spleen. This lesion may worsen rapidly due to development of a capno-thorax. A capno-thorax is different from a pneumothorax in that way that the underlying cause is not an injury to the lung itself. It can be controlled in two ways: intraoperatively by sealing the opening in the diaphragm over a placed suction catheter or postoperatively by temporary placement of a pleural drain. The pleural drain will be removed in the OR after full lung expansion is confirmed on a chest X-ray.

24.7.4 Miscellaneous Complications

Other complications reported with LS include

- Deep vein thrombosis
- Portal vein thrombosis
- Pulmonary embolus
- Wound infection

Recent reports have suggested a higher incidence of portal thrombosis when LS is performed [33, 34]. No clear relation to pneumoperitoneum has been stated, but close monitoring of postoperative thrombocytosis and preoperative anti-platelet therapy is warranted, especially in patients with additional risk factors such as myelofibrosis.

It is interesting to note that, particularly in larger series of LS, there is a remarkably low incidence of deep surgical infection or subphrenic abscess.

24.8 Final Remarks

Minimally invasive technique has been progressively accepted among surgeons as a safe approach to splenectomy. However, it is a complex laparoscopic procedure and most series in the literature understate its difficulty by including patients with benign disease and small spleens. LS for malignant disease is a greater challenge for the surgeon because of the size of the spleen and the patient's general medical condition. The clinical and anatomic characteristics of many disorders requiring splenectomy may influence the performance of LS. Patients with malignant hematological diseases are usually elderly, clotting abnormalities are not infrequent and large spleens present problems such as difficult manipulation and complicated removal from the abdomen [13–16].

24.8.1 The Challenging Spleen – Splenomegaly

A normal spleen weighs between 80 and 250 g, while those that surpass the costal margin weigh over 750–1,000 g. Splenomegaly can be defined by measuring the main diameters, but we prefer to use weight alone as we do not perform routine ultrasonographic or CT measurements. In open surgery, spleens over 400–500 g are considered splenomegalic, and some authors consider organs weighing over 1,000 or 1,500 g as massive splenomegaly. In the pre-laparoscopy era, substantial morbidity, greater transfusion requirements, and even death followed open splenectomy for malignancy. We classified our series of 327 patients into three groups according to spleen weight in order to analyze the impact of weight on outcome after laparoscopic splenectomy.

Table 24.4 The Barcelona data: perioperative outcome after LS: Stratified by spleen weight

	Overall	Spleen weight <400g	Spleen weight 400–1,000 g	Spleen weight >1,000 g
n	324	198	65	60
Benign/malignant	230/94	174/12	36/30	9/51
Sex (m/f)	207/117	65/133	35/30	33/27
Age (year)	48 (3–85)	39 (3–85)	53 (13–84)	60 (18–21)
OR time (min)	120 (35–400)	107 (35–360)	120 (65–400)	150 (45–300)
Length of stay (day)	3 (1–29)	3 (1–12)	4 (2–18)	5 (3–29)
Spleen weight	261 (40–6,100)	170 (35–179)	670 (400–1,000)	1,793 (1,000–6,100)
Conversion (*n*/%)	21/6.3	7/3.5	3/4.6	11/18.2
Morbidity (*n*/%)	63/18.9	23/11.5	19/29.1	19/31.5
Mortality (*n*/%)	20/0.6	1/0.5	0/0	1/1.7
Reoperation (*n*/%)	19/5.7	10/5	4/6.1	4/6.6
HALS (*n*/%)	44/13.2	4/2	11/16.8	30/50

LS was attempted in spleens up to 3,000 g and was completed in 111 of 126 patients who presented with a spleen size between 400 and 3,500 g. We included 60 patients with a spleen weight >1,000 g (range 1,000–3,500 g), and splenectomy was successfully completed laparoscopically in 49 (82%); the remaining 11 patients (spleen weight between 3,500 and 6,100 g) were converted because of difficulty with manipulation (Table 24.4). LS cannot be performed when intra-abdominal space is restricted due to a massive spleen [35]. Ongoing research is being conducted to preoperatively determine spleen volume and ratio spleen/abdominal cavity. This should allow predicting technical complexity and thus determining the best surgical approach in cases of splenomegaly [36].

24.8.2 Massive Splenomegaly

Massive splenomegaly is associated with higher postoperative morbidity – between 20% and 60% – in both open and laparoscopic surgery [32]. In a previous study, we were able to demonstrate that factors which predict complications after laparoscopic splenectomy are malignancy, advanced age, and splenomegaly [32]. These findings contrast with those of other surgeons who did not find differences when comparing laparoscopic splenectomy in patients with splenomegaly (>500 g) to a group with normal-sized spleen [7]. In our opinion; however, a spleen <1,000 g does not significantly increase the degree of difficulty, while a massive splenomegaly does.

The role of laparoscopic techniques for the treatment of massive splenomegaly (>3,000 g) remains controversial [37, 38] (Fig. 24.14). Obviously, this procedure depends on the expertise of the surgical team, the shape of the spleen, and the patient's body habitus.

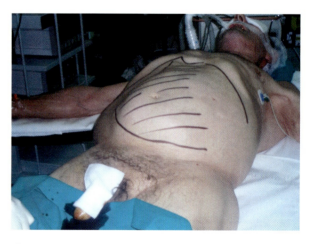

Fig. 24.14 Massive splenomegaly – Laparoscopic splenectomy could not be recommended

24.8.3 Splenectomy and Malignancy

Splenectomy for malignancy is currently limited mainly to treat symptomatic hypersplenism, to debulk patients with established disease, or to establish a diagnosis. Surgical staging of Hodgkin's disease has been replaced by noninvasive methods. Like other authors [15, 16], we found that patients with malignant hematological diseases were older and that operative time was longer than in benign cases, but the conversion rate remained low in spite of the relatively large size of the spleen. Even in absence of prospective randomized trials, results of comparing laparoscopic to open splenectomy for malignant cases favor LS, as the transfusion rates and major morbidity rates are reduced. Nelson and coworkers showed morbidity and mortality rates of 41% and 8%, respectively and a mean hospital stay of 13 days in an open series of 39 patients [39]. Most of these splenectomies were considered "high risk" because of non-Hodgkin's lymphomas and a mean spleen weight of 1,500 g. In similar series, LS showed reductions in major morbidity (18–23%), mortality, and stay [7, 8, 15, 40–45].

The laparoscopic technique used for splenomegaly is the same as that applied to small organs, but greater precision is required. Additional ports or endo-retractors are needed to raise the organ, especially when it is almost free, and when it is necessary to reach the upper pole to complete the dissection.

24.8.4 Approaching the Splenic Vessels

It is important to point out a few technical points concerning approach to the splenic artery, the full lateral approach and hand-assisted techniques. Prior to mobilization of the spleen, we routinely attempt to ligate the artery in the lesser sac in order to reduce spleen size, facilitate auto-transfusion, and to decrease the risk of hemorrhage. The full lateral approach aids in identifying the splenic pedicle. We prefer to transect the hilar vessels with an endostapler avoiding excessive intraoperative hemorrhage. In cases of non-Hodgkin lymphomas, we often encounter large lymph nodes in the hilum which makes it more difficult to identify the vascular structures. In this case, the endostapler is fired near the hilum, leaving the lymph nodes behind, avoiding unnecessary dissection and the risk of bleeding.

24.8.5 Role of Preoperative Splenic Embolization

Preoperative embolization of the spleen [29, 30] has been proposed to reduce intraoperative bleeding and the need for transfusion, but this practice has not gained wide acceptance. In our experience, there was no significant difference. Transfusion requirement in the subgroup of patients with enlarged spleen was 31%, compared to 16% in the group with normal-sized spleen. This may be due to higher intraoperative blood loss, but could possibly also be explained by more liberal use of transfusion in patients whose preoperative hematocrit values are lower.

24.8.6 Splenectomy and HALS

LS is clearly challenging when spleen size is significantly increased. In some cases the size of the spleen does not allow sufficient intra-abdominal space for manipulation and elevation of the organ, and conversion is inevitable. HALS may be justified when an accessory incision is needed to retrieve an intact organ or when there are major difficulties in inserting the spleen into a retrieval bag. Several non-randomized series have shown the potential advantages of HALS for splenectomy in cases of splenomegaly [7, 8, 40–48] (Table 24.5).

Our personal research interest is to compare HALS to standard LS in the same subset of patients, operated on by the same team. The main advantages in this series were shorter operative time and lower operative blood loss in the HALS group. One interesting observation in the HALS group is that general morbidity was lower when compared to conventional LS. This indicates that surgical trauma during HALS is less significant and potential advantages of a laparoscopic approach are maintained despite more intense intra-abdominal manipulation (Table 24.6).

In a previous multivariate analysis of factors related to complications after LS, we showed a significant correlation between malignancy and splenomegaly [32]. Reduced surgical trauma may be associated with a quicker and safer recovery, and fewer pulmonary and infectious complications. However, there are, as

Table 24.5 Laparoscopic and hand-assisted laparoscopic splenectomy: Selected comparative studies

	Year	Approach	N	Spleen weight median (g)	OR time (min)	Conversion rate (%)	Morbidity (%)	Mortality (%)	Length of stay (day)
Ailiwadi [40]	2002	LAP	19	740	212	37	32	16	4.5
		HALS	22	1,394	161*	14	18	0	3
Rosen [42]	2002	LAP	31	1,031	186	23	16	0	4.2
		HALS	14	1,516*	177	7	35	0	5.4
Targarona [45]	2005	LAP	40	1,576	165	18	38	0	6
		HALS	37	1,785	141*	8	20	1	6
Owera [44]	2006	OPEN	13	>1,000	95	–	30	7.7	10
		LAP	15	>1,000	175	7	13	0	3.8
Wang [46]	2007	LAP	16	>700	195	25	13	0	–
		HALS	20	>700	141	0	0	0	–

*$p < 0.05$

Table 24.6 The Barcelona data: Perioperative outcome after LS: Comparison between hand-assisted laparoscopic surgery (HALS) and pure laparoscopy in patients with a spleen weight >800 g

	Laparoscopy	HALS	p
n	43	42	ns
Benign/malignant	16/27	6/37	ns
Sex (m/f)	14/29	22/20	ns
Age (year)	55 ± 16	61 ± 24	ns
OR time (min)	161 ± 57	140 ± 66	0.01
Length of stay (day)	5 (2–14)	4 (2–29)	ns
Spleen weight (g)	1,683 ± 1,019	1,768 ± 1,097	ns
Conversion (n/%)	8/18.6	4/9.5	ns
Morbidity (n/%)	16/37.1	8/19	ns
Mortality (n/%)	1/2.3	0/0	ns

of yet, no prospective randomized studies comparing standard open splenectomy with a minimally invasive approach.

From a technical point of view, the main advantage of HALS is smoother retraction and exposure of the lower pole of the spleen. HALS also allows precise identification of the splenic artery and easier mobilization of the posterior aspect of the spleen. The introduced hand bluntly dissects the pancreatic tail and facilitates exact and careful placement of the endostapler. The spleen can be extracted intact or morcellated through the 7-cm incision.

24.8.7 Portal Vein Thrombosis

CT or ultrasonography in the immediate postoperative period suggests that the risk of portal thrombosis increases after laparoscopic splenectomy, and this has been directly related to the laparoscopic approach [33, 34]. Prolonged intra-abdominal pressure is associated with markedly lower portal blood flow and may trigger this complication, especially in cases of massive splenomegaly and hypercoagulability. Although there are only a few cases reported in the literature, this complication should be taken into account in the event of unexplained postoperative abdominal pain after LS.

24.9 Conclusion

Splenomegaly is not a contraindication to a laparoscopic approach. However, laparoscopic splenectomy in cases of splenomegaly requires advanced laparoscopic skills and is only necessary in a small subset of patients. Surgeons performing this procedure should be aware of the medical characteristics of each specific hematological disease and be familiar with hand-assisted techniques. However, further information from comparative studies is needed to determine the exact role of laparoscopy especially in the setting of massive splenomegaly. In selected patients, a single incision approach seems to be feasible but our preliminary results do not allow us to draw any conclusions as of yet.

Quick Reference Guide

1. Carefully evaluate
   - Anatomy of the spleen using a preoperatively obtained CT scan.
   - Patient chart paying attention to the coagulation parameters.
2. Volume and shape of the spleen determine position of the operating table: full lateral, semi-lateral, or supine.
3. Consider using the Hasson technique and avoid tearing the spleen when inserting the first trocar.
4. After completion of the initial diagnostic laparoscopy consider conversion to HALS if you think that the size of the spleen hampers its mobilization.
5. If HALS is used, place your hand-port in the subxiphoid area or below the costal margin as it permits conversion through a subcostal incision.
6. Control the artery first! It is easily located and simple clipping or ligature permits a reduction in spleen volume which greatly facilitates further dissection.
7. A large upper or lower pole located near the midline of the abdomen implies increased technical difficulty.
8. Locate the tail of the pancreas to avoid injury to it. Enlarged hilar lymph nodes may hamper its localization.
9. Assure hemostasis as it may be more difficult than in open surgery
10. Place a drain if
    - Preoperative clotting anomalies are present
    - Oozing surgical field
    - Intraoperatively recognized pancreatic injury

References

1. Bellows, C.F., Sweeney, J.F.: Laparoscopic splenectomy: present status and future perspective. Expert Rev. Med. Devices **3**, 95–104 (2006)
2. Park, A., Targarona, E.M., Trias, M.: Laparoscopic surgery of the spleen: state of the art. Langenbecks J. Surg. **386**, 230–239 (2001)
3. Habermalz, B., Sauerland, S., Decker, G., Delaitre, B., Gigot, J.F., Leandros, E., Lechner, K., Rhodes, M., Silecchia, G., Szold, A., Targarona, E., Torelli, P., Neugebauer, E.: Laparoscopic splenectomy: the clinical practice guidelines of the European Association for Endoscopic Surgery (EAES). Surg. Endosc. **22**(4), 821–848 (2008 Apr). Epub 2008 Feb 22
4. Weiss 3rd, C.A., Kavic, S.M., Adrales, G.L., Park, A.E.: Laparoscopic splenectomy: what barriers remain? Surg. Innov. **12**, 23–29 (2005)
5. Nicholson, I.A., Falk, G.L., Mulligan, S.C.: Laparoscopically-assisted massive splenectomy. A preliminary report of the technique of early hilar devascularization. Surg. Endosc. **12**, 73–75 (1998)
6. Terrosu, G., Baccarani, U., Bresadola, V., et al.: The impact of splenic weight on laparoscopic splenectomy for splenomegaly. Surg. Endosc. **16**, 103–107 (2002)
7. Todd, B., Park, A., Walsh, R.M., et al.: Laparoscopic splenectomy in patients with normal sized spleens vs splenomegaly: does the size matter? Am. Surg. **67**, 854–858 (2001)
8. Kercher, K.W., Matthews, B.D., Walsh, R.M., Sing, R.F., Backus, C.L., Heniford, B.T.: Laparoscopic splenectomy for massive splenomegaly. Am. J. Surg. **183**, 192–196 (2002)
9. Patel, A.G., Parker, J.E., Wallwork, B., et al.: Massive splenomegaly is associated with significant morbidity after laparoscopic splenectomy. Ann. Surg. **238**, 235–240 (2003)
10. Mahon, D., Rhodes, M.: Laparoscopic splenectomy: size matters. Ann. R. Coll. Surg. Engl. **85**, 248–251 (2003)
11. Kaban, G.K., Czerniach, D.R., Cohen, R., et al.: Hand-assisted laparoscopic splenectomy in the setting of splenomegaly. Surg. Endosc. **18**, 1340–1343 (2004)
12. Targarona, E.M., Balagué, C., Trias, M.: Is the laparoscopic approach reasonable in cases of splenomegaly? Semin. Laparosc. Surg. **11**, 185–190 (2004)
13. Swartz, S.I.: Splenectomy for haematological disorders. In: Hiatt, J.R., Phillips, E.H., Morgenstern, L. (eds.) Surgical Diseases of the Spleen, pp. 131–142. Spinger Verlag, Berlin (1997)
14. Giles, F.J., Lim, S.W.: Malignant splenic lesions. In: Hiatt, J.R., Phillips, E.H., Morgenstern, L. (eds.) Surgical Diseases of the Spleen, pp. 131–142. Springer Verlag, Berlin (1997)
15. Steiner, J.P., Liass, S., Phillips, E.H.: Laparoscopic splenectomy for malignant diseases. In surgical diseases of the spleen. Probl. Gen. Surg. **19**, 48–57 (2002)
16. Heniford Todd, Walsh, M.B.: Laparoscopic splenectomy for malignant disease. In: Greene, Fl, Todd Heniford, B. (eds.) Minimally Invasive Cancer Management. Springer, NY (2001)
17. ESMO guideline task form: ESMO minimal clinical recommendation for diagnosis, treatment and follow up of Hodgkin's disease. Ann. Oncol. **16**(S1), i54–i55 (2005)
18. Multani, P., White, C.A., Grillo, A.: Non-Hodgkin lymphoma: review of conventional treatments. Curr. Pharm. Biotechnol. **2**, 279–291 (2001)
19. NCCN Clinical practice Guidelines in OncologyTM. Non-Hodgkin's Lymphoma. V.3.2007, www.nccn.org
20. Palma, M., Kokhaei, P., Lundin, J., et al.: The biology and treatment of chronic lymphocytic leukemia. Ann. Oncol. **17**(10), x144–x154 (2006)
21. Wierda, W.G.: Current and investigational therapies for patients with CLL. Hematology Am. Soc. Hematol. Educ. Program **2006**, 285–294 (2006)

22. Hehlmann, R., Hochhaus, A., Baccarani, M.: European Leukemia Net. Chronic myeloid leukaemia. Lancet **370**, 342–350 (2007)
23. Hunter, T.: Treatment for chronic myelogenous leukemia: the long road to imatinib. J. Clin. Invest. **117**, 2036–2043 (2007)
24. Dingli, D., Mesa, R.A., Tefferi, A.: Myelofibrosis with myeloid metaplasia: new developments in pathogenesis and treatment. Intern. Med. **43**, 540–547 (2004)
25. Arana-Yi, C., Quintás-Cardama, A., Giles, F., et al.: Advances in the therapy of chronic idiopathic myelofibrosis. Oncologist **11**, 929–943 (2006)
26. Comperat, E., Bardier-Dupas, A., Camparo, P., et al.: Splenic metastases: clinicopathologic presentation, differential diagnosis, and pathogenesis. Arch. Pathol. Lab. Med. **131**, 965–969 (2007)
27. Silecchia, G., Raparelli, L., Perrotta, N., et al.: Accuracy of laparoscopy in the diagnosis and staging of lymphoproliferative diseases. World J. Surg. **27**, 653–658 (2003)
28. Cunneen, S.A., Lefor, A.T.: Lymphoma staging and nodal dissection. In: Greene, Fl, Todd Heniford, B. (eds.) Minimally Invasive Cancer Management. Springer, NY (2001)
29. Iwase, K., Higaki, J., Yoon, H.E., et al.: Splenic artery embolization using contour emboli before laparoscopic or laparoscopically assisted splenectomy. Surg. Laparosc. Endosc. Percutan. Tech. **12**, 331–336 (2002)
30. Poulin, E., Thibault, C., Mamazza, J., et al.: Laparoscopic splenectomy: clinical experience and the role of preoperative splenic artery embolization. Surg. Laparosc. Endosc. **3**, 445–450 (1993)
31. Targarona, E.M., Balagué, C., Trias, M.: Hand assisted laparoscopic splenectomy. Semin. Laparosc. Surg. **8**, 126–134 (2001)
32. Targarona, E.M., Cerdan, G., Trias, M.: Complications of laparoscopic splenectomy. Probl. Gen. Surg. **19**, 72–79 (2002)
33. Ikeda, M., Sekimoto, M., Takiguchi, S., Kubota, M., et al.: High incidence of thrombosis of the portal venous system after laparoscopic splenectomy: a prospective study with contrast-enhanced CT scan. Ann. Surg. **24**, 208–216 (2005)
34. Stamou, K.M., Toutouzas, K.G., Kekis, P.B., et al.: Prospective study of the incidence and risk factors of postsplenectomy thrombosis of the portal, mesenteric, and splenic veins. Arch. Surg. **141**, 663–669 (2006)
35. Targarona, E.M., Espert, J.J., Balague, C., et al.: Splenomegaly should not be considered a contraindication for laparoscopic splenectomy. Ann. Surg. **228**, 35–39 (1998)
36. Targarona, E.M., Balague, C., Pernas, J.C., Martinez, C., Berindoague, R., Gich, I., Trias, M.: Can we predict immediate outcome after laparoscopic rectal surgery? Multivariate analysis of clinical, anatomic, and pathologic features after 3-dimensional reconstruction of the pelvic anatomy. Ann. Surg. **247**(4), 642–649 (2008 Apr)
37. Boddy, A.P., Mahon, D., Rhodes, M.: Does open surgery continue to have a role in elective splenectomy? Surg. Endosc. **20**, 1094–1098 (2006)
38. Casaccia, M., Torelli, P., Cavaliere, D., et al.: Minimal-access splenectomy: a viable alternative to laparoscopic splenectomy in massive splenomegaly. JSLS **9**, 411–414 (2005)
39. Nelson, E.W., Mone, E.C.: Splenectomy in high-risk patients with splenomegaly. Am. J. Surg. **178**, 581–586 (1999)
40. Smith, L., Luna, G., Merg, A.R., McNevin, M.S., Moore, M.R., Bax, T.W.: Laparoscopic splenectomy for treatment of splenomegaly. Am. J. Surg. **187**, 618–620 (2004)
41. Borrazzo, E.C., Daly, J.M., Morrisey, K.P., et al.: Hand-assisted laparoscopic splenectomy for giant spleens. Surg. Endosc. **17**, 918–920 (2003)
42. Ailawadi, G., Yahanda, A., Dimick, J.B., et al.: Hand-assisted laparoscopic splenectomy in patients with splenomegaly or prior upper abdominal operation. Surgery **132**, 689–694 (2002)
43. Targarona, E.M., Balague, C., Cerdan, G., et al.: Hand-assisted laparoscopic splenectomy (HALS) in cases of splenomegaly: a comparison analysis with conventional laparoscopic splenectomy. Surg. Endosc. **16**, 426–430 (2002)
44. Rosen, M., Brody, F., Walsh, R.M., Ponsky, J.: Hand-assisted laparoscopic splenectomy vs conventional laparoscopic splenectomy in cases of splenomegaly. Arch. Surg. **137**, 1348–1352 (2002)
45. Grahn, S.W., Alvarez 3rd, J., Kirkwood, K.: Trends in laparoscopic splenectomy for massive splenomegaly. Arch. Surg. **141**, 755–761 (2006)
46. Owera, A., Hamade, A.M., Bani Hani, O.I., et al.: Laparoscopic versus open splenectomy for massive splenomegaly: a comparative study. J. Laparoendosc. Adv. Surg. Tech. A **16**, 241–246 (2006)
47. Targarona, E.M., Balague, C., Berindoague, R., et al.: Laparoscopic splenectomy in massive splenomegaly. Eur. Surg. **38**, 20–26 (2006)
48. Wang, K.X., Hu, S.Y., Zhang, G.Y., Chen, B., et al.: Hand-assisted laparoscopic splenectomy for splenomegaly: a comparative study with conventional laparoscopic splenectomy. Chin. Med. J. (Engl.) **120**, 41–45 (2007)

Part VIII

Special Topics: Endocrinology

Cancer of the Thyroid

Prashant Sinha and William B. Inabnet

25.1 Introduction

Thyroid cancer, in contrast to other surgically amenable tumors, has the distinct advantage of being relatively indolent in the majority of its presentations. Its management therefore has been relatively unchanged over the past several decades owing largely to the excellent results in terms of patient survival. Theodore Kocher reduced surgical mortality to 5% at the turn of the twentieth century, setting the stage for surgical resection as a mainstay of therapy. Since then, cancer-specific survival has steadily improved. As long-term prospective data have become available in the past several decades, interest in improving disease-free survival has prompted a critical evaluation of overall and initial management choices. In the past decade, gradual developments in molecular and pathological understanding of thyroid diseases as well as surgical technology have motivated a gradual paradigm shift towards more aggressive initial therapy in order to minimize secondary interventions and improve disease-free survival.

Long-term studies that have followed patients with differentiated thyroid cancer have shown late recurrences of 30 or more years with overall survival rates of 68–76%, recurrence rate of 13–30%, and cause-specific mortality at 30 years of 5–8% [1, 2]. Recurrence was managed with high doses of radioactive iodine (RAI), surgical resection or both. RAI today remains an important therapeutic and diagnostic tool; however, with better understanding of cancer physiology, it is recognized that a number of recurrent or residual cancers will not respond to it [3, 4]. Subsequently, there has been an increased interest in reducing or avoiding the use of RAI, while pursuing a more complete surgical resection. Total or near total thyroidectomy is now being advocated as the initial procedure for any stage of differentiated thyroid cancer in addition to RAI at lower doses or not at all [1, 2, 4–8]. Finally, lifelong patient follow-up is strongly advocated and a number of biochemical and imaging modalities are being used for increased surveillance in order to identify and treat any recurrences at earlier stages.

These changes occur at the same time as we see an increasing incidence of thyroid cancers in the USA, doubling over the past 15 years. This cannot be explained solely by improvements in detection or by radiation exposure in children born between 1930 and 1950 [9, 10]. Despite the rising incidence of cancer, mortality has not increased. Fortunately, the majority of thyroid cancer is follicular in origin, carrying a good prognosis with surgical resection. The shift in thyroid cancer management is focused on

- Reducing morbidity from operative interventions
- Applying more aggressive surgery to achieve R0 resections
- Reducing the rate of recurrences
- Preventing mortality if a recurrence occurs

Advances in pre- and postoperative management, diagnostic imaging, pathological analysis, as well as advances in surgical techniques have largely contributed to reducing morbidity, mortality, and length of hospitalization.

P. Sinha
St Anthony Surgical Associates, 74 North Main Street, Florida, NY 10921, USA

W.B. Inabnet (✉)
Division of Metabolic, Endocrine and Minimally Invasive Surgery, The Mount Sinai Medical Center, 5 East 98th Street, Box 1259, New York, NY 10029, USA
e-mail: william.inabnet@mountsinai.org

25.2 Thyroid Physiology

Thyroid tumors are often hormonally sensitive and an understanding of the endocrine hormone pathways provides the basis for diagnosis and treatment in a multidisciplinary setting. Two embryological cell lines contribute separate endocrine functions to the thyroid gland:

- Para-follicular C cells
- Follicular cells

The para-follicular C cells are of neural crest origin and responsible for the production of calcitonin. The pharyngeal ectoderm gives rise to the follicular cells that produce the primary thyroid hormones, thyroxine (T4), and triiodothyronine (T3). Calcitonin and thyroid hormone play important roles in the activity of thyroid tumors and interactions with the hypothalamus. It is important to understand the physiology of these hormones as they relate to tumor biology.

25.2.1 Thyroid Hormones – T3/T4

Thyroid hormone is synthesized within the thyroid follicles through uptake of inorganic iodine and subsequent iodination of tyrosine into T3 and T4. The shorter acting T3 is primarily synthesized by peripheral conversion of T4 and is relatively increased in states of iodine deficiency. T3 also plays an important role in feedback regulation through the important regulatory hormone, thyroid stimulating hormone (TSH).

25.2.2 Thyroid Stimulating Hormone (TSH)

TSH is secreted from the anterior pituitary gland in response to thyrotropin-releasing hormone (TRH) and is inhibited by T3. The hypothalamus synthesizes and secretes TRH to stimulate a basal level of TSH synthesis and secretion from the pituitary gland. TSH level changes inversely to thyroid hormone activity and is therefore a sensitive marker of thyroid hormone homeostasis. It is an important marker as well to guide therapeutic suppression of the thyroid using synthetic T4 (Levothyroxine). TSH also stimulates the production of thyroglobulin, the active substrate of the thyroid gland. Achieving suppression of TSH is an important component in the management of patients following surgery for differentiated thyroid cancer (DTC), as it can help to achieve hormonal and thyroid gland substrate suppression. Although it is seldom successful as monotherapy in the setting of residual or metastatic cancer, suppression of thyroid signaling may slow down or prevent transformation of residual thyroid tissue into carcinoma.

25.2.3 Role of Iodine and ^{131}Iodine

Iodine is a central component of thyroid hormone and plays a role in carcinogenesis as well as in diagnosis, and most importantly in therapy. Both deficiency and excess of iodine are associated with specific neoplastic changes. Goiter is primarily a result of iodine deficiency and may harbor follicular cancer cells, whereas iodine excess may promote autoimmune thyroiditis and papillary cancer. Purposeful iodine intake can suppress thyroid hormone production for several days (Wolff–Chaikoff effect), but this mechanism of suppression plays no role in the management of thyroid cancer. Iodine is most useful in its radioactive isotopes that can be used to ablate small amounts of remnant thyroid tissue or for imaging purposes. ^{131}I is used for ablation in doses of 30–200 mCi; a lower dose is usually required for imaging. A less radioactive variant, ^{123}I, can be used for thyroid scanning. Historically, the use of RAI as adjuvant therapy following surgery has led to an improved mortality and reduced recurrence rates in patients that have received a subtotal thyroidectomy. More recently, patients older than 45 years of age and those with tumors >4 cm were deemed of having higher risk for developing aggressive thyroid cancers. This group was shown to benefit from adjuvant RAI following near-total or even total thyroidectomy. RAI remains an important component of therapy when applied selectively to patients who need better control of residual disease and are at high risk for cancer recurrence. It increases the sensitivity of thyroglobulin, which is one of the most important markers for disease recurrence.

25.2.4 Thyroglobulin (Tg)

Thyroglobulin comprises the bulk of the matrix of thyroid tissue and acts as both a storage pool for thyroidal colloid and iodine, and as an active substrate for thyroid hormone synthesis and metabolism. Circulating Tg levels are useful to detect thyroid cancer recurrence or metastatic disease. While preoperative values are neither specific for thyroid cancer nor indicative of disease burden, the postoperative level, following total or near-total thyroidectomy and ^{131}I ablation, is a sensitive marker for cancer surveillance. Tg can be measured individually or in combination with RAI when scanning to screen for recurrence or metastatic disease. The major limitation in Tg screening is the need for complete or near-complete surgical removal or ablation of thyroid tissue in order to achieve a high sensitivity when used to detect early recurrence. As the number of total thyroidectomies has increased in recent years and the use of RAI has become more selective, Tg screening plays a more important role in the long-term surveillance for recurrence.

25.2.5 Calcitonin

Calcitonin is produced exclusively by para-follicular C cells and is responsible for osteoclast inhibition and downregulation of serum calcium. In the setting of medullary thyroid cancer (MTC), 1,000-fold elevations in serum calcitonin are seen. Calcitonin is used as a highly specific marker to establish a diagnosis and for post treatment follow-up in MTC arising purely from C cells. Given the counter regulatory mechanisms in calcium regulation, hypocalcemia is not always seen in medullary thyroid cancer, despite dramatic elevations in calcitonin. There has been some debate over the liberal use of calcitonin screening in the management of patients with clinically relevant thyroid nodules. The data have not supported the use of calcitonin screening in all cases, except when a clear familial syndrome is identified. Its utility is primarily in screening for local or distant recurrence. Calcitonin has no utility in the management of follicular or papillary thyroid cancer.

25.3 Thyroid Pathology

25.3.1 Differentiated Thyroid Cancers (DTC)

Differentiated cancers arising from the follicular cells of the thyroid include

- Papillary thyroid cancer (PTC)
- Follicular thyroid cancer (FTC)
- Follicular variant of papillary thyroid cancer (FvPTC)

Neoplasms of follicular cell origin are the most common form of thyroid cancer, representing approximately 90–95% of all newly diagnosed cases. Hürthle cell cancer is included in this group; however, its behavior varies enough that most segregate it into a separate group [11–13].

Of all these neoplasms of follicular origin, PTC is the most common and carries the best prognosis. PTC is common in areas with sufficient iodine intake and accounts for 80% or more of the thyroid cancer incidence in the USA and Japan.

Follicular thyroid cancer occurs at higher frequencies in iodine-deficient areas and carries a slightly worse prognosis than PTC. Its incidence is about 10–15%. FvPTC is more aggressive than FTC, accounting for 3% of follicular carcinomas.

25.3.2 Medullary Thyroid Cancer (MTC)

MTC originates from parafollicular C cells and its behavior and management varies significantly from the more common thyroid cancers. MTC is relatively rare, accounting for up to 5% of the DTC incidence. It occurs in 70% of the sporadic cases and in about 30% in association with multiple endocrine neoplasia type 2 (MEN 2). Ipsilateral or bilateral neck dissection is required as part of the treatment plan. MTC often presents bilaterally when associated with MEN 2, making a strong argument for frequent biochemical screening in families known to carry the MEN 2 gene mutation. Given its aggressive nature and its relative low incidence, it is not a well-adopted indication for a minimally invasive approach.

25.3.3 Anaplastic Thyroid Cancer

Anaplastic thyroid cancer has an incidence of 1%. It is an undifferentiated cancer that may result from de-differentiation of differentiated forms of thyroid cancer. The risk is increased with age >60 years, with a history of previous radiation exposure or with prior surgery for thyroid cancer. The prognosis is very poor and surgery plays only a limited role. All anaplastic carcinomas are T4 lesions, which can be further differentiated into resectable T4a and unresectable T4b lesions [14]. In the most recent AJCC TNM staging manual seventh edition, it is further subdivided into T4a being entirely intra-thyroidal and T4b being an anaplastic carcinoma with gross extra-thyroidal extension.

Some efforts at inducing re-differentiation of these cancers have been made in order to improve surgical and adjuvant therapies. Anaplastic thyroid cancer loses the ability to metabolize and take up iodine or to synthesize thyroglobulin. Adjuvant therapies, such as TSH suppression and radioiodine, are therefore ineffective for these malignancies. Re-differentiation aims at restoring these thyroid-specific functions. Patients diagnosed with anaplastic cancer are usually enrolled in clinical trials. Some chemotherapeutic agents showed promise for treatment in in vitro studies.

25.4 Workup of a Palpable Thyroid Mass

Palpable thyroid nodules >1 cm are present in 1.5% of men and 6% of women, and small thyroid cancers <1 cm in size have been found at autopsy in 5–10% of the population. Fortunately, clinically relevant thyroid cancer only affects approximately 4–16/100,000 [15]. A most recent estimate by the National Cancer Institute predicted about 37,200 new cases of thyroid cancer in 2009 with 1,630 deaths expected [16]. Increased use of high-resolution imaging has led to an increased detection rate of non-palpable nodes that some believe account for the rising incidence of thyroid cancer without a concurrent increase in mortality. Guidelines published by the American Thyroid Association Taskforce help guide the workup in this era of increased and improved imaging [17].

25.4.1 Definition, Risk Factors, and Clinical Presentation

A clinically relevant nodule is palpable, 1–1.5 cm in size, confirmed on ultrasound imaging, or found primarily on ultrasound examination. The workup of a thyroid nodule begins with a detailed history and physical focused on the thyroid gland and associated lymph node stations. Risk factors that should be elucidated include

- History of head and neck or total body irradiation
- Family history of thyroid malignancy in first-degree relatives
- Exposure to Chernobyl at a young age
- Rapid growth of the nodule
- Hoarseness

Classical physical findings are vocal cord paralysis, fixed nodule, and ipsilateral cervical lymphadenopathy.

25.4.2 "Hot" and "Cold" Nodules

Lab tests include TSH to assess for functional "hot" or nonfunctional "cold" nodules. Nuclear thyroid imaging helps to classify functional lesions as more or less suspicious for malignancy. Iso-active or hot nodules are less suspicious for cancer than inactive or "cold" nodules. Functional nodules are rarely malignant and may be followed clinically unless cytology or growth suggests otherwise.

25.4.3 Role of Ultrasound

Ultrasound evaluation is recommended for all palpable nodes to confirm their presence and to further examine the area of suspicion. It should be the first-line imaging before moving on to more extensive and invasive studies, such as scintigraphy or FNA. Characteristics suggestive of carcinoma include

- Irregular borders
- Solid vs. cystic areas
- Calcification within hypo-echogenic areas
- Lack of halo
- Extension into adjacent structures

25.4.4 Fine Needle Aspiration (FNA)

A fine needle aspiration of clinically relevant nodules is recommended and is the logical next step after ultrasound exam. The FNA may be performed with or without ultrasound guidance. Many groups found that ultrasound guidance provides higher FNA yields in addition to providing clues to malignancy by the imaging modality itself [18–20].

The technique of FNA has been refined in recent years and yields have improved. Cytological analysis is becoming more standardized and reliable in detecting carcinoma. More sophisticated cytological and molecular analytic methods are currently being investigated to improve this sensitivity and specificity [21, 22].

FNA results can be classified into four diagnostic categories:

- Insufficient
- Benign
- Indeterminate
- Malignant

Therapy is different for each of these diagnostic categories. Repeat FNA, with ultrasound guidance to improve the yield, is recommended for an *insufficient diagnosis*. Multiple negative attempts require an excisional biopsy. *Benign lesions* may be followed clinically unless functional aero-digestive compressive symptoms are present. *Malignant lesions* require appropriate surgical resection. *Indeterminate lesions* include several subcategories. The most common indeterminate lesion is the follicular neoplasm. These lesions are further evaluated by thyroid scans and cold nodules require either a lobectomy or total thyroidectomy. Other notable indeterminate lesions are "suspicious for papillary carcinoma" or "Hürthle cell neoplasm." These two subgroups do not require thyroid scanning and should be resected primarily. Clinical risk factors, enhanced cytological analysis, localization of the lesion, and patient's preference guide the initial surgical approach, lobectomy vs. total thyroidectomy.

25.4.5 Role of Molecular Testing

Reverse transcription polymerase chain reaction (RT-PCR) for circulating Tg and mRNA for circulating TSH receptors have been studied recently [23]. These molecular tests in conjunction with cytological results obtained by FNA are thought to increase the detection rate of DTC. The results are promising demonstrating sensitivity for carcinoma as high as 95% and specificity up to 83%. Combining these molecular tests with clinical findings and ultrasound features will enable the physician to offer a more accurate treatment plan to the patient. These molecular techniques are still being refined and as of yet do not constitute standard of care; however, as the body of evidence enlarges, this approach becomes compelling. Added molecular diagnostics may ultimately help to focus treatment on "clinically relevant" thyroid nodules.

25.5 Management of Specific Differentiated Thyroid Cancers

25.5.1 Papillary Thyroid Cancer

Papillary carcinoma is the most common thyroid malignancy representing 80% or more of the cancer incidence, and as much as 90% in iodine-rich areas. Originating from follicular cells, PTC is characterized by the organization of cells into papillae and the presence of psammoma bodies in about 40%. The usual clinical presentation is a solitary palpable thyroid nodule found on physical exam. Approximately 10–20% of patients with newly diagnosed PTC will present with palpable lymph nodes. Voice changes or neck pain herald locally extensive disease and carries a poorer prognosis.

Features unique to PTC include a propensity for multi-centricity and lymph node metastasis, but much less so for distant metastasis. Local invasion is more common than distant metastasis. Autopsy studies have demonstrated that 80% of clinically relevant PTC will have microscopic contralateral lobe involvement, and up to 80% will also have microscopic foci in ipsilateral lymph nodes [24, 25]. Survival studies showed that leaving these microscopic metastatic foci in place will not affect survival adversely. Recurrence however is problematic as demonstrated in a long-term follow-up of a Rochester, MN cohort, with 10- and 20-year recurrence rates of 7% and 14% following lobectomy in low-risk PTC and as high as 26% and

45% in high-risk PTC (AGES score >4), respectively. In those patients with recurrent disease, cancer-specific mortality was 48% and entirely due to cancer recurrence outside the remnant. Furthermore, bilateral total or near-total thyroidectomy significantly reduced loco-regional recurrence in multiple studies [5, 6, 8, 26].

25.5.1.1 An Argument for Early Thyroidectomy

Recent literature and trends have therefore indicated a change in paradigm to a more radical surgical approach in order to reduce mortality resulting from loco-regional recurrence. It is likely that lymph-node dissections and total thyroidectomy will also increase in frequency for lower risk papillary carcinomas.

Newer diagnostic modalities are molecular markers aiding FNA diagnosis and high-resolution ultrasound-guided biopsies of enlarged lymph nodes. Both advance the argument for an earlier total thyroidectomy and earlier lymph-node dissection replacing the older approaches of completion thyroidectomy and neck dissection only when palpable nodes were present.

25.5.1.2 Differentiating Low-risk from High-risk Patients

Several methods of differentiating low-risk from high-risk patients have been developed that take into account age, metastasis, extent, histologic grade, and size. AMES, AGES, TNM, and MACIS classifications are the scoring systems used to distinguish low-risk from high-risk patients [7, 27–30]. These scoring systems have been developed to guide the extent of initial surgery. However, there are patients classified as low-risk that present with clinically significant lymph nodes or even extra-cervical disease, requiring total thyroidectomy with clinically directed ipsilateral neck dissection.

25.5.1.3 Lobectomy vs. Total Thyroidectomy

There is some continued controversy regarding lobectomy vs. total thyroidectomy for patients that have tumors >1 cm in size. Most of the surgeons in the USA have adopted a more extensive initial approach as seen in a recent study of 1,500 US hospitals and over 5,584 patients with thyroid cancer [31, 32]. The majority (77.4%) of the patients in this study underwent total thyroidectomy irrespective of the tumor stage. While tumors <1 cm generally can be treated with thyroid lobectomy, some advocate total or near-total thyroidectomy with T4 suppression and ^{131}I ablation for all biopsy-proven PTC, irrespective of the size.

The arguments for total thyroidectomy are

- Definitive oncologic management given the odds of occult multifocal disease (10%)
- Acceptably low surgical morbidity of <1%
- Improved chances of successfully ablating remaining disease or metastasis with ^{131}I
- Improving the sensitivity of Tg measurements in detecting recurrent disease

For low-risk patients in whom the tumor is ≤1 cm and are ≤45 years of age, the 20-year mortality is as low as 1–4%. In older patients and in those with locally advanced tumors, the 20-year mortality rises to approximately 30–40%. With a generally favorable ratio (9:1) of low-risk to high-risk patients, a cumulative 20-year survival for all newly diagnosed PTCs is 80%.

Finally, there is some ongoing discussion of including a central neck dissection for PTC in order to remove microscopic nodal foci, while lateral neck dissection would be reserved for clinically relevant nodal disease.

25.5.1.4 The Mount Sinai Approach to PTC

Our practice is to perform a total thyroidectomy for preoperatively diagnosed PTC, perform a completion thyroidectomy for all PTC ≥1 cm that were diagnosed on lobectomy, and to perform a clinically directed lymph node dissection in the presence of suspicious nodes on physical exam, ultrasound, or intraoperatively during the course of the thyroidectomy. Thyroidectomy is deemed to be complete if either all tissues are removed, or no more than 1 g remains on the contralateral lobe.

25.5.1.5 Guidelines for Long-term Follow-up

Guidelines are focused on detecting recurrent disease early in order to be able to intervene surgically. Recurrent or metastatic disease is typically found in cervical lymph nodes, the surgical bed, mediastinum, or lungs. Aggressive and long-term close follow-up is necessary. Surveillance every 4–6 months is followed by annual surveillance once disease-free survival is established. Three common diagnostic modalities are used:

- High-resolution cervical ultrasound
- High-sensitivity thyroglobulin
- RAI scans

Ultrasound detects most of the recurrences and is the single-most sensitive modality, even for sub-centimeter cervical lesions. These account for most of the recurrences, with less than a third being distant metastasis identified by Tg levels and CT scans [8].

25.5.1.6 Management of Recurrent Disease

When recurrence is detected, surgical treatment is preferred. If unresectable, RAI ablation or radiation therapies for non-131I avid tumors are other options. When TSH-stimulated Tg levels are found to be between 1 and 10 ng/mL, TSH suppression is recommended in the absence of identifiable disease. However, if the Tg level is >10 ng/mL, RAI therapy is recommended even when imaging, including when PET is negative. Authors from MD Anderson further recommend CT scanning as a further imaging modality to locate recurrent disease in the presence of elevated unstimulated Tg levels of >1 ng/mL, and with negative cervical ultrasound and negative RAI scanning [8].

Finally, distant recurrence, particularly to bone or brain, may be difficult to treat. RAI may initiate cerebral edema and should be avoided in the presence of brain metastasis, while pulmonary metastases are amenable for local resection or ablation.

25.5.2 Follicular Thyroid Cancer

25.5.2.1 Pathological Features

Follicular cancer does not have papillomatous features or psammoma bodies. The histological organization of follicular carcinoma is spherical, surrounding a colloid-filled follicle. The cells often appear similar to normal follicular cells. The distinguished feature of follicular carcinoma is angio-invasion. Size can be variable, including smaller encapsulated carcinomas that can be indistinguishable from follicular adenomas, also referred to as minimally invasive follicular cancer, in contrast to larger, locally extensive cancers that can be seen grossly invading through their capsule. Capsular invasion, whether microscopic or gross, is a marker of advanced disease and carries prognostic value. Frozen-section examination is not particularly helpful due to the overall bland cellular characteristics. Detailed inspection of the entire capsule must be conducted on permanent pathology in order to find evidence of invasion.

Colloid content is also variable, but tends to be less than that in normal cells.

In addition to pure follicular carcinomas, there are also two other variants:

- Follicular variant of papillary thyroid cancer (FvPTC)
- Insular FTC

FvPTC are cancers that are predominantly follicular on histology, but which include some papillary features, such as psammoma bodies or papillary structures, or optically clear "Orphan Annie" nuclei. FvPTC behaves clinically more like PTC than FTC.

Insular FTC is more aggressive and distinguished histologically by areas that are nearly solid, devoid of colloid follicles, and consist of cells separated by capillaries.

25.5.2.2 Clinical Presentation and Prognosis

Clinically, FTC spreads hematogenously and is more likely to present with metastasis than PTC, which spreads via lymphatics first. FTC, when compared to PTC, is more likely to have signs of local invasion, such as pain, dysphonia, or dysphagia. Approximately 25% have local invasion and up to 33% will have distant metastasis at the time of first presentation.

The overall prognosis of FTC is slightly worse than PTC with most reports finding 70–90% 10-year survival depending on the mix of patients presenting with metastasis [33].

Surgical management should be a total thyroidectomy.

Similar to PTC, microcarcinomas <1 cm may also be managed without completion thyroidectomy. Furthermore, clinically positive nodes are removed when detected, but there is no rationale to support routine or prophylactic neck dissection in cases of microcarcinoma.

25.5.2.3 Management Dependent on FNA Result

Initial management of FTC is surgical and determined by the results of FNA or final pathology. A significant difference from PTC is that FTC is difficult to diagnose on FNA and suspicious biopsy results require lobectomy or total thyroidectomy to rule out malignancy on final pathology. Once a diagnosis of FTC is made, a completion thyroidectomy is performed for lesions ≥1 cm and but is optional for tumors <1 cm. Diagnosis of FTC by FNA may prompt more extensive preoperative evaluation to rule out distant disease and would include

- Chest X-ray
- CT/MRI
- Laryngoscopy

Voice changes, fixed lesions, and substernal lesions mandate same preoperative imaging assessment.

25.5.2.4 Guidelines for Long-term Follow-up

After initial surgery or completion thyroidectomy, surveillance and maintenance is achieved by maintaining TSH <1 ng/mL. Physical exam is performed and TSH, Tg, and Tg antibodies are measured at 4–6-month intervals and then annually. Similar to PTC, a TSH-stimulated Tg level is drawn yearly in the absence of ultrasound findings and an unstimulated Tg that is undetectable for T1-2, N0-1 initial-stage cancers. If the initial stage showed invasion of soft tissue or distant metastasis, or if Tg levels were elevated, an RAI scan is performed yearly until there is no more avidity. Postoperative management of FTC follows the above-mentioned guidelines for PTC, relying heavily on periodic high-resolution ultrasound and Tg levels as screening modalities. As is the case with PTC, recurrence should be resected whenever amenable and safe.

25.5.3 Anaplastic Thyroid Cancer

Surgery plays a very limited role in this type of cancer and most of the adjuvant therapies are a part of clinical trials with limited success. Some drugs that showed promising results in vitro are a part of these clinical trials these days.

25.5.3.1 Role of Retinoid Therapy

Retinoids have shown activity in a number of tumors by acting at cell cycle G0/G1 to cause arrest as well as causing some re-differentiation at a number of genes, including NIS, a sodium–iodide symporter that allows iodine uptake. Clinical trials did show some response in 38–50% of patients in restoring the ability to take up RAI; however, the amount of uptake was usually insufficient to cause ablation [22]. A small number of patients did have a clinical benefit and combination therapy may provide better results.

25.5.3.2 Role of Aromatic Fatty Acids

Aromatic fatty acids have been used in clinical trials for non-thyroid cancers and have shown in vitro that cell-cycle arrest and apoptosis can be induced as well as re-differentiation that restores NIS activity. Decreased responsiveness to TSH stimulation was noted as well. Fatty acids, such as phenylacetate and phenylbutarate, have demonstrated chemosensitizing activity in some forms of cancers. Clinical trials are yet to be done to address anaplastic thyroid cancer.

25.6 Minimally Invasive Approaches to Thyroid Cancer

25.6.1 General Considerations

Minimal access techniques for thyroid cancer have been carefully developed for a selected subset of thyroid pathologies. Consideration for minimal access surgery includes a detailed risk/benefit discussion, a thoughtful patient selection, and an intimate understanding of specific instrumentation and operative challenges.

Fortunately, a decade of evidence is available to help guide the surgeon and patient in this endeavor. Concerns that are ever present in traditional open thyroid surgery are even more so in minimal access techniques, particularly intra-operative injury to recurrent laryngeal nerves, parathyroid glands, and failure to achieve an appropriate oncologic resection. These risks are offset by the potential benefits from accelerated short-term recovery and reduction in postoperative pain. The benefits of minimal access techniques may be limited in some approaches to cosmesis [34]. Supporters of these new technologies appreciate improved visualization of nerves, parathyroid glands, or lymph nodes.

Careful patient selection is critical for surgical success. Most studies have found that the suitability of minimal access approaches is limited to a small subset of patients and ranges from 5% to 20%. The selection process includes consideration of

- Histology on FNA
- Preoperative imaging
- Patient demographics and preferences
- Likelihood of achieving oncologic control

Finally, various technical factors and surgeon experience affect significantly the learning curve of a given approach. Experience in endocrine surgery and minimal access techniques, including a familiarity with various energy-emitting dissecting tools, significantly enhances the learning curve, operative time, and patient safety.

There are a few randomized clinical trials that support the use of minimal incision size in reduction of postoperative pain and recovery [35–38]. There are no lasting benefits that have been measured, nor are there any practical benefits that impact the patient, such as earlier return to work or reduction in cost. With an increased detection rate of thyroid masses due to better screening, the perception of reduced harm from minimal access techniques may become increasingly important if treating small masses.

Several modalities of minimal access thyroid surgery have emerged over the past decade. The different techniques are classified as

- Minimal open incision
- Endoscopic approach
- Video-assisted open

25.6.2 Risks and Benefits

There are no long-term data yet to directly compare oncologic or survival endpoints of minimal access techniques with traditional approaches.

Miccoli et al. used thyroglobulin and RAI scanning as a technique to demonstrate surgical equivalence to traditional thyroidectomy, but cautioned that only T1, low-risk papillary cancers should be attempted until longer follow-up is available [39]. Most thyroid cancer management guidelines find that low-risk patients with locally confined disease are managed well by traditional surgical resection. Recurrence, morbidity, and mortality are exceedingly low in this group, all of which occur at frequencies near 1% or less. Fortunately, it is these patients with T1 thyroid carcinoma or small indeterminate FNA biopsies who do well with almost any approach, and are therefore the most appropriate candidates for minimal access techniques. Specimen extraction also places significant limitations on patient selection. Selection criteria will therefore require

- Limiting the procedure to early-stage cancers
- Smaller nodules
- Low gland weight and volumeparticularly when incisions as small as 15 mm are considered.

Novel surgical approaches are not without risk even when appropriate patients are selected. Consideration must also be given to general anesthesia time, which can be as long as 5 h using an endoscopic approach in comparison to 1.3 h of operating time under local anesthesia using conventional open thyroidectomy [40, 41]. Furthermore, even authors with a significant accumulated experience may encounter adverse events, including pneumothorax and esophageal or tracheal injury, and patients have to be counseled appropriately [42].

25.6.3 Patient Selection

Minimally invasive approaches to thyroid cancer begin with critical patient selection. Selection criteria are chosen to exclude those patients who would not benefit from these approaches either due to the risk of an incomplete resection or the risk of iatrogenic injury to vital structures. Locally advanced disease and re-operative thyroid beds present access challenges that preclude the current minimal access approaches. The presence of significant nodal disease may also present a challenge; however, there are series that report on concurrent and focused modified neck dissection [43–45]. Medullary thyroid cancer and anaplastic cancer are usually at an advanced stage at the time of first presentation in the majority of cases and will be excluded. Tumor size is a relative contraindication depending on the type of approach taken and the size of the incision available for specimen extraction. Morcelation cannot be applied to the thyroid due to the requirement for detailed structural analysis. In an analysis by Brunaud et al. in 2003, modern incision sizes for conventional open total thyroidectomy are discussed. They note a significant shift from classically described incisions of 6–8 cm to 4–7 cm incisions for thyroid cancer of all stages. Incisions smaller than this impose visual as well as extraction limits. When considering the variables of pain and scarring, the baseline for conventional open thyroidectomy should be an average incision length of 5–6 cm. It has also been suggested that the term "minimally invasive" should only be used for incisions of ≤3 cm. Consequently, with smaller incision sizes in minimal access approaches, most authors see the following measurements as limits: [35, 37, 42, 44, 46–50]

- Volume of the thyroid gland ≤30 mL
- Nodular diameter <3–4 cm
- Tumor size of <1–2 cm

The indications and selection criteria are slightly different among all described minimal access techniques (Table 25.1).

25.6.4 Minimally Invasive Adjunctive Techniques and Equipment

25.6.4.1 ElectroCautery and Sealing Devices

Instrumentations that have become invaluable to many endocrine surgeons are electrothermal cautery and different sealing devices, such as harmonic scalpel or Ligasure™ (Covidien-USA). These instruments are very effective in controlling vascular structures and in resecting the thyroid off the trachea, replacing traditional suture and knife technique. The primary concern in using these devices is the safety profile, particularly around the recurrent laryngeal nerve. While not extensively reported, the energy spread of thermosealing and ultrasonic devices is approximately 5 mm. Some time must be given to allow heat dissipation before dissecting near sensitive structures approximately 10–15 s.

25.6.4.2 Wall Lifting Devices

Wall lifting devices have been used in the early reports of minimal access thyroidectomy. Wall lifters have different shapes, including corkscrews or flat blades that are inserted under dissection flaps. Transcutaneous sutures that are retracted upwards by pulleys or siderail-mounted arms can be used as an alternative. The benefit of this approach has been in increasing the

Table 25.1 Types of minimally invasive thyroidectomy: Indications and selection criteria

	MIVAT	Mini Open[a]	Breast-Ax Endo	Cervical Endo	Axillary Endo
Anesthesia	Local or general	Local or general	General	General	General
Thyroid volume (mL)	<20–30	20–30+	<20–30	<20–30	<20–30
Incision	1.5–3 cm cervical	2.5–4 cm+ cervical	Four ports Total 3.4 cm Axillary and periareolar	Four ports Total 2.1 cm Cervical	Three to four ports Total 1.5–2 cm Axillary
Stage	Stage I, benign or indeterminate	Stage I–III	Stage I, benign or indeterminate	Benign or indeterminate	Stage I, benign or indeterminate
Node dissection	Central, lateral	Central	No	No	No
Duration of surgery	45–81	70–152	120–240	120–300	120–300
Reference	[35–39, 43–45, 48]	[41, 50–52, 56]	[42, 68, 69]	[40, 64, 72]	[47, 66, 73]

[a]Mini-open techniques may require extension of the incision to conventional open to allow removal of larger masses

operative working space without additional ports or instruments, or without subjecting the patient to high insufflation pressures and hypercarbia. Most surgeons have found that low insufflation pressures or improved retraction techniques allow efficient dissection without compromising on visualization, and therefore do not use wall lifting techniques.

25.6.4.3 Nerve Stimulator

Most endocrine surgeons do not routinely use nerve stimulators; however, they have been useful in difficult thyroid cases to identify proximity to nerves, especially when operating on recurrent disease. There are no reports of use of nerve stimulators in minimal access cases as of yet, mainly due to the low complexity of cases.

25.6.4.4 Regional Anesthesia

Regional anesthesia given preoperatively is an important adjunctive technique that provides significantly improved postoperative pain control, and allows rapid intra-operative vocal feedback for the assessment of recurrent and superior laryngeal nerves. Optimal pain control is achieved with long-acting Bupivicaine and Lidocaine, and a combination of deep cervical and superficial subplatysmal injection, and direct injection to the operative field. The benefits of regional anesthesia extend to cost savings from same day discharge and rapid recovery from intravenous sedation allowing faster room turnover. The patient benefit is significant for both awake and general anesthesia cases. Finally, in the management of the rare postoperative bleed, rapid access to the neck is facilitated by the long-acting anesthetic.

25.6.5 Minimally Invasive Open Technique (MIT)

25.6.5.1 General Aspects

Minimally invasive open thyroidectomy (MIT) is defined as a thyroidectomy performed without endoscopic assistance through an incision that is smaller than that used in conventional open surgery, and usually refers to incision sizes of 2.5–4 cm [41, 50–54]. Paul LoGerfo advanced the state of the art in thyroid surgery by transforming it into a same-day procedure. Over 80% of the thyroidectomies performed at our institution are now performed as outpatient procedures. This would not have been possible without two innovations. The first is the use of loco-regional anesthesia for most patients [55]. The second is the higher placement of the cervical incision, near the cricoid cartilage, allowing easier access to the upper pole, and reducing the length of incision to 2–4 cm for most patients. These modifications began in the late 1980s, becoming routine by the late 1990s, and with 18-year follow-up, has established itself as a safe standard at our institution.

25.6.5.2 Risks and Benefits

The benefits of reduced incision length and higher placement of cervical incision stem from a reduced need for subplatysmal flap dissection and reduced dissection trauma. Reduction in postoperative pain and length of stay is significant irrespective of the type of anesthetic used, allowing for same-day discharge on anti-inflammatory, non-narcotic medications for most of the patients [56]. The smaller incision, compared with a large 8–10-cm Kocher incisions, while more visible early in the postoperative period, fades nicely into natural skin folds with time. A recent report by Perigli et al. demonstrated that cosmetic results, scored by patients, found no difference between a 1.7- and 3.3-cm incision for video-assisted and MIT surgery, respectively [38]. There was a significant improvement in postoperative pain however between traditional, MIT, and video-assisted techniques. Series of minimal incision thyroidectomies have not demonstrated increases in major adverse events, such as postoperative bleeding, recurrent laryngeal nerve injury, or parathyroid-related hypocalcemia. Additionally, Gagner and Inabnet found that in comparison with an endoscopic transcervical approach, open 4–6-cm thyroidectomy patients did not have significantly different analgesic use when assessed at 3-week follow-up [57]. Our own data report an incidence of permanent hypocalcemia, vocal-cord paralysis, and reoperation for bleeding of 0%, 0.5%, and 0.5%, respectively. Temporary vocal cord paresis and temporary hypocalcemia occurred in 2% and 1.6%, respectively. Perigli, Ferzli, and Cavicci all have reported similar low rates of temporary and permanent injuries.

25.6.5.3 Patient Selection

Patient selection for MIT is similar to traditional thyroidectomy via a larger collar incision. Division of upper, middle, and lower pole vessels, identification, and preservation of laryngeal nerves and parathyroid glands are all performed similarly. Higher neck incisions are important as they allow access to the upper pole vessels that are divided early in the course of the dissection. Ferzli and Cavicchi both report on their series and limitations of MIT. Cavicchi recommends that only Stage I cancers with a volume of <20 mL should be removed via a 2.5–3-cm incision, whereas Ferzli did not preoperatively limit the sizes of the lesions. Both authors agree that this approach has the advantage of allowing extension of the incision as needed. Overall, Cavicchi performed MIT in 15.6% of their patients, while Ferzli used MIT in 28% of their cases. Of note, Ferzli did complete 91% of his operations through a 4-cm incision with a representative sample of pathologies, but the rate of total or near-total thyroidectomies was only 35%, compared with Cavicchi's rate of 82%. Our data report on 224 thyroidectomies with a 43% total thyroidectomy rate. In our recent study, thyroid weights but not incision size were reported, noting that general anesthesia was used for larger size cancers of 63.9 vs. 26.9 g, which were operated on under local anesthesia, and corresponding to papillary cancer sizes of 2.5 vs. 1.2 cm, and follicular cancers of 3.6 cm (local anesthesia only) [56]. Assuming that the density of thyroid tissue is approximately 1 g/cm^3, the data from these three studies suggest that thyroid weight or volume between 20 and 30 g or 30 cm^3 represent the upper limit of the size of the thyroid glands that may be managed with MIT through an incision <3 cm.

With a mandated incision size of <3 cm, the following criteria exclude the MIT approach:

- Re-operative fields
- Lymph node involvement outside the central compartment
- Thyroid size >30 cm^3

Long-term oncological results are not available in any of these series; however, the surgeons were not limited by impaired vision or access in achieving complete oncologic control. When mobilization of the thyroid gland is not possible within a 3-cm incision, the incision may be extended. Oncologic control should have the highest priority.

25.6.5.4 Surgical Technique of MIT – The Mount Sinai Approach

Required Instrumentation

We put a basic thyroid tray together, which includes a standard complement of fine-angled clamps, forceps, and retractors.

Electrocautery is used to divide the platysma, the plane between the strap muscles, and the thyroid capsule.

We use an almost suture-less approach by utilizing the low-profile LigaSure Precise™ (Valley Lab, Boulder, CO) to control vessels and to divide thyroid ligaments.

Fine clips, if needed, are used to control vessels in proximity to the laryngeal nerves.

Patient Positioning

The patient is placed supine and the neck is extended with a shoulder roll.

The arms are tucked on both the sides and the shoulders put on slight caudal traction.

Drapes are placed over an ether screen to allow the patient room to breathe and to allow rapid access to the airway in cases of regional anesthesia.

Regional Anesthesia – Technique

We use a mixture of 0.5% Lidocaine and 0.25% Bupivicaine in equal parts and prepare a volume of 60 mL. The transverse process of C2 and C4 are identified and palpated inferior and dorsal to the mastoid process. A 22-gauge needle is advanced until the transverse process of C2 is reached, and then retracted by ~2 mm. We aspirate to avoid intravascular injection and inject 10 cc at the level of C2 and C4. Another 10 cc is used to infiltrate the anterior border of the sternocleidomastoid muscle and superficially underneath the planned incision. An additional volume of 30 cc is injected at the opposite side. A volume of 10 cc is saved for direct injection at the superior poles, an area that is particularly sensitive and difficult to anesthetize pre-incision. Propofol provides adjunctive sedation and allows assessment of vocal cord function throughout the procedure. This technique of regional anesthesia provides excellent intra-operative and post-operative pain control. We utilize this technique for cases under general anesthesia as well.

Operative Steps

The incision is placed near the cricoid cartilage approximately 2–3 cm above the sternal notch. The strap muscles are separated at the midline with retraction. Blunt dissection is used to mobilize the lateral aspect of the target thyroid lobe until the carotid artery is exposed. The superior pole is identified, and the vessels ligated with electrothermal bipolar cautery taking care to preserve the external branch of the superior laryngeal nerve and the superior parathyroid gland. Once the superior pole vessels are divided, the thyroid gland is delivered through the incision and rotated medially to expose the area of the recurrent laryngeal nerve. This maneuver, in conjunction with a higher neck incision, allows for adequate visualization despite a small incision. The recurrent laryngeal nerve is traced along the tracheoesophageal groove into its insertion point. The inferior parathyroid gland is preserved, while the inferior thyroid artery and thyroid ligaments are divided using electrothermal bipolar cautery. The same maneuvers are used on the contralateral side in the event of total thyroidectomy. The strap muscles are re-approximated with a single suture allowing easy egress of blood and early identification of surgical bleeding. The platysma is closed with interrupted sutures and the skin is closed with a temporary Prolene™ 5–0 (Ethicon©, USA) suture and Collodion. The Prolene™ is removed after several hours following hardening of the Collodion.

Postoperative Management

Six hours of observation in the recovery area are mandatory. In the absence of technical difficulty, apparent invasion of the recurrent laryngeal nerve(s) with cancer, same-day discharge is safe. All patients are given 4 g of calcium daily for 5 days and then 2 g/day until follow-up in 2–3 weeks. Intermediate and long-term follow-up for thyroid cancer patients adheres to established guidelines.

25.6.6 Endoscopic Thyroid Surgery

25.6.6.1 Rationale for an Endoscopic Approach

Initially, endoscopic approaches to the neck were developed for focused approaches to preoperatively localized parathyroid adenomas [58–64]. Subsequently, this approach was expanded to the thyroid and further modified to avoid visible scars in the neck via

- Peri-areolar breast approach
- Subclavicular approach
- Transaxillary approach

Each of these approaches is described as follows. Benefits of focused endoscopic parathyroidectomy were readily apparent and the extension to thyroid disease, motivated by the increased incidence in early thyroid cancer and suspicious nodules, just a matter of time. The hope was to develop an approach that minimizes surgical trauma, scarring, and size of incision, treating early stage cancers. The cumulative experience is still small and suffers from short-term follow-up; however, the evidence demonstrates both technical difficulties and favorable benefits.

25.6.6.2 Risks and Benefits

Combination of small, strategically positioned incisions and a magnified view suggests that a finer dissection could be carried out resulting in fewer nerve or parathyroid injuries. Reduced dissection trauma directly translates into reduced postoperative pain.

Authors reporting on the benefits of an endoscopic approach generally refer to improved cosmetic, but vary in terms of length of stay, reduction in postoperative pain, and adverse events. No author has reported a reduction in operative time compared to traditional open or other minimal access approaches. Operating times range from 2 to 3 h. Insufflation pressure should be kept below 8–10 mmHg to avoid hypercarbia. Ikeda et al. published a small matched cohort study of 40 patients with FNA positive for follicular neoplasm. Twenty patients with a high-neck 5-cm incision were compared with 20 patients undergoing an endoscopic unilateral axillary approach. While early postoperative pain was more pronounced in the endoscopic group, the opposite was true on 3-month follow-up. One possible explanation to explain discomfort on swallowing in the open group might be the necessary division of the sternothyroid muscle.

Nerve or parathyroid injury and postoperative bleeding were not seen in the Ikeda study; similarly, Chantawibul [47] reported no complications as well, except one seroma. A few surgical groups have focused on the transaxillary approach, many in combination with peri-areolar ports [42, 47, 65–69]. The bilateral axillary and peri-areolar breast approach has gained recent popularity in the Eastern experience and has demonstrated minimal morbidity with an incidence of 1% or fewer for permanent nerve or parathyroid injuries. On the contrary, there was a high incidence of temporary nerve palsy with associated hoarseness in about 25% of the patients, but resolved over the course of 3 months [69]. Duncan et al. also reported, in a series of 32 patients operated with an ipsilateral axillary approach, no permanent nerve injury, but two temporary nerve palsies and one postoperative bleed, with the pectoralis muscle as a source, requiring minimal access re-exploration. Choe et al., in a large series of 110 patients, described one case of esophageal perforation and one pneumothorax. Axillary and breast approaches notably result in more pain, but ecchymosis and hematomas are not significantly increased. In a case of a transcervical endoscopic approach, Inabnet et al. experienced one permanent injury to the recurrent laryngeal nerve, which they found on postoperative laryngoscopy. They make the point to maintain a safe distance between the ultrasonic scalpel and the recurrent laryngeal nerve in order to avoid any damage, permanent or temporarily [64].

The benefits of proximal and distant endoscopic approaches vary significantly. Proximal ports used in a cervical location result in less tissue trauma and faster recovery, while distant ports cause increased pain but excellent cosmetic by avoiding any visible scar.

25.6.6.3 Oncological Outcome

All authors have demonstrated thyroglobulin levels below 1 ng/mL when total endoscopic thyroidectomy was compared with a similar cohort of patients undergoing traditional open surgery. There is still some disagreement in the literature about which approach to use for completion thyroidectomy – endoscopic or an open approach. The more recently described bilateral transaxillary approach can address the entire gland at the time of initial surgery. A central subclavicular approach has been described to achieve total thyroidectomy [70, 71]. No long-term data are available, but early follow-up data demonstrate appropriate oncologic control of early papillary and follicular cancers on postoperative screening ultrasound and by measuring thyroglobulin levels.

To adhere to oncological standards the ideal indications for these novel techniques are

- Indeterminate nodules
- Small T1 carcinomas

25.6.6.4 Patient Selection

There is little debate on the surgical community about the appropriate patient selection.

Indications

- Total gland volume <20–30 cm^3
- T1 microcarcinoma, age <50 years, no lymph node involvement
- Small nodules, indeterminate on FNA

Re-operative thyroid surgery is considered as a contraindication unless a completion thyroid lobectomy is approached from the contralateral side. Cosmetic preference should not be the driving force in ideal candidates. Given the novelty of this approach, sound judgment and a well-informed patient will lead to good outcomes in an appropriately selected patient group.

25.6.5.5 Endoscopic, Transcervical Approach

Huscher et al. first described a totally endoscopic approach to thyroid lobectomy using a set of three ports, two 5-mm and one 10-mm port, under low-pressure insufflation [40]. In his descriptive case report, the specimen, measuring 3 × 2 cm was extracted from the 10-mm port site in an operation lasting nearly 5 h. The three laparoscopic trocars were inserted under the platysma muscle at the anterior margin of the sternocleidomastoid muscle:

- 5-mm trocar at the jugular notch
- 5-mm trocar at the angle of the mandible
- 10-mm trocar, midway between the first two trocars, 4 cm above the clavicle

This trocar configuration corresponds to a lateral open incision when performing focused parathyroid or thyroid surgery. Special instrumentation included a 30° 5-mm camera, an ultrasonic scalpel, a wall lifting device, and an endoscopic pouch in order to maximize visualization and working space, and to remove the specimen that contained a focus of microcarcinoma on final pathology. The strap muscles were divided for exposure and both parathyroid glands and the recurrent laryngeal nerve were visualized. Clips were used to control upper and lower pole vessels. Notably, the patient had some subcutaneous emphysema, did not require postoperative analgesia, and was discharged on the second postoperative day.

Difficulties with the endoscopic transcervical approach in its early development included hypercarbia and limited working space with inadequate long instruments. Moving the ports to distances further away, reducing insufflation pressure, and using wall lifter instruments overcame these difficulties leading finally to development of the transaxillary approach. Henry et al. applied a lateral endoscopic approach adapted from focused parathyroidectomy to small, solitary indeterminate thyroid nodules [72]. The operative results were favorable but patient selection limited to, on FNA exam, indeterminate pathologies with thyroid volumes < 30 mL. Differences to Huscher's approach were the use of 2.5-mm ports instead of 5 mm, low insufflation pressure, and not utilizing any wall lifting devices. All 38 patients in this series had short operative times of 102 ± 27 min and were discharged on postoperative day 1.

Gagner and Inabnet developed an endoscopic transcervical approach using a 10-mm port, two 3-mm ports, and one 5-mm port with gas insufflation. The technique was modified to include an open partial dissection to allow a focused upper pole ligation through the 10-mm port prior to start gas insufflation up to a pressure of 10–12 mmHg. They reduced operating time greatly compared to their early experience and was reported with a median of 115 min. Dissection was performed with the help of gas insufflation and blunt dissection using the tip of a 0° camera. Vessels and thyroid ligaments were dissected and controlled with the ultrasonic scalpel. The 0° camera was switched during the course of the procedure to a 30° or 45° camera for improved visualization. The identification of parathyroid glands and recurrent laryngeal nerve was mandatory in their case series of 38 patients. Patients with carcinoma, identified on frozen section ($n = 3$), were treated with an open completion thyroidectomy, except for one case in which a 3-mm focus of papillary carcinoma was managed without completion thyroidectomy. There was one permanent, but asymptomatic ipsilateral recurrent laryngeal nerve injury detected on routine indirect laryngoscopy. This injury was thought to be due to the proximity of the ultrasonic scalpel to the nerve, while dissecting the lateral portion of the gland.

Elements common to different endoscopic transcervical approaches are

- Significant learning curve built on established expertise in open thyroid surgery
- Understanding of lateral approaches to thyroid-related structures
- Significant limitation on size and pathology of nodules that may be managed

All authors report decreased postoperative pain; however, meaningful long-term benefits, long-term oncological data, and a cost analysis are not available. Given the constraints on incision size, the endoscopic transcervical approach may be used only for lobectomies, for lesions <3 cm of low malignant potential.

Patient Positioning

The patient is placed supine with the neck extended using a shoulder roll.

The arms are tucked on both the sides with the shoulders under slight caudal traction.

Intubation is necessary given the potential for hypercarbia and subcutaneous emphysema in the neck area.

Necessary Instrumentation

A basic thyroid tray, which includes a standard complement of fine-angled clamps, forceps, and retractors, should always be available if conversion becomes necessary.

An advanced laparoscopic energy device with a 5-mm port profile will be required to control vessels and dissect the thyroid. My experience included, most authors have used an ultrasonic scalpel. As with all energy devices, a distance of 5 mm should be maintained from the nerves to avoid injury. When this is not possible, a low-profile clip applier is useful, particular at the middle thyroid vein.

Ports: Standard 5-mm ports (1), 3-mm (2), and 10-mm (1) ports are used for the approach used by Inabnet and Gagner, although smaller ports may replace the 5-mm port as described earlier.

Dissection and Retraction: Short-handled instruments are preferable. Curved- and round-tip dissecting instruments may be used interchangeably to grasp and dissect. Low-profile scissors are helpful, as is an endoscopic peanut.

Operative Steps

A lateral or central neck approach may be used. The lateral neck approach is described here; however, a fully endoscopic central neck approach may be used for total thyroidectomy [70, 71]. The operative steps for a central approach are similar to the description of video-assisted thyroid surgery in the next section.

As described by Gagner and Inabnet, the port placements are critical to facilitate dissection of the upper pole vessel, and to visualize the recurrent laryngeal nerve. A 10-mm port incision is placed near the level of the cricoid cartilage, but lateral to the carotid artery. A limited open dissection, through this incision, is carried down to the carotid sheath and medial to it. The space lateral and posterior to the superior thyroid gland is dissected, and ligation of the upper pole vessels is completed under direct vision using ultrasonic scalpel. Following this, the 10-mm trocar is placed, secured with a subcutaneous purse string and carbon dioxide insufflations started, which facilitates further dissection. Two 3-mm ports are placed inferior and medial to this 10-mm port. A 5-mm port is placed in the midline, below the medial 3-mm port, and will be used for the ultrasonic scalpel. The strap muscles are separated in their midline raphe or retracted medially, but are not transected. The inferior thyroid artery is located as a landmark to identify the recurrent laryngeal nerve. Once identified, the nerve is traced along its length to its insertion into the cricothyroid muscle. This allows safe dissection of the inferior pole vessels, parathyroid glands, and thyroid ligaments. A distance of >5 mm from the nerve, when using the ultrasonic scalpel, is recommended to avoid inadvertent injury from lateral energy spread. The inferior thyroid artery is ligated medial to its junction with the recurrent laryngeal nerve. This allows retraction of the thyroid away from the nerve in order to continue the dissection of the lobe and isthmus. The specimen is removed via the 10-mm port.

25.6.6.6 Endoscopic, Non-cervical Approaches

Patient preference for cosmetics was a motivating factor in the East-Asian experience leading to the development of non-cervical port techniques. In Korea and Japan, several groups moved laparoscopic ports to peri-areolar and axillary positions in order to primarily avoid the visible neck scar and secondarily to reduce instrument interference [67, 68, 73–77].

Bilateral Axillary-breast Approach (BABA)

This technique was described by Choe et al. [42], and by Chung et al. in a comparison of 109 BABA vs. open conventional surgery for malignant nodules <1 cm [69]. A total of four ports were placed in both axillae (two 5-mm ports) and bilateral in the peri-areolar area (two 12-mm ports).

Choe et al. reported an operating time of 165.3 min for 52 total and 53 subtotal endoscopic thyroidectomies. Seventy-seven cases of carcinoma were included in this series. There was one conversion for carcinoma because of subcapsular invasion and one conversion for tracheal perforation in the early experience. Preoperative selection was limited to neoplasms ≤3 cm, T1 carcinoma <1 cm, absence of nodal disease, and age <50 years. Breast malignancy was also ruled out preoperatively. Postoperative hospital stay was 4 days, compared to 3.7 days for their conventional thyroidectomies. A drain was placed and a surgical bra was used to compress the peri-areolar port sites. Thyroglobulin was ≤1 ng/mL at 2 months and ^{131}I whole body scanning found no residual disease. There was one nodal recurrence of papillary cancer managed by selective node dissection. There was one pneumothorax from barotrauma and one esophageal injury presenting 1 week postoperatively as infection, which was managed with exploration, inpatient local wound care, and antibiotics. Finally, the authors state a 15-case learning curve for an experienced thyroid surgeon.

Chung reported a higher rate of transient RLN injuries in his endoscopic series than Choe et al. – 25.2% vs. 2.5%, respectively. Permanent hypocalcemia was not significantly different – 4.5% in open thyroidectomies vs. 1.0% in the BABA group. Both the groups, Choe et al. and Chung, had reduction of postoperative thyroglobulin to <1.0 ng/mL in almost all patients (90.4% and 88.9% BABA). Incision size was 3.5–5 cm for the open group and length of stay was similar at 3.2 vs. 3.0 days (BABA). This cumulative experience has led both the authors to feel comfortable promoting this approach for microcarcinomas in the absence of nodal disease.

Transaxillary Approach

An axillary-only approach was used by Duncan [66], Ikeda [73], and Chantawibul [47] with success to manage ipsilateral thyroid lobe lesions. In comparison to BABA, fewer ports and less dissection is required; however, total thyroidectomy requires placement of bilateral axillary ports. Bilateral axillary approaches have the advantage of no interference between instruments, which is a problem described in the ipsilateral approach.

Planning an axillary approach to remove thyroid nodules or microcarcinoma should be done by experienced endocrine surgeons only. The approach is quite different from anterior or lateral neck exposures of the thyroid gland, and the cumulative experience in the literature demonstrates that significant complications can occur. The results demonstrate that this approach, when performed by experienced surgeons, is associated with minimal morbidity and complications and can be done as an outpatient procedure. Early postoperative pain is higher than in cervical approaches, late pain is nonexistent, and a high degree of patient satisfaction is reported. Long-term data are not available yet, but we suspect that there will be no difference in oncologic outcomes as long as stringent patient selection is maintained, including small microcarcinomas only without nodal involvement (Fig. 25.1).

25.6.6.7 Minimally Invasive Video-assisted Thyroidectomy

Video-assisted thyroidectomy was met with early enthusiasm by borrowing the techniques used for open thyroidectomy when performed through a high-neck incision. The reduction in the incision size to 15 mm was possible by using low-profile laparoscopic instruments, an endoscope for visualization, and ultrasonic scalpel for control of vessels. This approach is associated with

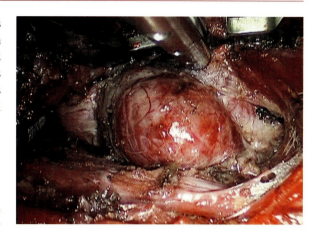

Fig. 25.1 View of right thyroid lobe during endoscopic transaxillary thyroidectomy

- Steep learning curve
- Minimal tissue dissection
- Ability to perform a total or completion thyroidectomy
- Excellent patient comfort
- Excellent cosmetic result

Furthermore, most of the few randomized trials in minimal access thyroid surgery have compared this technique to open surgery.

Miccoli et al. reported a similar approach to parathyroid surgery in 1997 and further developed this technique for thyroid surgery, which they described in 1999. They have gained the most experience with this technique with more than 600 cases reported as of 2004 [37, 60, 78, 79]. This technique incorporates features of both endoscopic technique and MIT, but is most similar to a mini-incision open thyroidectomy performed under magnification. The technique uses a 15-mm incision and insufflation of the subplatysmal plane with CO_2 to create the required working space. The dissection is performed after removing the trocar initially used for insufflations. Multiple instruments and a 5-mm 30° laparoscope are then inserted through the 15-mm incision. The major vessels are controlled with harmonic scalpel or clips, and the recurrent laryngeal nerve and parathyroid glands are routinely visualized.

This technique can be used efficiently to achieve operative times comparable to conventional open thyroidectomy, which is an important difference from endoscopic approaches that typically require 2 h. Miccoli's exceptional results with this approach include a mean operative time of 51.6 min for total thyroidectomy, overnight stay for all patients, and complication rates that are expected of experienced endocrine surgeons: 0.1% bleeding rate, 1.3% nerve palsy, and 0.2% permanent hypo-parathyroidism. The disadvantages of this approach are the requirement for a second assistant to hold the videoscope, a steep learning curve, and the inability to manage thyroid glands >20 mL in size or microcarcinomas >Stage I. Miccoli applied this technique to 11% of his patients after 5 years of experience, and 46% were total thyroidectomies. The three most common pathologies were follicular adenoma (28.1%), low-risk papillary cancer (27.4%), and multinodular goiter (25.7%).

While Miccoli's results are widely acknowledged as exceptional and the learning curve is somewhat steep, his results have been replicated by other endocrine surgeons. Bellantone's group, also in Italy, were able to achieve an 81-min total thyroidectomy time and modified Miccoli's approach by not using insufflation as a part of the dissection, and performing the procedures in loco-regional anesthesia using a superficial cervical block. Multiple authors have consistently found significantly reduced postoperative pain in randomized evaluations [35–38]. In terms of patient numbers, safety, and patient comfort, the literature clearly supports this technique.

25.6.7 Video-assisted Lateral Neck Dissection

Bellantone's group has extended their experience in managing thyroid cancer to include a pilot study in neck dissection. Reported as a feasibility study of two patients, Lombardi used the video-assisted approach in a lateral neck dissection for nodal papillary thyroid cancer [45]. Normally performed through a large, extended transverse cervicotomy, a 4-cm cervicotomy is reported when using a video-assisted approach. In this series, low-risk PTC (T1-T2, M0, age <45 years) with nodal disease was selected, and the thyroidectomy was performed in a mini-open fashion through a high cervicotomy of up to 4 cm in size. A 5-mm 30 scope and a combination of low-profile instruments adapted from plastic surgery and ENT were used, including scissors, spatulas, forceps, and a spatula-shaped aspirator. A combination of bipolar cautery, ultrasonic scalpel, and conventional suture ligature was used. The jugular nodes from level II to V were removed in between the standard landmarks

- Anterior – medial border of the sternocleidomastoid muscle (SCM)
- Medial – carotid sheet
- Lateral – anterior border of the trapezius muscle
- Posterior – scalenus anterior and scalenus medium
- Superior – posterior belly of the digastric muscle
- The clavicle and the subclavian vessels

Prior to this report, Bellantone, Tanaka Ikeda, and Miccoli have all reported selective node dissection of the central compartment [43, 44, 80, 81].

The results, as reported by Lombardi et al., were favorable with the video-assisted neck dissection adding approximately 1 h to the case, only transient hypocalcemia for both the patients, and the intra-operative recognition and control of a thoracic duct injury in one. Postoperative Tg levels were undetectable in both, and there was minimal RAI uptake and no evidence of disease on high-resolution ultrasonography. This pilot study was favorable and cautions a careful approach to malignant disease. The application of this technique to neck dissection holds promise in reducing the morbidity from modified radical neck dissection.

25.7 Future Trends

The treatment of early thyroid cancer has taken root in a number of flexible and highly individualized minimal access techniques. The early work in minimal access lymphadenectomy promises that these techniques may evolve to manage more advanced thyroid cancer. If current size limits on extraction can be overcome, larger cancers may be manageable through smaller incisions. The state of the art in cancer surveillance will continue to evolve and diagnostic accuracy promises to allow improved patient selection. Until then, we continue to be faced with a growing number of clinically relevant thyroid nodules that are suspicious or indeterminate. Minimal access techniques offer a kinder approach to the younger patient concerned with pain, return to work, and cosmetic outcomes, and reduce the surgical morbidity for older patients that present with more advanced cancers. The mini-open technique with its flexibility may become the default standard for open thyroid surgery. A shorter length of stay is facilitated in part by regional anesthesia. Finally, endoscopic and video assisted techniques provide individualized options to those wishing for minimal scarring or minimal pain. Surgeons wishing to add these techniques to their repertoire will face some learning curve challenges, but will find a growing body of literature and an ever increasing number of experienced endocrine surgeons willing to share their expertise.

Quick Reference Guide

1. **Patient selection for minimal access approaches**
   - Volume of the thyroid gland: ≤30 mL
   - Nodular diameter: <3–4 cm
   - Tumor size: <1–2 cm
2. **Exclusion criteria for minimal access approaches**
   - Re-operative fields
   - Lymph node involvement outside the central compartment
   - Thyroid size >30 mL
3. **Indications for endoscopic thyroid surgery**
   - Total gland volume <20–30 mL
   - T1 micro-carcinoma
   - Age <50 years
   - No lymphatic involvement
   - Small nodules, indeterminate on FNA
4. **Endoscopic trans-cervical approach**
   - **Port placement**
     - Critical step for accessing the upper pole vessels and to visualize the recurrent laryngeal nerve
     - A set of four ports is used
     - 10-mm port at the level of the cricoid cartilage, lateral to the carotid
     - Two 3-mm ports, inferior and medial to the 10-mm port
     - 5-mm port, midline, below the medial 3-mm port, used for harmonic scalpel
   - **Patient positioning**
     - Supine, neck extended over a shoulder roll
     - Arms tucked
     - Shoulders put on a slight caudal traction
   - **Operative steps**
     - Limited open dissection of the space lateral and posterior to the superior thyroid gland.
     - The upper pole vessels are divided under direct vision.
     - Placement of a 10-mm trocar through this initial incision and holding it in place with a purse string suture
     - Separate strap muscles in midline. Do not transect them!
     - If using the harmonic scalpel, keep a distance of at least 5 mm to the recurrent laryngeal nerve
     - Specimen will be removed through the 10-mm port
5. **Endoscopic non-cervical approaches**
   This approaches are still not routine procedures and a higher number of patients is needed to judge their value and to assess oncological adequacy.
   - **Bilateral axillary-breast-approach – BABA**
     - A set of four ports is used.
       - 5-mm port – one in each axilla
       - 12-mm port: one in each peri-areolar region of the breasts
   - **Trans-axillary approach**
     - Only ipsilateral lesions can be managed
     - "Sword fighting" – interference with instruments is a problem
6. **Mini-Incision Thyroidectomy – MIT**
   Operative technique
   Step 1: Incision
   - Transverse, near the cricoid cartilage
   - Use a natural skin crease
   - Do not exceed 2.5 cm

   Step 2: Thyroid exposure
   - Divide the platysma transversely with monopolar electrocautery.
   - Create subplatysmal flaps superiorly to the cricoid cartilage and inferiorly to the clavicle using both electrocautery and blunt dissection.
   - The strap muscles are separated in their midline using cautery.
   - Muscle fibers are removed off of the thyroid gland.

   Step 3: Superior pole dissection
   - Retractors are repositioned superiorly and laterally to expose the superior attachments of the thyroid gland.

- Avoid transection or traction on the external branch of the superior laryngeal nerve.
- An avascular plane between the trachea and the thyroid gland is demonstrated with spreading of an angled clamp directed dorsally.
- The thyroid gland in this location will be seen to be extending superiorly, and this portion of the gland will contain the superior pole vessels.
- These vessels should be dissected out and ligated individually.
- The superior pole of the thyroid gland can then be transected from its ligamentous attachment.

Step 4: Superior parathyroid gland
- The superior pole of the thyroid can now be rotated out of the skin incision.
- Lateral traction and blunt dissection dorsally will expose the carotid artery sheath.
- Superior extension of the blunt dissection along this lateral border will allow identification of the superior parathyroid gland. This should be gently dissected free from the thyroid gland.

Step 5: Exposure of the dorsal medial thyroid gland
- Blunt lateral dissection can be extended inferiorly to free the lateral edge of the thyroid gland.
- The thyroid gland may then be rotated medially and outside of the skin to a greater extent by placing Allis clamps on the lateral edge of the thyroid gland for traction.
- Gentle traction applied outwards and medially will elevate the middle thyroid vein, inferior thyroid artery, and recurrent laryngeal nerve.
- Ligation of the middle thyroid vein will give extra mobility to the gland. The middle thyroid vein should be ligated high on the thyroid gland to avoid inadvertent injury to the recurrent laryngeal nerve.
- Ligamentous attachments to the inferior pole will also allow more thyroid gland mobility out of the wound.
- The dorsal medial thyroid gland and tracheoesophageal groove are now easily visualized.

Step 6: Dissection of the recurrent laryngeal nerve
- The recurrent laryngeal nerve should then be carefully traced in an inferior to superior fashion along the tracheoesophageal groove up to its muscular insertion. Along this path, the nerve will be crossed by the inferior thyroid artery and sometimes parathyroid gland.
- By identifying the superior and inferior extent of the nerve, the artery may safely be ligated and the parathyroid gland safely preserved.
- Energy for dissection should be used until the nerve is clearly demonstrated.
- Clips, fine suture, or pressure should be used to control bleeding until the RLN is identified.
- A non-recurrent laryngeal nerve is rare, but is seen coursing lateral to medial and then into the muscle.
- The RLN can be confused with the middle thyroid vein or inferior thyroid artery, therefore any candidates for the RLN should not be directly grasped.
- By dissecting parallel on any candidate structure superiorly and inferiorly, the RLN can be ruled in or out.
- There may be branches of the RLN near its muscular insertion. These should be preserved.

Step 7: Inferior parathyroid gland
- The inferior parathyroid gland may be identified in step 5 or 6, and carefully removed off of the thyroid gland.
- The inferior parathyroid gland is highly variable and may descend into the thymus gland, along the trachea or esophagus or below the carotid.
- It is not necessary to definitively identify this gland if at least one or two glands are seen and preserved.
- Inadvertent devascularization of the parathyroid gland may be remedied by implantation into the forearm or strap muscles.

Step 8: Thyroid dissection
- The thyroid gland may now be dissected off the trachea by transecting its ligamentous attachments under full visualization of the RLN.

- By visualization of the nerve prior to transecting the ligament of Berry, nerve injury is virtually eliminated.
- A 5-mm minimum distance must be maintained from the nerve when using an energy source, such as a thermal sealing bipolar device or an ultrasonic scalpel.
- Traction upwards and medially will allow easy transection.
- The isthmus should be included in a thyroid lobectomy.
- Steps 1–8 may be repeated for the contralateral gland.
- The entire thyroid gland may be removed en bloc or in two halves.

Step 9: Completion
- Hemostasis should be evaluated at all quadrants.
- A Valsalva maneuver will sometimes identify potential sources of bleeding before closure.
- A final inspection for intact parathyroid glands should be made, and a final visualization of the RLN may be done, particularly if it was not identifiable prior to resection.

Step 10: Wound closure
- The strap muscles are re-approximated by one or two interrupted absorbable sutures, leaving the inferior aspect unopposed to allow deep bleed a route for egress.
- The platysma muscle edges are re-approximated with three to four interrupted sutures.
- The skin edges are approximated with a 5-0 Prolene running sub-cuticular suture without knots.
- With tension held at the suture ends, Collodion or other skin adhesive is applied.
- Once dry in several hours, the Prolene suture is pulled out, leaving only the adhesive for skin closure. This allows excellent healing with very fine, if any, scarring.

References

1. Mazzaferri, E.L., Jhiang, S.M.: Long-term impact of initial surgical and medical therapy on papillary and follicular thyroid cancer. Am. J. Med. **97**(5), 418–428 (1994)
2. Hay, I.D., et al.: Papillary thyroid carcinoma managed at the Mayo Clinic during six decades (1940-1999): temporal trends in initial therapy and long-term outcome in 2444 consecutively treated patients. World J. Surg. **26**(8), 879–885 (2002)
3. Schlumberger, M., et al.: Long-term results of treatment of 283 patients with lung and bone metastases from differentiated thyroid carcinoma. J. Clin. Endocrinol. Metab. **63**(4), 960–967 (1986)
4. Clark, O.H., et al.: Thyroid cancer: the case for total thyroidectomy. Eur. J. Cancer Clin. Oncol. **24**(2), 305–313 (1988)
5. DeGroot, L.J., et al.: Does the method of management of papillary thyroid carcinoma make a difference in outcome? World J. Surg. **18**(1), 123–130 (1994)
6. Grant, C.S., et al.: Local recurrence in papillary thyroid carcinoma: is extent of surgical resection important? Surgery **104**(6), 954–962 (1988)
7. Kjellman, P., et al.: Predictors of outcome in patients with papillary thyroid carcinoma. Eur. J. Surg. Oncol. **32**(3), 345–352 (2006)
8. Mittendorf, E.A., et al.: Followup of patients with papillary thyroid cancer: in search of the optimal algorithm. J. Am. Coll. Surg. **205**(2), 239–247 (2007)
9. Hodgson, N.C., Button, J., Solorzano, C.C.: Thyroid cancer: is the incidence still increasing? Ann. Surg. Oncol. **11**(12), 1093–1097 (2004)
10. Davies, L., Welch, H.G.: Increasing incidence of thyroid cancer in the United States, 1973-2002. JAMA **295**(18), 2164–2167 (2006)
11. D'Avanzo, A., et al.: Follicular thyroid carcinoma: histology and prognosis. Cancer **100**(6), 1123–1129 (2004)
12. Kushchayeva, Y., et al.: Comparison of clinical characteristics at diagnosis and during follow-up in 118 patients with Hurthle cell or follicular thyroid cancer. Am. J. Surg. **195**(4), 457–462 (2008)
13. Stojadinovic, A., et al.: Hurthle cell carcinoma: a 60-year experience. Ann. Surg. Oncol. **9**(2), 197–203 (2002)
14. Greene, F.L., American Joint Committee on Cancer., and American Cancer Society.: AJCC Staging Manual, 6th edn. Practice Guidelines in Oncology: Thyroid Carcinoma, vol. v.2.2007. 2002, xiv, 421 pp. Springer-Verlag, New York
15. United States Cancer Statistics: 1999–2003 Incidence and Mortality Web-based Report. 2007 8/23/2007]. www.cdc.gov/uscs. Accessed 23 Aug 2007
16. Thyroid Cancer Home Page - National Cancer Institute. 2007 8/23/2007]. www.cancer.gov/cancertopics/types/thyroid. Accessed 23 Aug 2007
17. Cooper, D.S., et al.: Management guidelines for patients with thyroid nodules and differentiated thyroid cancer. Thyroid **16**(2), 109–142 (2006)
18. Baskin, H.J., Duick, D.S.: The endocrinologists' view of ultrasound guidelines for fine needle aspiration. Thyroid **16**(3), 207–208 (2006)
19. Carmeci, C., et al.: Ultrasound-guided fine-needle aspiration biopsy of thyroid masses. Thyroid **8**(4), 283–289 (1998)
20. Papini, E., et al.: Risk of malignancy in nonpalpable thyroid nodules: predictive value of ultrasound and color-Doppler features. J. Clin. Endocrinol. Metab. **87**(5), 1941–1946 (2002)
21. Milas, M., et al.: The utility of peripheral thyrotropin mRNA in the diagnosis of follicular neoplasms and surveillance of thyroid cancers. Surgery **141**(2), 137–146 (2007). discussion 146

22. Wagner, K., et al.: Thyrotropin receptor/thyroglobulin messenger ribonucleic acid in peripheral blood and fine-needle aspiration cytology: diagnostic synergy for detecting thyroid cancer. J. Clin. Endocrinol. Metab. **90**(4), 1921–1924 (2005)
23. Karavitaki, N., et al.: Molecular staging using qualitative RT-PCR analysis detecting thyreoglobulin mRNA in the peripheral blood of patients with differentiated thyroid cancer after therapy. Anticancer Res. **25**(4), 3135–3142 (2005)
24. Russell, W.O., et al.: Thyroid Carcinoma. Classification, Intraglandular Dissemination, and Clinicopathological Study Based Upon Whole Organ Sections of 80 Glands. Cancer **16**, 1425–1460 (1963)
25. Noguchi, S., Noguchi, A., Murakami, N.: Papillary carcinoma of the thyroid. I. Developing pattern of metastasis. Cancer **26**(5), 1053–1060 (1970)
26. Chow, S.M., et al.: Local and regional control in patients with papillary thyroid carcinoma: specific indications of external radiotherapy and radioactive iodine according to T and N categories in AJCC 6th edition. Endocr. Relat. Cancer **13**(4), 1159–1172 (2006)
27. D'Avanzo, A., et al.: Prognostic scoring systems in patients with follicular thyroid cancer: a comparison of different staging systems in predicting the patient outcome. Thyroid **14**(6), 453–458 (2004)
28. Jukkola, A., et al.: Prognostic factors in differentiated thyroid carcinomas and their implications for current staging classifications. Endocr. Relat. Cancer **11**(3), 571–579 (2004)
29. Lo, C.Y., et al.: Optimizing the treatment of AMES high-risk papillary thyroid carcinoma. World J. Surg. **28**(11), 1103–1109 (2004)
30. Lo, C.Y., et al.: Follicular thyroid carcinoma: the role of histology and staging systems in predicting survival. Ann. Surg. **242**(5), 708–715 (2005)
31. Hundahl, S.A., et al.: Initial results from a prospective cohort study of 5583 cases of thyroid carcinoma treated in the united states during 1996. U.S. and German Thyroid Cancer Study Group. An American College of Surgeons Commission on Cancer Patient Care Evaluation study. Cancer **89**(1), 202–217 (2000)
32. Clark, O.H., Duh, Q.-Y., Kebebew, E.: Updates in Endocrine Surgery. In: Bewick C. (ed.) Facial Plastic Surgery Surgical Clinics of North America, vol. 84, xiv, 951 pp. W.B. Saunders Company, Philadelphia (2004)
33. Clark, O.H., Duh, Q.-Y., Kebebew, E.: Textbook of Endocrine Surgery. 2nd edn, xx, 828 pp. W.B. Saunders, Philadelphia (2006)
34. Ikeda, Y., et al.: Are there significant benefits of minimally invasive endoscopic thyroidectomy? World J. Surg. **28**(11), 1075–1078 (2004)
35. Bellantone, R., et al.: Video-assisted vs conventional thyroid lobectomy: a randomized trial. Arch. Surg. **137**(3), 301–4 (2002). discussion 305
36. Hegazy, M.A., et al.: Minimally invasive video-assisted thyroidectomy for small follicular thyroid nodules. World J. Surg. **31**(9), 1743–1750 (2007)
37. Miccoli, P., et al.: Comparison between minimally invasive video-assisted thyroidectomy and conventional thyroidectomy: a prospective randomized study. Surgery **130**(6), 1039–1043 (2001)
38. Perigli, G., et al.: Clinical benefits of minimally invasive techniques in thyroid surgery. World J. Surg. **32**(1), 45–50 (2008)
39. Miccoli, P., et al.: Minimally invasive video-assisted thyroidectomy. Am. J. Surg. **181**(6), 567–570 (2001)
40. Huscher, C.S., et al.: Endoscopic right thyroid lobectomy. Surg. Endosc. **11**(8), 877 (1997)
41. Spanknebel, K., et al.: Thyroidectomy using local anesthesia: a report of 1, 025 cases over 16 years. J. Am. Coll. Surg. **201**(3), 375–385 (2005)
42. Choe, J.H., et al.: Endoscopic thyroidectomy using a new bilateral axillo-breast approach. World J. Surg. **31**(3), 601–6 (2007)
43. Bellantone, R., et al.: Central neck lymph node removal during minimally invasive video-assisted thyroidectomy for thyroid carcinoma: a feasible and safe procedure. J. Laparoendosc. Adv. Surg. Tech. A **12**(3), 181–185 (2002)
44. Ikeda, Y., et al.: Minimally invasive video-assisted thyroidectomy and lymphadenectomy for micropapillary carcinoma of the thyroid. J. Surg. Oncol. **80**(4), 218–221 (2002)
45. Lombardi, C.P., et al.: Minimally invasive video-assisted functional lateral neck dissection for metastatic papillary thyroid carcinoma. Am. J. Surg. **193**(1), 114–118 (2007)
46. Bellantone, R., et al.: Minimally invasive, totally gasless video-assisted thyroid lobectomy. Am. J. Surg. **177**(4), 342–343 (1999)
47. Chantawibul, S., Lokechareonlarp, S., Pokawatana, C.: Total video endoscopic thyroidectomy by an axillary approach. J. Laparoendosc. Adv. Surg. Tech. A **13**(5), 295–299 (2003)
48. Lombardi, C.P., et al.: Video-assisted thyroidectomy under local anesthesia. Am. J. Surg. **187**(4), 515–518 (2004)
49. Ruggieri, M., et al.: The minimally invasive open video-assisted approach in surgical thyroid diseases. BMC Surg. **5**, 9 (2005)
50. Ferzli, G.S., et al.: Minimally invasive, nonendoscopic thyroid surgery. J. Am. Coll. Surg. **192**(5), 665–668 (2001)
51. Brunaud, L., et al.: Open minimally invasive parathyroid and thyroid surgery. Ann. Chir. **131**(1), 62–67 (2006)
52. Cavicchi, O., et al.: Minimally invasive nonendoscopic thyroidectomy. Otolaryngol. Head Neck Surg. **135**(5), 744–747 (2006)
53. Dieter, R.A.: Minimally invasive nonendoscopic thyroid surgery. J. Am. Coll. Surg. **193**(5), 585 (2001)
54. Ng, W.T.: Minimally invasive surgery of the thyroid and parathyroid glands (Br J Surg 2006; 93: 1-2). Br. J. Surg. **93**(5), 641 (2006)
55. Ross, D.E.: Thyroidectomy using local anesthesia. Am. J. Surg. **80**(2), 211–215 (1950)
56. Inabnet, W.B., et al.: Safety of same day discharge in patients undergoing sutureless thyroidectomy: a comparison of local and general anesthesia. Thyroid **18**(1), 57–61 (2008)
57. Gagner, M., Inabnet 3rd, W.B.: Endoscopic thyroidectomy for solitary thyroid nodules. Thyroid **11**(2), 161–163 (2001)
58. Brunt, L.M., et al.: Experimental development of an endoscopic approach to neck exploration and parathyroidectomy. Surgery **122**(5), 893–901 (1997)
59. Gagner, M.: Endoscopic subtotal parathyroidectomy in patients with primary hyperparathyroidism. Br. J. Surg. **83**(6), 875 (1996)

60. Miccoli, P., et al.: Minimally invasive, video-assisted parathyroid surgery for primary hyperparathyroidism. J Endocrinol Invest **20**(7), 429–430 (1997)
61. Norman, J., Chheda, H.: Minimally invasive parathyroidectomy facilitated by intraoperative nuclear mapping. Surgery **122**(6), 998–1003 (1997). discussion 1003-4
62. Gagner, M., Inabnet 3rd, B.W., Biertho, L.: Endoscopic thyroidectomy for solitary nodules. Ann. Chir. **128**(10), 696–701 (2003)
63. Inabnet, W.B., Gagner, M.: Endoscopic thyroidectomy. J. Otolaryngol. **30**(1), 41–42 (2001)
64. Inabnet 3rd, W.B., Jacob, B.P., Gagner, M.: Minimally invasive endoscopic thyroidectomy by a cervical approach. Surg. Endosc. **17**(11), 1808–1811 (2003)
65. Ikeda, Y., et al.: Clinical benefits in endoscopic thyroidectomy by the axillary approach. J. Am. Coll. Surg. **196**(2), 189–195 (2003)
66. Duncan, T.D., et al.: Endoscopic transaxillary approach to the thyroid gland: our early experience. Surg. Endosc. **21**(12), 2166–2171 (2007)
67. Shimizu, K., et al.: Video-assisted neck surgery: endoscopic resection of thyroid tumors with a very minimal neck wound. J. Am. Coll. Surg. **188**(6), 697–703 (1999)
68. Shimazu, K., et al.: Endoscopic thyroid surgery through the axillo-bilateral-breast approach. Surg. Laparosc. Endosc. Percutan. Tech. **13**(3), 196–201 (2003)
69. Chung, Y.S., et al.: Endoscopic thyroidectomy for thyroid malignancies: comparison with conventional open thyroidectomy. World J. Surg. **31**(12), 2302–2306 (2007)
70. Ikeda, Y., et al.: Total endoscopic thyroidectomy: axillary or anterior chest approach. Biomed. Pharmacother. **56**(Suppl 1), 72s–78s (2002)
71. Ikeda, Y., et al.: Endoscopic total parathyroidectomy by the anterior chest approach for renal hyperparathyroidism. Surg. Endosc. **16**(2), 320–322 (2002)
72. Henry, J.F.: Minimally invasive surgery of the thyroid and parathyroid glands. Br. J. Surg. **93**(1), 1–2 (2006)
73. Ikeda, Y., et al.: Endoscopic thyroidectomy by the axillary approach. Surg. Endosc. **15**(11), 1362–1364 (2001)
74. Ohgami, M., et al.: Scarless endoscopic thyroidectomy: breast approach for better cosmesis. Surg. Laparosc. Endosc. Percutan. Tech. **10**(1), 1–4 (2000)
75. Shimizu, K.: Minimally invasive thyroid surgery. Best Pract. Res. Clin. Endocrinol. Metab. **15**(2), 123–137 (2001)
76. Shimizu, K., et al.: Video-assisted minimally invasive endoscopic thyroid surgery using a gasless neck skin lifting method–153 cases of benign thyroid tumors and applicability for large tumors. Biomed. Pharmacother. **56**(Suppl 1), 88s–91s (2002)
77. Yamashita, H., et al.: Video-assisted thyroid lobectomy through a small wound in the submandibular area. Am. J. Surg. **183**(3), 286–289 (2002)
78. Miccoli, P.: Minimally invasive surgery for thyroid and parathyroid diseases. Surg. Endosc. **16**(1), 3–6 (2002)
79. Miccoli, P., et al.: Minimally invasive video-assisted thyroidectomy: five years of experience. J. Am. Coll. Surg. **199**(2), 243–248 (2004)
80. Kitagawa, W., et al.: Endoscopic neck surgery with lymph node dissection for papillary carcinoma of the thyroid using a totally gasless anterior neck skin lifting method. J. Am. Coll. Surg. **196**(6), 990–994 (2003)
81. Miccoli, P., et al.: Video assisted prophylactic thyroidectomy and central compartment nodes clearance in two RET gene mutation adult carriers. J. Endocrinol. Invest. **27**(6), 557–561 (2004)

Cancer of the Parathyroid

Paolo Miccoli, Gabriele Materazzi, and Piero Berti

26.1 Introduction

Parathyroid carcinoma was described for the first time by de Quervain in 1904 as a nonfunctioning tumor. In 1933, Sainton and Mille described the first functioning carcinoma of the parathyroid gland [1].

With an estimated incidence of 0.015 per 100,000 people and an estimated prevalence of 0.005% in the USA, parathyroid carcinoma is one of the rarest of all human cancers [1].

The incidence of hyperparathyroidism (HPT) has increased since 1974. After the introduction of multichannel auto-analyzers, HPT got diagnosed more frequently in asymptomatic individuals [2], but in comparison to the benign causes of HPT, the incidence of parathyroid carcinoma is essentially unchanged. However, there has been a small increase in the proportion of patients presenting with mildly symptomatic parathyroid carcinoma following the detection of hypercalcemia on biochemical screening [2, 3].

In Europe, the USA, and Japan, parathyroid carcinoma has been estimated to cause HPT in 0.017–5.2% of the cases. Various series show that the incidence of parathyroid carcinoma among patients with primary hyperparathyroidism (PHP) is probably around 1%. However, the nationwide survey of parathyroid disease in Japan has documented an incidence of nearly 5% [4]. The cause for this is unclear and may represent either an *absolute* increase – due to genetic or environmental factors – or a *relative* increase – due to large numbers of patients with mildly symptomatic HPTN. In a recent Italian study, 5.2% of patients operated for HPT were found to have parathyroid carcinoma [5].

26.2 Etiology of Parathyroid Cancer and Risk Factors

The etiology of parathyroid carcinoma is unknown. Previous cervical neck radiation is an important risk factor for thyroid carcinoma; however, only few cases of parathyroid carcinoma in patients with a history of previous cervical radiation have been reported [6–9]. This malignancy has been reported in 9–30% of patients with benign HPT. Chronic renal failure leading to secondary HPT can be considered a risk factor for parathyroid carcinoma as well [6, 7].

Parathyroid carcinoma has been reported in families with multiple endocrine neoplasia 1 (MEN 1) and with autosomal dominant familial isolated HPT [6]. Hereditary hyperparathyroidism-jaw tumor syndrome (HPT-JT) is associated with an increased risk of developing the disease. Germ-line inactivating HRPT2 mutations have been found in HPT-JT and there is evidence that they may be of pathogenic importance in sporadic parathyroid carcinoma [10–12]. In addition, 3% of cases of parathyroid carcinoma have been reported in patients aged less than 20 years, indicating that genetic factors may play an important role in this cancer [1, 6, 7].

P. Miccoli (✉), G. Materazzi, and P. Berti
Department of Surgery, University of Pisa, Via Roma 67, 56100 Pisa, Italy
e-mail: pmiccoli@dc.med.unipi.it

26.3 Molecular Pathogenesis

26.3.1 Cyclin D1/PRAD1

Cyclin D1 or PRAD1 (parathyroid adenoma1) is an oncogene located on chromosome 11, on the band 11q13. A chromosomal rearrangement of the Cyclin D1 gene, involving the regulatory region of the parathyroid hormone (PTH) gene, has been reported in 5% of parathyroid adenomas. In addition, the Cyclin D1 oncoprotein is overexpressed in 18–40% of parathyroid adenoma [1, 7, 13].

Overexpression of Cyclin D1 protein is strikingly frequent in parathyroid carcinomas. Many authors showed allelic deletions of the 13q12–14 region involving both the RB gene and the BRCA2 gene. These data strongly support the presence of a tumor suppressor gene on the long arm of chromosome 13, which is critical to parathyroid carcinogenesis [14, 15].

Tumor-specific gains or losses of chromosomal material suggest that oncogenes at location 1q, 5q, 9q, 16p, 19p, and Xq and tumor suppressor genes at locations 1p, 3q, 4q, 13q, and 21q may be involved in the pathogenesis of parathyroid carcinoma [13, 15, 16]. Interestingly, a number of genes commonly lost in adenomas were rarely lost in carcinomas. This supports the hypothesis that parathyroid carcinomas tend to arise *de novo* rather than from pre-existing adenomas [7].

26.4 Clinical Features and Laboratory Findings

Parathyroid carcinomas are typically slow-growing tumors. They have a tendency to recur locally and metastasis occurs late. Ninety-five percent of parathyroid carcinomas are functioning tumors and they secrete parathyroid hormone (PTH) [7]. Almost all the patients are symptomatic at presentation and features of parathyroid carcinoma are primarily due to the effects of excessive secretion of PTH by the functioning tumor, rather than due to infiltration of vital organs by the tumor mass. Male to female ratio is 1:1. Mean age of the patients is 45 years. Parathyroid carcinoma usually presents with a palpable mass in the neck and features of severe hypercalcemia, which is usually severe. Serum calcium levels >14 mg/dL are seen in

Table 26.1 Clinical findings suspicious for parathyroid carcinoma [26]

Hypercalcemia is >14 mg/dL
Serum PTH levels are greater than twice the normal value
A cervical mass is palpable in a hypercalcemic patient
Hypercalcemia associated with unilateral vocal cord paralysis
Concomitant renal and skeletal diseases are observed in a patient with a markedly elevated serum PTH

about two thirds of the patients as compared to less than 10% of the patients with benign HPT. Hoarseness with recurrent laryngeal nerve palsy is rare, but when present, very suggestive of parathyroid carcinoma [1]. The prevalence of bone disease is much greater in patients with parathyroid carcinoma than it is in patients with parathyroid adenoma with ≤70% of patients showing symptoms related to calcium absorption with osteoporosis and bone pain [17, 18]. Both renal and bone-related symptoms are present simultaneously at the time of diagnosis in ≤50% of patients with parathyroid cancer [6]. In contrast, simultaneous renal and overt skeletal involvement is distinctly unusual in primary HPT [19].

Anemia is more common when compared to benign disease (80% vs 10%, respectively). Other laboratory features include hypophosphatemia, hypercalciuria, and hyperphosphaturia [6, 7]. Hypomagnesemia, hypokalemia, and hyperuricemia are seen in some cases [6].

Elevated levels of intact PTH (iPTH) are virtually diagnostic and can be very high (3–10 times above the upper limit of normal for the assay employed) in cases of functioning parathyroid carcinoma [7, 17].

Diagnosing parathyroid cancer needs a high suspicion if certain clinical findings are present (Table 26.1).

26.5 Histology

The histological distinction between benign and malignant parathyroid tumors is difficult to make [19]. Although the cell type is not known to be of prognostic significance, histological cell types associated with parathyroid cancer include chief cells, transitional clear cells, and mixed cell types. Macroscopic and microscopic infiltrations often do not correlate, and adhesions to surrounding structures do not necessarily imply malignancy. Features which have been classically associated with carcinomas have also been found in parathyroid adenomas. They include: [20–22]:

- Dense fibrous trabeculae
- Trabecular growth pattern
- Mitoses
- Capsular invasion

Capsular and vascular invasion appears to correlate best with tumor recurrence [23].

The type well-differentiated carcinoma was described in approximately 80% of a study population of 286 patients when looking at pathological features [24].

An aneuploid DNA pattern is more common, and mean nuclear DNA content is greater in carcinomas than in adenomas. Aneuploidy appears to be associated with a poorer prognosis when present in a carcinoma [25, 27]. As a downside, aneuploidy occurs too frequently in parathyroid adenomas to be of significance in differentiating a benign from a malignant parathyroid lesion [27–29].

In general, the clinical course and the gross pathology observed at the time of surgery are as important as the histological findings in defining a lesion as a parathyroid carcinoma.

26.6 Diagnostic Modalities

26.6.1 High Resolution Ultrasound and Color Doppler

High-resolution and color Doppler neck ultrasound is considered an excellent diagnostic tool in detecting the tumor, showing dimensions of the mass and its relationships with the surrounding structures. However, ultrasound accuracy is highly operator dependent and it cannot completely assess the retro-esophageal, retro-tracheal, and mediastinal areas. Computed tomography (CT), radionuclide scintigraphy (Thallium/Technetium scintigraphy or Sestamibi scan), and MRI are other imaging modalities frequently used.

CT scan appears to be the best investigation for detecting the primary tumor, its local extent, and metastases. Bear in mind that none of the imaging modalities has a sensitivity of more than 50% for small tumors [30–34].

26.6.2 Flow Cytometry

Use of flow cytometric analysis to determine aneuploidy, S-phase fraction, and proliferation index values to distinguish parathyroid carcinoma from adenoma or hyperplasia has yielded conflicting results. Production of human chorionic gonadotropin (hCG) subunits alpha and beta has been observed in parathyroid carcinoma and not in benign tumors [19, 35].

26.6.3 Venography

Venography with venous sampling for iPTH from thyroid, vertebral, thymic, and internal mammary veins remains one of the most sensitive techniques. A unilateral gradient is in favor of a single adenoma or carcinoma, whereas a bilateral gradient usually indicates diffuse hyperplasia [35]. It is a time-consuming but relatively safe procedure.

26.6.4 Arterial Angiography

Selective or super-selective angiography requires experienced personnel. Instances of severe neurological complications (e.g. quadriplegia, and even death) can occur due to inadvertent injection of contrast material into spinal branches of the thyro-cervical or costo-cervical trunk. Safer but less-sensitive techniques include nonselective intra-arterial or intravenous digital subtraction angiography [35].

In summary, the diagnosis of PHP is essentially clinical and biochemical. Localization of the tumor is achieved by ultrasound, targeting a mass that is usually firm and palpable. Biopsy is not necessary before surgery and is in fact contraindicated for either benign or malignant parathyroid tumors [36].

26.7 TNM Staging

Shaha and Shah have proposed a staging system, because interestingly the American Joint Committee on Cancer/International Union Against Cancer (AJCC/UICC) has not yet developed a TNM staging system for parathyroid carcinoma [37] (Table 26.2).

Table 26.2 Proposed TNM classification and stage grouping for parathyroid cancer

T	
T1	Primary tumor < 3 cm
T2	Primary tumor > 3 cm
T3	Primary tumor of any size with invasion of the surrounding soft tissues
T4	Massive central compartment disease invading the trachea and esophagus or recurrent parathyroid carcinoma
N	
N0	No regional lymph node metastases
N1	Regional lymph node metastases
M	
M0	No evidence of distant metastases
M1	Evidence of distant metastases
STAGES	
Stage I	T1 N0 M0
Stage II	T2 N0 M0
Stage III a	T3 N0 M0
Stage III b	T4 N0 M0
Stage III c	Any T, N1, M0
Stage IV	Any T, any N, M1

26.8 Surgical Treatment

26.8.1 Role of Surgery

Surgery is the only potentially curative treatment for parathyroid carcinoma. Early surgery at a point when extensive local invasion and distal metastases are less likely is the most important factor for optimal outcome. For these reasons, both *preoperative suspicion* and *intraoperative recognition* of the malignant nature of the tumor are of paramount importance. Patients whose clinical presentation is suggestive of parathyroid carcinoma warrant thorough exploration of all the four parathyroid glands, as parathyroid carcinoma has been reported to coexist with parathyroid adenoma or hyperplasia [24].

26.8.2 Intraoperative Findings

Parathyroid cancers may be distinguished from adenomas by their firm, stony-hard consistency and lobulation; adenomas tend to be soft, round, or oval in shape, and of a reddish-brown color. In most series, the median maximal diameter of parathyroid carcinoma is between 3.0 and 3.5 cm compared with approximately 1.5 cm for benign adenomas [1]. In approximately 50% of the patients, the malignant tumor is surrounded by a dense, fibrous, grayish-white capsule that infiltrates adjacent tissues. Histopathologically, as with other endocrine neoplasms, the distinction between benign and malignant parathyroid tumors is difficult to make [1, 7, 35].

The extent to which capsular and vascular invasion appears to be unequivocally correlated with tumor recurrences and metastases makes a strong case for these findings to be considered the sole pathognomonic markers of malignancy [35].

26.8.3 Operative Strategy in Parathyroid Cancer

26.8.3.1 Minimally Invasive Approaches

Endoscopic, video-assisted, radioguided, and every recently introduced minimally invasive parathyroidectomy techniques are absolutely contraindicated. Traditional cervicotomy is strongly recommended when approaching a parathyroid mass suspicious for carcinoma.

26.8.3.2 Extent of Resection

After opening the midline, when the gross pathological findings suggest malignancy, e*n bloc* resection of the tumor is mandatory. The extent of the resection includes the ipsilateral thyroid lobe and isthmus, along with all areas of local adherence. The trachea should be skeletonized and the tumor removed without violating the capsule.

26.8.3.3 Involvement of the Recurrent Nerve

If the recurrent laryngeal nerve is involved, it should be sacrificed, as failure to do so may lead to local recurrence.

26.8.3.4 Role of Intraoperative Biopsy and Frozen Section

Simple biopsy with or without frozen section should not be attempted due to the inability to distinguish between benign and malignant lesions as well the fear of seeding malignant cells to surrounding tissues [17]. Often, the surgeon might have to rely on the gross appearance of the lesion to determine its nature.

26.8.4 Outcome After en-bloc Resection

Ninety percent of all patients undergoing en bloc resection are long-term survivors and the local failure rate is only 10%. On the contrary, incomplete resection leads to a local recurrence rate of 50% and disease-related mortality of 46% [6, 17, 35].

26.8.5 Surgery and the Incidentally Found Parathyroid Cancer

A difficult situation may arise when the diagnosis of the malignancy is done in the early postoperative period on the basis of pathology. It is particularly complex given the notorious uncertainty surrounding the histology of parathyroid carcinoma. If the gross findings were suggestive of a parathyroid cancer and the subsequent pathology appears to be aggressive or the patient remains hypercalcemic, re-exploration of the neck is indicated. If none of these features is present, but the diagnosis is made on the basis of the microscopic characteristics; immediate reoperation may not always be necessary. Such patients must be observed carefully with frequent measurements of PTH and serum calcium levels [6, 17]. There is no role for prophylactic neck dissection [34].

26.8.6 Recurrent and Metastatic Parathyroid Cancer

Parathyroid carcinoma grows slowly and metastasizes late. Early recurrence is an unfavorable prognostic factor. Most recurrences usually occur within 2–3 years of initial surgery. Local recurrences (30%) as well as metastases to cervical lymph nodes (30–40%) are fairly common. Distal metastases commonly involve the lungs (20–40%) [6, 35]. Other sites like mediastinum, bone, pleura, pericardium, and pancreas may also be affected.

The disease is usually indolent and most patients die of metabolic complications rather than the disease itself. Even a very small metastasis may produce significant PTH to cause severe hypercalcemia. Significant palliation may be achieved from the resection of the recurrent or residual disease in patients with recurrent hypercalcemia. Localization studies should be performed before reoperation. Thallium 201–technetium 99 m scanning is useful in locating tumors in the neck area and the mediastinum. Intraoperative localization of the parathyroid may be achieved with the help of technetium 99 m-sestamibi scan used concurrently with a handheld, ã-detecting probe [31, 32, 35]. CT scan and MRI may be useful adjuncts to ultrasonography in evaluating the disease process in the neck and are better modalities to detect distant metastases in the chest or abdominal cavity. If noninvasive testing does not localize the tumor, selective venous sampling or arteriography may help.

26.8.7 Postoperative Surveillance

Close postoperative monitoring is essential to detect hungry bone syndrome. It should be regarded as sign for successful surgery and is caused by deposition of calcium and phosphate into the bones. Hypocalcemia may be severe, protracted, and needs to be anticipated. It might require large dosages of intravenous calcium and calcitriol [34].

26.9 Systemic Therapy

26.9.1 Radiotherapy

Parathyroid carcinoma is traditionally considered to be resistant to radiotherapy; only isolated reports of long-term control exist [35, 38]. The recommended dose of radiation is 40–50 Gy in patients with high risk for recurrence. The radiation field should:

- Include the tumor bed
- Extend superiorly to the hyoid bone
- Extend inferiorly to the clavicle
- Include paratracheal and perithyroidal areas

The radiation target volume should include all cervical lymph nodes, including the superior mediastinum if lymph node involvement is present. Radiation has also a role in palliating patients with metastatic disease [9, 38, 39].

26.9.2 Chemotherapy

There are no large, randomized clinical trials involving chemotherapy due to a very low incidence of parathyroid carcinomas. The experience of use of various chemotherapeutic agents is limited to anecdotal cases [35]. Several regimens have been tried and found to be ineffective [1, 6, 17, 38].

- Nitrogen mustards
- Vincristine + Cyclophosphamide + Actinomycin D
- Adriamycin + Cyclophosphamide + 5-Flurouracil
- Adriamycin alone

Partial and temporary remissions have been reported with estrogen and testosterone [1]. A single patient with pulmonary metastases responded to treatment with Dacarbazine, 5-Flurouracil, and Cyclophosphamide with a decrease in PTH and normalization of serum Ca^{++} for a duration of 13 months [1]. Another patient responded to Dacarbazine alone with a brief but significant decline in serum calcium level. The MACC (**M**ethotrexate, **A**driamycin, **C**yclophosphamide, **C**CNU) regimen produced a dramatic regression of a large mediastinal mass and malignant pleural effusion, lasting 18 months. Another case of a nonfunctioning carcinoma was treated with a modified MACC (Mitoxantrone used instead of Adriamycin) protocol and had a partial response for 10.1 months. Over the last few decades, many new drugs with novel mechanisms of action and better toxicity profile have become available. However, there have been no studies evaluating the efficacy of these agents in parathyroid carcinoma. Thus, the role of chemotherapy in this disease entity is not well defined and needs further investigations [35].

26.10 Treatment of Hypercalcemia

At the clinical stage, when parathyroid carcinoma becomes widely disseminated and surgical resection is no longer effective, the prognosis is generally poor [6]. The therapeutic goal at this point is to control hypercalcemia and its symptoms. The treatment is the same as for hypercalcemia due to any other cause. Management will include infusion of saline solution, loop diuretics, and various hypocalcemic agents like bisphosphonates, plicamycin, calcitonin, and gallium nitrate. Recently, a novel calcimimetic agent (NPS R568) has been developed as an allosteric modulator of the calcium receptor [40, 41]. Other agents like WR-2721 and octreotide have been used in some cases [6, 7]. Bradwell et al. proposed a new approach to resistant hypercalcemia by immunization with human and bovine PTH peptides. The T-cells recognize foreign antigens (bovine PTH) and help B cells to produce antibodies against self-PTH, which are detectable after 4 weeks. A rapid improvement in the symptoms without significant adverse effects is described by the authors [42].

26.11 Nonfunctioning Carcinomas

Only 1.9–5% of parathyroid carcinomas are nonfunctioning. The factors responsible for the lack of HPT may be

- Lack of hormone synthesis
- Impaired or reduced secretion of the hormone
- Synthesis of an abnormal hormone

Nonfunctioning carcinomas are treated the same way we would treat functioning carcinomas and carry a similar prognosis with a median survival of 2 years (range: 9 months to 5 years) [6, 7].

26.12 Outcome and Prognosis

Prognosis of patients with parathyroid carcinoma is variable. Early recognition and R0 resection at the time of initial surgery carries the best prognosis. The average time between initial surgery and first recurrence is approximately 3 years with a recurrence free survival of 30%. Once the tumor recurs, complete cure is unlikely. However, palliative surgery and/or chemotherapy may prolong survival and increase the quality of life. In such cases, the 5-year overall survival is about 50% and 10-year survival varies from 13% to 49% [6, 7, 35].

Quick Reference Guide

1. *En bloc – R0* resection is the key therapeutic step and mandatory
2. Addressing parathyroid cancer needs a high clinical suspicion
3. The clinical course and the gross pathology observed at the time of surgery are as important as the histological findings in defining a lesion as a parathyroid carcinoma
4. *Diagnosis of PHP*: done clinically in combination with biochemical studies
5. **The two most important key points in defining the lesion as cancer**:
   - Preoperative suspicion
   - Intraoperative recognition of the malignant nature of the mass
6. **Preoperative biopsy**
   Not necessary, even contraindicated for either benign or malignant parathyroid tumors
7. Parathyroid carcinoma is traditionally considered to be resistant to radiotherapy and chemotherapy is of limited use
8. Minimally invasive parathyroidectomy techniques are absolutely contraindicated, if parathyroid cancer is suspected *preoperatively*
9. **Extent of resection**
   Ipsilateral thyroid lobe and isthmus, and all areas of local adherence. Skeletonize the trachea and do not violate the tumor capsule!
10. **Incidental parathyroid cancers**:
    Intraoperative findings were suggestive of cancer and the subsequent pathology appears to be aggressive or the patient remains hypercalcemic → re-explore the neck
    No pathologic features were present at the time of surgery and the diagnosis is made on the basis of microscopic characteristics → immediate re-operation may not always be necessary

References

1. Koea, J.B., Shaw, H.F.: Parathyroid cancer: biology and management. Surg. Oncol. **8**, 155–165 (1999)
2. Bilezikian, J.P., Silverberg, S.J.: Asymptomatic primary hyperparathyroidism. N Engl J. Med. **350**, 1746–1751 (2004)
3. Wermers, R.A., Khosla, S., Atkinson, E.J., Hodgson, S.F., O'Fallon, W.M., Melton III, J.: The rise and fall of primary hyperparathyroidism: a population based study in Rochester, Minnesota, 1965-1992. Ann. Intern. Med. **126**, 433–440 (1997)
4. Cordeiro, A.C., Montenegro, F.L., Kulcsar, M.A., Dellanegra, L.A., Tavares, M.R., Michaluart, P., et al.: Parathyroid carcinoma. Am. J. Surg. **175**, 52–55 (1998)
5. Dionisi, S., Minisola, S., Pepe, J., Geronimo, S.D., Paglia, F., Memeo, L.: Concurrent parathyroid adenomas and carcinoma in the setting of multiple endocrine neoplasia type 1: presentation as hypercalcemic crisis. Mayo Clin. Proc. **77**, 866–869 (2002)
6. Fraker, D.L.: Parathyroid tumors. In: DeVita Jr., V.T., Hellman, S., Rosenberg, S.A. (eds.) Cancer: Principles and Practice of Oncology, 6th edn, pp. 1763–1769. Lippincott Williams and Wilkins, Philadelphia (2001)
7. Shane, E., Bilezikian, J.P.: Parathyroid carcinoma: a review of 62 patients. Endocr. Rev. **3**, 218–226 (1982)
8. Christmas, T.J., Chapple, C.R., Noble, J.G., Milroy, E.J., Cowie, A.G.: Hyperparathyroidism after neck irradiation. Br. J. Surg. **75**, 873 (1988)
9. Chow, E., Tsang, R.W., Brierley, J.D., Filice, S.: Parathyroid carcinoma – The Princess Margret hospital experience. Int. J. Radiat. Oncol. Biol. Phys. **41**, 569–572 (1998)
10. Howell, V.M., Haven, C.J., Kahnoski, K., Khoo, S.K., Petillo, D., Chen, J., et al.: HRPT2 mutations are associated with malignancy in sporadic parathyroid tumors. J. Med. Genet. **40**, 657–663 (2003)
11. Weinstein, L.S., Simonds, W.F.: HRPT2, a marker of parathyroid cancer. N. Engl. J. Med. **349**, 1691–1692 (2003)
12. Shattuck, T.M., Valimaki, S., Obara, T., Gaz, R.D., Clark, O.H., Shoback, D., et al.: Somatic and germ-line mutations of the HRPT2 gene in sporadic parathyroid carcinoma. N Engl J. Med. **349**, 1722–1729 (2003)
13. Kytola, S., Farnebo, F., Obara, T., Isola, J., Grimelius, L., Farnebo, L.V., et al.: Patterns of chromosomal imbalances in parathyroid carcinomas. Am. J. Pathol. **157**, 579–586 (2000)

14. Cryns, V.L., Thor, A., Xu, H.J., Hu, S.X., Wierman, M.E., Vickery, A.L., et al.: Loss of the retinoblastoma tumor suppressor gene in parathyroid carcinoma. N. Engl. J. Med. **330**, 757–761 (1994)
15. Dotzenrath, C., Teh, B.T., Farnebo, F., Cupisti, K., Svensson, A., Toell, A., et al.: Allelic loss of the retinoblastoma tumor suppressor gene: a marker for aggressive parathyroid tumors? J. Clin. Endocrinol. Metab. **81**, 3194–3196 (1996)
16. Arnold, A., Kim, H.G., Gaz, R.D., Eddy, R.L., Fukushima, Y., Byers, M.G., et al.: Molecular cloning and chromosomal mapping of DNA rearranged with the parathyroid hormone gene in a parathyroid adenoma. J. Clin. Invest. **83**, 2034–2040 (1989)
17. Lafferty, F.W.: Primary hyperparathyroidism. Changing clinical spectrum, prevalence of hypertension, and discriminant analysis of laboratory tests. Arch. Intern. Med. **141**(13), 1761–1766 (1981)
18. Nikkilä, M.T., Saaristo, J.J., Koivula, T.A.: Clinical and biochemical features in primary hyperparathyroidism. Surgery **105**, 148–153 (1989)
19. Shane, E.: Clinical review 122: parathyroid carcinoma. J. Clin. Endocrinol. Metab. **86**(2), 485–493 (2001)
20. Schantz, A., Castleman, B.: Parathyroid carcinoma. A study of 70 cases. Cancer **31**(3), 600–605 (1973)
21. Levin, K.E., Galante, M., Clark, O.H.: Parathyroid carcinoma versus parathyroid adenoma in patients with profound hypercalcemia. Surgery **101**(6), 649–660 (1987)
22. Bondeson, L., Sandelin, K., Grimelius, L.: Histopathological variables and DNA cytometry in parathyroid carcinoma. Am. J. Surg. Pathol. **17**(8), 820–829 (1993)
23. Iacobone, M., Lumachi, F., Favia, G.: Up-to-date on parathyroid carcinoma: analysis of an experience of 19 cases. J. Surg. Oncol. **88**(4), 223–228 (2004)
24. Hundahl, S.A., Fleming, I.D., Fremgen, A.M., et al.: Two hundred eighty-six cases of parathyroid carcinoma treated in the U.S. between 1985–1995: a National Cancer Data Base Report. The American College of Surgeons Commission on Cancer and the American Cancer Society. Cancer **86**(3), 538–544 (1999)
25. Levin, K.E., Chew, K.L., Ljung, B.M., et al.: Deoxyribonucleic acid cytometry helps identify parathyroid carcinomas. J. Clin. Endocrinol. Metab. **67**(4), 779–784 (1988)
26. Obara, T., Fujimoto, Y.: Diagnosis and treatment of patients with parathyroid carcinoma: an update and review. World J. Surg. **15**(6), 738–744 (1991 Nov–Dec)
27. Sandelin, K., Auer, G., Bondeson, L., et al.: Prognostic factors in parathyroid cancer: a review of 95 cases. World J. Surg. **16**(4), 724–731 (1992 Jul–Aug)
28. Mallette, L.E.: DNA quantitation in the study of parathyroid lesions. A review. Am. J. Clin. Pathol. **98**(3), 305–311 (1992)
29. Obara, T., Okamoto, T., Kanbe, M., et al.: Functioning parathyroid carcinoma: clinicopathologic features and rational treatment. Semin. Surg. Oncol. **13**(2), 134–141 (1997 Mar–Apr)
30. Lumachi, F., Zucchetta, P., Varotto, S., Polistina, F., Favia, G., D'Amico, D.: Noninvasive localization procedures in ectopic hyperfunctioning parathyroid tumors. Endocr. Relat. Cancer **6**, 123–125 (1999)
31. Mariani, G., Gulec, S.A., Rubello, D., Boni, G., Puccini, M., Pelizzo, M.R., et al.: Preoperative localization and radioguided parathroid surgery. J. Nucl. Med. **44**, 1443–1458 (2003)
32. Johnston, L.B., Carroll, M.J., Britton, K.E., Lowe, D.G., Shand, W., Besser, G.M., et al.: The accuracy of parathyroid gland localization in primary hyperparathyroidism using sestamibi radionuclide imaging. J. Clin. Endocrinol. Metab. **81**, 346–352 (1996)
33. Lumachi, F., Tregnaghi, A., Zucchetta, P., Marzola, M.C., Cecchin, D., Marchesi, P., et al.: Technetium-99 m sestamibi scintigraphy and helical CT together in patients with primary hyperparathyroidism: a prospective clinical study. Br. J. Radiol. **77**, 100–103 (2004)
34. Even-Sapir, E., Keidar, Z., Sachs, J., Engel, A., Bettman, L., Gaitini, D., et al.: The new technology of combined transmission and emission tomography in evaluation of endocrine neoplasms. J. Nucl. Med. **42**, 998–1004 (2001)
35. Kvols, L.K.: Neoplasms of the diffuse endocrine system. In: Kufe, D.W., Pollock, R.E., Weichselbaum, R.R., Bast, R.C., Holland, J.F., Frei, E. (eds.) Cancer Medicine, 6th edn, pp. 1295–1299. BC Decker, Hamilton (2003)
36. Spinelli, C., Bonadio, A.G., Berti, P., Materazzi, G., Miccoli, P.: Cutaneous spreading of parathyroid carcinoma after fine needle aspiration cytology. J. Endocrinol. Invest. **23**(4), 255–257 (2000 Apr)
37. Shaha, A.R., Shah, J.P.: Parathyroid carcinoma. A diagnostic and therapeutic challenge. Cancer **86**, 378–380 (1999)
38. Clayman, G.L., Gonzalez, H.E., El-Naggar, A., Vassilopoulou-Sellin, R.: Parathyroid carcinoma: evaluation and interdisciplinary management. Cancer **100**, 900–905 (2004)
39. Munson, N.D., Foote, R.L., Northcutt, R.C., Tiegs, R.D., Fitzpatrick, L.A., Grant, C.S., et al.: Parathyroid carcinoma: is there a role for adjuvant radiation therapy? Cancer **98**, 2378–2384 (2003)
40. Collins, M.T., Skarulis, M.C., Bilezikian, J.P., Silverberg, S.J., Spiegel, A.M., Mark, S.J.: Treatment of hypercalcemia secondary to parathyroid carcinoma with a novel Calcimimetic agent. J. Clin. Endocrinol. Metab. **33**, 1083–1088 (1998)
41. Cohen, A., Silverberg, S.: Calcimimetics: therapeutic potential in hyperparathyroidism. Curr. Opin. Pharmacol. **2**, 734–739 (2003)
42. Bradwell, A.R., Harvey, T.C.: Control of hypercalcemia of parathyroid carcinoma by immunization. Lancet **353**, 370–373 (1999)

27 Cancer of the Pancreas: Distal Resections and Staging of Pancreatic Cancer

Vivian E. Strong, Joshua Carson, and Peter J. Allen

27.1 Diagnostic Laparoscopy in Pancreatic Cancer

27.1.1 Laparoscopic Staging

27.1.1.1 A Historical Perspective

Though often perceived as a recent innovation, laparoscopic staging of pancreatic cancer dates back nearly a century. In fact, cancer staging provided the impetus for the first (although somewhat primitive) application of laparoscopy in 1911 when Bernheim described a patient with pancreatic cancer who underwent "cystoscopy of the abdominal cavity" [1]. Shortly after laparoscopy in its modern form was established, with fiber-optics and controlled pneumoperitoneum, laparoscopic staging became the standard of care for pancreatic cancer in Europe during the 1980s. The subsequent emergence of high-resolution radiographic technologies restored the use of the noninvasive workup. However, with further experience demonstrating the limitations of even the most modern scanning techniques in detecting pancreatic metastases, a new push for laparoscopic staging has emerged.

27.1.1.2 Context-dependent Approach to Laparoscopic Staging

As with all procedures, the role and efficacy of laparoscopic staging depends on the pretest scenario. In all cases, a patient with the presumed diagnosis of pancreatic cancer should have an abdominal CT scan with intravenous contrast, ideally with a pancreas-based protocol. The evolution of CT has facilitated this imaging modality as a valuable tool for staging patients. Conventional CT is now replaced by dynamic thin section CT, spiral CT, multidetector CT, and three-dimensional reconstructions, all of which have improved the ability to detect distant metastases and vascular invasion. Velanovich et al. and later Prokesch et al. demonstrated that whereas conventional CT had a 45% sensitivity and 92% specificity for correcting differentiating local and distant metastases for patients with pancreas cancer, the use of multidetector CT alone increased that sensitivity to 86% [2, 3].

Thus, patients now can be better stratified into three basic groups based on imaging

1. Clear radiographic evidence of metastases
2. Evidence of advanced local, but not metastatic, disease
3. Workup detects contained local disease only

Except for the case in which radiographically identified metastasis cannot be accessed percutaneously for confirmatory biopsy, laparoscopic staging has no role in group 1 because of stage IV disease. In groups 2 and 3, however, the question becomes more complex.

V.E. Strong (✉)
Division of Gastric and Mixed tumors, Memorial Sloan-Kettering Cancer Center, 1275 York Avenue, New York, NY 10065, USA
e-mail: strongv@mskcc.org

J. Carson
Memorial Sloan-Kettering Cancer Center, 1275 York Avenue, New York, NY 10065, USA

P.J. Allen
Division of Hepato-Pancreato-Biliary Surgery, Memorial Sloan-Kettering Cancer Center, 1275 York Avenue, New York, NY 10065, USA
e-mail: allenp@mskccc.org

27.1.1.3 Laparoscopic Staging of Known Unresectable Disease

Laparoscopic staging of pancreatic adenocarcinoma has traditionally been performed with the objective of confirming feasibility of resection prior to definitive surgical treatment. At some centers, however, the practice has been extended to cases of known locally advanced disease, for the purpose of further stratifying nonsurgical experimental treatment protocols. Proponents of laparoscopy in the setting of disease known to be unresectable argue that the increased sensitivity of laparoscopic staging in detecting metastatic disease both increases the precision of experimental clinical trials for unresectable disease and spares patients with occult metastatic disease from the morbidity and burden of futile treatments [4]. In addition, for those patients experiencing severe pain, during the time of laparoscopy to define locally advanced versus metastatic disease, it is possible to simultaneously perform a laparoscopic celiac plexus block for pain relief [5].

27.1.1.4 Laparoscopic Staging of Disease Deemed Resectable by Preoperative Imaging

The most common use of laparoscopic pancreatic staging, and the most frequently debated, is in the setting of disease staged as resectable on preoperative workup. Here, the objective is to further stratify presumed operative candidates in order to avoid unnecessary laparotomy. Operative staging is performed in patients for whom curative resection is attempted, to allow thorough assessment of the abdomen for previously undetected metastases. While the advent of high-resolution helical CT imaging has greatly improved the sensitivity of radiographic staging for detection of metastatic and locally advanced disease, many patients are deemed resectable by preoperative radiographic imaging, only to be reclassified as unresectable on open inspection. This may be somewhat dependent on the quality of preoperative CT imaging and the radiological review. In the study by Shoup et al. from 2004, a series of 100 patients with radiographically staged locally advanced adenocarcinoma of the pancreas underwent staging laparoscopy. Laparoscopy identified metastatic disease in 37% of these patients, increasing the sensitivity and appropriate treatment of these patients with a minimally invasive approach [4]. This also improves the quality of clinical studies, and by improving patient selection, it improves the patient care provided within these studies to improve the overall treatment for these patients. Proceeding with laparotomy only to abort an operative resection subjects the patient to morbidities and risks associated with laparotomy, such as a significant delay in the administration of medical treatments, risk of incisional infection or hernia in addition to the disappointment of not having a definitive resection.

27.1.1.5 Accuracy of Laparoscopic Staging

The utility of staging laparoscopy depends on its relative efficacy compared to standard preoperative diagnostics. Contemporary imaging technology is highly specific for unresectable disease, such that laparoscopy is rarely indicated to confirm inoperability. However, using open exploration as the gold standard, CT staging frequently fails in sensitivity. The rate of false negatives depends on the resolution of imaging equipment, but even using contrast-enhanced high-resolution spiral CT scanning, preoperative imaging at best offers a sensitivity for unresectable disease up to 95% [6–8]. While the sensitivity of the preoperative workup can be improved with adjuvant diagnostic techniques such as endoscopic ultrasound, this still leaves significant false negatives. Studies assessing the impact of laparoscopic staging before laparotomy have found as many as 25–40% of patients with disease deemed resectable by imaging to have occult metastases or local advancement identified on laparoscopy [9–20]. In such cases, laparoscopy ultimately avoided unnecessary laparotomy for many patients falsely determined to be resectable on preoperative imaging. It should be noted that even laparoscopy carries a rate of false negatives, with some patients deemed resectable at laparoscopy who are subsequently not resectable at laparotomy.

27.1.1.6 Efficacy of Laparoscopic Staging

The yield of laparoscopic staging can be increased, by augmenting the pretest probability of detecting unresectable disease on laparoscopy through careful patient selection. For instance, Jimenz et al. report a nearly twofold risk of radiographically occult metastasis in patients with tumors located in the body or tail of the pancreas as compared to those with tumors of the pancreatic head [10]. Interestingly, a similar correlation between location and occult metastasis was not identified in patients undergoing laparoscopy with radiographically detected locally advanced disease [4]. Serum markers have also proven helpful, with a serum concentration of Ca19-9 < 100 U/mL associated with an extremely low risk of occult metastasis [21]. The value of such patient selection should not be underestimated, as cost-benefit analyses of laparoscopic staging without pretest stratification leads to an overall increase in OR time and expense [10].

27.1.1.7 Patient Selection

The selection of patients for preoperative staging depends largely on the practice setting and clinical situation. In a tertiary care setting where patients are often extensively evaluated prior to presentation and are expecting an aggressive treatment plan, one might be inclined to reserve preoperative laparoscopy for situations with a high pretest likelihood such as distal tumors. Alternatively, in a community-oriented setting, when patients are seen early in the course of disease detection and a positive laparoscopy might save a patient laparotomy, more liberal use of this diagnostic procedure may be warranted.

27.1.1.8 Points of Controversy

Beyond the ongoing question of cost-effectiveness, two other criticisms have been raised in discussions of laparoscopic staging – both of which have lost considerable ground in light of recent studies. Many clinicians avoided laparoscopic procedures in the setting of adenocarcinoma following early reports of tumor recurrence at port-sites [22]. Studies now confirm that port-site recurrences are rare, and likely associated with advanced peritoneal disease [23]. Another argument raised against laparoscopic staging was the claim that patients with unresectable disease required open biliary bypass procedures for prophylactic palliation. Again, subsequent studies have demonstrated endoscopic stenting to be an effective and minimally invasive approach to palliating the subset of patients who need this intervention [24].

27.1.1.9 A Sophisticated Approach to Staging Laparoscopy

While most objections to laparoscopic staging have been addressed, there is still no consensus regarding the precise role for this diagnostic approach in the workup of pancreatic adenocarcinoma. Nonetheless, the general principles of diagnostic utility remain. Ultimately, the value of laparoscopic staging in any setting depends on the likelihood that it will alter the course of treatment. Thus, before considering laparoscopy, one must clarify two issues:

1. Which treatment options is the patient willing to consider if the test is negative?
2. What is the pretest probability that the test will be positive?

Weighing these two factors against the known cost of laparoscopy should lead to a reasonable assessment of diagnostic laparoscopy's utility in any given scenario.

27.2 Interventional Laparoscopy in Pancreatic Cancer

27.2.1 Laparoscopic Distal Pancreatectomy

With the gradual introduction of laparoscopic technique into ever-expanding applications over the past several decades, pancreatic surgery has assumed a unique status to explore and extend the applications of laparoscopic surgery. Particular aspects of pancreatic resection make it challenging technically, but with the potential benefits of a laparoscopic approach such as improved intra-operative visualization and avoidance of a large incision, decreased postoperative pain, ileus, and shorter hospital stay [25].

Pancreatic resections performed for neoplastic indications fit into two fundamental categories:

1. Pancreaticoduodenectomies – The Whipple procedure
2. Partial pancreatic resections

The laparoscopic pancreaticoduodenectomy carries a distinct set of indications and concerns separate from those involved in partial pancreatic resections, and as such it will be discussed separately in Chap 28. In this chapter, we address factors specific to laparoscopic partial pancreatic resections – specifically, laparoscopic distal pancreatectomy and laparoscopic pancreatic enucleation.

27.2.1.1 Patient Selection

Patient selection begins by addressing the disease process via a thorough understanding of the indication for resection since laparoscopic resection largely mirrors that for open procedures, with certain exceptions. Unless the operating surgeon is prepared to perform a laparoscopic Whipple procedure, proximal duct involvement and adenocarcinoma should be ruled out in patients with proximal lesions. Also, particularly in the setting of a suspected endocrine neoplasm, a thorough attempt to rule out multiple neoplasms should be undertaken prior to surgery. Most critically, Multiple Endocrine Neoplasm Syndrome (MEN) must be ruled out to avoid an invasive resection that leaves behind multiple occult tumors. Given the likelihood of multiple small tumors in patients with MEN, if the disease is detected on workup, a painstaking search for occult nonpancreatic lesions should be undertaken before proceeding with pancreatic resection. If none are found, laparoscopic enucleation of a single identified lesion, with close follow-up, is a reasonable approach. Careful consideration should also be paid to the possibility of adenocarcinoma. Currently, resections of known adenocarcinoma of the pancreas at our institution are performed via an open approach. While we acknowledge the advantage of open palpation to improve evaluation of the extent of disease in the treatment of known adenocarcinoma, evolving technologies in laparoscopic imaging and technology may soon expand even these current limitations. Alternatively, Hand-Assisted Laparoscopic resection provides the benefit of manual palpation with a less-invasive incision until improved technology becomes available.

For other neoplastic pancreatic pathologies, the indications and contraindications for laparoscopic versus open resection are essentially the same as for any other laparoscopic intervention.

The relative indications are essentially

- Patient preference
- Surgeon familiarity and comfort with the procedure

Relative contraindications are

- Lack of adequate anatomic visualization
- Multiple previous abdominal operations
- Suspicion for extensive adhesions
- Significant untreated diaphragmatic hernia
- Advanced pulmonary disease

27.2.1.2 Preoperative Workup

Role of Preoperative Tumor Localization

The current trend in clinical practice is toward less-aggressive attempts at preoperative localization in preparation for open resection of pancreatic neoplasms. Proponents of this approach argue that in cases where the suspicion for an extra-pancreatic lesion is low, the ease and efficacy of a thorough intraoperative exploration obviate the need for costly and often tedious attempts to identify and localize the precise lesion preoperatively.

This approach may not be as useful in the setting of anticipated laparoscopic surgery. Laparoscopic exploration is more likely than open exploration to fail to identify the lesion intended for resection. Furthermore, synchronous lesions are more likely to be missed if localization is limited to the intraoperative exploration. Finally, since tumor location may impact the feasibility of laparoscopic resection, there is reason to confirm exact location before beginning a laparoscopic procedure.

The methodology of the localizing workup depends on several factors including likely pathology, surgeon preference, and institutional imaging technology. For instance, a lesion discovered as an incidental radiographic finding and scheduled for resection to rule out malignancy may not require any further imaging should a systemic workup fail to identify any signs of an endocrine syndrome. On the other hand, any patient undergoing resection for a hyperfunctioning endocrine neoplasm merits a thorough attempt at localization, as a failure to identify and resect all functioning lesions can lead to a complete treatment failure.

Multiple Endocrine Neoplasia (MEN)

Finally, when treating endocrine or neuroendocrine pancreatic lesions, specific attention must be paid to the possibility of an underlying MEN syndrome. All patients with suspected endocrine or neuroendocrine lesions should undergo basic screening, regardless of family history. Cost-effective and sensitive, a serum calcium measurement is just one basic test for the patient with no known family history of endocrine neoplasia. In a patient with a positive family history, and thus a higher pretest probability, genetic testing, when available, is likely in order.

27.2.1.3 Surgical Technique

Patient Positioning and Trocar Placement

After induction of general anesthesia, the patient is placed in the supine position in the split leg position with the operating surgeon positioned between the patient's legs and the assistant surgeon on the patient's right. A Veress needle in the left lateral subcostal space, or an umbilical Hassan trocar, is utilized to gain entry into the peritoneal space and place the first trocar. A complete evaluation of the peritoneal cavity is performed. Any suspicious peritoneal nodules or liver lesions are biopsied before beginning dissection. If the decision is made to proceed with resection, we will place a set of another three trocars: 5 mm subcostal left and right and a 12 mm trocar in the left mid-clavicular line (Fig. 27.1).

Mobilization and Dissection

The resection starts with placement of a Nathanson retractor to allow cephalad retraction of the liver. This allows the view seen in Fig. 27.2. Entry into the lesser sac is accomplished via the gastrocolic ligament (Fig. 27.3), avoiding injury to the gastroepiploic vessels. The posterior stomach is then retracted anteriorly and the short gastric vessels ligated (Fig. 27.4). This exposes the anterior body and tail of the pancreas (Fig. 27.5). To allow optimal exposure of the tail of the pancreas, the splenic flexure may need to be mobilized.

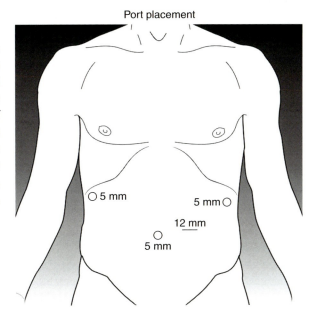

Fig. 27.1 Typical placement of port sites used for laparoscopic distal pancreatic resection

If the lesion is not readily visible, a laparoscopic ultrasound may be performed. If the tumor is close to or involving the splenic vessels, or if there is associated fibrosis or inflammation, the decision may be made, at this time, to remove the spleen as well. The dissection of the pancreas proceeds via mobilization of the inferior border of the pancreas (Fig. 27.6), using a cautery device such as Sonosurg™ or the harmonic scalpel to ligate all small peri-pancreatic branches. This dissection is carried out to the tail of the pancreas, allowing mobilization that provides a complete view of the posterior tail of the pancreas. The splenic vessels are thus identified from both the posterior and anterior views and once dissected free from the pancreas, stapled with an Endo-GIA stapler, vascular load (Fig. 27.7), either individually or with both the artery and vein together. For splenic-preserving resections, the peripancreatic vessels are sequentially ligated along the length of the splenic artery and vein to facilitate complete pancreatic tail mobilization. This frees the distal pancreas, which can then be stapled with a blue or green load universal Endo-GIA with Seamguard™ attachment, if desired (Figs. 27.8 and 27.9). The transected specimen is then placed in an endocatch bag and removed via the left mid-quadrant port site that is slightly enlarged to

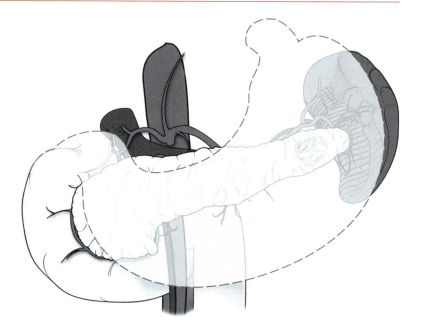

Fig. 27.2 Relationship of surrounding structures to the pancreas prior to dissection

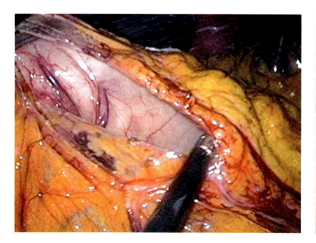

Fig. 27.3 View of the posterior stomach after entry into the lesser sac via the gastrocolic ligament

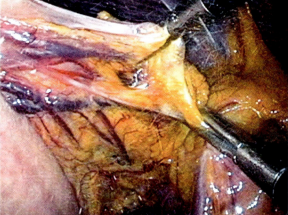

Fig. 27.4 Ligation of the short gastric vessels needed to provide optimal exposure of the lesser sac

facilitate specimen extraction. The final anatomic view is shown in Fig. 27.10. We do not routinely leave a Jackson–Pratt drain.

27.2.2 Specific Resections

27.2.2.1 Central Pancreatectomy

The relative indications for laparoscopic distal pancreatectomy over laparoscopic enucleation (or vice versa) are no different than for the corresponding open procedures. Laparoscopic distal pancreatectomy is reserved for distal lesions. Central pancreatectomies have been reported in the treatment of pancreatic neoplasms [26–28]; the benefit of retaining the salvaged distal segment must be weighed against the theoretical risks of a prolonged procedure and anastomotic failure. Given the good functional reserve of the healthy pancreas, significant evidence of compromised reserve should be established before electing to reattach the distal segment.

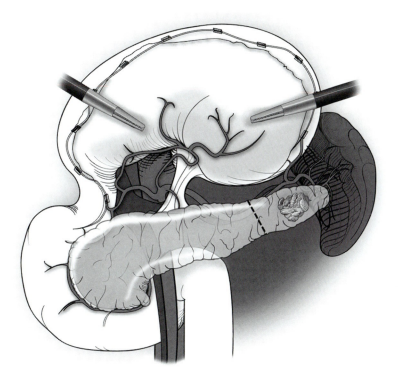

Fig. 27.5 View of the pancreas after entering the lesser sac via the gastrocolic ligament and ligation of short gastric vessels

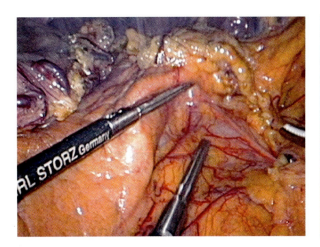

Fig. 27.6 View of the inferior border of the pancreas and associated retroperitoneal attachments

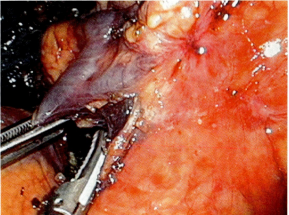

Fig. 27.7 View of the splenic vessels after dissection of the superior border of the pancreas and creation of a window to allow stapling

27.2.2.2 Enucleation of a Pancreatic Lesion

When feasible and appropriate, enucleations are generally preferred to allow tissue sparing and minimalism. Despite the theoretical appeal of the lesser resection of enucleations, reported morbidity rates are actually comparable with those found in distal pancreatectomies [29–31]. Of course, the more proximal the lesion, the greater the advantage offered by enucleation. However, in order to safely treat a lesion with enucleation, one must confirm that the lesion is separate from the pancreatic duct with little to no suspicion of malignant potential (Table 27.1).

Fig. 27.8 Positioning of the universal Endo-GIA stapling device once dissection is complete and the pancreas is prepared for transection

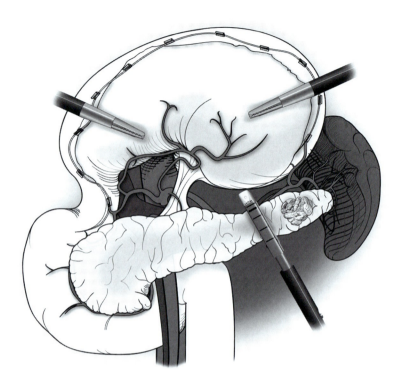

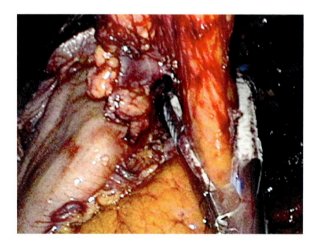

Fig. 27.9 Tail of the pancreas lifted upward after complete mobilization in preparation for transection with a stapling device

27.2.3 Splenic Preservation

The classic distal pancreatectomy, first reported by Mayo in 1913, involves an associated splenectomy [32]. In 1943, Mallet-Guy and Vachon introduced the first splenic preservation technique for distal pancreatectomy [33]. Preserving the splenic artery and vein in the described paper proved an involved technique, which was ultimately not feasible in most cases and cumbersome at best. In 1988, Warshaw demonstrated that splenic preservation could be accomplished far more expeditiously by sacrificing the splenic artery and vein, and relying on the short gastric vessels for splenic perfusion [34, 35]. In the late 1990s, Brennan and Shoup showed that this same principle could be applied to distal pancreatectomies in the setting of "low-grade" malignancies, with improved perioperative outcomes and no compromise in disease-free survival. While splenectomy is advocated by some, it should not be considered an essential component to a good oncologic procedure [36]. It is our practice to attempt splenic preservation for all laparoscopic distal pancreatectomies, except when invasion is detected. The literature suggests that failure of splenic preservation is one of the most common reasons causing conversion from laparoscopic to open pancreatectomy.

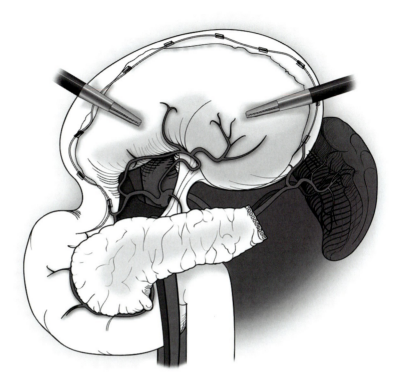

Fig. 27.10 View of the stapled pancreas (spleen-preserving technique) after extraction of the specimen

27.2.4 Laparoscopic Resection of Specific Pathologies

27.2.4.1 Neuroendocrine Lesions

The most common neoplastic indications for laparoscopic pancreatic resections are neuroendocrine neoplasms. These lesions are distinctly suited to laparoscopic resection in the sense that they typically do not require extended lymphatic dissections and frequently present with symptoms before growing to cumbersome dimensions.

The literature contains numerous reports of laparoscopic enucleations of insulinomas, nearly all with excellent results. These lesions are almost uniformly benign, recurrence (in the absence of MEN syndrome) is rare, and symptomatic improvement is the rule. If sufficient space is found between the lesion and the pancreatic duct, enucleation is preferred over distal pancreatectomy as it offers a far lower risk of postoperative fistula formation. However, should enucleation prove infeasible, these lesions can be successfully managed with laparoscopic distal resections, provided they lie in the distal pancreas. In either case, intraoperative ultrasound is recommended to rule out the presence of synchronous tumors [37]. Even in the absence of MEN, multiple lesions are not uncommon, and as a major goal of resection is to eliminate associated symptoms, failure to excise a second functional lesion represents a significant treatment failure.

Laparoscopic resections have proven feasible for a variety of additional endocrine neoplasms. Good results have been reported for laparoscopic resections of gastrinomas, VIPomas, glucagonomas, and polypeptidomas [37]. These lesions are more frequently malignant and, as such, require a low threshold for conversion to an open procedure. As such, even in cases of low suspicion of malignancy, a clear margin should be attempted, and specimens should be removed in protective specimen bags. When suspecting lesions with greater risk of malignancy such as gastrinomas and glucagonomas, the initial resection should be a distal pancreatectomy, and should include adequate margins and intraoperative frozen section analysis should be employed to ensure adequate resection. While more extensive

Table 27.1 Laparoscopic distal pancreatectomy and enucleation ($n > 9$ patients): *Characteristics, Indications, Procedures*

	Patients, n (male)	Age, years	Diagnosis	Procedure	DP w/ spleen preserved, n (%)	Hand assisted, n (%)	EBL	Conversion
Pierce et al. 2007	22	56.3 ± 15	Cyst (1), glucagonoma (1), gastrinoma (2), insulinoma (3), metastasis (2), IPTMT (4), nonfunctioning NE tumor (3), cystadenoma (6)	LDP (18), LEn (4)		4	244 ± 516	1
Giger et al. 2006	15		Serous cystadenoma (1), pseudocysts (2), NETs (11)	LDP (6), LEn (3)				6
Toniato et al. 2006	12		Insulinoma (12)	LDP (7), LEn (4)	5			
Root et al. 2005	11		NET (7), unspecified (1), cystic neoplasm (3)	LDP (8), LEn (3)	4 (43%)	2		1
Mabrut et al. 2005	122	52 (8–80)	Benign (87%), malignancy (13%)	LDP (98), LEn (24)	61/98 (62%)	6 (5%)	<300 CC	17 (41%)
Ayav et al. 2005	34	48 (20–77)	Insulinoma (34)	LDP (15), LEn (19)	12/15 (80%)	0	NA	10 (29%)
Dulucq et al. 2002	21 (6)	58 ± 12	NE (1), cystadenoma (12), pseudopapillary tumor (1), lymphangioma (1), CP (3), adenocarcinoma (3)	LDP (21)	16/21 (76%)	0	162	1 (5%)
Lebedyyev et al. 2004	12 (3)	59	NE (2), cystadenoma (6), adenocarcinoma (2)	LDP (12)	7/12 (58%)	0	NA	3 (25%)
Fernandez-Cruz et al. 2005	13 (1)	40 (22–66)	Sporadic insulinoma (11), multiple insulinomas (2)	LDP (5), LEn (8)	5/5 (100)	0	DP: 360, EN: 200	1 (8%)

27 Cancer of the Pancreas: Distal Resections and Staging of Pancreatic Cancer

Study	N	Age	Diagnosis	Procedure			EBL	Complications
Edwin et al. 2004	27	56 (21–81)	NE (14), cystadenoma (2), adenocarcinoma (4), other (7)	LDP (20), LEn (7)	5/20 (25%)	1 (4%)	DP: 400, EN: 100	4 (15%)
Shimizu et al. 2004	11 (6)	DP: 44–68, En: 51–65	NE (4), non-NE (2), cystadenoma (2), CP (3)	LED (9), LEn (2)	2/9 (22%)	0	DP: 213 ± 227, EN: 75 ± 35	2 (18%) (DP: 2, EN: 0)
Fernandez-Cruz et al. 2004	19 (2)	55 (34–70)	Cystadenoma (17), borderline mucinous cystic tumor (1)	LDP (19)	11/19 (58%)	0	400 ± 210	0
Fabre et al. 2002	13 (2)	60 (32–85)	NE (1), cystic tumors (6), CP (9), adenocarcinoma (1)	LDP (13)	10/13 (77%)	0	NA	2 (15%)
Park and Heniford 2002	25 (9)	46 (36–73)	NE (9), cystadenoma (6), CP (4), simple cyst (4), other (2)	LDP (23), LEn (2)	12/23 (52%)	2 (8%)	274	2 (8%)
Fernandez-Cruz et al. 2002	18 (3)	53 (25–72)	NE (10), Cystic tumors (8)	LDP (13), LEn (5)	12/13 (92%)	0	DP: 515, EN: 200	2 (11%)
Patterson et al. 2001	19 (6)	53 (22–83)	NE (7), benign cystic lesions (9), adenocarcinoma (2), Schwanoma (1)	LDP (15), LEn (4)	3/15 (20%)	1 (5%)	200	2 (11%)
Berends et al. 2000	10 (2)	42 (16–72)	Insulinoma (10)	LDP (1), LEn (9)	NA	0	<100	4 (40%)
Cuschieri and Jakimowicz 1998	13	49 (38–66)	NE (6), cystadenoma (1), CP (7)	LDP (9), LEn (3), NA (1)	0	0	400	1 (8%)
Gagner and Pomp 1997	13 (6)	46.5 (27–75)	NE (9), CP (1), cystadenocarcinoma (1), R/O NE tumor (2)	LDP (9), LEn (4)	NA	0	NA	4 (31%)

CP pancreatic cyst, *DP* distal pancreas, *EBL* estimated blood loss, *EN* enucleation, *IPTMT* intrapapillary tumor/mucinous tumor, *LDP* laparoscopic distal pancreatectomy, *LEn* laparoscopic enucleation, *NA* not applicable, *NE* neuroendocrine, *NET* neuroendocrine tumor, *R/O* ruled/out, *UTI* urinary tract infection resection is frequently indicated in MEN, the patient should be made aware that occult, symptomatic lesions may be missed, despite careful preoperative and intraoperative investigations.

27.2.4.2 Pancreatic Cystic Lesions

Laparoscopic resection has an important role in the management of certain cystic lesions of the pancreas. As the identification of pancreatic cysts is increasing with improved imaging, the management of these lesions becomes increasingly challenging. Mucinous lesions such as intraductal papillary mucinous neoplasms (IPMN) and mucinous cystadenomas have premalignant potential, although the time to development of malignancy is not known [38]. Serous cystadenomas are benign and other than growth in size, which may lead to symptoms that could ultimately result in surgery, these lesions do not require resection. Some centers have recommended routine resection of all pancreatic cysts [39–41]. However, others, including our institution, recommend a selective approach to resection [42–44], which includes radiographic monitoring for those with lack of a solid component and small cyst diameter and potential resection for good operative candidates with suspected mucinous lesions over 3 cm in size. Obstruction implies ductal involvement, and suspicion of malignancy warrants distal pancreatectomy. Laparoscopic distal pancreatectomies have been reported in both scenarios with good results, and is an appropriate consideration for the well-selected patient [45–50] and the literature contains multiple reports of successful treatment of both mucinous and serous-type cysts with laparoscopic distal resections [38, 46, 47, 51, 52].

27.3 Reported Results

In practice, laparoscopic partial pancreatic resections have been performed successfully at a variety of centers for over a decade. Given both the rarity of the indicating disease states and the unique surgical expertise required, the bulk of the literature reporting results from these procedures involves small, low-powered case series. One of the largest studies, however, is a multicenter study by Mabrut et al. of 127 patients, representing the largest and most complete series of laparoscopic pancreatic resections reported in the English literature to date. They confirm the findings of smaller studies demonstrating laparoscopic distal pancreatectomy to be feasible, effective, and well tolerated when compared to the open approach for a wide variety of pathologies. Overall, they reported a median postoperative hospital stay of 7 days, a conversion rate to an open procedure of 14%, a complication rate of 31%, a fistula rate of 17%, and 0% perioperative deaths. The rest of the literature when viewed in sum appears generally in keeping with these results (Table 27.2).

These studies likely bias toward an underappreciation of the efficacy and safety of laparoscopic methods since a large portion of these small series included cases performed early in the operating surgeon's learning curve, and thus do not perfectly reflect the efficacy of these procedures in fully trained hands. In open pancreatic surgery, surgeons performing pancreaticoduodenectomies, a classic and nearly universal procedure among surgical training programs, have been found to have a clearly appreciable learning curve over their first 60 cases [53]. Likewise, the learning curve phenomenon has also been documented for various laparoscopic procedures [54–56], and is a generally accepted fact among practicing surgeons. One can only expect a similar, if not more pronounced, learning curve exists for laparoscopic pancreatic surgery, which is generally extremely technically demanding and, at least in the current era, rarely encountered in surgical training programs. Thus, reports documenting the results of surgeons' and/or institutions' early experience with such procedures cannot be expected to reflect the full potential of such procedures.

27.4 Complications and Recovery

Complications associated with laparoscopic pancreatic resections are similar to those associated with open resections. Given the smaller incisions, wound complications are less of a concern in laparoscopic surgery. As mentioned above, the initial application of laparoscopic technique to oncologic surgery raised some concerns about port-site seeding and metastases, but subsequent investigations have shown this phenomenon to be quite rare, and almost uniformly associated with previous metastatic disease.

Table 27.2 Laparoscopic distal pancreatectomy and enucleation: *Outcomes*

	OR time, n (Male)	Complications, PF	Reoperation	Postoperative stay	Op Mortality	Follow up	Recurrence
Pierce et al. 2007	236 ± 60	36.4% (pancreas related) UTI (1), PE (1), infection (1), pseudocyst (1), PF: 6 (27%)	4.5%	4.5 ± 2	0		
Giger et al. 2006	268 ± 74			8 ± 2	0		
Toniato et al. 2006	170				0		
Root et al. 2005	304	Infected hematoma: 1, PF: 0	0	5	0		
Mabrut et al. 2005	LDP: 200, LEn: 120	19 (16%), PF: 17 (14%)	21 (17%)	7 (3–67)	0	15 (3–47) in malignant cases	3 (23%)
Ayav et al. 2005	156 (50–420), LDP: 175, LEn: 115	<13 (<38%), PF: 5 (15%)	2 (6%)	11.9 (5–39)	0	26 (2–87)	1 (3%)
Dulucq et al. 2003	154 ± 63	5 (23%), PF: 1 (5%)	2 (9.5%)	10.8 (6–15)	0	Benign: 50, malignancy: 19	0
Lebedyvev et al. 2004	354 (74–805)	6 (50%)	0	NA	0	NA	NA
Fernandez-Cruz et al. 2005	LDP: 240, LEn: 180	3 (23%)	1 (18%)	LDP: 7 ± 4, LEn: 5	0	28 (6–42)	0
Edwin et al. 2004	LDP: 235, LEn: 120	≥9 (≤33%), PF: 1 (4%)	1 (4%)	5.5 (2–22)	2 (7.4%)	NA	NA
Shimizu et al. 2004	LDP: 293 ± 58, LEn: 185 ± 4	2 (18%), PF: 2 (18%)	0	NA	0	NA	NA
Fernandez-Cruz et al. 2004	198 ± 58	6 (23%), PF: 3 (16%)	1 (5%)	DP: 5.5 ± 1	0	22 (6–42)	0
Fabre et al. 2002	280	4 (30%), PF: 1 (8%)	1 (8%)	NA (5–22)	0	NA	NA
Park and Heniford 2002	222	4 (16%), PF: 1 (4%)	0	4.1	0	NA	NA
Fernandez-Cruz et al. 2002	270	6 (33%), PF: 5 (28%)	1 (6%)	5	0	NA	NA
Patterson et al. 2001	264	5 (26%), PF: 3 (16%)	0	7.6 (1–26)	0	NA	NA
Berends et al. 2000	NA	5 (50%), PF: 2 (20%)	1 (10%)	7 (3–21)	0	18 (3–36)	0
Cuschieri and Jakimowicz 1998	240–300	3 (23%), PF: 1 (8%)	0	7.1 (5–10)	0	NA	NA
Gagner and Pomp 1997	LDP: 270, LEn: 180	5: (38%), PF: NA	0	LDP: 5, LEn: 4	0	27 (15–28)	3 (23%)

CP pancreatic cyst, *DP* distal pancreas, *EBL* estimated blood loss, *EN* enucleation, *IPTMT* intrapapillary tumor/mucinous tumor, *LDP* laparoscopic distal pancreatectomy, *LEn* laparoscopic enucleation, *NA* not applicable, *NE* neuroendocrine, *NET* neuroendocrine tumor, *OR* operating room, *PE* pulmonary embolism, *PF* pancreatic fistula *R/O* ruled/out, *UTI* urinary tract infection

As already established in the laparoscopic treatment of other organ malignancies, the superior visualization afforded by laparoscopic technology may compensate for the corresponding loss of tactile feedback for surgeons comfortable with the techniques. While the existing data are not comprehensive, the limited reports do not suggest an increase in recurrence rates associated with laparoscopic resection.

Ultimately, the complication most likely to delay the patient's recovery in laparoscopic pancreatic resections, as in open resections, is the development of a pancreatic fistula. Unfortunately, imprecise and inconsistent definitions of pancreatic fistula make it difficult to draw firm comparisons between various studies, let alone between approaches. However, the vast majority of studies reporting results from series of laparoscopic pancreatic resections include a report of fistula rate. While the range is wide, meta-analysis of the studies yields a mean fistula rate of 13% [57]. These rates are within the range reported for open pancreatic resections.

Along with improved pain control, the outcome most frequently offered as justification for laparoscopic surgery is quicker recovery, frequently assessed in terms of length of hospital stay. Here, data are misleading. Overall, the mean length of stay for laparoscopic pancreatic resections ranges from 4 to 6 days, just barely shorter than those found in open series [58]. However, these data do not reflect the bimodal distribution of postoperative course of pancreatic resection patients. The occurrence of a pancreatic fistula and/or anastomotic leak greatly prolongs recovery from pancreatic resection. As the leak rate is similar in open and laparoscopic series, both open and laparoscopic series report hospital course rates that are skewed by the prolonged stays of patients with postoperative leaks. Comparing the overall hospital stay rates fails to account for the more rapid recovery associated with laparoscopic resection who do not leak. Thus, the impact of the shortened stay experienced by the majority of the patients is statistically overwhelmed by the vastly longer stays experienced by those patients who suffer from a leak.

Quick Reference Guide

1. Patient positioning:
   - Supine with split leg setup
   - Bump under the left shoulder blade

2. Enter the lesser sac via the gastro-colic ligament and be sure to provide adequate exposure of the pancreas by taking several of the lower short gastric vessels.
3. Once the pancreas is visualized, begin with mobilization of the inferior pancreas using meticulous hemostasis technique with cautery device to avoid unnecessary bleeding that may impair visualization of the appropriate planes.
4. Facilitate a complete mobilization of the pancreas out to the tail, taking the posterior attachments with good hemostasis technique.
5. Evaluate the pancreatic lesion, if not readily visible use laparoscopic ultrasound.
6. Identify and carefully dissect the splenic artery and vein.
   If any concerns regarding proximity to the lesion exist, plan to remove the spleen as well.
7. Added splenectomy

   - Dissect and isolate splenic artery and vein
   - Staple the vessels with one firing of a gray load GIA stapler

   Spleen preserving

   - Dissect splenic artery and vein off the pancreas
   - Careful hemostasis technique is crucial!

8. Use a stapling device or electro-cautery to transect the pancreas

   - Obtain a good margin
   - Assure hemostasis

9. Remove the specimen via an endocatch bag
10. If there are any concerns about safety and resectability of the lesion with a laparoscopic approach, have a low threshold for conversion to an open approach

References

1. Bernheim, B.M.: IV. Organoscopy: cystoscopy of the abdominal cavity. Ann. Surg. **53**(6), 764–767 (1911 Jun)
2. Velanovich, V., Wollner, I., Ajlouni, M.: Staging laparoscopy promotes increased utilization of postoperative therapy for unresectable intra-abdominal malignancies. J. Gastrointest. Surg. **4**(5), 542–546 (2000 Sep)
3. Prokesch, R.W., Chow, L.C., Beaulieu, C.F., Nino-Murcia, M., Mindelzun, R.E., Bammer, R., et al.: Local staging of pancreatic carcinoma with multi-detector row CT: use of curved planar reformations initial experience. Radiology **225**(3), 759–765 (2002 Dec)

4. Shoup, M., Winston, C., Brennan, M.F., Bassman, D., Conlon, K.C.: Is there a role for staging laparoscopy in patients with locally advanced, unresectable pancreatic adenocarcinoma? J. Gastrointest. Surg. **8**(8), 1068–771 (2004 Dec)
5. Strong, V.E., Dalal, K.M., Malhotra, V.T., Cubert, K.H., Coit, D., Fong, Y., et al.: Initial report of laparoscopic celiac plexus block for pain relief in patients with unresectable pancreatic cancer. J. Am. Coll. Surg. **203**(1), 129–131 (2006 Jul)
6. Freeny, P.C., Traverso, L.W., Ryan, J.A.: Diagnosis and staging of pancreatic adenocarcinoma with dynamic computed tomography. Am. J. Surg. **165**(5), 600–606 (1993 May)
7. Fuhrman, G.M., Charnsangavej, C., Abbruzzese, J.L., Cleary, K.R., Martin, R.G., Fenoglio, C.J., et al.: Thin-section contrast-enhanced computed tomography accurately predicts the resectability of malignant pancreatic neoplasms. Am. J. Surg. **167**(1), 104–111 (1994 Jan)
8. Gulliver, D.J., Baker, M.E., Cheng, C.A., Meyers, W.C., Pappas, T.N.: Malignant biliary obstruction: efficacy of thin-section dynamic CT in determining resectability. AJR Am. J. Roentgenol. **159**(3), 503–507 (1992 Sep)
9. Conlon, K.C., Brennan, M.F.: Laparoscopy for staging abdominal malignancies. Adv. Surg. **34**, 331–350 (2000)
10. Jimenez, R.E., Warshaw, A.L., Rattner, D.W., Willett, C.G., McGrath, D., Fernandez-del, C.C.: Impact of laparoscopic staging in the treatment of pancreatic cancer. Arch. Surg. **135**(4), 409–414 (2000 Apr)
11. Cuschieri, A.: Laparoscopy for pancreatic cancer: does it benefit the patient? Eur. J. Surg. Oncol. **14**(1), 41–44 (1988 Feb)
12. Catheline, J.M., Turner, R., Rizk, N., Barrat, C., Champault, G.: The use of diagnostic laparoscopy supported by laparoscopic ultrasonography in the assessment of pancreatic cancer. Surg. Endosc. **13**(3), 239–245 (1999 Mar)
13. Reddy, K.R., Levi, J., Livingstone, A., Jeffers, L., Molina, E., Kligerman, S., et al.: Experience with staging laparoscopy in pancreatic malignancy. Gastrointest. Endosc. **49**(4 Pt 1), 498–503 (1999 Apr)
14. Warshaw, A.L., Tepper, J.E., Shipley, W.U.: Laparoscopy in the staging and planning of therapy for pancreatic cancer. Am. J. Surg. **151**(1), 76–80 (1986 Jan)
15. Warshaw, A.L., Gu, Z.Y., Wittenberg, J., Waltman, A.C.: Preoperative staging and assessment of resectability of pancreatic cancer. Arch. Surg. **125**(2), 230–233 (1990 Feb)
16. Fernandez-del, C.C., Rattner, D.W., Warshaw, A.L.: Further experience with laparoscopy and peritoneal cytology in the staging of pancreatic cancer. Br. J. Surg. **82**(8), 1127–1129 (1995 Aug)
17. John, T.G., Greig, J.D., Carter, D.C., Garden, O.J.: Carcinoma of the pancreatic head and periampullary region. Tumor staging with laparoscopy and laparoscopic ultrasonography. Ann. Surg. **221**(2), 156–164 (1995 Feb)
18. Nieveen van Dijkum, E.J., Romijn, M.G., Terwee, C.B., de Wit, L.T., van der Meulen, J.H., Lameris, H.S., et al.: Laparoscopic staging and subsequent palliation in patients with peripancreatic carcinoma. Ann. Surg. **237**(1), 66–73 (2003 Jan)
19. Menack, M.J., Spitz, J.D., Arregui, M.E.: Staging of pancreatic and ampullary cancers for resectability using laparoscopy with laparoscopic ultrasound. Surg. Endosc. **15**(10), 1129–1134 (2001 Oct)
20. Conlon, K.C., Dougherty, E., Klimstra, D.S., Coit, D.G., Turnbull, A.D., Brennan, M.F.: The value of minimal access surgery in the staging of patients with potentially resectable peripancreatic malignancy. Ann. Surg. **223**(2), 134–140 (1996 Feb)
21. Karachristos, A., Scarmeas, N., Hoffman, J.P.: CA 19-9 levels predict results of staging laparoscopy in pancreatic cancer. J. Gastrointest. Surg. **9**(9), 1286–1292 (2005 Dec)
22. Alexander, R.J., Jaques, B.C., Mitchell, K.G.: Laparoscopically assisted colectomy and wound recurrence. Lancet **341**(8839), 249–250 (1993 Jan 23)
23. Shoup, M., Brennan, M.F., Karpeh, M.S., Gillern, S.M., McMahon, R.L., Conlon, K.C.: Port site metastasis after diagnostic laparoscopy for upper gastrointestinal tract malignancies: an uncommon entity. Ann. Surg. Oncol. **9**(7), 632–636 (2002 Aug)
24. Siddiqui, A., Spechler, S.J., Huerta, S.: Surgical bypass versus endoscopic stenting for malignant gastroduodenal obstruction: a decision analysis. Dig. Dis. Sci. **52**(1), 276–281 (2007 Jan)
25. Soper, N.J., Brunt, L.M., Kerbl, K.: Laparoscopic general surgery. N. Engl. J. Med. **330**(6), 409–419 (1994 Feb 10)
26. Ayav, A., Bresler, L., Brunaud, L., Boissel, P.: Laparoscopic approach for solitary insulinoma: a multicentre study. Langenbecks Arch. Surg. **390**(2), 134–140 (2005 Apr)
27. Cuschieri, S.A., Jakimowicz, J.J.: Laparoscopic pancreatic resections. Semin. Laparosc. Surg. **5**(3), 168–179 (1998 Sep)
28. Orsenigo, E., Baccari, P., Bissolotti, G., Staudacher, C.: Laparoscopic central pancreatectomy. Am. J. Surg. **191**(4), 549–552 (2006 Apr)
29. Ammori, B.J., El-Dhuwaib, Y., Ballester, P., Augustine, T.: Laparoscopic distal pancreatectomy for neuroendocrine tumors of the pancreas. Hepatogastroenterology **52**(62), 620–624 (2005 Mar)
30. Edwin, B., Mala, T., Mathisen, O., Gladhaug, I., Buanes, T., Lunde, O.C., et al.: Laparoscopic resection of the pancreas: a feasibility study of the short-term outcome. Surg. Endosc. **18**(3), 407–411 (2004 Mar)
31. Fernandez-Cruz, L., Saenz, A., Astudillo, E., Martinez, I., Hoyos, S., Pantoja, J.P., et al.: Outcome of laparoscopic pancreatic surgery: endocrine and nonendocrine tumors. World J. Surg. **26**(8), 1057–1065 (2002 Aug)
32. Mayo, W.J.: I. The surgery of the pancreas: I. Injuries to the pancreas in the course of operations on the stomach. II. Injuries to the pancreas in the course of operations on the spleen. III. Resection of half the pancreas for tumor. Ann. Surg. **58**(2), 145–150 (1913 Aug)
33. Mallet-Guy, P., Vachon, A.: Pancreatites Chroniques Gauches. Masson, Paris (1943)
34. Warshaw, A.L.: Conservation of the spleen with distal pancreatectomy. Arch. Surg. **123**(5), 550–553 (1988 May)
35. Rodriguez, J.R., Madanat, M.G., Healy, B.C., Thayer, S.P., Warshaw, A.L., Fernandez-del, C.C.: Distal pancreatectomy with splenic preservation revisited. Surgery **141**(5), 619–625 (2007 May)
36. Shoup, M., Brennan, M.F., McWhite, K., Leung, D.H., Klimstra, D., Conlon, K.C.: The value of splenic preservation with distal pancreatectomy. Arch. Surg. **137**(2), 164–168 (2002 Feb)
37. Takaori, K., Matsusue, S., Fujikawa, T., Kobashi, Y., Ito, T., Matsuo, Y., et al.: Carcinoma in situ of the pancreas associated with localized fibrosis: a clue to early detection of neoplastic lesions arising from pancreatic ducts. Pancreas **17**(1), 102–105 (1998 Jul)

38. Maitra, A., Fukushima, N., Takaori, K., Hruban, R.H.: Precursors to invasive pancreatic cancer. Adv. Anat. Pathol. **12**(2), 81–91 (2005 Mar)
39. Horvath, K.D., Chabot, J.A.: An aggressive resectional approach to cystic neoplasms of the pancreas. Am. J. Surg. **178**(4), 269–274 (1999 Oct)
40. Siech, M., Tripp, K., Schmidt-Rohlfing, B., Mattfeldt, T., Widmaier, U., Gansauge, F., et al.: Cystic tumours of the pancreas: diagnostic accuracy, pathologic observations and surgical consequences. Langenbecks Arch. Surg. **383**(1), 56–61 (1998 Mar)
41. Ooi, L.L., Ho, G.H., Chew, S.P., Low, C.H., Soo, K.C.: Cystic tumours of the pancreas: a diagnostic dilemma. Aust. N. Z. J. Surg. **68**(12), 844–846 (1998 Dec)
42. Walsh, R.M., Vogt, D.P., Henderson, J.M., Zuccaro, G., Vargo, J., Dumot, J., et al.: Natural history of indeterminate pancreatic cysts. Surgery **138**(4), 665–670 (2005 Oct)
43. Spinelli, K.S., Fromwiller, T.E., Daniel, R.A., Kiely, J.M., Nakeeb, A., Komorowski, R.A., et al.: Cystic pancreatic neoplasms: observe or operate. Ann. Surg. **239**(5), 651–657 (2004 May)
44. Allen, P.J., D'Angelica, M., Gonen, M., Jaques, D.P., Coit, D.G., Jarnagin, W.R., et al.: A selective approach to the resection of cystic lesions of the pancreas: results from 539 consecutive patients. Ann. Surg. **244**(4), 572–582 (2006 Oct)
45. Fabre, J.M., Dulucq, J.L., Vacher, C., Lemoine, M.C., Wintringer, P., Nocca, D., et al.: Is laparoscopic left pancreatic resection justified? Surg. Endosc. **16**(9), 1358–1361 (2002 Sep)
46. Fernandez-Cruz, L., Martinez, I., Gilabert, R., Cesar-Borges, G., Astudillo, E., Navarro, S.: Laparoscopic distal pancreatectomy combined with preservation of the spleen for cystic neoplasms of the pancreas. J. Gastrointest. Surg. **8**(4), 493–501 (2004 May)
47. Han, H.S., Min, S.K., Lee, H.K., Kim, S.W., Park, Y.H.: Laparoscopic distal pancreatectomy with preservation of the spleen and splenic vessels for benign pancreas neoplasm. Surg. Endosc. **19**(10), 1367–1369 (2005 Oct)
48. Khanna, A., Koniaris, L.G., Nakeeb, A., Schoeniger, L.O.: Laparoscopic spleen-preserving distal pancreatectomy. J. Gastrointest. Surg. **9**(5), 733–738 (2005 May)
49. Klingler, P.J., Hinder, R.A., Menke, D.M., Smith, S.L.: Hand-assisted laparoscopic distal pancreatectomy for pancreatic cystadenoma. Surg. Laparosc. Endosc. **8**(3), 180–184 (1998 Jun)
50. Maruyama, M., Kenmochi, T., Asano, T., Saigo, K., Miyauchi, H., Miura, F., et al.: Laparoscopic distal pancreatectomy as the total biopsy of the pancreas: tool of minimally invasive surgery. J. Hepatobiliary Pancreat. Surg. **11**(4), 290–292 (2004)
51. Matsumoto, T., Kitano, S., Yoshida, T., Bandoh, T., Kakisako, K., Ninomiya, K., et al.: Laparoscopic resection of a pancreatic mucinous cystadenoma using laparosonic coagulating shears. Surg. Endosc. **13**(2), 172–173 (1999 Feb)
52. Watanabe, Y., Sato, M., Kikkawa, H., Shiozaki, T., Yoshida, M., Yamamoto, Y., et al.: Spleen-preserving laparoscopic distal pancreatectomy for cystic adenoma. Hepatogastroenterology **49**(43), 148–152 (2002 Jan)
53. Tseng, J.F., Pisters, P.W., Lee, J.E., Wang, H., Gomez, H.F., Sun, C.C., et al.: The learning curve in pancreatic surgery. Surgery **141**(4), 456–463 (2007 Apr)
54. Archer, S.B., Brown, D.W., Smith, C.D., Branum, G.D., Hunter, J.G.: Bile duct injury during laparoscopic cholecystectomy: results of a national survey. Ann. Surg. **234**(4), 549–558 (2001 Oct)
55. Bennett, C.L., Stryker, S.J., Ferreira, M.R., Adams, J., Beart Jr., R.W.: The learning curve for laparoscopic colorectal surgery. Preliminary results from a prospective analysis of 1194 laparoscopic-assisted colectomies. Arch. Surg. **132**(1), 41–44 (1997 Jan)
56. Tekkis, P.P., Senagore, A.J., Delaney, C.P., Fazio, V.W.: Evaluation of the learning curve in laparoscopic colorectal surgery: comparison of right-sided and left-sided resections. Ann. Surg. **242**(1), 83–91 (2005 Jul)
57. Ammori, B.J., Baghdadi, S.: Minimally invasive pancreatic surgery: the new frontier? Curr. Gastroenterol. Rep. **8**(2), 132–142 (2006 Apr)
58. D'Angelica, M., Are, C., Jarnagin, W., DeGregoris, G., Coit, D., Jaques, D., et al.: Initial experience with hand-assisted laparoscopic distal pancreatectomy. Surg. Endosc. **20**(1), 142–148 (2006 Jan)

Cancer of the Pancreas: The Whipple Procedure

28

Michael L. Kendrick

28.1 Introduction

Cancer of the pancreas accounts for only 3% of all new cancer cases in the USA, yet it remains the fourth leading cause of death from cancer [1]. This remarkable statistic emphasizes the lethality of pancreas cancer and our current inability to identify it early and therefore our inability to effectively treat the majority of patients. Surgical resection currently provides the only realistic opportunity for cure in patients with pancreatic adenocarcinoma. Unfortunately, less than 20% of patients are candidates for resection based on locally unresectable or metastatic disease at presentation. Advances in preoperative imaging, operative techniques, and perioperative care have led to improvements in patient selection and operative morbidity as well mortality. In high-volume centers, operative mortality is frequently reported to be less than 3%. Pancreaticoduodenectomy, also known as the "Whipple procedure," is the operation of choice for lesions of the pancreatic head, neck, and uncinate process. Recent large series from centers specializing in pancreatic cancer have reported 5-year survival rates of 15–30% in patients undergoing surgical resection of pancreatic adenocarcinoma. These findings underscore the need for earlier detection and useful neoadjuvant or adjuvant treatment modalities to improve the outcomes of these patients.

28.2 Role of Adjuvant/Neoadjuvant Therapy

Several trials have demonstrated a modest survival advantage for patients receiving adjuvant chemotherapy following resection. Utilizing a predominantly neoadjuvant treatment approach, actual 5-year survival of up to 27% has been reported following pancreatic resection with the use of multimodality therapy [2]. Critics of the neoadjuvant approach attribute the potential survival advantage to patient selection bias, as patients who have progression of disease or clinical deterioration during treatment are "selected-out" of the typical cohort of patients undergoing resection. Without a randomized, controlled trial or identification of more effective treatment modalities, the use of neoadjuvant approaches will likely remain controversial.

28.3 Vascular Resection – *Yes or No?*

Vascular resection in patients with locally advanced pancreatic adenocarcinoma is now performed in several centers. Current data support resection of the portal or superior mesenteric vein when necessary to achieve a gross (R2) and microscopic (R1) negative margin. Survival is not reduced by the need for vascular resection as long as a curative resection is performed. It is superior to patients with locally advanced disease who are treated nonoperatively [3].

M.L. Kendrick
Department of Surgery, Mayo Clinic, Mayo Clinic College of Medicine, 200 First Street, SW, Rochester, MN 55905, USA
e-mail: kendrick.michael@mayo.edu

28.4 Significance of IPMN

Perhaps the greatest opportunity to impact outcomes of pancreatic ductal adenocarcinoma is to identify it in an early or premalignant stage. Pancreatic intraductal papillary mucinous neoplasm (IPMN) is a cystic, neoplastic disease of the ductal epithelium considered to be a precursor of ductal adenocarcinoma. It is broadly classified into three categories depending upon the pattern of involvement

- Branch duct IPMN
- Main duct IPMN
- Mixed IPMN

Branch duct IPMN harbors invasive adenocarcinoma in approximately 15% of patients if it is >3 cm in size, symptomatic, or contains mural nodules. In the absence of these factors, branch duct IPMN harbors malignancy in less than 5% and observation is recommended. Conversely, invasive malignancy is present in approximately 50% of patients with main duct IPMN and resection is warranted.

28.5 Evolution of "The Whipple Procedure"

Pancreaticoduodenectomy is a standardized oncologic procedure based on anatomic (vascular, biliary, and intestinal) and tumor-related (lymphatic drainage, contiguous organ) factors of the pancreatic head. Several modifications have been described over time including preservation of the pylorus, differences in anastomotic reconstruction (pancreatico-jejunostomy versus pancreatico-gastrostomy), and pancreatic anastomotic technique (duct-to-mucosa versus invagination). Few of these modifications have had significant impact on overall patient outcomes and surgeon preference guides the technique utilized. Reduction in morbidity and mortality can be largely attributed to improved patient selection, surgeon experience, technical ability, and the advances in postoperative management of complications. Improved imaging, endoscopic, and percutaneous interventional techniques have allowed nonoperative management of postoperative hemorrhage and anastomotic leakage in the majority of patients with these serious postoperative complications.

28.6 Minimally Invasive Approach

28.6.1 Historic Review

The first description of laparoscopic pancreaticoduodenectomy (LPD) was published by Gagner and Pomp in 1994 [4]. Unlike minimally invasive cholecystectomy, colectomy, or bariatric surgery, this has not lead to a rapid or widespread acceptance. Pessimism was fostered by early reports of long operative times, the need for advanced laparoscopic skills, and the lack of apparent advantages over open approaches [5]. To reduce operative time and avoid the need for advanced skills of reconstruction, several authors have reported hybrid techniques such as laparoscopic resection with open reconstruction and hand-assisted approaches [6, 5]. More recently, a renewed interest in LPD has arisen as a result of advances in high definition optics, improved laparoscopic equipment, robotics, and more widespread acquisition of minimally invasive skills.

28.6.2 The Challenges

The complexity of a pancreaticoduodenectomy can be attributed to

- Retroperitoneal location of the pancreas
- Vascular, biliary, and intestinal integration of the pancreas
- Need for both a complex resection and reconstruction

These factors and the textural characteristics of the pancreas itself set the stage for potential major postoperative morbidity and mortality. Thus, it has been with significant reservation that minimally invasive approaches have been utilized for pancreaticoduodenectomy.

28.6.3 Patient Selection

Selecting the appropriate patient for a minimally invasive approach is based on the advanced laparoscopic skills and oncologic experience of the surgeon. Early

28 Cancer of the Pancreas: The Whipple Procedure

Table 28.1 Suggested selection criteria for laparoscopic pancreaticoduodenectomy in the early experience

Ideal patient criteria for resection and reconstruction
Body mass index (kg/m²) <35
Small tumor (<5 cm)
Dilated pancreatic duct
Dilated extrahepatic bile duct
Clinical suspicion of firm pancreas (chronic obstruction)
No previous major upper abdominal surgery
No suspicion of portal or mesenteric venous involvement
Tumor distant from uncinate margin

in a surgeon's experience, nonobese patients with an obstructing lesion (firm pancreas with large pancreatic duct) are the best candidates. Suggested criteria for patients early in the surgeon's experience are listed in Table 28.1. While patients with nonobstructing lesions and absence of inflammation (small pancreatic duct and soft pancreas) may allow for an easier dissection, they require a more tenuous, difficult reconstruction, in the author's opinion.

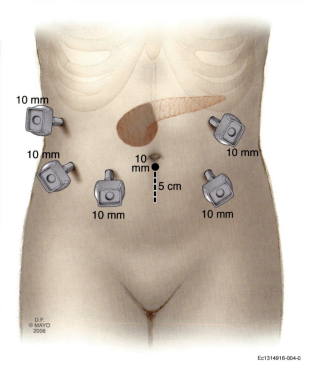

Fig. 28.1 Trocar positioning for total laparoscopic pancreaticoduodenectomy (©Mayo Clinic, with permission)

28.7 Surgical Technique

28.7.1 Positioning of the Patient and Trocar Placement

The procedure is performed with the patient in supine position and legs together. A total of six (12 mm, bladeless) trocars are used and are placed in a semicircular line (Fig. 28.1). The first is an optical trocar placed in the left subcostal region in the anterior axillary line. A CO_2 pneumoperitoneum is established at a pressure of 14 mmHg and an initial diagnostic laparoscopy is performed. The five remaining trocars are then placed in the left midclavicular line, infraumbilical region, right midclavicular line, right anterior axillary line (lower abdomen), and the right anterior axillary line subcostally. A thorough diagnostic laparoscopy is performed inspecting all visible peritoneal and visceral surfaces. A 7.5-MHz laparoscopic ultrasound probe is used to perform ultrasonography of the liver and pancreas.

28.7.2 Resection

Using ultrasonic shears, the gastrocolic ligament is divided and the lesser sac widely exposed. The hepatic flexure of the colon is mobilized inferiorly and a Kocher maneuver is performed (Fig. 28.2). The portal vein (PV) is identified at the superior border of the pancreatic neck and the superior mesenteric vein (SMV) at the inferior border. A tunnel is dissected posterior to the pancreatic neck, anterior to the SMV and PV. The gastro-duodenal artery and right gastric arteries are ligated, clipped, and divided (Fig. 28.3). At this point, exposure is adequate to assess for tumor invasion into the anterior aspect of the portal or SMV (Fig. 28.4). An "umbilical" tape is placed around the neck of the pancreas to facilitate exposure and allow a "no-touch" technique during resection. The right gastroepiploic vessels are ligated and divided. The first portion of the duodenum is dissected and transected with a linear stapler 2–3 cm distal to the pylorus. The bile duct at the superior border of the pancreatic head is dissected, ligated distally, and divided (Fig. 28.5). A cholecystectomy is performed. The fourth portion of the duodenum and proximal jejunum are

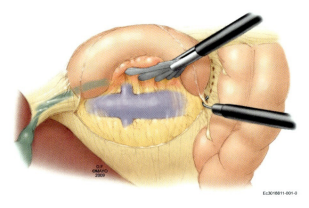

Fig. 28.2 Full Kocherization of the duodenum (©Mayo Clinic, with permission)

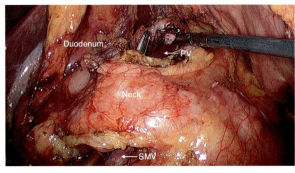

Fig. 28.4 Intraoperative photograph of the pancreatic neck dissection with reticulating grasper passed posterior (©Mayo Clinic, with permission)

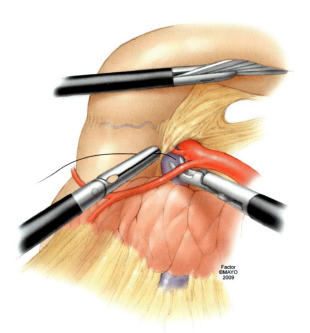

Fig. 28.3 Dissection and ligation of the gastroduodenal artery (©Mayo Clinic, with permission)

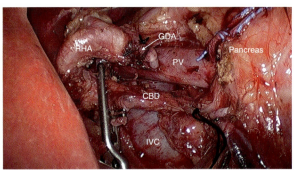

Fig. 28.5 Intraoperative photograph of the bile duct dissection and preparation for transection (©Mayo Clinic, with permission)

mobilized and the jejunum is transected 15 cm distal to the ligament of Treitz with the linear stapler. The jejunal mesentery is divided back to the uncinate process using Ligasure (Tyco Healthcare Group, Dublin, Ireland) (Fig. 28.6). The jejunal stump is passed into the supramesocolic compartment. The pancreatic neck is divided with the ultrasonic shears with exception of the duct which is divided sharply with scissors (Fig. 28.7a). Dissection of the pancreatic head and uncinate process off the PV, SMV, and superior mesenteric artery is typically performed using Ligasure. Larger tributary vessels

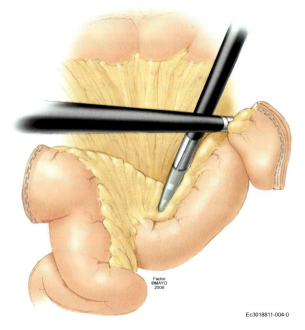

Fig. 28.6 Transection of the jejunum and division of the jejunal mesentery with Ligasure (©Mayo Clinic, with permission)

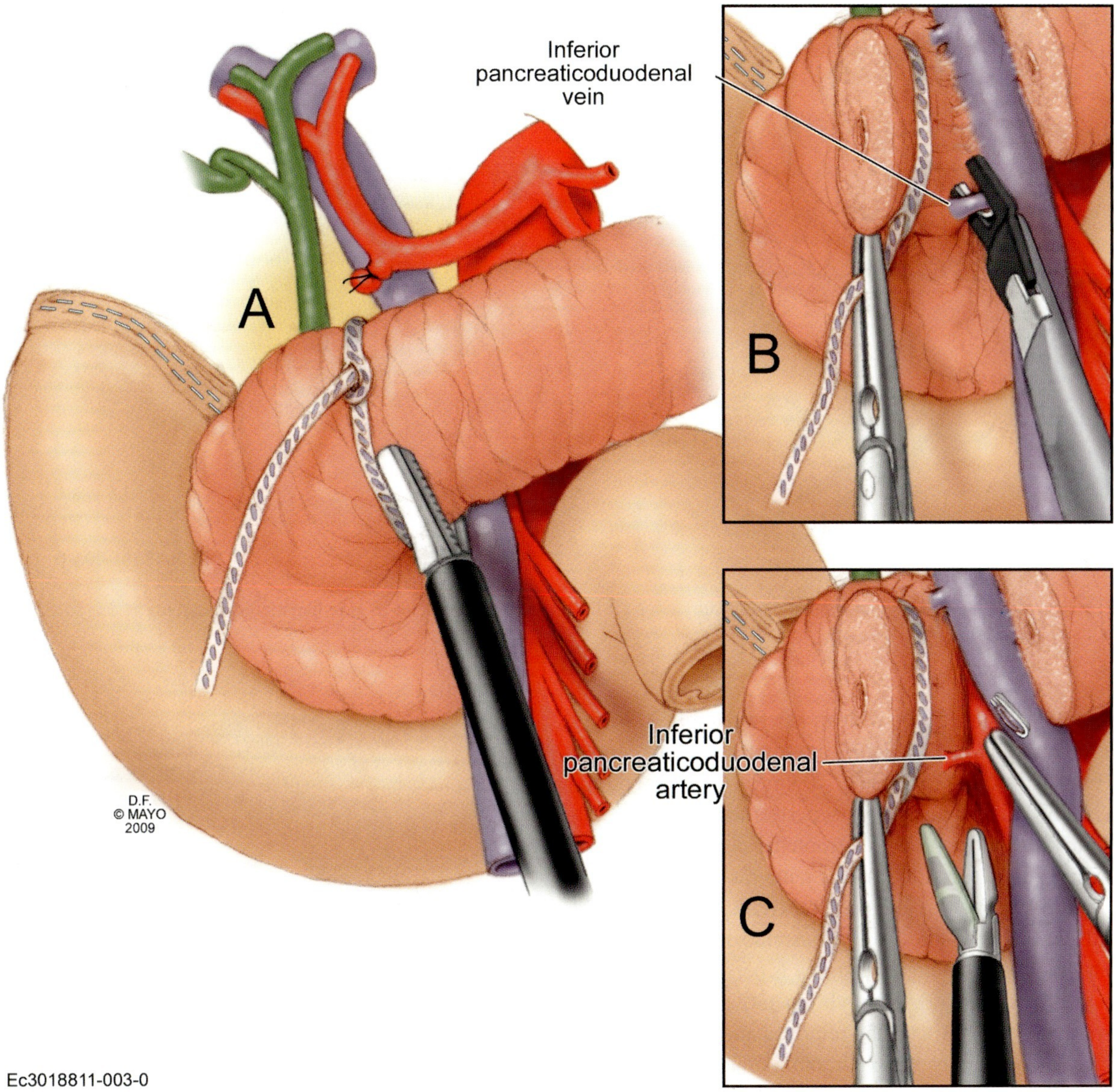

Fig. 28.7 (**a**) Transection of the pancreatic neck and (**b**, **c**) resection of the head and uncinate process (©Mayo Clinic, with permission)

(pancreaticoduodenal vessels) are ligated or clipped (Fig. 28.7b, c). Again, note how the umbilical tape facilitates a no-touch technique during resection. All peripancreatic lymphatic tissue is taken en bloc with the specimen. The specimen is then removed in an endosac via the infraumbilical trocar site extended to accommodate the specimen (typically 4–7 cm). The PV groove and retroperitoneal/uncinate margin on the specimen are inked and separate bile duct and pancreatic neck margins are obtained prior to sending the specimen for frozen section analysis. After fascial closure of the extraction site, the pneumoperitoneum is reestablished.

28.7.3 Reconstruction

- Pancreaticojejunostomy, end-to-side
- Hepaticojejunostomy, end-to-side
- Duodenojejunostomy, end-to-side

Intracorporeal reconstruction is begun once margin status is confirmed on histology. The jejunum is brought through the duodenal resection bed, posterior to the superior mesenteric vessels into the supramesocolic compartment. An end-to-side, pancreaticojejunostomy, duct-to-mucosa type anastomosis is performed over an

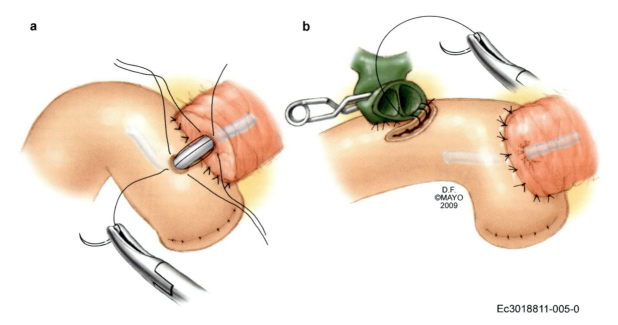

Fig. 28.8 (**a**) End-to-side pancreaticojejunostomy over a Silastic stent and (**b**) end-to-side hepaticojejunostomy (©Mayo Clinic, with permission)

8 cm long Silastic tube with an inner layer of 5-0 Vicryl suture and an outer layer of interrupted 3-0 silk suture (Fig. 28.8a). Approximately 10 cm distally, an end-to-side hepaticojejunostomy is performed with running (bile duct >5 mm) or interrupted (bile duct ≤5 mm) Vicryl suture (Fig. 28.8b). The jejunum is secured, closing the defect at the ligament of Treitz. Approximately 40 cm distal to the biliary anastomosis, an antecolic, end-to-side duodenojejunostomy is performed with two layers of running 3-0 Vicryl. Operative drains are not routinely used. Trocars are removed and trocar sites are closed with an absorbable, monofilament, subcuticular suture. The completed reconstruction is depicted in Fig. 28.9.

28.7.4 Perioperative Care

After anesthesia recovery, patients are admitted to a general surgical floor unless significant medical comorbidities or intraoperative hemodynamics warrant continuous monitoring overnight. Perioperative prophylactic antibiotics (preincision and two postoperative doses) and subcutaneous unfractionated heparin (preincision and 3 times a day during hospitalization) are given. On

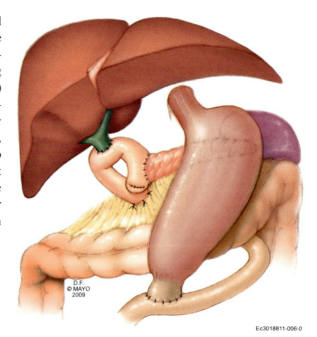

Fig. 28.9 Completed reconstruction of laparoscopic pylorus-preserving pancreaticoduodenectomy (©Mayo Clinic, with permission)

postoperative day 1, the NG tube is removed, and the patient is not given any food or water orally. A clear liquid diet is begun postoperative day 2, and oral diet is advanced as tolerated. Analgesia consists of scheduled intravenous Ketorolac and supplemental intravenous morphine via a patient-controlled analgesia pump. Once tolerating oral intake, patient-controlled analgesia is discontinued and oral narcotic analgesics are given as needed. Patients are discharged after postoperative day 5 if tolerating oral intake and there are no signs or symptoms of complications.

as various technical approaches and diagnoses. Further, while hybrid approaches make the procedure more feasible for the surgeon, it may limit the maximal benefit achievable with a "total" laparoscopic approach. To date, there are only three series in the peer-reviewed literature that contain more than ten patients undergoing total LPD [7, 10, 11], and only nine with more than five patients (including hybrid approaches and excluding conversions) [5, 6, 8, 9, 12, 13] (Table 28.2).

28.8 Outcomes

28.8.1 Perioperative Outcomes

As with most novel techniques or approaches, initial outcome assessment is limited by insufficient number of patients, short-term follow-up, and outcomes within the surgeon's learning curve. Data from these early reports also represent an inherent selection bias as well

The current reports of LPD contain insufficient data to validate the typical advantages of minimally invasive approaches such as decreased pain, reduced wound-related complications, shorter hospitalization, and

Table 28.2 Laparoscopic pancreaticoduodenectomy: Series with >5 patients

Author	Year	Patients	Surgical approach	TLPD	OR time (min)	EBL (cc)	Morbidity (%)	Mortality (n/%)	Length of stay (day)
Kendrick [7]	2010	62	PL n=54	62	368	240	42	1(1.6)	7
			RA n=8						
Cho [6]	2009	15	OR n=15	0	338	445	27	0	16
Pugliese [8]	2008	19	CO n=6	6	461	180	37	0	18
			OR n=7						
			RA n=1						
			PL n=5						
Gumbs [9]	2008	35	NR	NR	360	300	NR	0	NR
Palanivelu [10]	2007	42	PL n=42	42	370	65	31	1(2)	10
Dulucq [11]	2006	25	CO n=3	13	287	107	32	1(5)	16
			OR n=9						
			PL n=13						
Lu [12]	2006	5	PL n=5	5	528	770	60	1	NR
Guilianotti [13]	2003	8	RA n=8	8	490	NR	37	1(12.5)	NR
			No pancreatic anastomosis (stump sutured closed)						
Gagner [5]	1997	10	CO n=4	4	510	NR	50	0	22
			HA n=2						
			PL n=4						

PL pure laparoscopic, *RA* robotic-assisted, *CO* converted to open, *OR* laparoscopic resection with open reconstruction, *HA* hand assisted, *NR* not recorded quicker recovery, which have been demonstrated for many other procedures. Based on an increasing body of literature with regard to other laparoscopic procedures, it is reasonable to assume that the typical laparoscopic benefits will be realized for patients undergoing LPD. For distal pancreatectomy, advantages of reduced blood loss and complication rate, and shorter hospitalization have been demonstrated for the laparoscopic approach [14]. There are currently no comparative trials of total laparoscopic versus open pancreaticoduodenectomy. Cho and colleagues recently reported a comparison of laparoscopic-assisted (laparoscopic resection with conversion to open for reconstruction) to open pancreaticoduodenectomy. The mean operative time, blood loss, complication rate, and length of hospital stay was similar between the two groups [6]. Despite the potential advantages of minimally invasive approaches, the major morbidity of pancreatic resection is pancreatic fistula and delayed gastric emptying. Whether the laparoscopic approach can reduce either of these complications remains speculative. Current series of LPD, however, suggest that even within the initial learning curve, these complication rates are comparable with those reported in open series, and outcomes beyond the learning curve are eagerly awaited.

Despite these favorable outcomes, operative time and length of hospital stay should not be the determining factor in the success and acceptance of LPD. While admittedly these are of some benefit, they are of least concern to the patient. Rather, the patient is far more concerned about a successful oncologic procedure, an uncomplicated recovery, and an acceptable quality of life. A prospective assessment, measuring quality of life in patients undergoing laparoscopic and open pancreaticoduodenectomy is currently underway and results are forthcoming.

28.8.2 Adequacy of Oncologic Resection

While LPD is clearly feasible, the oncologic adequacy and outcomes of this approach have not been adequately evaluated. Existing series lack sufficient number of patients and length of follow-up to accurately assess the definitive oncologic outcomes such as disease free or overall survival. Palanivelu and colleagues reported 40 patients with malignancy undergoing LPD. Median survival for the total group was 49 months and 5-year survival of 30.7% and 19.1% for ampullary and pancreatic ductal adenocarcinoma respectively. Until large series containing long-term follow-up are available to assess disease-free and overall survival, potential surrogates to assess the quality of the oncologic resection may include the extent of resection, resection margin status, and number of lymph nodes harvested. Based on these outcomes, early results of LPD are comparable to those reported for open pancreaticoduodenectomy suggesting at least the possibility of noninferiority. Table 28.3 shows the oncologic outcomes of the largest series of LPD to several series of open pancreaticoduodenectomy for adenocarcinoma [2, 15, 16]. Acknowledging that these studies are not directly comparable due to the heterogeneity of the patients undergoing LPD, it appears that outcomes are comparable. A randomized, controlled trial is needed to substantiate any potential outcome advantages of laparoscopic over open approaches. It is unlikely that this will be done in the near future given the lack of enough expertise with such a complex procedure, few centers performing the procedure, and the number of patients required to make a valid statistical comparison.

28.9 Future Considerations

28.9.1 Robotic Whipple

Recently, robotic-assisted approaches for LPD appear to be attracting more enthusiasm and several centers are beginning to gather preliminary experience. This technology may facilitate the widespread application of minimally invasive pancreaticoduodenectomy as dissection and suturing more closely approximate the skills of open surgery. However, these potential advantages may be balanced by the disadvantage of lack of haptic feedback, especially in pancreatic resection and reconstruction. Controlled trials performed by those experienced with both approaches will be necessary to establish any potential advantages of robotic assistance over purely laparoscopic approaches.

Table 28.3 Selected series of laparoscopic and open pancreaticoduodenectomy

Author	Laparoscopic approach			Open approach		
	Kendrick [7]	Palanivelu [10]	Dulucq [11]	Katz [2]	Sohn [16]	Schnelldorfer [15]
Publication year	2010	2007	2006	2009	2000	2008
Patients (n)	62	42	22[a]	329	526	357
Operative data						
Operative time (min)	368	370	287	NR	NR	353
Estimated blood loss (mL)	240	65	107	950	750	889
Clinical diagnosis						
Invasive cancer diagnosis (%)	73	95	82	100	100	100
Pancreatic adenocarcinoma (%)	50	21	50	100	100	100
Pathology data						
Mean tumor size (cm)	3	2.9	2.8	3	3.1	3.2
Lymph nodes retrieved (n)	15	13	18	15	NR	NR
Regional LN metastases (%)	60	NR	NR	48	73	49
R0 resection (%)	89	100	100	84	70	77
Postoperative data						
Major complication (%)	42	31	32	NR	31	39
Mortality n (%)	1(1.6)	1(2)	1(8)	4(1%)	12(2.3)	5(1.4)
LOS (d)	7	10	16	12	13.7	14.7

LN lymph node, LOS length of stay, d day
[a] Includes patients undergoing laparoscopic resection with open reconstruction (n=9)

28.9.2 Training

Several studies have demonstrated improved outcomes of pancreatic resection when performed by experienced surgeons in high-volume centers [17]. If this is valid for open surgery, it would seem to apply even more so for LPD. Currently, many experienced hepatobiliary surgeons have little experience in advanced laparoscopic surgery. Laparoscopic cholecystectomy, splenectomy, distal pancreatectomy, and minor liver resection require little in the way of advanced laparoscopic skills and require no reconstruction. Conversely, surgeons with advanced laparoscopic skills in other areas are not typically experienced in hepatobiliary oncology. The subject of training for such advanced laparoscopic hepatobiliary procedures is an important one. In the author's opinion, the safe broad expansion of LPD will require modification of current training models in hepatobiliary surgical fellowships to have advanced laparoscopic training as a prerequisite or as an integrated part of the fellowship.

Quick Reference Guide

1. Six 12-mm trocars are placed in a semicircular line to allow versatility of all instruments to improve exposure and access throughout the procedure
2. Perform a thorough exploration to rule out metastases and assess local resectability. A Kocher maneuver and dissection around the pancreatic neck facilitates assessment of local tumor invasion. Intraoperative laparoscopic ultrasound is also helpful
3. Pass an umbilical tape around the pancreatic neck to assist with retraction, exposure, and maintenance of a "no-touch" technique. Transect the gastroduodenal artery, duodenum (pylorus preservation), and bile duct

4. Dissect the distal duodenum and proximal jejunum from the left side of the patient. Transect the jejunum and divide the jejunal mesentery back to the uncinate process using the Ligasure. Pass the jejunal stump into the supramesocolic compartment
5. Transect the inferior aspect of the pancreatic neck with ultrasonic shears up to the pancreatic duct. Divide the pancreatic duct sharply with scissors and then complete the parenchymal transection with the ultrasonic shears
6. Dissect the pancreatic head and uncinate process off mesenteric vessels and portal vein using Ligasure. Specifically identify and ligate or clip superior and inferior pancreaticoduodenal vessels
7. Extract the specimen in an endobag through the infraumbilical port site, extending this incision just enough to accommodate the specimen
8. The end-to-side pancreaticojejunostomy is facilitated by a Silastic stent during placement of sutures. This can be removed prior to tying sutures, or left in place to pass spontaneously. All anastomotic reconstruction is performed from the patient's right side
9. An end-to-side hepaticojejunostomy is created with a single layer of either running or interrupted Vicryl suture
10. For the pylorus-preserving procedure, an end-to-side duodenojejunostomy is created with two layers of running Vicryl

References

1. Jemal, A., Siegel, R., Ward, E., et al.: Cancer statistics 2008. CA Cancer J. Clin. **58**, 71–96 (2008)
2. Katz, M.H.G., Wang, H., Fleming, J.B.: Long-term survival after multidisciplinary management of resected pancreatic adenocarcinoma. Ann. Surg. Oncol. **16**, 836–847 (2009)
3. Tseng, J.F., Chandrajit, P.R., Lee, J.E., et al.: Pancreaticoduodenectomy with vascular resction: margin status and survival duration. J. Gastrointest. Surg. **8**, 935–950 (2004)
4. Gagner, M., Pomp, A.: Laparoscopic pylorus-preserving pancreaticoduodenectomy. Surg. Endosc. **8**, 408–410 (1994)
5. Gagner, M., Pomp, A.: Laparoscopic pancreatic resection: is it worthwhile? J. Gastrointest. Surg. **1**, 20–26 (1997)
6. Cho, A., Yamamoto, H., Nagata, M.: Comparison of laparoscopy-assisted and open pylorus-preserving pancreaticoduodenectomy for periampullary disease. Am. J. Surg. **198**, 445–449 (2009)
7. Kendrick, M.L., Cusati, D.: Total laparoscopic pancreaticoduodenectomy: feasibility and outcome in an early experience. Arch. Surg. **145**, 19–23 (2010)
8. Pugliese, R., Scandroglio, I., Sansonna, F.: Laparoscopic pancreaticoduodenectomy: a retrospective review of 19 cases. Surg. Laparosc. Endosc. Percutan. Tech. **18**, 13–18 (2008)
9. Gumbs, A.A., Gayet, B.: The laparoscopic duodenopancreatectomy: the posterior approach. Surg. Endosc. **22**, 539–550 (2008)
10. Palanivelu, C., Jani, K., Senthilnathan, P., et al.: Laparoscopic pancreaticoduodenectomy: technique and outcomes. J. Am. Coll. Surg. **205**, 222–230 (2007)
11. Dulucq, J.L., Wintringer, P., Mahajna, A.: Laparoscopic pancreaticoduodenectomy for benign and malignant diseases. Surg. Endosc. **20**, 1045–1050 (2006)
12. Lu, B., Cai, X., Lu, W.: Laparoscopic pancreaticoduodenectomy to treat cancer of the ampulla of Vater. JSLS **10**, 97–100 (2006)
13. Giulianotti, P.C., Coratti, A., Angelini, M.: Robotics in general surgery. Arch. Surg. **138**, 777–784 (2003)
14. Kooby, D.A., Gillespie, T., Bentrem, D., et al.: Left-sided pancreatectomy: a multicenter comparison of laparoscopic and open approaches. Ann. Surg. **428**(3), 438–446 (2008)
15. Schnelldorfer, T., Ware, A.L., Sarr, M.G., et al.: Long-term survival after pancreaticoduodenectomy for pancreatic adenocarcinoma: is cure possible? Ann. Surg. **247**, 456–462 (2008)
16. Sohn, T.A., Yeo, C.J., Cameron, J.L., et al.: Resected adenocarcinoma of the pancreas – 616 patients: results, outcomes, and prognostic indicators. J. Gastrointest. Surg. **4**, 567–579 (2000)
17. Eppsteiner, R.W., Csikesz, N.G., McPhee, J.T., et al.: Surgeon volume impacts hospital mortality for pancreatic resection. Ann. Surg. **249**, 635–640 (2009)

Cancer of the Adrenal Gland

Ronald Matteotti, Luca Milone, Daniel Canter, and Michel Gagner

29.1 Introduction

The adrenal glands are small but vital structures for homeostasis. This chapter reviews the approach to evaluating adrenal masses, discusses indications for adrenalectomy perioperative management, and provides an overview of surgical techniques for adrenalectomy. A surgeon emabarking on care of a patient needing adrenalectomy should be familiar with adrenal physiology, the anatomy of the retroperitoneum, as well as be conversant in imaging modalities to view the adrenal gland.

29.2 Clinical Indications for Adrenal Surgery

29.2.1 Suspected Malignancy

Greater than 85% of incidentally-discovered adrenal lesions are benign adenomas [1, 2]. The incidence of adrenocortical carcinomas (ACC) is approximately 1 per million [3–5].

Three factors will help the surgeon differentiate between adrenocortical carcinomas and a benign adenoma:

- Size of the mass
- Radiologic characteristics
- Rate of growth of the mass

29.2.1.1 Influence of Size of the Adrenal Mass on Surgical Decision Making

The medium diameter of an adrenal mass incidentally discovered at the time of imaging for other reasons is 3 cm [6]. Large masses, typically those greater than 6 cm, should automatically be removed since >30% will prove to be cancerous [7] unless imaging reveals macroscopic fat. Macroscopic fat suggests a myelolipoma [8]. Masses indentified incidentally that are less than 4 cm in diameter require a metabolic evaluation and close follow-up with imaging but automatic resection is not necessary [9, 10]. On the other hand, the incidence of malignancy in masses between 4 and 6 cm is approximately 6%, and the consensus is to resect these masses in individuals who are at an acceptable risk for surgery [1, 2, 6, 11, 12]. Following these guidelines, a surgeon will have a 93% sensitivity and 42% specificity for identifying a malignant adrenal lesion [6].

R. Matteotti
Surgical Oncologist/Minimally Invasive Surgeon,
263 Osborn Street, Philadelphia, PA 19128, USA
e-mail: ronald.matteotti@gmail.com

L. Milone
Department of Surgery, Staten Island University Hospital,
475 Seaview Avenue,
Staten Island, NY 10305, USA
e-mail: lucamilone@gmail.com

D. Canter
Fellow Urologic Oncology, Fox Chase Cancer Center,
Philadelphia, PA, USA
e-mail: daniel.canter@fccc.edu

M. Gagner
Department of Surgery, Florida International University,
Mount Sinai Medical Center
e-mail: gagner.michel@gmail.com

29.2.1.2 Radiographic Assessment of an Adrenal Lesion

Radiologic findings of a large, heterogeneous, poorly-circumscribed mass should immediately raise concern. The majority of adrenal lesions are small, homogeneous, and have regular contours [13]. Adrenal masses that are less than 4 cm and are hormonally inactive belong to the subgroup that needs the closest attention to the imaging morphology in determining whether resection is warranted.

In addition to assessment of size, homogeneity, and contours, lesion density is helpful in determining the etiology of an adrenal mass. Adenomas are differentiated from other lesions by assessment of intracytoplasmic lipid content. A diagnosis of an adrenal adenoma on a CT without contrast is almost 100% specific [14]. Lesions that exhibit attenuation of <10 HU on unenhanced CT are typically adenomas [9]. It is important to note, however, that 30% of adrenal adenomas will demonstrate attenuation above this level [15–17]. Such lesions will be read as indeterminate. The majority of these lipid-poor adenomas that exhibit a density above 10 HU can still be differentiated from other adrenal pathology using "washout" imaging technique. The specificity for lesions that lose more than 40–60% of gained enhancement on delayed contrast-enhanced CT imaging (i.e. those that "washout") is close to 100% and so these lesions should be managed as adenomas [15–18].

Magnetic resonance imaging is a newer modality for characterizing adrenal neoplasms. The intracellular fat content of adrenal lesions can be evaluated by opposed phase chemical-shift strategies [19]. The presence of abundant cytoplasmic lipid demonstrated by the loss of signal intensity on out-of-phase sequences when compared to in-phase images predicts the presence of an adenoma [13, 20]. MR chemical-shift imaging is arguably superior to unenhanced CT in characterizing indeterminate lesions [21, 22], CT washout studies are however the gold standard in characterizing lipid-poor adenomas [19, 23–25]. MR-based washout techniques are not clinically useful, since gadolinium contrast agents do not possess the dose-dependent signal intensity properties that are inherent in iodinated contrast agents (i.e. gadolinium contrast agents do not "washout") [19] (Fig. 29.1).

29.2.1.3 Observing Growth Kinetics of an Adrenal Lesion

Malignant transformation of adrenal incidentalomas is low, in the range of 1 in 1,000 [7]. If based on the above criteria, an adrenal mass is managed conservatively, and current recommendations are that they be followed 6, 12, and as possible at 24 months with imaging studies [2, 9]. Approximately 5% to 9% of adrenal masses grow at least 1 cm in diameter upon interval follow-up [7, 26] and, typically, growth in the follow-up period should result in a recommendation for resection [2]. These patients should, however, be counseled that the chances of uncovering malignant pathology based on interval growth are low [2].

29.2.2 Functional Adrenal Mass

Hormonal testing should be conducted on all adrenal incidentalomas, since over 11% will show metabolic activity [9]. Cortisol-producing adenomas are found in 5.3% of cases, while aldosteronomas uncovered in approximately 1% and 5.1% of incidentalomas will prove to be pheochromoctyomas [1, 2]. Those lesions that are hypermetabolic should typically be resected.

29.2.3 Isolated Adrenal Metastasis

Retrospective series suggest that in patients with a history of previous malignancy, 50% of new adrenal lesions are metastatic [27, 28]. Isolated metastases to the adrenal are at times resected; however, such cases require a thoughtful multidisciplinary approach [27, 29–33]. Common primary tumors metastasizing to the adrenal include (Fig. 29.2).

- Small cell lung cancer
- Renal cell carcinoma
- Melanoma
- GI – cancer
- Breast – CA
- Hepatocellular – CA

29.2.4 Cushing's Syndrome

Cushing's Syndrome is caused by non-ACTH-dependent production of cortisol most commonly by an adrenal tumor [83]; Cushing's disease is usually produced by an ACTH-secreting pituitary tumor. In addition to treatment of Cushing's syndrome, by resecting the adrenal tumor, the surgeon is at times called upon to treat patients with ACTH-dependent conditions. Trans-sphenoidal pituitary

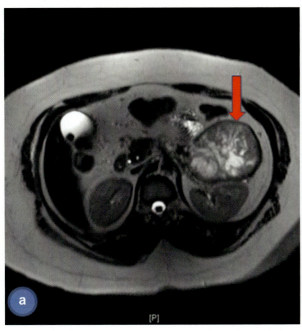
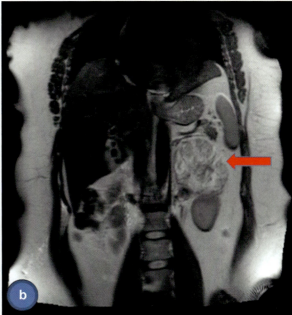

Fig. 29.1 Left adrenal mass: *MRI* (**a**) coronal and (**b**) sagittal

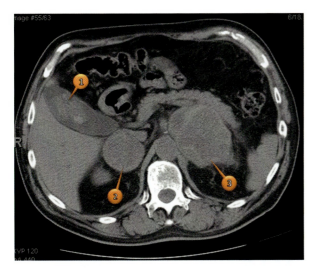

Fig. 29.2 Bilateral adrenal metastasis. *1* – primary gallbladder cancer, *2* – simple metastasis *right* adrenal gland, and *3* – complex, multilobulated metastasis *left* adrenal gland

adenoma resection fails in 20–40% of patients with Cushing's disease [34, 35]. Even in the group of patients deemed to have a successful pituitary adenoma resection, the recurrence of Cushing's disease is 25% [36]. When at least one attempt at neurosurgical correction has failed, bilateral adrenalectomy may be considered by the multidisciplinary team treating the patient. Although rapid resolution of hypercortisolism can be expected, the adrenal surgeon must counsel the patient regarding the life-long need for both glucocorticoid and mineralocorticoid replacement, and a 10–30% chance of developing Nelson–Salassa syndrome [37–40]. The syndrome is characterized by complications such as ocular chiasm compression, oculomotor deficiencies, and rarely a rise in intracranial pressure due to progressive growth of the pituitary adenoma in the absence of appropriate glucocorticoid feedback [40]. Also, it is wise to warn the patient of the remote possibility of leaving residual functional adrenal tissue at the time of the bilateral adrenalectomy [41].

Approximately 10% of all incidence of Cushing's Syndrome is caused by ectopic secretion of ACTH by malignant tissue [42]. Although resection of the primary ACTH-producing tumor is ideal, such approach is possible in only ~10% of patients [43]. Bilateral adrenalectomy is a therapeutic option in the appropriately selected patient [42].

29.3 Work-up of an Adrenal Incidentaloma

29.3.1 General Considerations

All adrenal incidentalomas need a metabolic evaluation, since over 10% secrete hormones [9]. Cortisol and catecholamine levels should be evaluated in all new patients, while patients with hypertension also need to have an evaluation of their aldosterone levels [2, 9]. Collaboration with an endocrinologist is helpful, especially with the nuances of further evaluating abnormal levels of these steroid hormones.

29.3.2 Initial Evaluation for Hypercortisolism

Approximately 5–8% of adrenal masses will exhibit autonomous cortisol hypersecretion (Cushing's syndrome) upon evaluation [1, 7]. In clinical practice, the evaluation of hypercortisolism involves evaluation of exogenous steroid use and once that is excluded, one of the following tests:

- Overnight low-dose dexamethasone suppression test – OST
- Late-night salivary cortisol test
- 24-h urinary-free cortisol evaluation – UFC

All three tests provide relatively equivalent test characteristics [44], though UFC may have a lower sensitivity [45–47].

29.3.3 Initial Evaluation for Hyperaldosteronism – Conn's Syndrome

Hyperaldosteronism as a result of an adrenal mass occurs only 1% of the time in adrenal incidentalomas [1, 48]. First-line screening for Conn's syndrome consists of obtaining a morning plasma aldosterone to renin ratio (ARR). In the setting of an aldosterone level of ≥15 ng/mL, an ARR of ≥20 is suspicious. Five percent of patients with newly diagnosed hypertension will be found to have an alodosterone-secreting adenoma upon work-up [49]. Therefore, all patients with a history of hypertension who are found to have adrenal incidentaloma should be tested for aldosterone hypersecretion. Confirmatory testing is mandatory and consultation with an endocrinologic expert advisable [48, 50]. Adrenal vein sampling is often performed if all other tests are inconclusive [51].

29.3.4 Initial Evaluation for Catecholamine Hypersecretion

Pheochromocytoma occurs in 5% of patients with an adrenal mass [2]. As a result a diagnosis of pheochromocytoma must be entertained and appropriate evaluation performed in all patients with an adrenal mass, even in those in whom metastatic disease is strongly suspected [52]. Arguments that the work-up can be omitted in patients with masses that exhibit a density less than 10 HU are weakened by isolated reports of rare low-density pheochromocytomas that possess an unenhanced attenuation of <10 HU and demonstrate brisk contrast washout [53, 54].

Screening for a pheochromocytoma should include either free fractionated plasma metanephrines or 24-h urinary fractionated metanephrine levels [55, 56]. There is currently some debate regarding which test is superior, though both tests demonstrate excellent sensitivity and specificity. Collaboration with endocrinology is essential for this evaluation [2, 57].

29.3.5 Follow-up Metabolic Testing

Experts suggest that all patients with metabolically inactive adrenal incidentalomas, who are expectantly managed, undergo annual metabolic screening for 3–4 years following diagnosis [9]. The percentage of patients who will develop metabolic activity in subsequent screening exams is in the range of 2% [7].

29.4 Perioperative Considerations

29.4.1 Preventing Postoperative Adrenal Insufficiency

Up to one-fifth of patients have biochemical adrenal insufficiency following adrenalectomy although clinically significant adrenal insufficiency appears to be rare. Patients with Cushing's syndrome in whom the contralateral gland can be suppressed are at an especially high risk and should be monitored closely [45]. Even though the incidence of clinically significant adrenal insufficiency is rare it can be catastrophic. Prior to bilateral adrenalectomy, proactive therapy must be appropriately instituted, since Addisonian crises may result in death [58].

29.4.2 Preoperative Catecholamine Blockade

Patients undergoing resection of pheochromocytoma also require thoughtful perioperative management. The common practice is to employ prophylactic preoperative catecholamine blockade in all patients with pheochromocytoma [59]. With this practice perioperative mortality has decreased from 50% to less than 3% [60, 61].

Alpha-blockade with or without alpha-methyltyrosine, an inhibitor of catecholamine biosynthesis, is the most widely recommended preoperative regimen [59]. Calcium channel blockade alone for patients with mild symptomatology has also been favored by some authors [62]. Catecholamine-induced cardiomyopathy should be evaluated by preoperative echocardiography [63]. Patients should be encouraged to vigorously hydrate themselves once catecholamine blockade is started in order to have an adequate intravascular volume. Some institutions routinely preadmit patients for intravenous fluid administration the day before surgery [60].

29.4.3 Postoperative Management

The lasting effects of the preoperative catecholamine blockade can result in hypotension. Hypoglycemia can also be caused by inhibition of insulin release due to increased catecholamine levels [61, 63]. Some centers routinely admit patients to the intensive care unit following removal of a pheochromocytoma to monitor for these conditions [60].

29.5 Laparoscopic Adrenalectomy for Cancer

The role of laparoscopy in the management of large or malignant adrenal tumors is still controversial. Laparoscopy to remove tumors as large as 15 cm, although reported in the literature [70], is technically challenging mainly due to size, increased vascularity, and difficulty with tumor manipulation.

Adrenal glands are relatively common sites for metastatic disease, but more so if enlarged or malfunctioning, a manifestation of a systemic process [64, 67]. A selective literature review of large series of adrenalectomies reports out of a total of 1,838 cases, an incidence of malignant pathology of 6.5% and of those 40.3% were metastatic disease. Most of the time, the diagnosis of malignancy was made upon final pathology. There was no difference in operative time, complication rate, and morbidities between adrenalectomy for malignant or benign tumors [66, 77] (Table 29.1).

Marangos et al. reported 41 laparoscopic adrenalectomies for metastatic diseases. The medium tumor size was 6 cm with a range of 1.5–15 cm. Only one conversion and one case with a positive margin were reported, and the authors concluded that laparoscopy for metastatic adrenal tumors is feasible, regardless of their size [75].

Table 29.1 Laparoscopic adrenalectomy: Selected reports of malignancy

	Year	Procedures (n)	Malignancy (n)	Metastasis (n)
Naya [78]	2005	126	1	–
Kercher [71]	2005	81	2	–
Palazzo [79]	2006	19	3	–
Walz [81]	2006	560	7	12
Lee [72]	2008	358	48	8
Lezoche [73]	2008	214	10	9
Meyer-Rochow [76]	2008	36	8	3
Humphrey [68]	2008	30	1	–
Berber [65]	2009	172	17	–
Kazaryan [69]	2009	242	22	16
Total		1,838	119	48

29.6 Choosing the Best Surgical Approach to the Adrenal Gland

Despite the abundant literature, the best laparoscopic approach to adrenals is still controversial. The three most commonly performed laparoscopic approaches are

- Lateral transabdominal – LTA
- Retroperitoneal adrenalectomy – REA
- Anterior transabdominal – ATA
  and all have specific advantages and disadvantages (Table 29.2).

29.6.1 Lateral Transabdominal Approach (LTA)

The lateral transabdominal approach is clearly the most commonly used, whereas an anterior transabdominal approach is the least practiced. As no prospective randomized clinical trial has been done on this issue there is no evidence that one approach is superior to the other. LTA is more universally used as it may be applied in the vast majority of adrenalectomies when tumor size poses a limitation in using REA [80]. Another advantage of LTA is the possibility of exploring the entire abdomen and to localize extra-adrenal tissue using intraoperative ultrasound. This aspect is especially important in treating a patient with pheochromocytoma. Also, the supine position allows diagnosing and treating other disease processes, planned or when incidentally found [73].

29.6.2 Retroperitoneal Adrenalectomy (REA)

Retroperitoneal adrenalectomy in the hands of a surgeon familiar with this approach, could result in less blood loss mainly due to the high pressure, 20–28 mmHg, necessary to establish a capno-retroperitoneum and is generally associated with less operative

Table 29.2 The three most common laparoscopic approaches to the adrenal: Advantages and disadvantages

Lateral Trans-abdominal Approach (LTA)	
Advantages	*Disadvantages*
Less dissection	Bilateral adrenalectomy: change of position needed
Less retraction	Certain difficulty in the presence of dense adhesions
Better exposure	More intra-abdominal injuries?
Other intra-abdominal pathologies may be diagnosed and treated	
Retroperitoneal Approach (REA)	
Advantages	*Disadvantages*
Bilateral adrenalectomy: no need for position change if already in Jack-knife position	Small operative field

Potential advantage in:
  Previous abdominal surgery
  Obese patients
  Pregnant patients
	Appropriate only for small tumors <5–6 cm

Avoids intraperitoneal injury?	Inability to diagnose and treat concurrent intra-abdominal pathology
	Lack of familiar landmarks to the average abdominal surgeon
Anterior Trans-abdominal Approach (ATA)	
Advantages	*Disadvantages*
Bilateral adrenalectomy: no need for position change	Difficult exposure
Appropriate for large tumors	More dissection is needed
Other intra-abdominal pathologies may be diagnosed and treated	Longer operative time?

time [65, 68, 69, 71–74, 76, 78–81]. Only three trocars are needed while 4–5 trocars are used for LTA to gain exposure.

REA could be performed through a single posterior access as well. Walz et al. described their experience with single access retroperitoneoscopic adrenalectomy (SARA) using two ports only in a recent series of five patients. A 1.5-cm incision was utilized to remove five adrenal tumors with a maximum diameter of 4 cm. Operative times ranged from 35 to 70 min and no conversion to standard laparoscopy was necessary [82].

29.6.3 Anterior Transabdominal Approach (ATA)

The ATA is abandoned by many surgeons due to difficult dissection involving

- Left adrenal
  - Take down of the left colonic flexure
  - Vicinity of spleen and pancreatic tail with possible injury and high morbidity
- Right adrenal
  - Vicinity of the duodenum
  - Adrenal vein is posterior to the inferior vena cava, and difficult to dissect and control

However, this approach does not require a change of position for bilateral adrenalectomy or if any other intra-abdominal procedure is performed.

29.7 Surgical Anatomy

The adrenal glands are a pair of organs, triangular-shaped, situated at the upper pole of the kidneys. They are located below the 11th rib at the level of the first lumbar vertebrae.

29.7.1 Macroscopic Landmarks

The left adrenal gland has a close relationship to vital structures

- Medial – Aorta and left diaphragmatic crus
- Posterior – Splenic vessels and pancreatic tail
- Anterior – Peritoneum

The right gland lies in a narrow space bordered by

- Inferior vena cava
- Right kidney
- Duodenum
- Right hepatic lobe
- Right diaphragmatic crus

29.7.2 Arterial Supply

The adrenal gland receives its blood supply from three distinct arterial branches
- Superior adrenal artery – Take off at inferior phrenic artery
- Middle adrenal artery – Take off at the aorta
- Inferior adrenal artery – Take off at the renal artery

29.7.3 Venous Drainage

Both adrenal glands are usually drained by a single adrenal vein, referred as well as suprarenal vein. The suprarenal vein on the right side drains into the posterior lateral aspect of the IVC, and the suprarenal vein on the left side drains into the left renal vein or inferior phrenic vein. In 10% of the patients you will encounter accessory veins on the right side draining into the inferior subhepatic vein or inferior phrenic vein. As an anatomical variation, the right adrenal could present itself with two branches of the main vein (Fig. 29.3).

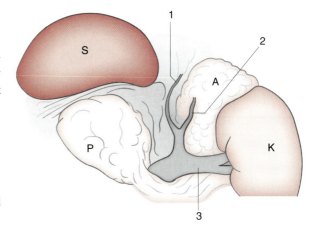

Fig. 29.3 Laparoscopic left adrenalectomy: Exposure of the adrenal vessels. *A* – left adrenal, *P* – pancreas, *K* – kidney, *S* – spleen, *1* – phrenic vein, *2* – adrenal vein, and *3* – renal vein. (Drawing by Hippmann GbR, Schwarzenbruck, Germany)

29.8 Surgical Technique

29.8.1 Lateral Transabdominal Adrenalectomy – LTA Left Side

29.8.1.1 Operating Room Setup and Patient Positioning

Patients are placed in lateral decubitus position with the left side up. A cushion is placed under the patient's right flank and the table is flexed so that the left side is hyperextended. The left arm is extended and suspended. The skin should be prepped extending from the nipple to the anterior superior iliac spine and from the abdominal midline anteriorly to the spine posteriorly. The surgeon and the assistant are positioned on the contralateral side of the lesion. Two monitors are placed one on each side of the patient's head at the top of the operating table (Figs. 29.4 and 29.5).

29.8.1.2 Trocar Placement

We always use an open technique to access the abdominal cavity and do so in the left subcostal area at the level of the anterior axillary line. The first trocar placed is a 10-mm trocar and will be used for the laparoscope. After safe insertion of this first trocar, we establish a pneumoperitoneum at 15 mmHg. A 30°, 10-mm camera is then inserted and a full diagnostic laparoscopy performed, to assess the abdominal cavity

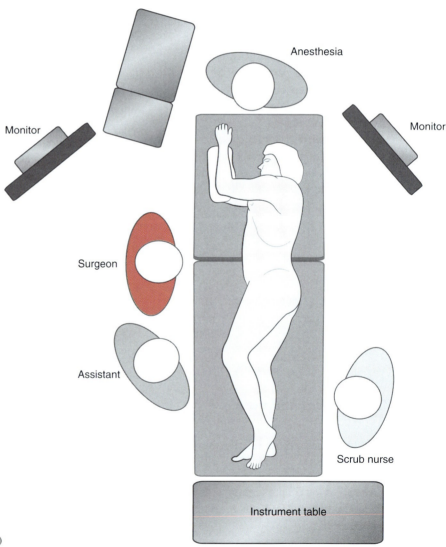

Fig. 29.4 Laparoscopic left adrenalectomy: Operating room setup. (Drawing by Hippmann GbR, Schwarzenbruck, Germany)

29 Cancer of the Adrenal Gland

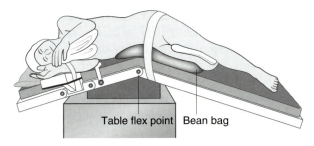

Fig. 29.5 Laparoscopic left adrenalectomy: Patient positioning. (Drawing by Hippmann GbR, Schwarzenbruck, Germany)

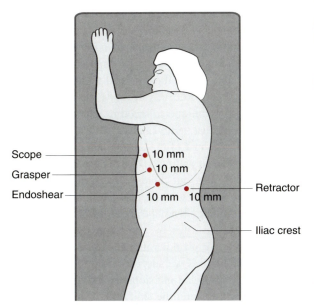

Fig. 29.6 Laparoscopic left adrenalectomy: Trocar placement. (Drawing by Hippmann GbR, Schwarzenbruck, Germany)

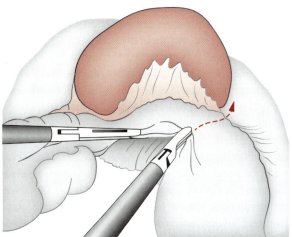

Fig. 29.7 Laparoscopic left adrenalectomy: Division of lieno-renal ligament. (Drawing by Hippmann GbR, Schwarzenbruck, Germany)

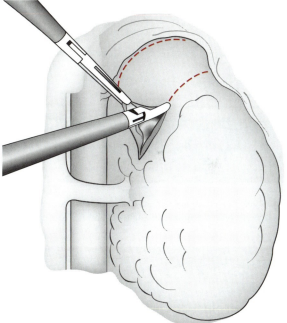

Fig. 29.8 Laparoscopic left adrenalectomy: Inferio–superior dissection line. (Drawing by Hippmann GbR, Schwarzenbruck, Germany)

for adhesions, metastatic disease, or organ abnormality. If the diagnostic laparoscopy excludes local invasion or distant disease, then we will go ahead with further trocar placement. Two more trocars, 5 or 10 mm, are then inserted in the flank, one right below the 11th rib and the second slightly more anterior and medial to the first trocars. Sometimes a fourth trocar is needed for retraction and will be inserted at the costovertebral junction. The camera is now repositioned to the most anterior trocar and the other two trocars are used as working ports (Fig. 29.6).

29.8.1.3 Dissection of the Left Adrenal Gland

Working with hot laparoscopic scissors, the ultrasonic scalpel or Ligasure™ (Covidien-USA) in the right hand, the splenic flexure is mobilized medially and the colon separated from the inferior pole of the adrenal gland to expose the lineo-renal ligament (Fig. 29.7). Next, the lineo-renal ligament is incised infero-superiorly approximately 1 cm away from the spleen (Fig. 29.8). The dissection is carried up to the diaphragm and stopped when the short gastric vessels are encountered posteriorly behind the stomach. This step of the dissection moves the spleen medially and exposes the retroperitoneal space for further dissection (Fig. 29.9). The lateral edge and anterior portion of the adrenal gland will become visible in the perinephric fat superiorly and medially. If necessary, the fourth 5-mm trocar will be used to retract large-sized spleens. In the event that the adrenal gland is not easily identified by now, we will use laparoscopic ultrasound. This will be helpful as well to identify the site of disease within the adrenal gland and the adrenal vein. To avoid fracture of the adrenal capsule, we leave a little periadrenal fat on the adrenal which is used to retract and manipulate the gland instead of grasping the gland itself. Grasping the perinephric fat, dissection of the lateral and anterior part of the adrenal gland is carried out using the hook cautery or Ligasure™ (Fig. 29.10). Once the lateral portion of the gland has been exposed, the dissection is continued inferiorly, to expose and clip the left adrenal vein at the beginning of the dissection. Alternatively, the dissection can be continued superiorly and the vein will be secured at the end. The decision about which route to take, inferior or superior, depends on the exposure gained after mobilizing the spleen and on the size of the adrenal gland. In case of big glands, >5 cm, the superior approach will help obtain a better visualization of the adrenal vein. When the vein is visualized it will be dissected free in its circumference to facilitate the insertion of the clips or secure placement of a sealing device. It is not necessary to identify the confluence of adrenal and renal vein. The adrenal vein should be clipped about 1 cm from the renal vein and then divided with straight laparoscopic scissors. Recently we have started to use a total clip-less technique, dissecting and dividing the adrenal vein by just using Ligasure™ (Covidien-USA) (Fig. 29.11). The rest of the adrenal dissection is now completed with the sealing device of choice, Ligasure™ (Covidien-USA) in our hands. After obtaining complete hemostasis, the gland is inserted into an endobag and extracted in total from the abdomen through one of the 10-mm trocar sites by spreading the abdominal wall muscles. We do not routinely place a drain but will not hesitate to if we suspect an injury to the pancreatic tail. The fascial incisions are closed with a 2-0 absorbable sutures and the skin with 4-0 subcuticular absorbable sutures.

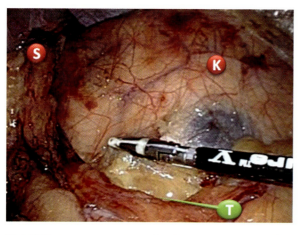

Fig. 29.9 Laparoscopic left adrenalectomy: Dissection line. *T* – line of Toldt, *S* – spleen, medialized, and *K* – kidney

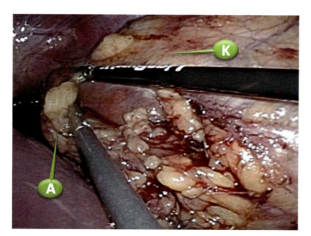

Fig. 29.10 Laparoscopic left adrenalectomy: Developing the plane between *K* left kidney and *A* left adrenal gland

29.8.2 Lateral Transabdominal Adrenalectomy – LTA Right Side

29.8.2.1 Patient Positioning and Trocar Placement

The patient is positioned in the same way as described for a left-sided lesion. Pneumoperitoneum is established using an open technique. A 10-mm trocar is inserted 2 cm below and parallel to the costal margin and a 30°, 10 mm, laparoscope is inserted. Under direct vision three additional 10-mm trocars are positioned. The second trocar is placed in the right flank, inferior and posterior to the tip of the 11th rib just above the hepatic flexure of the colon. In contrast to a left-sided

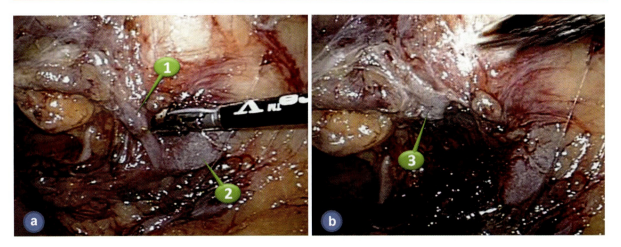

Fig. 29.11 Laparoscopic left adrenalectomy: Dissection of adrenal vein. (**a**) Before dissection and (**b**) after dissection with Ligasure™, *1* – left adrenal vein, *2* – left renal vein, and *3* – left adrenal vein after dissection

adrenal lesion it is usually not necessary to mobilize the hepatic flexure. The third trocar is inserted in the most anterior position of the subcostal area between the epigastrium and anterior axillary line, lateral to the edge of the ipsilateral rectus muscle. The last trocar is introduced either at the tip of the 12th rib or at the costo-vertebral subcostal angle. Before doing so the peritoneal reflection of the lateral edge of the right kidney has to be dissected to avoid injury to the kidney. Four trocars are necessary because the right lobe of the liver must be retraced (Fig. 29.12).

29.8.2.2 Dissection of the Right Adrenal Gland

With upward retraction of the liver we expose the medial aspect of the adrenal gland. The liver retractor should be positioned in the most anterior port. It is often unavoidable to mobilize the liver in order to obtain the best exposure of the junction between the adrenal gland and the inferior vena cava. The right lateral hepatic attachments and the triangular ligament are dissected using ultrasonic scalpel or Ligasure™ (Covidien-USA). This dissection will permit more effective retraction to push the liver medially. This is the key step of the dissection to provide adequate exposure of the confluence of right adrenal vein and inferior vena cava (Fig. 29.13). The dissection of the right gland is now started from the infero-lateral edge and continued medially and upward along the lateral edge of the inferior vena cava. This dissection exposes the adrenal vein that is often short. If the vein is too big to

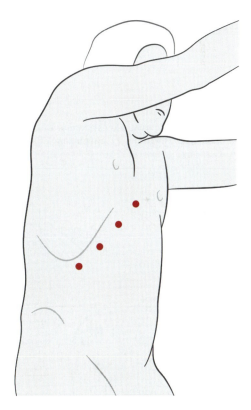

Fig. 29.12 Laparoscopic right adrenalectomy: Trocar placement. (Drawing by Hippmann GbR, Schwarzenbruck, Germany)

be clipped or a sealing device proves to be unsafe we will use an EndoGIA with a vascular cartridge. The superior pole of the gland is then dissected free. Small branches from the inferior phrenic vessels will be clipped or ligated with Ligasure™ (Fig. 29.14). The

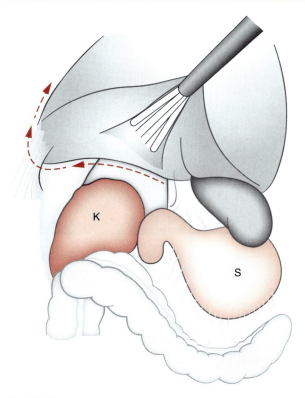

Fig. 29.13 Laparoscopic right adrenalectomy: Liver retraction and dissection line. (Drawing by Hippmann GbR, Schwarzenbruck, Germany)

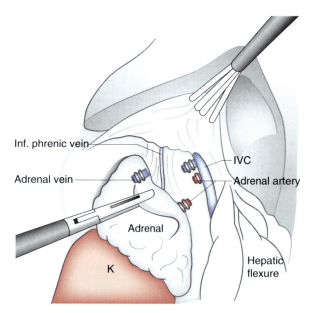

Fig. 29.14 Laparoscopic right adrenalectomy: Right adrenal vessel dissection and control. (Drawing by Hippmann GbR, Schwarzenbruck, Germany)

dissection is concluded on the lateral side. The gland is placed in an endobag and removed from the most anterior trocar site. The laparoscopic wounds are closed the same way as described for left-sided lesions.

29.8.3 Anterior Transabdominal Adrenalectomy (ATA)

29.8.3.1 Patient Positioning and Trocar Placement

Patients are placed in a supine position. The first assistant, holding the camera, stands on the right side of the patient, while the primary surgeon positions her/himself on the left side. We establish a pneumoperitoneum of 13 mmHg using an open technique. The first trocar, 10 mm, is placed at the umbilicus and is used for the camera. We routinely use 30°, 10-mm laparoscope. A diagnostic laparoscopy is performed to assess operability. Once extensive or local invasive disease is excluded we proceed with placement of the remaining trocars. Three 5- or 10-mm trocars are placed under direct vision: one in the epigastrium, the next in the left subcostal area on the semiclavicular line, and the last right in the middle between trocar two and three in the subcostal area.

29.8.3.2 Dissection of the Adrenal Gland

The operation begins by lifting up the transverse meso colon to expose the ligament of Treitz and identifying the inferior mesenteric vein (IMV). In thin patients, it is often possible to see the left renal vein shining through the retro peritoneum. The posterior peritoneum is opened laterally to the IMV and close to inferior border of the pancreas. This maneuver allows clear visualization of the left renal vein and the left middle adrenal vein.

The adrenal vein is then isolated, clipped, or divided with Ligasure™. The dissection of the left adrenal gland is done with a combination of blunt dissection and sealing devices in a medial to lateral direction. After complete dissection of the adrenal gland, it will be placed into a specimen retrieval bag and extracted through the umbilical port site. We do not routinely place a drain but will do so if an injury to the pancreatic tail is suspected or if we experience diffuse slow ooze from the resection site. All port sites are closed in two layers – fascia and skin – with absorbable sutures.

29.8.4 RetroPeritoneal Adrenalectomy (REA)

29.8.4.1 Patient Positioning and Trocar Placement

The patient is positioned prone, lying on a rectangular support that allows the ventral abdominal wall to hang through. A 1.5-cm transverse incision just below the tip of the 12th rib is performed and the retroperitoneal space is reached using blunt and sharp dissection. A small cavity is digitally formed for insertion of one 5-mm trocar 4–5 cm lateral and beneath the 11th rib. This initial trocar is placed under finger guidance. The same technique is applied to a 10-mm trocar inserted 4–5 cm medial to the initial incision and about 3 cm below the 12th rib. This trocar should be pushed into the retroperitoneal space and directed cranially at an angle of 45°. A blunt balloon trocar and an adjustable sleeve is introduced through the initial incision and locked in place by inflating the balloon. The capno-retroperitoneum is created and maintained at a pressure of 20–28 mmHg. The higher insufflations pressure chosen, when compared to regular laparoscopy, help both in creating and maintaining the retroperitoneal space necessary to perform the dissection. The high pressure decreases as does the bleeding rate. A 10-mm/30° endoscope is used, which is initially introduced into the middle trocar and, after creating the retroperitoneal space, will be placed into the trocar nearest to the spine.

29.8.4.2 Dissection of the Adrenal Gland

The first step of the operation is to create a retroperitoneal space below the diaphragm by pushing down the adipose tissue. This allows visualization of the upper pole of the kidney which is then mobilized. By these two simple steps, often done bluntly, we accomplish exposure of the adrenal gland. One of the instruments is now used to retract the mobilized upper pole of the kidney. Sometimes it is necessary to place a fourth trocar below the first line of ports to facilitate retraction of the kidney. Mobilization of the adrenal gland begins medial and caudal between the diaphragmatic branch and adrenal gland. In this area on the right side, the arteries of the adrenal gland run posterior to the inferior vena cava. These vessels are traditionally secured by electro-coagulation, clips, or at our institution by Ligasure™ (Covidien-USA) only. By lifting up the adrenal gland, the inferior vena cava is visualized posteriorly in its retroperitoneal-cranial segment. The short supra-renal vein thus becomes clearly visible running postero-laterally. This vessel is followed to a length of 1 cm and divided with Ligasure™. Dissection of the right adrenal gland is completed by lateral and cranial dissection. For left-sided adrenal lesions, the adrenal gland vein must be dissected in the space between the adrenal gland and the diaphragmatic branch medial to the upper pole of the kidney. After dissection of the main vein lateral to the confluence with the diaphragmatic vein, dissection of the adrenal gland is continued medially, laterally, and cranially until the entire gland is freed circumferentially. The golden-brown adrenal gland is placed in a nonpermeable retrieval bag and extracted through one of the trocar sites. We do not place drains routinely. The wounds are then closed in layers with absorbable sutures.

Quick Reference Guide

1. Preoperative work-up is key to successful adrenal surgery
2. Every newly diagnosed adrenal mass requires a functional evaluation to rule out hormone-secreting lesions
3. Preoperative conditioning includes
   - Two weeks prior to surgery: α – Blockade with Phenoxybenzamine 30–60 mg/day
   - 3 days prior to surgery: β-Blockade with Inderal 10 mg p.o. TID
   - 1–2 days prior to surgery: start to hydrate the patient

4. Choose the surgical approach most appropriate to treat the pathology and which matches your skill set
    - Lateral transabdominal – LTA (The most practiced approach)
    - Anterior transabdominal – ATA
    - Retroperitoneal adrenalectomy – REA
5. Avoid injury to the capsule of the adrenal gland and maintain good oncological practice at all times
6. Always perform a diagnostic laparoscopy first to exclude local invasion or distant disease and base your further surgical decision on your findings
7. Knowledge about surgical anatomy is absolutely mandatory!
    - Arteries: can be divided between clips or clipless using Ligasure™
    - Veins: Ligasure is usually sufficient; be aware that the adrenal vein on the right side could be large and will require an EndoGIA vascular load

    Keep in mind that the right adrenal vein could have two main branches and be prepared
8. Macroscopic landmarks:

    Left adrenal gland:
    - Medial – Aorta and left diaphragmatic crus
    - Posterior – Splenic vessels and pancreatic tail
    - Anterior – Peritoneum

    Right adrenal gland:
    - Inferior vena cava
    - Right kidney
    - Duodenum
    - Right hepatic lobe
    - Right diaphragmatic crus
9. Always remove the specimen using an impermeable endobag to avoid spillage of tumor cells
10. We do not routinely place a drain except if we suspect an injury to the pancreatic tail or encounter diffuse oozing without obvious source

References

1. Young Jr., W.F.: Management approaches to adrenal incidentalomas. A view from Rochester, Minnesota. Endocrinol. Metab. Clin. North Am. **29**, 159–185 (2000). x
2. Young Jr., W.F.: The incidentally discovered adrenal mass. N Engl J. Med. **356**, 601–610 (2007)
3. Aubert, S., Wacrenier, A., Leroy, X., et al.: Weiss system revisited: a clinicopathologic and immunohistochemical study of 49 adrenocortical tumors. Am. J. Surg. Pathol. **26**, 1612–1619 (2002)
4. Fassnacht, M., Allolio, B.: Clinical management of adrenocortical carcinoma. Best Pract. Res. Clin. Endocrinol. Metab. **23**, 273–289 (2009)
5. Roman, S.: Adrenocortical carcinoma. Curr. Opin. Oncol. **18**, 36–42 (2006)
6. Mantero, F., Terzolo, M., Arnaldi, G., et al.: A survey on adrenal incidentaloma in Italy. Curr. Opin. Oncol. **85**(2), 637–644 (2000)
7. Barzon, L., Sonino, N., Fallo, F., et al.: Prevalence and natural history of adrenal incidentalomas. Eur. J. Endocrinol. **149**, 273–285 (2003)
8. Han, M., Burnett, A.L., Fishman, E.K., et al.: The natural history and treatment of adrenal myelolipoma. J. Urol. **157**, 1213–1216 (1997)
9. Grumbach, M.M., Biller, B.M.K., Braunstein, G.D., et al.: Management of the clinically inapparent adrenal mass ("Incidentaloma"). Ann. Intern. Med. **138**, 424–429 (2003)
10. Cicala, M.V., Sartorato, P., Mantero, F.: Incidentally discovered masses in hypertensive patients. Best Pract. Res. Clin. Endocrinol. Metab. **20**, 451–266 (2008)
11. Barry, M.K., van Heerden, J.A., Farley, D.R., et al.: Can adrenal incidentalomas be safely observed? World J. Surg. **22**, 599–604 (1998)
12. Thompson, G.B., Young Jr., W.F.: Adrenal incidentaloma. Curr. Opin. Oncol. **15**, 84–90 (2003)
13. Korobkin, M., Giordano, T.J., Brodeur, F.J., et al.: Adrenal adenomas: relationship between histologic lipid and CT and MR findings. Radiology **200**, 743–747 (1996)
14. Hamrahian, A.H., Ioachimescu, A.G., Remer, E.M., et al.: Clinical utility of noncontrast computed tomography attenuation value (hounsfield units) to differentiate adrenal adenomas/hyperplasias from nonadenomas: Cleveland clinic experience. J. Clin. Endocrinol. Metab. **90**, 871–877 (2005)
15. Szolar, D.H., Korobkin, M., Reittner, P., et al.: Adrenocortical carcinomas and adrenal pheochromocytomas: mass and enhancement loss evaluation at delayed contrast-enhanced CT. Radiology **234**, 479–485 (2005)
16. Korobkin, M., Brodeur, F.J., Francis, I.R., et al.: CT time-attenuation washout curves of adrenal adenomas and nonadenomas. Am. J. Roentgenol. **170**, 747–752 (1998)
17. Pena, C.S., Boland, G.W.L., Hahn, P.F., et al.: Characterization of indeterminate (lipid-poor) adrenal masses: use of washout characteristics at contrast-enhanced CT. Radiology **217**, 798–802 (2000)
18. Heinz-Peer, G., Memarsadeghi, M., Niederle, B.: Imaging of adrenal masses. Curr. Opin. Urol. **17**, 32–38 (2007)
19. Hussain, H.K., Korobkin, M.: MR imaging of the adrenal glands. Magn. Reson. Imaging Clin. N. Am. **12**, 515–544 (2004). vii
20. Namimoto, T., Yamashita, Y., Mitsuzaki, K., et al.: Adrenal masses: quantification of fat content with double-echo chemical shift in-phase and opposed-phase FLASH MR images for differentiation of adrenal adenomas. Radiology **218**, 642–646 (2001)
21. Israel, G.M., Korobkin, M., Wang, C., et al.: Comparison of unenhanced CT and chemical shift MRI in evaluating lipid-rich adrenal adenomas. Am. J. Roentgenol. **183**, 215–219 (2004)

22. Haider, M.A., Ghai, S., Jhaveri, K., et al.: Chemical shift MR imaging of hyperattenuating (>10 HU) adrenal masses: does it still have a role? Radiology **231**, 711–716 (2004)
23. Caoili, E.M., Korbkin, M., Francis, I.R., et al.: Delayed enhanced CT of lipid-poor adrenal adenomas. Am. J. Roentgenol. **175**, 1411–1415 (2000)
24. Park, B.K., Kim, C.K., Kim, B., et al.: Comparison of delayed enhanced CT and chemical shift MR for evaluating hyperattenuating incidental adrenal masses. Radiology **243**, 760–765 (2007)
25. Boland, G.W., Blake, M.A., Hahn, P.F., et al.: Incidental adrenal lesions: principles, techniques, and algorithms for imaging characterization. Radiology **249**, 756–775 (2008)
26. Libe, R., Dall'Asta, C., Barbetta, L., et al.: Long-term follow-up study of patients with adrenal incidentalomas. Eur. J. Endocrinol. **147**, 489–494 (2002)
27. Lenert, J.T., Barnett, C.C., Kudelka, A.P., et al.: Evaluation and surgical resection of adrenal masses in patients with a history of extra-adrenal malignancy. Surgery **130**, 1060–1067 (2001)
28. Frilling, A., Tecklenborg, K., Weber, F., et al.: Importance of adrenal incidentaloma in patients with a history of malignancy. Surgery **136**, 1289–1296 (2004)
29. Tanvetyanon, T., Robinson, L.A., Schell, M.J., et al.: Outcomes of adrenalectomy for isolated synchronous versus metachronous adrenal metastases in non-small-cell lung cancer: a systematic review and pooled analysis. J. Clin. Oncol. **26**, 1142–1147 (2008)
30. Mercier, O., Fadel, E., de Perrot, M., et al.: Surgical treatment of solitary adrenal metastasis from non-small cell lung cancer. J. Thorac. Cardiovasc. Surg. **130**, 136–140 (2005)
31. Collinson, F.J., Lam, T.K., Bruijn, W.M., et al.: Long-term survival and occasional regression of distant melanoma metastases after adrenal metastasectomy. Ann. Surg. Oncol. **15**, 1741–1749 (2008)
32. Mittendorf, E.A., Lim, S.J., Schacherer, C.W., et al.: Melanoma adrenal metastasis: natural history and surgical management. Am. J. Surg. **195**, 363–368 (2008). discussion 368–369
33. O'Malley, R.L., Godoy, G., Kanofsky, J.A., et al.: The necessity of adrenalectomy at the time of radical nephrectomy: a systematic review. J. Urol. **181**, 2009–2017 (2009)
34. Pivonello, R., De Martino, M.C., De Leo, M., et al.: Cushing's syndrome. Endocrinol. Metab. Clin. North Am. **37**, 135–149 (2008). ix
35. Newell-Price, J., Bertagna, X., Grossman, A.B., et al.: Cushing's syndrome. Lancet **367**, 1605–1617 (2006)
36. Patil, C.G., Prevedello, D.M., Lad, S.P., et al.: Late recurrences of Cushing's disease after initial successful transsphenoidal surgery. J. Clin. Endocrinol. Metab. **93**, 358–362 (2008)
37. Chow, J.T., Thompson, G.B., Grant, C.S., et al.: Bilateral laparoscopic adrenalectomy for corticotrophin-dependent Cushing's syndrome: a review of the Mayo clinic experience. Clin. Endocrinol. (Oxf) **68**, 513–519 (2008)
38. Vella, A., Thompson, G.B., Grant, C.S., et al.: Laparoscopic adrenalectomy for adrenocorticotropin-dependent Cushing's syndrome. J. Clin. Endocrinol. Metab. **86**, 1596–1599 (2001)
39. Lacroix, A.: Evaluation of bilateral laparoscopic adrenalectomy in adrenocorticotropic hormone-dependent Cushing's syndrome. Nat. Clin. Pract. Endocrinol. Metab. **4**, 310–311 (2008)
40. Assie, G., Bahurel, H., Coste, J., et al.: Corticotroph tumor progression after adrenalectomy in Cushing's disease: a reappraisal of Nelson's syndrome. J. Clin. Endocrinol. Metab. **92**, 172–179 (2007)
41. Kemink, L., Hermus, A., Pieters, G., et al.: Residual adrenocortical function after bilateral adrenalectomy for pituitary-dependent Cushing's syndrome. J. Clin. Endocrinol. Metab. **75**, 1211–1214 (1992)
42. Porterfield, J., Thompson, G., Young, W., et al.: Surgery for Cushing's syndrome: an historical review and recent ten-year experience. World J. Surg. **32**, 659–677 (2008)
43. Aniszewski, J.P., Young Jr., W.F., Thompson, G.B., et al.: Cushing syndrome due to ectopic adrenocorticotropic hormone secretion. World J. Surg. **25**, 934–940 (2001)
44. Elamin, M.B., Murad, M.H., Mullan, R., et al.: Accuracy of diagnostic tests for Cushing's syndrome: a systematic review and metaanalyses. J. Clin. Endocrinol. Metab. **93**, 1553–1562 (2008)
45. Tsagarakis, S., Vassiliadi, D., Thalassinos, N.: Endogenous subclinical hypercortisolism: diagnostic uncertainties and clinical implications. J. Endocrinol. Invest. **29**, 471–482 (2006)
46. Mitchell, I.C., Auchus, R.J., Juneja, K., et al.: "Subclinical Cushing's syndrome" is not subclinical: improvement after adrenalectomy in 9 patients. Surgery **142**, 900–905 (2007). discussion 905 e1
47. Nieman, L.K., Biller, B.M., Findling, J.W., et al.: The diagnosis of Cushing's syndrome: an Endocrine Society Clinical Practice Guideline. J. Clin. Endocrinol. Metab. **93**, 1526–1540 (2008)
48. Young, W.F.: Primary aldosteronism: renaissance of a syndrome. Clin. Endocrinol. (Oxf) **66**, 607–618 (2007)
49. Rossi, G.P., Bernini, G., Caliumi, C., et al.: A prospective study of the prevalence of primary aldosteronism in 1, 125 hypertensive patients. J. Am. Coll. Cardiol. **48**, 2293–2300 (2006)
50. Mulatero, P., Stowasser, M., Loh, K.-C., et al.: Increased diagnosis of primary aldosteronism, including surgically correctable forms, in centers from five continents. J. Clin. Endocrinol. Metab. **89**, 1045–1050 (2004)
51. Young, W.F., Stanson, A.W., Thompson, G.B., et al.: Role for adrenal venous sampling in primary aldosteronism. Surgery **136**, 1227–1235 (2004)
52. Tsvetov, G., Shimon, I., Benbassat, C.: Adrenal incidentaloma: clinical characteristics and comparison between patients with and without extraadrenal malignancy. J. Endocrinol. Invest. **30**, 647–652 (2007)
53. Blake, M.A., Krishnamoorthy, S.K., Boland, G.W., et al.: Low-density pheochromocytoma on CT: a mimicker of adrenal adenoma. Am. J. Roentgenol. **181**, 1663–1668 (2003)
54. Blake, M.A., Kalra, M.K., Sweeney, A.T., et al.: Distinguishing benign from malignant adrenal masses: multi-detector row CT protocol with 10-minute delay. Radiology **238**, 578–585 (2005)
55. Pacak, K., Eisenhofer, G., Ahlman, H., et al.: Pheochromocytoma: recommendations for clinical practice from the First International Symposium. Nat. Clin. Pract. Endocrinol. Metab. **3**, 92–102 (2007). October 2005

56. Grossman, A., Pacak, K., Sawka, A., et al.: Biochemical diagnosis and localization of pheochromocytoma: can we reach a consensus? Ann. NY Acad. Sci. **1073**, 332–347 (2006)
57. Eisenhofer, G., Siegert, G., Kotzerke, J., et al.: Current progress and future challenges in the biochemical diagnosis and treatment of pheochromocytomas and paragangliomas. Horm. Metab. Res. **40**, 329–337 (2008)
58. Asari, R., Scheuba, C., Kaczirek, K., et al.: Estimated risk of pheochromocytoma recurrence after adrenal-sparing surgery in patients with multiple endocrine neoplasia type 2A. Arch. Surg. **141**, 1199–1205 (2006)
59. Pacak, K.: Preoperative management of the pheochromocytoma patient. J. Clin. Endocrinol. Metab. **92**, 4069–4079 (2007)
60. Lenders, J.W., Eisenhofer, G., Mannelli, M., et al.: Phaeochromocytoma. Lancet **366**, 665–675 (2005)
61. Pacak, K., Linehan, W., Eisenhofer, G., et al.: Recent advances in genetics, diagnosis, localization, and treatment of pheochromocytoma. Ann. Intern. Med. **134**, 315–329 (2001)
62. Ulchaker, J.C., Goldfarb, D.A., Bravo, E.L., et al.: Successful outcomes in pheochromocytoma surgery in the modern era. J. Urol. **161**, 764–767 (1999)
63. Kinney, M.A.O., Narr, B.J., Warner, M.A.: Perioperative management of pheochromocytoma. J. Cardiothorac. Vasc. Anesth. **16**, 359–369 (2002)
64. Abrams, H.L., Spiro, R., Goldstein, N.: Metastases in carcinoma; analysis of 1000 autopsied cases. Cancer **3**(1), 74–85 (1950)
65. Berber, E., et al.: Comparison of laparoscopic transabdominal lateral versus posterior retroperitoneal adrenalectomy. Surgery **146**(4), 621–625 (2009). discussion 625–626
66. Eto, M., et al.: Laparoscopic adrenalectomy for malignant tumors. Int. J. Urol. **15**(4), 295–298 (2008)
67. Greene, F.L., et al.: Minimal access cancer management. CA Cancer J. Clin. **57**(3), 130–146 (2007)
68. Humphrey, R., et al.: Laparoscopic compared with open adrenalectomy for resection of pheochromocytoma: a review of 47 cases. Can. J. Surg. **51**(4), 276–280 (2008)
69. Kazaryan, A.M., et al.: Laparoscopic adrenalectomy: Norwegian single-center experience of 242 procedures. J. Laparoendosc. Adv. Surg. Tech. A **19**(2), 181–189 (2009)
70. Kebebew, E., et al.: Results of laparoscopic adrenalectomy for suspected and unsuspected malignant adrenal neoplasms. Arch. Surg. **137**(8), 948–951 (2002). discussion 952–953
71. Kercher, K.W., et al.: Laparoscopic curative resection of pheochromocytomas. Ann. Surg. **241**(6), 919–926 (2005). discussion 926–928
72. Lee, J., et al.: Open and laparoscopic adrenalectomy: analysis of the National Surgical Quality Improvement Program. J. Am. Coll. Surg. **206**(5), 953–959 (2008). discussion 959–961
73. Lezoche, E., et al.: Flank approach versus anterior sub-mesocolic access in left laparoscopic adrenalectomy: a prospective randomized study. Surg. Endosc. **22**(11), 2373–2378 (2008)
74. Lin, Y., et al.: Experience of retroperitoneoscopic adrenalectomy in 195 patients with primary aldosteronism. Int. J. Urol. **14**(10), 910–913 (2007)
75. Marangos, I.P., et al.: Should we use laparoscopic adrenalectomy for metastases? Scandinavian multicenter study. J. Surg. Oncol. **100**(1), 43–47 (2009)
76. Meyer-Rochow, G.Y., et al.: Outcomes of minimally invasive surgery for phaeochromocytoma. ANZ J. Surg. **79**(5), 367–370 (2009)
77. Moinzadeh, A., Gill, I.S.: Laparoscopic radical adrenalectomy for malignancy in 31 patients. J. Urol. **173**(2), 519–525 (2005)
78. Naya, Y., et al.: Laparoscopic adrenalectomy in patients with large adrenal tumors. Int. J. Urol. **12**(2), 134–139 (2005)
79. Palazzo, F.F., et al.: Long-term outcome following laparoscopic adrenalectomy for large solid adrenal cortex tumors. World J. Surg. **30**(5), 893–898 (2006)
80. Rubinstein, M., et al.: Prospective, randomized comparison of transperitoneal versus retroperitoneal laparoscopic adrenalectomy. J. Urol. **174**(2), 442–445 (2005). discussion 445
81. Walz, M.K., et al.: Posterior retroperitoneoscopic adrenalectomy – results of 560 procedures in 520 patients. Surgery **140**(6), 943–948 (2006). discussion 948–950
82. Walz, M.K., Alesina, P.F.: Single access retroperitoneoscopic adrenalectomy (SARA) – one step beyond in endocrine surgery. Langenbecks Arch. Surg. **394**(3), 447–450 (2009)
83. Kutikov, A., Morgan, T.: www.urologymatch.com (2010). Accessed on 4th June

Part IX

Special Topics: Gynecology

30. Minimally Invasive Management of Gynecologic Malignancies

Farr Reza Nezhat, Jennifer Eun Sun Cho, Connie Liu, and Gabrielle Gossner

30.1 Introduction

Laparoscopy was used for a second-look assessment in ovarian cancer patients back in the 1970s. However, it is only with the advent of new developments in equipment in the late 1980s and early 1990s, along with the vision of pioneers in laparoscopic surgery that has made operative laparoscopy in gynecologic oncology feasible. Laparoscopy has multiple benefits in the cancer patient, including image magnification to visualize metastatic or recurrent disease in the deep pelvis, anterior abdominal wall, and upper abdomen, improved dissection, and fewer injuries in challenging areas such as the retro peritoneum. There is decreased bleeding from small vessels due to the pressure from pneumoperitoneum, shorter hospital stay, and faster recovery. Postoperative complications such as ileus and small bowel obstruction, wound infection and separation, and thrombo-embolic events are less with laparoscopy than laparotomy. Postoperative chemotherapy or radiation can be initiated earlier, and radiation complications from bowel adhesions are minimized. Significant progress has been made in the last two decades in gynecologic malignancy. In this chapter, the application of laparoscopy in cervical, endometrial, and ovarian cancer are presented.

F.R. Nezhat (✉), J.E.S. Cho, C. Liu, and G. Gossner
Department of Minimally Invasive Surgery, St. Luke's Roosevelt Hospital, 425 West 59th Street, Suite 9B, Yew York, NY 10021, USA
e-mail: fnezhat@chpnet.org

30.2 Laparoscopy and Applications in Cervical Carcinomas

Cervical cancer is the most common gynecologic cancer in the world, and has been diagnosed in approximately 11,070 women in 2008 in the USA [1]. Nearly 4,000 individuals succumbed to the disease in the same year. As familiarity with laparoscopy has increased and surgical skills have improved over the years, it has been actively utilized in staging and surgical treatment of cervical cancer.

30.2.1 Indications for Laparoscopy in Cervical Cancer

Laparoscopy has been used in the management of both early and advanced stages of cervical cancer in a number of different applications. In early cervical cancer, laparoscopy has been utilized to perform pelvic and para-aortic lymphadenectomy along with a laparoscopic-assisted radical vaginal hysterectomy or vaginal trachelectomy, total laparoscopic radical hysterectomy or a radical trachelectomy. In advanced stages, pretreatment surgical staging with pelvic and para-aortic lymphadenectomy has become a useful way to direct treatment. Laparoscopy has also been applied prior to a pelvic exenteration, laparoscopic ovarian transposition, and laparoscopically guided interstitial radiation implant placement, although the data are limited in these clinical scenarios.

30.2.2 Surgical Technique

30.2.2.1 General Considerations and Required Instruments

Appropriate preoperative counseling and written informed consent is obtained. All patients receive perioperative prophylactic antibiotics, and the procedure is performed under general anesthesia in the dorsal lithotomy position with Allen stirrups and sequential compression devices on both lower extremities (Fig. 30.1). Patients are prepped and draped in the usual sterile fashion, and a Foley catheter is placed prior to incision and remains in position for the duration of the procedure. An intrauterine manipulator is placed if possible. Different instruments can be used for desiccation such as the bipolar device, harmonic shears (©Ethicon Endo-Surgery, Inc), Ligasure™ (©ValleyLab), Gyrus™ (©Gyrus ACMI), or Enseal™ (Ethicon). Additional instruments can be used for grasping and dissection such as the Nezhat-Dorsey suction irrigator (©Davol), atraumatic graspers, endoshears, and bowel graspers. Our preferred method is to use the harmonic shears and endo-shears for fine dissection, and the Ligasure for dessication of big vessels [2, 3] (Fig. 30.2).

30.2.2.2 Laparoscopic Radical Hysterectomy

This method describes the technique that can be performed via traditional laparoscopy or robotic-assisted laparoscopy using the DaVinci™ (Intumed) system which consists of the surgeon's console, surgical cart, and video cart (Fig. 30.3).

Trocar Placement

The four trocar approach is utilized, with entry into the abdomen obtained in the standard fashion using the Veress needle or direct trocar entry technique. The initial 5–10 mm trocar is placed in the periumbilical area (Fig. 30.4). CO_2 is used to insufflate the abdomen to maintain an intra-abdominal pressure of 15 mmHg. Two 5-mm trocars are placed in the bilateral lower quadrants 2–3 cm above the anterior superior iliac spine and a 10-mm trocar is placed in the suprapubic area under direct visualization (Fig. 30.5).

Diagnostic Laparoscopy

Exploration of the abdomen and pelvis is performed. Any lesions suspicious for malignancy are biopsied and sent to pathology. If there is any evidence of endometriosis or severe adhesions, these would be treated first. Perfect knowledge of pelvic anatomy is essential (Fig. 30.6).

Recto-aginal Space

The radical hysterectomy is started by developing the recto-vaginal space. The uterus is anteverted, and a moist sponge on a forceps is placed into the posterior fornix to assist in the visualization of the appropriate surgical plane. The peritoneum between the uterosacral ligaments is incised using the harmonic shears, and the rectum gently dissected away from the vagina (Fig. 30.7).

Vesico-aginal Space

The attention shifts to the pelvic side wall dissection where the round ligaments are desiccated and cut using the harmonic shears. The anterior leaf of the broad ligament is opened, and the bladder flap developed using both sharp and blunt dissection. The bladder is pushed off the lower uterine segment, cervix, and

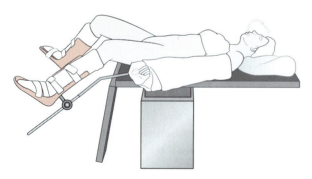

Fig. 30.1 Patient positioning: lithotomy position with legs in Allen stirrups, arms tucked, and patient securely strapped. (Drawing by Hippmann GbR, Schwarzenbruck, Germany)

Fig. 30.2 Operating room setup. (Drawing by Hippmann GbR, Schwarzenbruck, Germany)

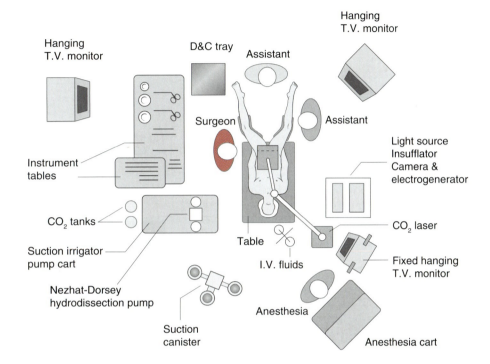

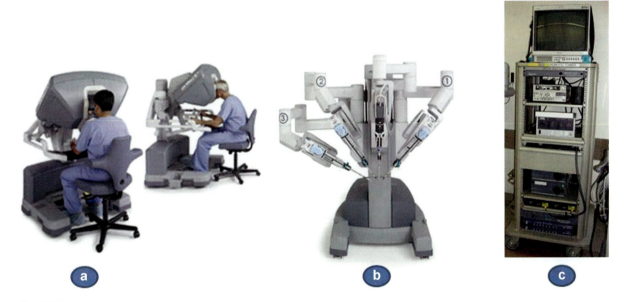

Fig. 30.3 Robotic equipment. (**a**) The console (**b**) the robot, and (**c**) the video cart

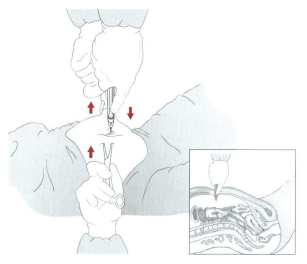

Fig. 30.4 Trocar placement. Insertion of first trocar: abdominal wall is lifted up and trocar inserted perpendicularly. (Drawing by Hippmann GbR, Schwarzenbruck, Germany)

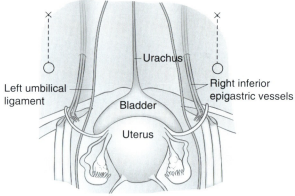

Fig. 30.6 Pelvic anatomy. (Drawing by Hippmann GbR, Schwarzenbruck, Germany)

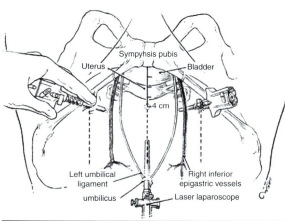

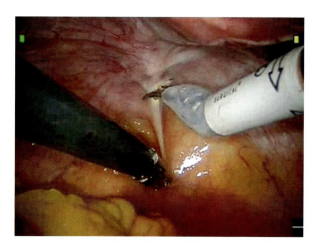

Fig. 30.7 Laparoscopic radical hysterectomy: development of recto-vaginal space

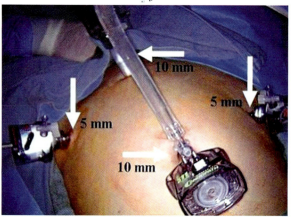

Fig. 30.5 Trocar placement. Laparoscopic procedure: 10-mm trocars placed in the umbilicus and the suprapubic area, 5-mm trocars placed in the lateral lower abdomen

upper vagina. A sponge on a forceps is again inserted into the anterior vaginal fornix to facilitate development of the vesico-vaginal space (Figs. 30.8 and 30.9).

Addressing the Adnexa

If the adnexa are to be removed, the infundibulo-pelvic ligament is isolated, desiccated, and cut. If the adnexa are preserved, the utero-ovarian ligament and the proximal portion of the fallopian tube is desiccated using available blood vessel sealing devices and divided.

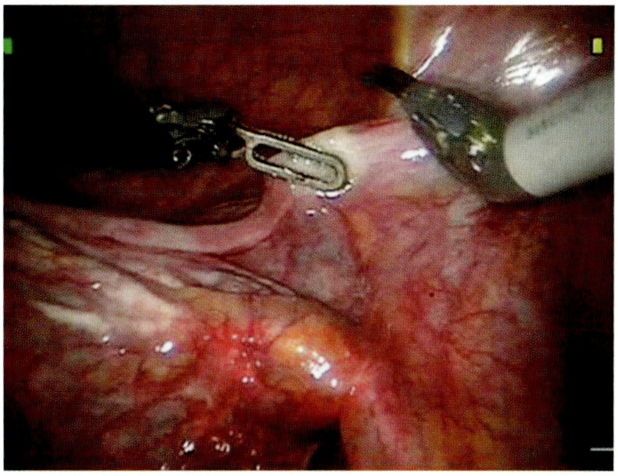

30 Minimally Invasive Management of Gynecologic Malignancies

Fig. 30.8 Laparoscopic radical hysterectomy: opening of pelvic sidewall

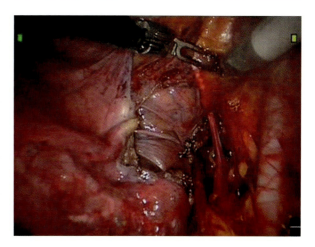

Fig. 30.10 Laparoscopic radical hysterectomy: dissection of obturator fossa

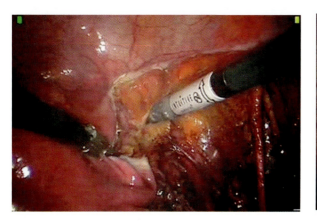

Fig. 30.9 Laparoscopic radical hysterectomy: development of vesico-vaginal space

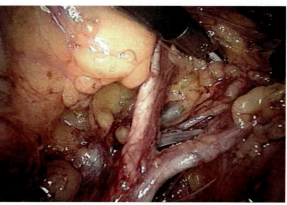

Fig. 30.11 Laparoscopic radical hysterectomy: transection of uterine artery

The posterior broad ligament is opened using the harmonic shears, and the para-vaginal and para-rectal spaces developed by blunt dissection.

Para-vesicle Space

The para-vesicle space is then developed by placing tension on the obliterated hypogastric artery using the tip of the suction irrigator and grasping forceps, between the iliac vessels laterally and obliterated hypogastric artery and bladder medially. The dissection is carried inferior to the iliac vessels, and the obturator nerve is identified. At this time the lymphadenectomy is carried out (Fig. 30.10).

Para-rectal Space and Uterine Artery

The obliterated hypogastric artery (superior vesical artery) is placed on upward tension, and the origin of the uterine artery from the internal iliac vessels is identified. The para-rectal space is developed by blunt dissection between the following borders:

- Medial – rectum
- Lateral – ureter
- Anterior – uterine artery
- Posterior – sacrum

The uterine artery is desiccated or divided between clips (Fig. 30.11).

Dissection of the Ureter

The uterine vessels are placed on medial tension, and the ureter is identified and unroofed. The curved tip of the endoshears is used to dissect the ureter out of the tunnel all the way to the bladder (Fig. 30.12).

Transection of the Uterus and Removal of Specimen

The complete uterosacral-cardinal ligament complex and vagina are then divided using harmonic shears, Ligasure™, or a laparoscopic stapling device. The laterality of the dissection is decided based on the size of the cervical lesion. The uterus is then completely separated from the vagina and removed through the vagina (Figs. 30.13 and 30.14).

Closure of Vaginal Cuff

The vaginal cuff is closed either vaginally or laparoscopically using 0 Polyglactin or Polydiaxanone monofilament sutures in figure-of-eight technique or running fashion (Fig. 30.15).

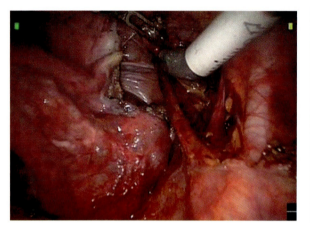

Fig. 30.12 Laparoscopic radical hysterectomy: unroofing of ureters

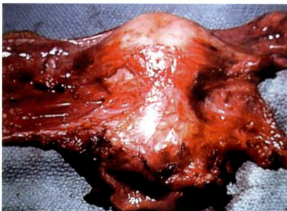

Fig. 30.14 Laparoscopic radical hysterectomy: surgical specimen: uterus, cervix, and 2–3 cm of vaginal tissue

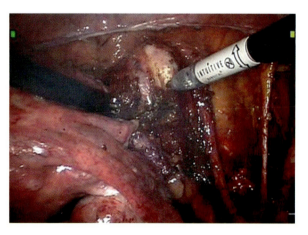

Fig. 30.13 Laparoscopic radical hysterectomy: colpotomy

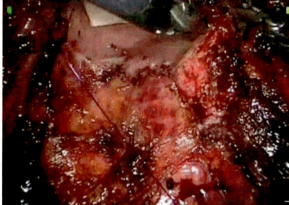

Fig. 30.15 Laparoscopic radical hysterectomy: vaginal cuff closure

30.2.2.3 Lymphadenectomy

Trocar Placement

The technique of lymphadenectomy involves resection of the pelvic and para-aortic nodes in a manner similar to that performed in open surgery. The port placement is important in ensuring adequate accessibility to the lymph nodes and is similar to that of the hysterectomy, as described above, if a pelvic lymphadenectomy is planned. In a para-aortic lymphadenectomy up to the inferior mesenteric artery (IMA), the port placement is the same except another 5-mm trocar is placed in the right or left midabdomen, at the same level of the lower trocar to allow traction on the bowel for optimal exposure. In robotic-assisted procedures, a 10-mm port is placed at the umbilicus and two 8-mm ports are inserted under direct vision about 4 fingerbreadths lateral and inferior to the umbilical port. If para-aortic lymphadenectomy is planned, the 10-mm midline port is placed 4–8 cm above the umbilicus, and the 8-mm ports positioned accordingly. A 5–10-mm accessory port is placed in between the umbilical midline port and one of the lateral ports. An additional accessory port can be placed in the suprapubic area. There needs to be enough space between port sites to prevent interference from nearby trocars and instruments. Instruments commonly used include atraumatic graspers and an electrocautery device such as the harmonic shears or the Ligasure™ [2].

Pelvic Lymphadenectomy

- Pelvic wall dissection is performed as described before, and para-vesical and para-rectal spaces are developed.
- Lymph nodes from the midcommon iliac vessels and external iliac vessels down to the level of the deep circumflex veins are removed using the harmonic shears.
- The obturator nerve and vessels are identified, and the lymph nodes between the obturator nerve and external iliac vessels are removed. The iliac vessels are retracted laterally for this portion of the procedure. Care is taken to avoid injury to the obturator nerve and the hypogastric vein which runs below the hypogastric artery.
- The lymph nodes are removed either through the vagina, or through an endocatch bag, which can be removed through any of the 10–12-mm trocars (Fig. 30.16).

Para-aortic Lymph Node Dissection

- We usually start by elevating and incising the peritoneum overlying the right common iliac artery, extending the incision over the sacral promontory and above the IMA, exposing the vessels underneath.

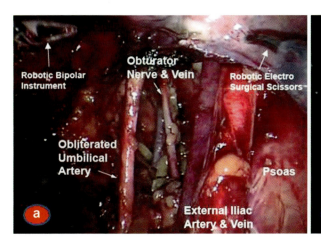
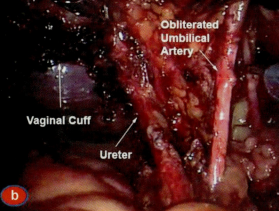

Fig. 30.16 Pelvic Lymphadenectomy. (**a**) Lymph nodes are removed from the common external iliac vessels, hypogastric vessels, and obturator fossa. (**b**) The obturator nerve and ureter are identified before dissection occurs

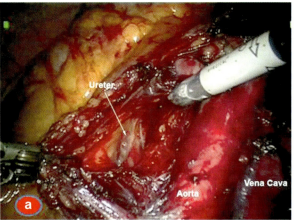

Fig. 30.17 Para-Aortic Lymphadenectomy. (**a**) The ureter is identified during dissection. The lymph nodes left of the aorta are dissected. A similar procedure is done on the right side of the aorta. (**b**) Anatomy after completed lymphadenectomy: Aorta, inferior mesenteric artery, inferior vena cava

- The underlying retro peritoneum is developed by sharp and blunt dissection. The right ureter is identified, and the lymph nodes along the right side of the aorta are carefully separated, being cautious to avoid injury to the inferior vena cava lying directly underneath.
- The left side may be more difficult because of the proximity and location of the IMA and sigmoid colon. The left ureter is identified, and the lymph nodes between the IMA and the left common iliac vessels are carefully detached. If indicated, the lymph chain above the IMA and below the renal vessels is removed as well.
- The peritoneal incision over the sacral promontory is extended, exposing the presacral nodes, lying between the aortic bifurcation. They are firmly grasped, and excised using the harmonic shears. Small vessels are coagulated to assure perfect hemostasis.
- The lymph nodes are removed either through the vagina, or via an endocatch bag (Fig. 30.17).

Retroperitoneal Lymphadenectomy – The Technique

The patient is placed in the dorsal lithotomy position or supine on the operating table. The surgeons stand on the left side of the patient and the monitor is positioned on the right side.

- The operation starts as a standard diagnostic laparoscopy as described above. A 5- or 10-mm trocar is placed at the umbilicus to survey the abdominal cavity for any metastatic disease. If none is noted, the lymphadenectomy is initiated.
- A 15-mm incision is made 3–4 cm medial to the left iliac spine, and extended down through the fascia. The peritoneum is not incised. The surgeon bluntly dissects the peritoneum from the abdominal muscles under laparoscopic visualization. The dissection is extended into the iliac fossa, and then more medially over the left common iliac artery. The more blunt dissection that is done with the finger, the faster the endoscopic dissection that follows.
- When dissection is sufficient to introduce two trocars into the newly created space, a 10-mm trocar superior and posterior to the first incision (on the mid-axillary line), and a 5-mm trocar on the anterior axillary line, approximately 5 cm below the ribs, will be inserted. A balloon trocar is placed into the 15-mm incision, with the balloon carefully positioned in the extraperitoneal space under laparoscopic guidance, inflated with saline, and secured to the abdominal wall. The camera is inserted through this trocar, while the other two trocars accommodate instruments to carry out the lymphadenectomy.
- The peritoneal cavity is now deflated while the retroperitoneal space is inflated. The left psoas muscle, left ureter, and left common iliac artery are identified before any dissection is started. Further dis-

section of the space is then accomplished using grasping forceps, monopolar scissors, harmonic shears, and bipolar cautery to control any bleeding.
- After enough dissection is completed, attention is drawn to the right lateral common iliac nodes and presacral nodes which are identified and dissected off the inferior vena cava. The right lateral caval nodes are then removed as well, taking care not to injure the vena cava.
- The left side requires caution and clear knowledge of the normal anatomy. The IMA, ovarian vessels, and the ureter are identified, and the lymph nodes below the renal vessels are dissected and removed first. The removal continues with the left lateral retro-caval and retro-aortic lymph nodes.
- The surgical field is examined and checked for hemostasis. After the procedure is completed, the peritoneum is fenestrated to the abdominal cavity to drain a possible lymphocele that may occur. The extraperitoneal space is deflated, and the incisions closed.

30.2.3 Early Stage Cervical Carcinoma

The standard treatment for early stage cervical cancer, Stage IA2 to Stage IIA is a radical hysterectomy, along with pelvic and possible para-aortic lymphadenectomy. Advanced stages are treated with chemo/radiation. The radical hysterectomy has been traditionally accomplished through a generous abdominal incision. Over the last two to three decades, there has been much incorporation of minimally invasive techniques in the surgical management of the early stage cervical cancer patient, from total laparoscopic hysterectomies to trachelectomies.

30.2.3.1 Radical Vaginal Hysterectomy

Radical vaginal surgery has been performed in the past, with two distinct forms described in the literature:

- Schauta–Amreich – *more radical*
- Schauta–Stoeckel – *less radical*

In either form, the hysterectomy is completed through the vagina, with care taken to identify the ureters and uterine vessels. The procedure was initially described by Anton Pawlik, but was popularized by Frederik Schauta [2].

Schauta–Amreich

The patient is positioned in the dorsal lithotomy position, prepped and draped in usual sterile fashion with preoperative antibiotics administered. After a dilute solution of Pitressin (1 ampoule in 60–100 cc of normal saline) is injected into the left medio-lateral perineum, a Schuchardt incision is made, which is a type of enlarged medio-lateral episiotomy which enlarges the operative field and increases access to the left para-rectal space. Kocher forceps are then placed onto the vaginal mucosa at the junction between the upper and middle thirds, and traction is exerted on the forceps resulting in an internal prolapse of the vaginal wall around the cervix, forming a vaginal cuff. Layers of mucosa are separated by injecting Pitressin circumferentially between the placed forceps. Using a scalpel, an incision is made circumferentially in the vaginal mucosa beyond the tips of the Kocher clamps. A full thickness incision through three layers of the vaginal wall is made on the anterior and posterior aspects of the developed vaginal cuff with a scalpel. Only the mucosal layer is incised in the dorso-lateral aspects, between the 3–4 o'clock and 8–9 o'clock areas so as to preserve the relationship between the vaginal cuff and para-cervical ligaments. The vaginal cuff is separated from the rest of the vagina, and folded over the cervix with strong grasping clamps. It is then strongly retracted dorsally to allow the ventral aspect of the uterus and surrounding tissues to be freed from the vagina. Care must be taken to identify the bladder and the terminal ureter, which is attached to the para-cervical and parametrial ligaments and must be separated carefully. The vesico-vaginal space must be identified and dissected before the bladder pillars are approachable. Once the left para-vesical space is developed, the ureter can be isolated, and the bladder pillar can be divided. The uterine artery can then be located, dissected, and ligated close to its origin. The right para-vesical space is opened and the right ureter and uterine artery are performed in a similar manner. Attention is then directed posteriorly, where the posterior peritoneal fold is opened, the intestines are packed away, and the rectum displaced posteriorly with a retractor. The rectal pillars are now identified and transected close to the rectum. The cardinal ligaments can then be divided. Care must be taken to retract the bladder away. The anterior peritoneum is then opened and the uterine fundus is delivered through it. The round ligaments and infundibulo-pelvic ligaments can be divided if the ovaries are to be removed. The peritoneum and vaginal cuff can then be closed according to the preference of the surgeon. The Schuchardt incision is then repaired.

Schauta–Stoeckel

A Schauta–Stoeckel radical vaginal hysterectomy is less radical than its counterpart, with major differences being that the Schauta–Stoeckel operation does not involve a Schuchardt incision and the cardinal ligaments are divided at its midpoint.

The Schauta hysterectomy became less popular due to the inherent inability of the technique to perform a lymphadenectomy, which was partially overcome with the onset of laparoscopy and the ability to perform lymphadenectomy. The two techniques of laparoscopy and vaginal hysterectomy evolved over time into laparoscopically assisted radical vaginal hysterectomy and total laparoscopic radical hysterectomy. The largest series to date was reported by Hertel et al., who performed a laparoscopically assisted vaginal radical hysterectomy on 200 patients. The average operating time was 333 min, with a mean of 22 pelvic lymph nodes removed. Intraoperative complications included 1 bowel injury, four blood vessel injuries, 7 ureteral injuries, and 14 bladder injuries. The median follow-up was 40 months, with an estimated 5-year survival of 83% [4]. With advancement of new instrumentation and technology, laparoscopic-assisted radical vaginal hysterectomy has not been widely used around the world for the management of cervical cancer. Instead, total laparoscopic or robotic-assisted total laparoscopic radical hysterectomy gained more and more acceptance.

30.2.3.2 Total Laparoscopic Radical Hysterectomy

The first total laparoscopic radical hysterectomy with pelvic and para-aortic lymphadenectomy was performed by Nezhat et al. in June 1989 and was published in the early 1990s [2]. Since then, numerous authors have reported their experience with laparoscopic radical hysterectomy (Table 30.1). One cohort study comparing laparoscopy and laparotomy is published by Zakashansky et al. [3]. There were a total of 60 women in the study; 30 individuals underwent a laparoscopic radical hysterectomy, 30 patients underwent laparotomy. Compared to the laparotomy group, the laparoscopic group had less blood loss (200 vs 520 mL), more nodes retrieved (31 vs 21.8 pelvic nodes), and a shorter hospital stay (3.8 vs 5.6 days). Intra- and postoperative complications and recurrence rates were similar in both groups and not statistically significant. These findings illustrate that laparoscopy leads to superior surgical outcomes when compared to traditional open surgery.

There is currently a multicenter, international, randomized study done by Obermair et al., comparing laparoscopy and robotic techniques to laparotomy [5]. If completed, the study will be the first blinded, randomized clinical trial comparing laparoscopy and robotic-assisted laparoscopy versus laparotomy.

30.2.3.3 Robotic Radical Hysterectomy

Enhanced robotic technology has been utilized to complete more radical cases in patients with cervical cancers than any other gynecologic malignancy. Much of the literature is in the form of case series and case reports. The largest studies comparing robotic-assisted radical hysterectomy to laparoscopy were conducted by Nezhat et al. and Magrina et al. Nezhat et al. prospectively compared robotic-assisted laparoscopy to traditional laparoscopy in patients with early stage cervical carcinoma in a fellowship program [6]. His group found that the robotic technique was equivalent to the laparoscopic approach. No statistical difference was observed regarding operative time (323 vs. 318 min), pelvic lymph node retrieval (24.7 vs. 31 nodes), estimated blood loss (157 vs. 200 mL), or hospital stay (2.7 vs. 3.8 days) between the robotic-assisted laparoscopy and traditional laparoscopy groups, respectively. None of the robotics or laparoscopic procedures required conversion to laparotomy and postoperative complications were comparable.

Magrina et al. compared three groups, robotic-assisted laparoscopy, traditional laparoscopy, and laparotomy and concluded that the robotic and laparoscopic groups were very similar in their surgical outcomes, and were preferable over laparotomy [7]. Blood loss and length of hospital stay were similar for laparoscopy and robotics and reduced significantly when compared to laparotomy. Blood loss was 133 vs. 208 vs. 443.6 mL between the robotic, laparoscopy, and laparotomy groups, respectively. The hospital days were 1.7 vs. 2.4 vs. 3.6 days respectively. There were no significant differences in complication rates among the three groups.

30.2.3.4 Laparoscopic Lymphadenectomy

In cervical cancer, one of the most important prognostic factors is the status of the lymph nodes. Approximately 7–15% of all patients with early invasive cervical carcinoma are found to have lymphatic spread. Removal and assessment of the pelvic and para-aortic lymph nodes are an important part of the surgical staging procedure, and resection of bulky nodes has also been shown to have a therapeutic benefit. Lymphadenectomy can be approached transperitoneally or retro-peritoneally as described above. Numerous surgeons have performed laparoscopic lymphadenectomy with acceptable morbidity rates.

The first case of laparoscopic retroperitoneal pelvic lymphadenectomy in the literature was reported by Dargent and Salvat in a case report of a retroperitoneal lymphadenectomy in 1989 [8]. The first laparoscopic transperitoneal pelvic lymphadenectomy was published by Querleu et al., and the initial laparoscopic transperitoneal para-aortic lymphadnectomy was reported by Nezhat et al. [9, 10]. Since then, lymphadenectomy has been performed in cervical cancer patients as an adjunct to surgical staging, and has been proven to be a safe and accurate procedure. Not only does laparoscopy provide magnification of the operative field, the pneumoperitoneum decreases venous bleeding and assists in identification of small accessory vasculature leading to better visualization and hemostasis of the surgical field (Table 30.2).

A recent study by Tillmanns et al. summarized findings of laparoscopic retroperitoneal lymphadenectomy, and found that the procedure had an overall detection rate of 13% of occult metastasis in the aortic lymph nodes in the 299 reported cases in the literature [11]. They performed their surgery as an outpatient procedure, and reported median blood loss to be 25 mL, with an average operating time of 108 min.

Whether or not laparoscopic lymphadenectomy has an established role in patients suffering from advanced cervical cancer is debatable, but it should be considered given the low morbidity, fast recovery, and potential useful information obtained.

30.2.3.5 Sentinel Lymph Node Sampling

The thinking behind sentinel lymph node sampling is to identify and evaluate the first lymphatic nodes that the cancer would most likely metastasize to, and then use its status to chart further treatment, avoiding complete lymphadenectomy because of its associated complications. The sentinel lymph node was initially identified using angiography. This technique led to side effects such as phlebitis and allergic reactions due to dye injection. Currently, there are two different approaches being practiced. The first is the use of isosulfan blue dye to identify the lymphatic ducts that drain the lymph nodes. The second is the use of radiotracers and a handheld gamma probe to visualize the sentinel lymph nodes. Combination of both provides the highest yield.

Laparoscopy in sentinel lymph node sampling has several obvious advantages including faster recovery period, faster return to normal activities, shorter hospital stay, decreased requirement for pain medications, and faster return of bowel function.

The largest case series, to date, on this technique is by Plante et al., who reported 70 patients undergoing surgery for early cervical cancer [12]. In 42%, preoperative lympho-scintiography and intracervical blue dye injection were used. Intracervical blue dye injection was done in the remaining participants. Overall, sentinel node detection was 87%, with blue dye alone 79% and with blue dye plus lympho-scintiography 93%. The sentinel lymph node detection rate was 56% among patients with macroscopically involved lymph nodes.

Gynecologic Oncology Group (GOG) protocol 206 involves lymphatic mapping and sentinel lymph node biopsy, investigating the sensitivity of the sentinel lymph nodes in predicting lymph node metastasis in patients with invasive cervical carcinoma using laparoscopy or laparotomy. The study is currently being conducted.

Table 30.1 Laparoscopic radical hysterectomy and pelvic lymphadenectomy with or without para-aortic lymphadenectomy – selected reports

	Year	n	PLN	OR time (min)	Blood loss (mL)	LOS (day)	Complications
Nezhat et al. [9, 13]	1992 1993	7	22	315	30–250	2.1	None
Sedlacek et al. [14]	1994	14	16	420	334	5.5	1 VVF; 1 ureteral injury
Ting et al. [15]	1994	4	8	330–480	150–500	–	None
Ostrzenski et al. [16]	1996	6	–	280	–	2.0–6.0	1 hydronephrosis
Kim et al. [17]	1998	18	22	363	619	–	None
Hsieh et al. [18]	1998	8	–	–	–	6.5	None
Spirtos et al. [19]	2002	78	23.8	205	250	2.9	3 cystotomies; 1 UVF; 1 DVT; 5 conversions
Lee et al. [20]	2002	12	19.2	235	428	6.8	2 transfusions
Lin et al. [21]	2003	10	16.8	159	250	4.1	None
Obermair et al. [22]	2003	55	–	210	200	5.0	3 vascular; 1 nerve
Pomel et al. [23]	2003	50	13.2	258	200	7.5	1 bladder; 1 nerve; 1 hernia
Abu-Rustum et al. [24]	2003	19	25.5	371	301	4.5	2 conversions; 1 fever
Gil-Moreno et al. [25]	2005	27	19.1	285	400	5.0	None
Ramirez et al. [26]	2006	20	13	332.5	200	1	1 cystotomy; 1 PE; 1 pneumomediastinum; 1 vaginal dehiscence; 1 lymphocyst
Li et al. [27]	2007	90	21.3	263	370	13.8	4 vascular; 4 cystotomy; 29 urinary retention; 1 UVF, 1 VVF; 1 bowel obstruction; 4 lymphocyst

Table 30.1 (continued)

	Year	n	PLN	OR time (min)	Blood loss (mL)	LOS (day)	Complications
Magrina et al. [7]	2008	31	25.9	220	208	2.4	1 rectotomy
							1 fever
							1 trocar site infection
							1 UTI
							1 corneal abrasion
							1 lymphorrhea
Chen et al. [28]	2008	295	22	162	230	10.3	5 conversion (3 bleeding, 1 bowel injury, 1 hypercapnia)
							5 UVF
							4 VVF
							3 ureteral stenosis
							9 DVT
							4 lymphocyst
							5 lymphedema
Nezhat et al. [6]	2008	30	31	318	200	3.8	2 cystotomy
							1 ileus
							2 PE, DVT
							1 urinary retention
							2 *C. Difficile* colitis
Pellegrino et al. [29]	2008	57	24	310	200	–	1 cystotomy
							2 ureteral stenosis
							2 vaginal cuff diastasis
							1 conversion
Malzoni et al. [30]	2009	127	23.5	196	55	4	1 bladder injury (intraop)
							1 UVF
							6 fever
Total		958					Total Complications: 137
							Urinary: 51 (37.2%)
							Fistula: 14 (10.2%)
							Vascular: 9 (6.6%)
							Infectious: 8 (5.8%)
							Intestinal: 5 (3.6%)
							Hematological: 3 (2.2%)
							Wound dehiscence: 3 (2.2%)

PLN pelvic lymph nodes, *OR time* mean operating room time, *LOS* length of hospital stay, *VVF* vesico-vaginal fistula *UVF* uretero-vaginal fistula, *DVT* deep venous thrombosis, *PE* pulmonary embolism

Table 30.2 Laparoscopic pelvic and para-aortic lymphadenectomy: selected series in gynecologic oncology

	Year	Modality of dissection	n	PLND (mean)	PALND (mean)	Complications (n)
Childers et al. [31]	1993	Electrosurgery	29	–	–	1 ureteral 1 cystotomy 1 pneumothorax 3 minor
Chu et al. [32]	1997	–	67	26.7	8	1 vascular
Dottino et al. [33]	1999	Electrosurgery	94	11.9	3.7	1 vascular 2 minor
Vidaurretta et al. [34]	1999	Electrosurgery	84	18.5	–	1 vascular 2 lymphocele
Altgassen et al. [35]	2000	–	99	21-24.3	5.1-10.6	3 vascular, 1 hemorrhage 1 enterotomy 3 intestinal obstruction 1 ureteral 2 nerve impingement 5 minor
Scribner et al. [36]	2001	–	103	23.2	6.8	1 vascular (fatal) 1 DVT 2 pulmonary embolus (1 fatal) 2 ureteral 1 bladder laceration
Schlareth et al. [37]	2002	Electrosurgery and ABC	67	32.1	12.1	7 vascular 2 hematomas 8 infectious 1 ureteral 2 lymphoceles
Holub et al. [38]	2002	Ultrasonic LDS Electrosurgery	27 32	17.5 13.7	–	1 injury to epigastric artery 1 febrile morbidity 1 inflammation of obturator nerve
Abu-Rustum et al [39]	2003	Monopolar and ABC	114	10.3	5.3	1 vascular 1 DVT 3 intestinal 1 enterotomy 1 cystotomy 4 infectious 1 uterine perforation

Table 30.2 (continued)

	Year	Modality of dissection	n	PLND (mean)	PALND (mean)	Complications (n)
Köhler et al. [40]	2004	Electrosurgery	650	18.8	10.8	19 (2.9%) intraoperative
						(7 vascular, 3 bowel)
						35 (5.8%) postoperative
						(16 irritation of nerves, 6 lymphedema, 3 symptomatic lymphoceles, 3 chylascos)
Nezhat et al. [41]	2005	Ultrasonic LDS	100	20	15	2 vascular
						1 DVT
						1 bowel obstruction minor
						1 cystotomy
						1 trocar-site hernia
						1 port site metastasis
Nagao et al. [42]	2006	Electrosurgery	76	–	14	8 conversions to laparotomy
						(3 vascular, 2 obesity, 2 peritoneal tears leading to loss of pneumoperitoneum)
Thavaramara et al. [43]	2008	Electrosurgery	31	12	1	2 vascular
						1 enterotomy
						1 bowel minor
Total			1573			144
						Vascular/hematological: 36 (25.0%)
						Neurological: 19 (13.2%)
						Bowel: 14 (9.7%)
						Infectious: 13 (9.0%)
						Lymphocele: 13 (9.0%)
						Urinary: 8 (5.6%)
						Pulmonary: 3 (2.1%)

ABC Argon beam coagulation, *LDS* Laparoscopic dissection shears, *PLND* pelvic lymph node dissection, *PALND* para aortic lymph node dissection

30.2.3.6 Trachelectomy

Due to the widespread use of early screening procedures, there have been more cases of early cervical cancers detected, bringing up a dilemma in treating younger patients diagnosed with invasive carcinoma. Laparoscopy has enabled new options for these women who, in the past, would have received radical treatment. Laparoscopic-assisted vaginal trachelectomy or total laparoscopic or robotic-assisted trachelectomy has been an attractive alternative to those desiring preservation of fertility.

There are certain criteria when to consider laparoscopic trachelectomy

- Childbearing age with the desire to preserve fertility
- Reasonable ability to conceive
- FIGO Stage Ia2 to Ib1, with lesions less than 2 cm
- Limited endo-cervical involvement on colposcopy
- Negative lymph nodes
- Absence of lymphovascular space invasion

Preoperative Considerations

Preoperative assessment includes the location and size of the tumor, and its distance from the isthmus and upper endo-cervical canal. The length of the endo-cervical canal and the length of the uterine cavity to the fundus should be measured on an MRI such that the correct length of the cervix is resected. Ideally a 1 cm margin of normal tissue surrounding the area of concern should be obtained. All patients should be counseled carefully with regard to complications of the treatment, including the risk of failure of the procedure, risk of adverse pregnancy outcomes, and the need for careful observation if pregnancy is achieved after completion of surgery [2].

If a combined laparoscopic and vaginal surgical approach is planned, first, laparoscopic pelvic and possible para-aortic lymphadenectomies are carried out and sent to pathology for frozen section. Trachelectomy is initiated only if the lymph nodes are negative for metastatic spread. Attention is then shifted to the vaginal surgical field to complete the rest of the procedure transvaginally, dissecting the distal cervix, para-cervical tissue, and the upper vagina as it would be performed in a Schauta vaginal hysterectomy.

Surgical Technique

A laparoscopic pelvic lymphadenectomy is performed in usual fashion. Any suspicious nodes are sent for analysis, and the procedure is continued in absence of distant metastasis. After injecting pitressin into the paracervical and vaginal tissues, a 2-cm cuff is outlined around the cervix using elecrocautery. The para-vesical and para-vaginal spaces are incised, and the bladder reflected away from the cervix and lower uterine segment. The bladder pillars, lateral cardinal ligaments, and utero-sacral ligaments are identified. The descending branch of the cervical artery is located and divided. It is essential to dissect up the complete length of the endocervical canal, particularly with glandular adenocarcinomas avoiding opening the peritoneum. The recto-vaginal septum is dissected and pushed cranially. With squamous cell carcinoma, a strip of proximal cervical tissue may be conserved at the isthmus, which will aid in future pregnancies by providing some cervical competency. A Hegar dilator is inserted into the endo-cervical canal, and the cervix is removed depending on the type of carcinoma. Once the specimen is removed, a nonabsorbable isthmic or upper cervical cerclage is placed using number 1-Nylon with care taken to prevent stitching across the isthmus causing possible synechiae. A vagino-isthmic anastomosis is then performed using mattress sutures of number 1-Vicryl along with two interrupted sutures laterally close to the edges of the anastomosis. A Foley catheter is placed into the endometrial cavity through the isthmus and cerclage to prevent stenosis and synechiae. The bladder catheter is left in place for 5 days, and the vaginal pack for 24 h [2].

Review of the Literature

Multiple case reports and series have been published regarding laparoscopic lymphadenectomy along with radical vaginal trachelectomy, and more recently, total laparoscopic lymphadenectomy combined with trachelectomy. The latest review has been published by Milliken and Shepherd, who reported that a total of 790 patients worldwide had radical vaginal trachelectomy procedures between 1994 and 2008. There have been 29 cases of recurrence (4%) and 16 reported deaths after recurrence (2%) [44]. There were 302 pregnancies with 190 live births. Twenty seven women (9%) delivered prematurely at 32 weeks. In their own case series, Milliken and Shepherd examined 158 women treated with radical, vaginal trachelectomy. Thirteen patients (8%) experienced perioperative complications, and four recurrences were reported. There were 88 pregnancies, with 44 live births in 31 women. Nineteen pregnancies in 14 women miscarried in the first trimester, there were 12 midtrimester abortions in 9 women, and one stillbirth. Sonoda et al. reported on 43 women with early stage cervical cancer who underwent radical vaginal trachelectomy with lymphadenectomy [45]. The mean operating time was 330 min, with a median pelvic lymph node count of 25 and median hospital stay of 3 days. Eleven (79%) of 14 women who were trying to conceive were able to conceive. Four (36%) required assisted reproductive technologies. Four patients delivered full-term babies via cesarean sections, one patient miscarried, and two patients had elective abortions. Four women were pregnant at the time of publication. The median follow-up was 21 months, and there was only one recurrence.

In the last few years, a few case reports were published reporting on total laparoscopic-assisted trachelectomies or robotic-assisted trachelectomies. Chuang et al. described a successful robotic-assisted radical trachelectomy with lymphadenectomy for a young patient with early cervical carcinoma [46]. The total operative time was 345 min, blood loss 200 mL, with 43 lymph nodes retrieved and a hospital stay of 2 days. To date, there was no evidence of residual disease. The patient has not yet conceived.

30.2.4 Advanced Stage Cervical Carcinoma

In advanced stage cervical carcinoma, the standard therapeutic options include chemo-radiation and occasionally exenteration for stage IVa disease, a radical procedure associated with a high morbidity and mortality. In this setting, laparoscopy has been utilized in ways to optimize treatments by pretreatment surgical staging.

30.2.4.1 Pretreatment Surgical Staging with Pelvic and Para-aortic Lymphadenectomy

Cervical cancer is usually staged clinically. However, since clinical exams and imaging studies have been associated with high false-negative rates, especially for evaluation of the status of lymph node metastasis, surgical staging will allow more precise assessment of the intraperitoneal cavity and retro-peritoneal lymph nodes. It allows as well removal of bulky pelvic and/or para-aortic lymph nodes which could be associated with improved survival. PET/CT has been used to evaluate the status of lymph node involvement; overall sensitivity and specificity were 73% and 97%, respectively, to detect nodal metastasis [47]. Neither PET nor CT is an effective method for reliably detecting nodal disease [58]. Surgical staging of cervical cancer remains controversial and has been debated for decades. Lagasse et al. published a series of 95 patients back in the 1970s who underwent surgical staging prior to radiation therapy [48]. Eighteen patients (19%) were found to have unsuspected metastases to the common iliac or peri-aortic lymph nodes. Several studies have shown improved outcomes in surgically staged patients. In Holcomb et al., 89 patients underwent pretreatment staging via laparotomy versus treatment planning based on clinical staging [49]. The median survival of patients in the pretreatment laparotomy group was statistically longer than in the control group with clinical staging only, 29 months versus 19 months, respectively. This suggested that surgical staging may be beneficial in patients with locally advanced cervical carcinoma. The impact of pretherapy surgical staging in advanced cervical cancer has been shown to be favorable particularly with minimally invasive methods, as noted in Odunsi et al., and Denschlag et al. Odunsi et al. examined 51 women, surgically staging by an extraperitoneal approach [50]. Lymph node metastasis was found in 30 of 51 patients (59%). There were no significant treatment delays because of surgery, and all patients received radio-sensitization with chemotherapy, and radiation therapy based on the results. The procedure allowed for a more precise individualization of treatment. Denschlag et al. also supports pretreatment surgical staging by performing an extraperitoneal lymphadenectomy prior to initiation of adjuvant therapy, with a low complication rate [51].

30.2.4.2 Laparoscopic Ovarian Transposition

In patients who are younger, the ovarian function can be preserved by ovarian transposition prior to the initiation of radiation to minimize damage from necessary therapy. The largest series reported is by Pahisa et al., which included 28 patients who were 45 years of age or younger with stage Ib1 cervical cancer [52]. There was no intraoperative or postoperative morbidity related to the operation and no cases of ovarian metastasis. Twelve patients received adjuvant pelvic radiotherapy. The mean follow-up time was 44 months. Ovarian preservation was performed in 64% of those receiving radiation and 93% of the patients receiving no radiation. Two patients developed benign ovarian cysts requiring surgery, but there were no other long-term adverse effects from the operation. Laparoscopy has been shown to lead to shorter recovery times and decreased hospitalizations, all of which are beneficial to a patient facing additional steps in her treatment plan.

30.2.4.3 Laparoscopy Prior to Pelvic Exenteration

Pelvic exenteration is a radical procedure that is offered to patients with centrally recurrent, or rarely locally advanced cervical carcinoma. It is performed with curative intent. Approximately 50% of patients undergoing laparotomy for pelvic exenteration have intra- or retro-peritoneal metastasis and are not candidates for this procedure and it has to be abandoned [53]. Laparoscopy is a useful tool used to examine the intraabdominal and retro-peritoneal cavity prior to embarking on this radical procedure to ensure absence of any distant metastasis. There are a few case series in the literature addressing the occurrence of laparoscopy prior to exenteration with variable but acceptable results. Plante and Roy explored 11 patients with laparoscopy prior to exenteration, and found that 3 were eligible for exenteration and the remaining 8 were not [54]. Similarly, in Köhler et al., 41 patients underwent laparoscopy and 20 were deemed ineligible for exenteration [55].

Several case series are in the literature describing experience with laparoscopically assisted pelvic exenteration procedures. Ferron et al. reported a series of seven patients, two with a total exenteration, three with an anterior/middle exenteration, and two with a posterior/middle exenteration [56]. The mean operating time was 6.5 h, blood loss was <500 mL, with an average hospital stay of 27 days. The follow-up period was 14 months with two patients free of disease, one patient with local recurrence, and four patients who passed away, of which three had metastatic disease. Pumtambekar et al. reported 12 patients who underwent an anterior pelvic exenteration, with a mean operating time of 1.5 h, blood loss of 100–500 mL [57]. Hospital stay averaged 3 days, and the follow-up period was 15 months.

30.2.4.4 Laparoscopically Guided Interstitial Radiation Implant

In selected patients, particularly those with advanced stage disease, interstitial brachytherapy offers an alternative to intracavitary therapy. Traditionally, placement of interstitial needles is performed without the visualization within the pelvic cavity. This treatment is associated with high complication rates (5–48%). Laparoscopy may provide verification and guidance of needle placement thus decreasing treatment-related morbidity. A pilot study of 15 patients with locally advanced cervical carcinoma demonstrated the utility of laparoscopy in verifying placement of the interstitial radiation needles. In Choi et al., 15 patients received radiation therapy for cervical carcinoma. Interstitial needle placement was confirmed by laparoscopy [58]. The technique was considered safe, and the needles were withdrawn under laparoscopic guidance. In Recio et al., a total of 98 needles were placed under laparoscopic guidance [59]. Eleven perforations of the pelvic peritoneum and/or bladder were identified intraoperatively in five of the six patients, leading to repositioning of the needles. More recently, Engle et al. reported 42 women who underwent interstitial brachytherapy, with 28 patients undergoing traditional interstitial brachytherapy and 14 patients undergoing laparoscopic-assisted interstitial brachytherapy [60]. Overall, the laparoscopic-assisted procedure appeared safe, but increased the operating time, with a mean time of 177 min compared to 91 min in the traditional group. The laparoscopic procedure allowed for lysis of adhesions, identification of carcinomatosis, and was useful in visualizing accurate placement of the needles.

30.3 Laparoscopy and Applications in Endometrial Cancer

30.3.1 Introduction

Endometrial cancer is the most common gynecologic malignancy in the USA with an estimated 40,100 cases diagnosed in 2008 [1]. Fortunately, the majority of these cases is diagnosed at an early stage and can be successfully treated and often cured with surgery. Traditionally, this surgical approach has been a total abdominal hysterectomy, bilateral salpingo-oophorectomy, cytologic washings, and selective pelvic and para-aortic lymphadenectomy. Though the complication rate of this type of surgery is not extraordinarily high, a significant number of women diagnosed with endometrial cancer also have other comorbidities such as older age, diabetes, hypertension, and obesity. These conditions have been well documented to increase surgical risk and confer a higher perioperative morbidity and mortality. Therefore, the adoption and utilization of minimally invasive surgical techniques to treat this patient population is an attractive option for optimizing surgical and oncologic outcomes. Laparoscopy has been used for endometrial cancer in three conditions

- Primary staging with hysterectomy, bilateral salpingo-oophorectomy, lymphadenectomy, washings
- Patients after prior hysterectomy without previous staging
- Evaluation and management of recurrence

30.3.2 Patient Positioning and Technique

Perhaps, the two most important components of a successful and safe minimally invasive procedure in women with newly diagnosed gynecologic cancers are proper patient positioning and careful intraoperative management and coordination with anesthesia. These components are especially important with regard to the endometrial cancer patient population, as the majority of these women are obese or morbidly obese. Therefore, the operating table should be electric and have a weight capacity of at least £500, ensuring a surgical profile that accommodates all patients and allows for maximal maneuverability. Most importantly, the surgical bed should be able to achieve steep Trendelenburg in order to maximize surgical exposure when needed. Patients should be placed in dorsal lithotomy position utilizing either Yellow fin or Allen stirrups. The patient's arms are properly padded protecting the elbow and wrist regions and then tucked at her side. Shoulder braces, foam, or a beanbag are used to ensure that the patient does not slide when placed in Trendelenburg.

Simple interventions by anesthesia can help minimize surgical complications. We advocate all patients having an oro-gastric tube placed before placing a Veress needle or attempting abdominal access. This decreases the chance of an inadvertent gastric injury. Intraoperative fluid restriction helps reduce postoperative edema, fluid-overload, and nerve injury. Pressure-controlled ventilation helps reduce peak airway pressures in obese patients or in patients requiring steep Trendelenburg. It also minimizes diaphragmatic excursion while performing the para-aortic lymphadenectomy portion of the staging procedure.

A recent prospective study of lymphatic metastasis in endometrial cancer patients by Mariani et al. highlights the importance of adequate surgical exposure in patients requiring para-aortic lymphadenectomy [61]. Of 281 patients undergoing lymphadenectomy, 22% had positive lymph nodes. Fifty-one percent had both, pelvic and para-aortic lymph node metastasis, 33% had pelvic involvement only, and 16% had para-aortic involvement only. Interestingly, 77% of patients with para-aortic node metastasis had involvement above the IMA. Of those patients, 60% had negative ipsilateral nodes below the IMA, and 71% had negative ipsilateral common iliac nodes. The authors suggest that the para-aortic lymph node dissection be carried out to the level of the renal vessels in patients requiring definitive comprehensive surgical staging. Similar findings were also noted in a study by Malzoni et al. in which 46% of patients had positive nodes above the IMA with ipsilateral negative nodes below the IMA [30]. The specific setup and technique of the surgery are described in a prior section.

30.3.3 Laparoscopic Surgical Staging

In 1993, Childers et al. were the first to report on laparoscopic lymphadenectomy with LAVH in a series of 59 patients with clinical Stage I disease [31]. Lymphadenectomy was performed based on risk factors of tumor grade and depth of invasion. One patient required laparotomy for hysterectomy, while laparoscopic lymphadenectomy was not possible in 6% because of limited exposure secondary to obesity. Complications occurred in 5%, including ureteral transection, cystotomy, and development of a pneumothorax in a woman with congenital diaphragm defects. Since the report of this first case series, numerous studies in the literature have subsequently documented the feasibility and safety of laparoscopy for the staging and treatment of endometrial cancer.

A significant portion of the literature has recently focused more on surgical and oncologic outcomes with regard to survival in patients treated by laparoscopy versus laparotomy (Table 30.3). In a retrospective cohort study by Nezhat et al., 67 patients underwent laparoscopy and 127 underwent laparotomy for clinical Stage I or II endometrial cancer [62]. The complication rates between the two groups were comparable. Women undergoing laparoscopy had a shorter hospital stay and less morbidity related to infection. The median follow-up for the laparoscopy and laparotomy group was 36.3 months and 29.6 months, respectively. The 2- and 5-year estimated recurrence-free survival rates for the laparoscopy and laparotomy groups were 93 % vs. 91.7% and 88.5% vs. 85%, respectively. The 2- and 5-year overall survival rates (100% vs. 99.2% and 100% vs. 97%) were also similar between the two groups.

Prospective randomized trials comparing laparotomy with laparoscopy for the treatment of endometrial cancer are more limited, especially with regard to survival outcomes. Tozzi et al. were the first to report on survival outcomes from a prospective randomized controlled clinical trial of 122 women with endometrial cancer [63]. Sixty-three patients were randomized to the laparoscopy arm and 59 to the laparotomy arm. Evaluation of treatment-related morbidity showed a significant reduction in intraoperative complications, such as blood loss (241.3 vs. 586.1 mL, $P=.02$) and required transfusions (3 vs. 12, $P=.037$). Reductions in mean duration of return of bowel function (2 vs. 2.3 days, $P=.02$), and mean length of hospital stay (7.8 vs. 11.4 days, $P=.001$) were also seen in the laparoscopic arm when compared to the laparotomy arm. The long-term (>7 days) postoperative complications including wound infections, wound dehiscence, and hernia formation were significantly higher

Table 30.3 Endometrial cancer: comparison of disease-free survival between laparoscopy and laparotomy

	Year	Disease-free survival	
		Laparoscopy (n/%)	Laparotomy (n/%)
Malur et al. [64]	2001	37 (97.3)	37 (93.3)
Langebrekke et al. [65]	2002	27 (100)	24 (95.9)
Holub et al. [66]	2002	177 (93.7)	44 (93.2)
Eltabbakh et al. [67]	2002	100 (90)	86 (92)
Kuoppala et al. [68]	2004	40 (100)	40 (95)
Tozzi et al. [69]	2005	63 (91.2)	59 (93.8)
Zapico et al. [70]	2005	31 (81.6)	30 (81.1)
Gil-Moreno et al. [71]	2006	54 (98.2)	276 (87.6)
Cho et al. [72]	2007	165 (95.5)	144 (96.5)
Kalogiannidis et al. [73]	2007	69 (91)	100 (84)
Nezhat et al. [62]	2008	67 (88.5)	127 (85)
Malzoni et al. [74]	2009	81 (91.4)	78 (88.5)
Total		911 (93.2)	1045 (87.1)

in the laparotomy group (12% vs. 34%, $P=.02$). The conversion rate to laparotomy due to complications was 1.4%. Most importantly, the interim survival analysis revealed no significant difference in overall or disease-free survival between the two groups at a median follow-up of 44 months.

Another recent study by Malzoni et al. compared total laparoscopic hysterectomy to abdominal hysterectomy, with lymphadenectomy in 159 patients with clinical Stage I endometrial cancer [30]. Similar to other studies comparing laparoscopic-assisted vaginal hysterectomy to laparotomy, there was a significantly longer mean operative time in the total laparoscopic arm compared to the laparotomy arm. However, there was less mean operative blood loss, shorter duration of postoperative ileus, and shorter length of hospital stay in the laparoscopic arm. Overall, para-aortic lymph node dissection was performed with a similar frequency between the two groups. The mean number of pelvic and para-aortic lymph nodes removed was not significantly different between the two groups.

After a mean duration of follow-up of 38.5 months (range 2–81 months) the total recurrence rate was approximately 10%. Seven (8.6%) of 81 patients in the laparoscopic group had a recurrence versus 9 (11.5%) of 78 patients of the laparotomy group ($p>0.05$).

The Gynecologic Oncology Group (GOG) has completed a large Phase III randomized study (LAP-2) comparing laparoscopy to laparotomy in patients with clinical Stage I or II endometrial carcinoma or sarcoma [75].

Nine hundred and twenty patients were randomized to laparotomy and 1,696 to laparoscopy. The conversion rate was 24%, and the main reason was poor exposure. Laparoscopy patients had similar rates of intraoperative injuries as had the laparotomy patients (9.5% vs. 7.6%, $p=0.11$), fewer postoperative adverse events (27.5% vs. 36.9%, $p<0.001$), and shorter duration of hospitalization (median 3 vs. 4 days, $p<0.001$). Analysis of oncologic outcomes data is not yet available.

30.3.4 Robotic-assisted Endometrial Cancer Staging

Multiple studies have confirmed the benefits of laparoscopy compared to laparotomy with comparable survival outcomes in small prospective randomized trials. There are certain factors however, which have limited its widespread adoption by gynecologic oncologists. These include the long learning curve associated with surgical training and experience in advanced laparoscopy, and the heavy reliance of the surgeon on skilled operative assistants. Certain patient-related factors may also impede the success of a comprehensive laparoscopic staging procedure, including obesity, adhesive disease, uterine size, and inability of the patient to tolerate steep Trendelenberg positioning (Fig. 30.18).

The DaVinci™ robotic system (Intuitive Surgical Corporation, Sunnyvale, CA, USA) is being utilized

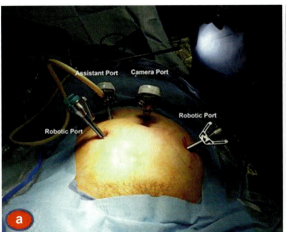
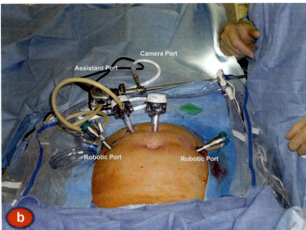

Fig. 30.18 Trocar placement. Robotic procedure: 12-mm port in the umbilicus, 8-mm trocars about 4-cm inferior and lateral to the umbilical site. Accessory ports: 5-mm port in between the 12 and 8 mm trocars, 10-mm trocar in the suprapubic area. (**a**) standard port placement (**b**) trocar placement for para-aortic lymphadenectomy

by an increasing number of gynecologic oncologists to facilitate comprehensive laparoscopic staging in patients with endometrial, cervical, and early ovarian cancers. In a recent study by Mabrouk et al. which surveyed members of the Society of Gynecologic Oncologists, 91% of respondents reported performing laparoscopic surgery in their practices. Twenty-four percent of respondents reported that they perform robotic-assisted surgery in their oncology practices, and 66% planned on increasing their utilization in the next year [76]. The DaVinci™ robotic surgical interface system may be considered an advanced laparoscopic tool. It allows the surgeon to overcome some of the limitations conferred by conventional laparoscopy. It provides the surgeon with improved visualization including a three-dimensional image screen and magnification for intricate tissue dissection. The articulated instruments provide the surgeon with enhanced dexterity, precision, and control compared to conventional laparoscopy. Use of robotics in gynecologic oncology is a rapidly evolving phenomenon, and recent reports in the literature have focused on its feasibility, safety, and outcomes when compared to conventional laparoscopy and laparotomy.

Boggess et al., in a retrospective cohort study of 322 women undergoing comprehensive surgical staging for endometrial cancer, compared outcomes for 3 different surgical techniques [77]. Women underwent either a laparotomy (TAH), laparoscopy (TLH) or robotic-assisted (TRH) procedure. The robotic cohort had a higher lymph node yield, decreased blood loss, and shorter hospital stay when compared to the other two cohorts. The TRH and TLH cohorts had comparable conversion rates to laparotomy (2.9% and 4.9%, respectively) and fewer postoperative complications.

A prospective cohort study by Seamon et al. including 181 patients with clinical Stage I or occult Stage II endometrial cancer, compared outcomes of robotic versus laparoscopic hysterectomy and lymphadenectomy [78]. The robotic cohort had a reduced estimated blood loss (100 vs. 250 mL, $P<0.001$), transfusion rate (3% vs. 18%, $P=0.002$), and median length of hospital stay (1 night vs. 2 nights, $P<0.001$) compared to the laparoscopy cohort. Although the patients in the robotic arm had a higher mean body mass index (34 vs. 29, $P<0.001$), the laparotomy conversion rate was lower (12% vs. 26%, $P=0.017$). The reason for conversion to laparotomy in the majority of these patients was poor exposure. Despite a longer set-up time in the robotic arm, the overall room and operative times were significantly reduced.

One should keep in mind a significant bias in these studies – the surgeon's prior experience. In some investigations, the surgeries are performed by people skilled in conventional laparoscopy first and have now learned the robotic-assisted technique. Subsequently, their results could be misleading when compared to those physicians who have become acclimated to robotic-assisted laparoscopy initially without first mastering the conventional laparoscopic skills.

30.3.5 Completion of Staging

Patients who have received a total hysterectomy and found to have a subsequent uterine carcinoma unfortunately need a reoperation for completion of the staging procedure. Laparoscopy has been evaluated as an effective means to complete surgical staging. Childers et al. reported on 13 patients with incompletely staged adenocarcinoma of the endometrium who underwent laparoscopic staging [79]. All patients had inspection of the entire peritoneal cavity, pelvic washings, and/or pelvic or para-aortic lymphadenectomy, and two had their ovaries removed. The average interval between the initial surgery and laparoscopic staging was 47 days. There were no intraoperative complications. The estimated blood loss was less than 50 mL on average, and mean hospital stay was 1.5 days. The average number of lymph nodes removed was 17.5. Extrauterine disease was found in three patients, one with intraperitoneal washings positive for adenocarcinoma, and two with pelvic lymph nodes positive for microscopic disease.

The Gynecologic Oncology Group (GOG) protocol 9402 determined the feasibility of laparoscopic staging in 58 patients with incompletely staged cancers of the uterus, ovary, fallopian tube, and primary peritoneum [80]. These patients had a laparoscopic bilateral para-aortic lymphadenectomy. The procedures were individualized based on the extent of the initial surgery, and laparotomy was performed for resectable disease. There were initially 95 eligible patients, of whom 9 (10%) women were incompletely staged and 17 patients (20%) underwent a laparotomy. The hospital stay was significantly shorter (3 vs. 6 days, $p=0.4$). Of those with a laparoscopy, 6% had bowel complications, and 11% was found to have more advanced disease than initially expected. A subgroup analysis of endometrial cancer patients was not performed.

These studies conclude that laparoscopy is a safe and effective procedure in patients who require restaging after initial surgery, but conversion to laparotomy may result due to adhesions or more advanced disease than expected.

30.3.6 Management of Recurrences

The possibility of recurrence from operative tumor dissemination in patients with Stage 1, grade 1 or 2 disease is 4% (7 of 150); those with grade 3 and superficial disease had a 14% recurrence in conventional abdominal surgery, as reported by DiSaia and Creasman [81]. Several studies have examined the recurrence rates after laparoscopic staging, and found equivalence in the laparoscopic group when compared to laparotomy groups. Most recently, Zullo et al. reported long-term efficacy rates and safety rates of laparoscopic surgery and laparotomy approaches in endometrial cancer [82]. After a follow-up period of 78 and 79 months for the laparoscopic and laparotomy group, respectively, there was no difference in the cumulative recurrence rate (20% vs. 18.4%) and death (17.5% vs. 15.8%). There was no significant difference in overall and disease-free survival observed.

When endometrial cancer recurrences do occur, management is tailored to the individual condition. Those that are located in the vagina occur in over 18% of recurrent cases and are traditionally treated with pelvic radiation and brachytherapy [83]. Surgical excision is limited to cases with central pelvic recurrence after radiotherapy failure. However, this treatment is associated with significant morbidity and mortality and not ideal for some patients. Alternative treatment options have been explored in the laparoscopic realm. Nezhat et al. reported a case of an endometrial cancer recurrence at the vaginal apex, treated successfully with laparoscopic radical parametrectomy and partial vaginectomy [ ]. The operative time was 315 min with an estimated blood loss of 100 mL. The patient was discharged on postoperative day 3 with no complications. The final pathology revealed grade two endometrioid adenocarcinoma with margins free of tumor. She remained free of disease 12 months after the procedure. Further reports remain to be examined on a larger population to determine the efficacy of laparoscopy to manage recurrent cases.

30.3.7 Special Considerations

30.3.7.1 Obesity

Results from the 2005–2006 National Health and Nutrition Examination Survey (NHANES) estimates that 32.7% of US adults are overweight, 34.3% are obese, and 5.9% are extremely obese [84]. Obesity is related to higher surgical morbidity, including longer operative times, higher blood loss, more postoperative wound complications, and an increased risk of venous thrombo-embolism. With 68% of patients diagnosed with endometrial cancer meeting criteria for obesity, the development of a surgical approach which provides comparable staging adequacy with decreased morbidity is essential [85].

Development of and improvement in technology which utilizes a minimally invasive surgical approach in these patients is of paramount importance. In a retrospective cohort study by Scribner et al., a successful laparoscopic staging procedure was completed in 63.6% of the obese population [36]. Obesity was the primary reason in 23.6% of patients for conversion to laparotomy. Eisenhauer et al. performed a retrospective analysis comparing surgical outcomes in obese women undergoing surgical staging by laparotomy, laparoscopy, or laparotomy with panniculectomy [86]. Both, laparotomy with panniculectomy and laparoscopy alone were associated with higher total lymph node retrieval ($p=.002$), and decreased incisional complications ($p=.002$). The median para-aortic lymph node counts were not significant between the three groups.

With the evolution of robotic surgery, many are looking toward this new technology as a means to overcome some of the technical challenges inherent in conventional laparoscopy and the obese patient. Gehrig et al. compared TRH with TLH in a retrospective cohort study of 79 obese and morbidly obese patients [87]. Complete surgical staging was accomplished in 92% of the robotic patients and in 84% of the laparoscopic cohort. There were no differences between the two groups with regard to conversion to laparotomy.

For both the obese and morbidly obese patients, robotic surgery was associated with a shorter operative time (189 vs. 215 min, $P=0.0004$), less blood loss (50 vs. 150 mL, $P<0.0001$), and shorter hospital stay (1.02 vs. 1.27 days, $P=0.0119$). There was a significant difference in mean para-aortic (10.3 vs. 7.03, $P=0.01$) and total lymph node counts (31.4 vs. 24, $P=0.004$) for the two groups. The difference became nonsignificant when only morbidly obese patients were taken into account, suggesting, as the authors stated, that robotic technology may not overcome all of the technical difficulties in this patient population.

30.3.7.2 Elderly

The majority of women diagnosed with endometrial cancer are postmenopausal. Older patients often have comorbidities which place them at increased surgical risk. Therefore, demonstration of the safety of laparoscopy in this patient population has been essential. Fortunately, Scribner et al., in a retrospective analysis, evaluated a total of 125 women ≥65 years of age with clinical Stage I endometrial cancer [88]. Laparoscopy was completed in 52/67 (77.6%) attempted procedures. Conversion to laparotomy was secondary to obesity (10.4%), bleeding (6%), intraperitoneal cancer (4.5%), and adhesions (1.5%). Pelvic, common iliac, and para-aortic lymph node counts were similar between the two groups. Although the operative time was significantly longer for the laparoscopic group (236 vs. 148 min), there was no increased morbidity attributable to longer duration under anesthesia. They had a shorter length of hospitalization, less blood loss, less postoperative ileus, and less wound complications when compared to the laparotomy group. Quicker recovery times allow elderly patients to maintain their independence and therefore may positively impact their quality of life (QoL).

30.3.8 Quality of Life Assessment

Zullo et al. performed a prospective randomized comparison of QoL as the primary endpoint between laparoscopy and laparotomy for the treatment of early stage endometrial cancer [89]. QoL was assessed by the Italian version of the Short-Form Healthy Survey (SF-36). The baseline QoL at study entry was similar in both treatment groups. At 1, 3, and 6 months after surgery, QoL was significantly higher in the laparoscopy group compared to the laparotomy group. Although QoL was the primary study endpoint, they also noted less intraoperative blood loss, lower drop in hemoglobin levels, less postoperative pain, shorter mean hospitalization, and fewer postoperative complications in the laparoscopy group. The incidence of intraoperative complication was similar between the two groups (7.5% vs. 7.9%), as was the mean number of pelvic and para-aortic lymph nodes removed.

In the GOG LAP-2 trial, QoL was evaluated in 782 patients. Patient's QoL was assessed using the Functional Assessment of Cancer Therapy-General (FACT-G), a measure of patients' physical, emotional, and social well-being before and after surgery [90]. Postsurgical QoL was higher at 1, 3, and 6 weeks postoperatively for patients undergoing laparoscopy. However, observed differences were not significant by 6 months.

30.4 Laparoscopy and Applications in Ovarian, Fallopian Tubal, and Primary Peritoneal Carcinomas

30.4.1 Introduction

Approximately, 21,650 new ovarian cancer cases and 15,520 deaths are estimated in the USA in 2008 [1]. Currently, the lifetime risk of developing ovarian cancer in the USA is approximately 1 in 70 with over 65% diagnosed with advanced stage disease. Although five-year survival rates of greater than 90% have been reported in patients with early stage disease, patients with more advanced distant disease have 5-year survival rates closer to 25%. Fallopian tubal carcinoma is rare with less than 0.2% of cancer diagnoses among women annually. Primary peritoneal carcinoma is also quite rare with rates reported as 0.03 per 100,000 [1]. Given the rarity of these two cancers, there are limited studies describing the current statistics of these malignancies. However, they have been demonstrated to share a similar biologic behavior with ovarian cancer and are treated with the same surgical and chemotherapeutic approach. Thus, the application of laparoscopy in the management of these cancers is comparable to that described for ovarian cancer.

According to the International Federation of Obstetrics and Gynecology (FIGO), surgical staging for these cancers includes

- Hysterectomy
- Bilateral salpingo-oophorectomy
- Pelvic washings for cytology
- Pelvic and para-aortic lymph node dissection
- Peritoneal and diaphragmatic biopsies
- Infracolic omentectomy

In early stage disease, this procedure has been successfully performed laparoscopically in select cases with preliminary data suggesting comparable results to laparotomy [91–94]. In addition to complete surgical staging, dependent on the patient's risk factors that may alter prognosis, patients with localized disease may consider fertility-sparing surgical staging.

In advanced ovarian cancer, surgical optimal cytoreduction has been associated with a significant survival advantage. A laparoscopic approach in the treatment of advanced ovarian cancer may confer several benefits. First, laparoscopy may serve not only as a tool for proper diagnosis, but also as a triage tool for resectability. The decision to attempt primary cytoreduction has come to question due to increasing research assessing the benefit of neoadjuvant chemotherapy with interval debulking among patients who cannot be optimally debulked or patients with other comorbidities that may limit optimal cytoreductive surgery. Second-look laparoscopy has been implemented to assess clinical response in patients enrolled in clinical trials to assess the efficacy of chemotherapy protocols. Third, complete laparoscopic cytoreduction has been reported in limited studies.

Laparoscopy offers all the obvious advantages and in addition to that a shorter interval to adjuvant therapy which is very important for patients with ovarian cancer requiring further treatment.

30.4.2 Surgical Technique

The traditional surgical approach to an adnexal mass has been via laparotomy. However, regardless of the index of suspicion for malignancy, laparoscopic evaluation of adnexal masses is appropriate in the hands of a skilled laparoscopic surgeon. The sequence of events should parallel those implemented in laparotomy:

- Thorough evaluation of the abdomen and pelvis
- Peritoneal washings for cytology
- Ovarian cystectomy or oophorectomy as indicated
- Biopsies of suspicious lesions
- Frozen section evaluation

The incidence of malignancy ranges from 0.4% to 14% in patients undergoing laparoscopic evaluation for adnexal masses [95].

When an obvious epithelial ovarian malignancy is encountered, a complete staging protocol must be performed as outlined above. In select cases involving women with limited, early stage, low-grade ovarian cancers, a fertility-sparing procedure may be considered. In some cases, resections of small bowel or colon may be necessary; therefore, preoperative bowel preparation may be warranted, as is a discussion about possible colostomy or other bowel changes. Although in

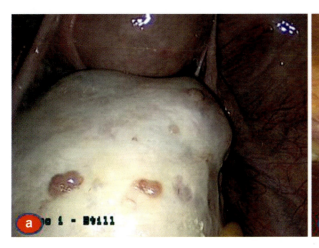 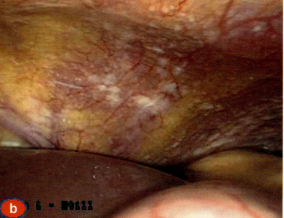

Fig. 30.19 Suspicious adnexal mass. (**a**) Surface ovarian excrescences positive for malignant implants. (**b**) Metastatic implants in the upper abdomen and anterior abdominal wall

the past, the conventional method was via laparotomy, advancements in technology has made it possible to complete tumor debulking laparoscopically, utilizing instruments such as the carbon dioxide laser, PlasmaJet™ (Plasma Surgical Ltd.), and Argon Beam Coagulator (Beacon Laboratories Inc., Valleylab Inc.) (Fig. 30.19).

30.4.3 Low Malignant Potential or Borderline Ovarian Tumors

Borderline ovarian tumors represent 10–20% of epithelial ovarian cancers and typically have an excellent prognosis. Survival rates for all borderline ovarian tumors range from 92% among those with advanced stage disease to 98% in those with Stage I disease [96]. Borderline ovarian tumors occur predominantly in a premenopausal population with the highest frequency occurring in patients aged 30–50 with 50–85% diagnosed as Stage I. The two most frequent histologic subtypes of borderline ovarian tumors are serous or mucinous tumors. Serous tumors are bilateral in 30% of patients with concurrent peritoneal implants in 35% [96]. Tempfer et al. conducted a pooled analysis of 317 patients with borderline ovarian tumors of varying histology and found that up to 30% of patients diagnosed with borderline tumors at the time of frozen section are subsequently found to have invasive ovarian cancer on final pathology [97]. The majority of these patients were of serous histology with 129 serous, 8 endometrioid, and 11 mixed tumors. In addition to preventing the need for reoperation in the event that invasive cancer is diagnosed on final pathology, surgical staging provides the patient with important prognostic information. Mucinous tumors are malignant in only 5% of cases with rare case reports of nodal metastases, thus complete staging may not be necessary in these patients [96, 98]. However, appendiceal primaries are quite common among the mucinous tumors, thus we routinely perform an appendectomy in these patients. At our institution, we recommend routine surgical staging to patients found to have borderline nonmucinous ovarian tumors at the time of frozen section.

An additional consideration unique to the treatment of borderline ovarian tumors is that the incidence of borderline tumors is predominantly among reproductive age patients. Fertility-sparing options may range from ovarian cystectomy to adnexectomy. Recurrence rates vary regardless of the surgical approach [96]:

- After adnexectomy 0–20%
- After ovarian cystectomy 12–58%
- After radical surgery 2.5–5.7%

Laparoscopic staging in borderline ovarian tumors has become increasingly common with advances in endoscopic techniques and instruments. The first case reports of laparoscopic treatment in borderline ovarian tumor were reported by Reich et al. in 1990 and Nezhat et al. in 1992 [99, 100]. In these reports, the procedure included a laparoscopic hysterectomy, bilateral adnexectomy, peritoneal sampling, peritoneal cytology, and partial omentectomy. Subsequently, multiple case series have emerged to further evaluate the clinical outcomes and feasibility of laparoscopic treatment of borderline ovarian tumors (Table 30.4). The largest case series, to date, was conducted by Fauvet et al. where 107 patients underwent laparoscopic treatment of borderline ovarian tumors. The mean follow-up was 27.5 months with 100% survival and only four patients with evidence of disease [101]. Brosi et al. have the longest documented follow-up (78 months) with a survival rate of at least 83% and the remaining patients lost to follow-up [102]. No difference in overall or progression-free survival has been reported. Thus, to date, the preliminary data regarding borderline ovarian tumors suggest that laparoscopic management of borderline ovarian tumors is feasible and efficacious.

30.4.4 Early Stage Invasive Ovarian Cancer

Early stage invasive ovarian cancer requires complete surgical staging to obtain important prognostic information which dictates postoperative management. Understaging of patients should be avoided. Surgical staging traditionally involves total abdominal hysterectomy, bilateral salpingo-oophorectomy, omentectomy, peritoneal biopsies, pelvic and para-aortic lymph node dissection, and peritoneal washings. If complete staging was not performed at the initial time of diagnosis, a restaging procedure that may be accomplished via laparoscopy or laparotomy is typically recommended to stage these patients.

The first case report of laparoscopic staging in early stage invasive ovarian cancer was reported by Querleu and LeBlanc in 1994 which included complete pelvic and infrarenal para-aortic retroperitoneal lymph node dissection in a case series of nine patients undergoing

Table 30.4 Borderline ovarian tumors: laparoscopic management

	Year	n	Mean follow-up (m)	Survival (n)	Recurrence (n)	Complication (n)	Conversion (n)
Darai et al. [103]	1998	25	41	23[c]	3	None	7 Presumption of cancer and failure of laparoscopic procedure
Seracchioli et al. [104]	2001	19[b]	42	19	1	None	0
Querleu et al. [105]	2003	30[c]	29	30	1	3	0
Camatte et al. [96]	2004	19 4[c] 11	45	34	6	0	0
Desfeux et al. [106]	2005	14 34[b]	29	47	2	–	16
Fauvet et al. [101]	2005	107	27.5	103 ANED 4 AWED	13	None	42 for suspected cancer of large tumor volume
Romagnolo et al. [107]	2006	52	44	51	7	–	0
Brosi et al. [102]	2007	21 20[b]	78	35[a]	0	None	0
Total		356		346	33	3	65

ANED alive with no evidence of disease, *AWED* alive with evidence of disease
[a] missing patients were lost to follow-up
[b] Conservative treatment (cystectomy or unilateral adnexectomy)
[c] Restaging cases, recurrent cases

restaging procedures for either ovarian or fallopian tube cancers. This case series demonstrated a mean blood loss of <300 cc and average hospital stay of only 2.8 days [94]. This study was among the first to demonstrate the feasibility of a complete laparoscopic staging procedure in early ovarian cancer.

Nezhat et al. reported the longest mean follow-up in a case series of 36 patients with invasive ovarian carcinoma managed with laparoscopic staging/restaging. Mean duration of follow-up time was 55.9 months, and there was a demonstrated 100% overall survival rate. Importantly, this study had the largest number of primary staging procedures [92]. Few retrospective case series have compared laparoscopy to laparotomy regarding the feasibility and overall outcomes. Chi et al. conducted a case control study of staging in early ovarian cancer with 20 patients staged by laparoscopy compared to 30 patients staged by laparotomy [108].

There were no differences in the omental specimen size or number of lymph nodes obtained. Blood loss and hospital stay was lower for the laparoscopy group, but operating time was longer. There were no conversions to laparotomy or other intraoperative complications in the laparoscopy group. It was concluded that laparoscopy was safe and efficacious in staging early ovarian cancer (Table 30.5).

Due to the rarity of early ovarian cancer, diagnosis, and challenges with preoperative diagnosis, a randomized control trial has not been feasible. Alternative evaluations of accuracy can be inferred by comparing upstaging rates between laparoscopic and laparotomy cases. In restaging procedures, the current literature suggests that the rate of upstaging among complete laparoscopic staging procedures is in the range of 11–19% [80]. The upstaging rate among patients who had a complete laparotomy

Table 30.5 Early ovarian and fallopian tube malignancy: laparoscopic staging

	Year	n	Operative time (min)	Blood loss (mL)	Length of stay (day)	Complications (n)	Upstaged (%)	Follow-up (m)	Current status
Querleu et al. [94]	1994	9	227	<300	2.8	1	n/a	n/a	n/a
Pomel et al. [23]	1995	8	313	n/a	4.75	2	12.5%	n/a	8 NED
Childers et al. [91]	1995	14	n/a	n/a	1.6	2	40%	n/a	n/a
Amara et al. [98]	2000	8	215	n/a	2.5	5	33%	n/a	7 NED, 1 expired
Leblanc et al. [109]	2004	42	238	n/a	3.1	3	19	54	4 expired
Tozzi et al. [63]	2004	24	176	n/a	7	1	0	46.4	36 NED
Chi et al. [108]	2005	20	312	235	3.1	0	n/a	n/a	n/a
Ghezzi et al. [110]	2007	15	377	n/a	3	2	27	16	20 NED
Park et al. [93]	2008	17	303.8	231.2	9.4	2	5.8	19	1 expired, 16 NED
Nezhat et al. [92]	2009	36	229	195	2.37	5	17.6	55.9	36 NED
Total or average		193	265.6		3.96	23			123 NED, 6 expired

NED no evidence of disease

restaging procedure has been reported to be as high as 36%. The feasibility of completion staging by laparoscopy in patients with incompletely staged ovarian, fallopian tube, endometrial, and primary peritoneal cancers was demonstrated in Gynecologic Oncology Group protocols 9302 and 9402 [80]. A total of 84 patients were eligible, of which 74 had ovarian, fallopian tube, or primary peritoneal cancers. Fifty-eight patients underwent complete laparoscopic staging, confirmed with photographic documentation. Nine patients were incompletely staged laparoscopically due to lack of peritoneal biopsies, cytology, or bilateral lymph nodes. Seventeen patients underwent laparotomy: 13 due to lack of exposure from adhesions, 3 due to complications, and 1 due to metastatic macroscopic disease. Complications associated with laparoscopically treated patients included five bowel injuries, one cystotomy, one small bowel obstruction, one venotomy, and two patients with extensive blood loss requiring transfusion. In comparing patients managed laparoscopically with those managed with laparotomy, the laparoscopic group demonstrated significant less blood loss, shorter hospital stay, and Quetlet index as well as comparable nodal yields.

As suggested by Childers et al., these studies support that laparoscopy may offer an advantage in the management of early ovarian cancer by allowing better visualization of difficult areas such as the subdiaphragmatic region, obturator spaces, anterior and posterior cul-de-sacs, as well as magnification and detection of smaller lesions that may be missed during a laparotomy [91].

30.4.5 Advanced Stage Invasive Ovarian Cancer

The majority of patients with ovarian cancer are diagnosed with either FIGO Stage III or IV disease. The mainstay of treatment includes optimal surgical cytoreduction followed by platinum-based combination chemotherapy. Clinical risk factors that contribute to poor prognosis include

- FIGO Stage IV disease
- ≥5 cm residual tumor
- ≥20 residual lesions
- 1 L of ascites
- Poor performance status
- Older age
- Poor histology
- High tumor grade
- High postoperative CA-125

As the use of laparoscopy has increased in gynecologic oncology, three applications in advanced ovarian cancer have emerged in the literature:

- Determination of resectability
- Second look evaluation
- Primary or recurrent cytoreduction

30.4.5.1 Determination of Resectability

A recent meta-analysis, including 6,885 patients in total, conducted by Bristow et al. found that maximal cytoreduction is one of the most powerful determinants of cohort survival among patients with Stage III or IV ovarian cancer. They found that each 10% increase in maximal cytoreduction was associated with a 5.5% increase in median survival time [111]. This data supports the suggestion that optimal cytoreduction be defined as no macroscopic residual tumor left behind. However, depending on individual institutions, surgical skills, and aggressiveness, the percentage of patients with no measurable tumor after debulking surgery ranges from 8% to 85%.

In cases where primary, optimal cytoreduction is not possible, the option of neo-adjuvant chemotherapy with interval debulking has been proposed. A randomized study by Vergote et al. further explores the clinical outcomes of conventional therapy (primary surgery followed by chemotherapy) with neo-adjuvant chemotherapy [112]. This study consisted of 718 patients with biopsies suggestive of ovarian cancer and metastatic lesions at other sides than the pelvis, measuring at least 2 cm. The patients were randomized to undergo either conventional therapy or neo-adjuvant chemotherapy followed by interval debulking. Seventy-six percent of patients in each group had Stage IIIc disease and 24% had Stage IV disease. Median progression-free survival was noted to be 11 months in both groups and median overall survival was noted to be 29 and 30 months, respectively. However, the neo-adjuvant chemotherapy group had significantly less morbidity. Their conclusion was that "due to the lower morbidity neo-adjuvant chemotherapy can be considered as the preferred treatment."

A review of the current literature suggests that survival after neo-adjuvant chemotherapy with interval cytoreductive surgery does not differ significantly from those treated with primary debulking surgery and adjuvant chemotherapy. The advantages of this approach include increased rate of optimal cytoreduction, less extensive surgery, lower blood loss, lower morbidity, shortened hospital stay, and a diagnostic tool to select platinum-resistant patients. The challenges to this approach include the limitations of current diagnostics such as CA-125 and CT scanning to predict resectability.

Laparoscopy has been demonstrated to have a higher sensitivity than these other tools. Vergote et al. reported a series of 285 patients in 1998 utilizing laparoscopy to determine whether the patient could be optimally debulked. They found a 96% accuracy of resectability [113]. Fagotti et al. described 64 patients that underwent laparoscopy followed by immediate laparotomy and compared the intraoperative findings. They found that no patients deemed unresectable on laparoscopy were found to be candidates for optimal debulking on subsequent laparotomy, yielding a negative predictive value of 100%. In fact, 87% of patients categorized as resectable on the laparoscopic assessment were optimally debulked [114]. Overall, rates in the literature suggest that the accuracy of laparoscopy in predicting resectability ranges from 80% to 96%. More recently, laparoscopy-based scoring models have been reported to further enhance accuracy in predicting resectability. Fagotti et al. incorporated eight laparoscopic features as potential indicators of surgical outcome:

- Presence of ovarian masses – unilateral or bilateral
- Omental cake
- Peritoneal carcinomatosis
- Diaphragmatic involvement
- Mesenteric retraction
- Bowel infiltration
- Liver metastases

They found that an overall predictive index score of ≥8 identified patients undergoing suboptimal cytoreduction with a specificity of 100% and negative predictive value of 70% [115].

30.4.5.2 Second-look Laparoscopy

The second-look procedure consists of a systematic pathologic assessment of the abdominal/pelvic cavity in a patient who is clinically without evidence of disease following the completion of primary staging and front-line chemotherapy. Although controversial in the clinical setting of ovarian carcinoma, this procedure can provide important prognostic information for the patient and represents the most accurate method to evaluate the efficacy of adjuvant chemotherapy protocols. There is also some suggestion that in patients with suboptimal debulking in Stage III ovarian cancer who have achieved a complete clinical response to platinum-based combination chemotherapy, there appears to be a distinct survival benefit from second-look surgical procedures.

Littell et al. conducted a study directly comparing second-look laparoscopy with laparotomy evaluations [116]. This study consisted of 70 patients who underwent second-look laparoscopy with a plan for immediate laparotomy if the laparoscopic impression was negative for disease. The authors found that a negative second-look laparoscopy with negative cytology carries a 91.5% prediction of negative laparotomy. Laparotomy was associated with a higher morbidity including two small bowel injuries, small bowel obstruction, fever, cardiac ischemia, wound cellulites, and pneumonia. The laparoscopy only group had three vaginal cuff dehiscence intraoperatively during vaginal preparation prior to the initiation of surgery. No other complications intraoperatively or postoperatively were noted. Thus while laparotomy may offer a small increase in sensitivity and negative predictive value, this study concluded that it does not warrant the increased morbidity [116].

30.4.5.3 Cytoreductive Surgery for Primary Advanced or Recurrent Ovarian Cancer

To date, limited studies have been published describing laparoscopic advanced ovarian cancer debulking. Amara et al. first reported a small case series that included complete laparoscopic management of advanced or recurrent ovarian cancer [35]. In this series, three patients underwent primary staging or cytoreductive procedures: one Stage Ia borderline tumor, one Stage IIIc papillary serous cancer, and one unstaged patient who had completed neo-adjuvant chemotherapy. Three cases of staging completion were performed to yield Stage Ia, IIa, and Ic malignancies. Finally, four cases of second-look laparoscopy with interval debulking were performed. All patients did well postoperatively except one patient who expired due to recurrent disease, declining further treatment. We have recently reported our initial experience in laparoscopic primary and secondary debulking for advanced ovarian cancer [35]. Nezhat et al. evaluated a total of 32 patients who were subdivided into two groups: Group 1 consisted of 13 patients who underwent primary cytoreduction, and Group 2 consisted of 19 patients who underwent secondary/tertiary cytoreduction [117]. Procedures performed included ascites aspiration, radical/simple hysterectomy, salpingo-oophorectomy, pelvic- and para-aortic lymphadenectomy, omentectomy, appendectomy, trachelectomy, upper vaginectomy, ureteral resection and uretero-neocystostomy, splenectomy, liver and bowel resection, and ablation/resection of peritoneal and diaphragmatic lesions. Optimal debulking was feasible in 10 patients in Group 1, and 16 patients in Group 2. Operative time and mean blood loss in Group 1 compared to Group 2 were 277 min and 240 mL, and 191 min and 126 mL, respectively. No patient required blood transfusion or developed subsequent port-site metastases. The average hospital stay was 5.5 days for Group 1 and 3 days for Group 2. Two patients in Group 1 had ureteral transection, one unintentionally, and one performed intentionally to achieve optimal cytoreduction. Both were repaired laparoscopically. In addition, one patient developed a vesico-vaginal fistula while receiving intraperitoneal chemotherapy. This patient underwent a fistula repair during her laparoscopic second-look procedure. Other complications included postoperative vaginal cuff bleeding ($n=1$), lymphoceles ($n=2$), and vaginal dehiscence ($n=1$), sepsis ($n=1$), subclavian vein thrombosis ($n=1$), and diverticular perforation ($n=1$). In Group 1, after 13.7 months of mean follow-up, two patients who had suboptimal debulking procedures had expired, nine patients were alive with no evidence of disease (NED) and two patients were alive with disease (AWD). In Group 2, after 26.9 months mean follow-up, six patients had expired, ten patients were NED, and three patients were AWD. These results are encouraging and the role of laparoscopy in managing advanced ovarian cancer will continue to expand. More long-term studies are needed to fully appreciate the role of this technology in advanced ovarian cancer staging.

Laparoscopic primary or secondary cytoreduction has also been described with the introduction of hand-assisted laparoscopic surgery (HALS). This technique permits introduction of a hand intraperitoneally during traditional laparoscopy, retaining tactile sensation for the surgeon. The initial report of HALS uses in advanced ovarian cancer was in a patient undergoing splenectomy for an isolated metastasis. Krivak et al. described a case series of 25 patients for whom 22 were successfully optimally cytoreduced with HALS with a median hospital stay of 2 days and only 1 intraoperative complication of a small bowel enterotomy that was immediately repaired extracorporeally with HALS [118]. The remaining three patients were converted to laparotomy: one for extensive upper abdominal disease, one for extensive adhesions, and finally, one for disease requiring posterior exenteration to achieve optimal cytoreduction. No hand-port recurrences have been reported to date. HALS has been associated with shorter operative times that are similar to open surgery, while maintaining the lower blood loss and short hospital stay associated with laparoscopic patients.

30.4.6 Pitfalls of Laparoscopic Management in Ovarian Cancer

Several main concerns have limited the widespread use of laparoscopy in ovarian cancer: the potential for inadequate staging, tumor cell peritoneal dissemination with carbon dioxide pneumoperitoneum, possibly a higher incidence of cyst rupture, and port-site metastases. These "pitfalls of laparoscopy" are discussed below.

30.4.6.1 Inadequate Staging

Inadequate staging may occur in cases with low intraoperative suspicion for malignancy, inaccurate frozen section evaluation, or in institutions where gynecologic oncology support may be limited. However, in cases where frozen section examination confirms cancer, complete laparoscopic staging should be possible in the hands of an experienced gynecologic oncologist. Adequacy of staging may be defined by nodal yield Table (30.6).

30.4.6.2 Cyst Rupture

The adverse effect of cyst rupture in laparoscopy and laparotomy approaches is conflicting. In general, tumor rupture rates have been reported from 10.5% to 41.8%. Currently, the largest study addressing the effect of cyst rupture consists of a retrospective, multicenter study of over 1,500 patients. Vergote et al. found that a cyst or mass rupture was an independent predictor of disease-free survival. However, this study is limited as a majority of patients had incomplete staging procedures which may influence disease-free survival [119]. In contrast, Sjövall et al. found no difference in survival in a retrospective review of 394 patients [120]. An additional confounding variable is the use of iatrogenic controlled cyst decompression. This technique may include a controlled drainage of the mass while contained in the endoscopic bag to prevent spillage. Importantly, studies that compare tumor rupture rates do not account for those that may have occurred in such a controlled fashion. Regardless of these study limitations, one should aim to maintain oncologic principles and avoid spillage of cancer cells during extraction of an ovarian mass.

30.4.6.3 Port-site Metastases

Port-site metastases have been largely reported as case reports in the literature for both borderline and early invasive pathologies. The etiology of port-site metastases is uncertain. Several hypotheses include tumor cell entrapment, direct spread from instrumentation, direct spread from the trocar where instruments are exchanged, and the "chimney effect." The tumor cell entrapment theory poses that free floating tumor cells implant on the raw surface of incisional sites that are later protected by

Table 30.6 Ovarian cancer: comparison of nodal yields between laparoscopy and laparotomy

	Year		Laparoscopy	Laparotomy	p value
Chi et al. [108]	2005	Total pelvic lymph nodes (mean)	11.14	14.7	>0.05
		Total para-aortic lymph nodes (mean)	6.7	9.2	>0.05
		Omental size (cm^3)	186	347	1.00
Park et al. [93]	2008	Total pelvic lymph nodes (mean)	13.7	19.3	0.052
		Total para-aortic lymph nodes (mean)	6.4	8.9	0.187

the fibrinous exudates that forms as result of healing. Direct contamination by instruments or exchanging instrumentation does not explain the many reported port-site metastases that have occurred in sites where no tissue manipulation takes place, such as a Veress needle puncture site or the camera trocar site. The "chimney effect" suggests that tumor cells travel along the sheath of the trocars with the leaking gas. However, multiple studies that have attempted to assess for aerosolized tumor cells have been inconclusive.

In cases of borderline ovarian tumors, only a few cases of port-site metastases have been reported. Of the nine reported cases, surgical excision was performed with a 100% overall survival at 6–72 months follow-up [121]. In contrast, invasive ovarian cancer has port-site metastases reported in up to 16% of cases. In one study, the risk of port-site metastases was highest (5%) in patients with recurrence of ovarian or primary peritoneal malignancies undergoing procedures in the presence of ascites. The overall prognosis has not been affected with these metastatic lesions as they tend to respond to chemotherapy without relapse. In fact, one study reported no survival differences among patients with port-site metastases, compared to patients without port-site metastases. Techniques that may minimize the likelihood of port-site metastases include removal of an intact specimen in an impermeable retrieval bag and layered closure of the trocar sites [122].

30.5 Conclusion

Laparoscopy was initially applied in gynecology as a diagnostic tool in many cases of ovarian cancer. Currently, laparoscopy has emerged as the most commonly

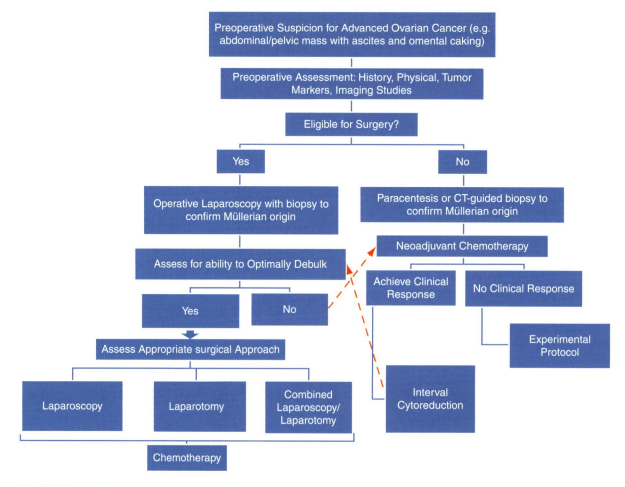

Fig. 30.20 Laparoscopic management of ovarian cancer: algorithm

performed procedure for gynecologists in the evaluation of an adnexal mass. In ovarian tumors with low malignant potential, several case-series and case-control studies suggest similar overall survival rates of 98% and progression-free survival among patients who underwent laparoscopic treatment compared with those who underwent traditional laparotomy. In invasive ovarian cancer, studies support laparoscopy as a feasible alternative to laparotomy with some suggestion of lower complication rates while maintaining comparable survival and disease-free survival rates. In advanced ovarian cancer, the current literature suggests feasibility in select cases. With the continued expansion of endoscopic techniques and instruments, laparoscopy has emerged as a feasible alternative to laparotomy in managing gynecologic malignancies. Our group created a potential algorithm to incorporate the current applications of laparoscopy in the management of advanced ovarian cancer (Fig. 30.20).

Quick Reference Guide

1. **Operating room setup**: usually at least two monitors are used, one on each side of the patient, allowing the surgeon to switch sides if necessary.
2. **Patient positioning**: dorsal lithotomy with legs placed in Allen stirrups. The patient should be securely strapped to the table, allowing steep Trendelenburg for optimal exposure in the pelvis.
3. **Laparoscopic radical hysterectomy – *Trocar placement:*** 4-trocar approach is advisable and all trocars should be placed in a way to facilitate not only the radical hysterectomy, but as well the necessary lymphadenectomy.
4. **Laparoscopic radical hysterectomy – *Rectovaginal space***
   Incise the peritoneum between the utero-sacral ligaments using the harmonic scalpel and gently dissect the rectum off the vagina. Avoid any rectal injury!
5. **Laparoscopic radical hysterectomy – *Vesicovaginal space/opening of the pelvic sidewall***
   Transect the round ligaments using the harmonic scalpel and open the anterior leaf of the broad ligament. Develop the bladder flap with a combination of blunt and sharp dissection.
6. **Laparoscopic radical hysterectomy – *Paravesicle space***
   Place tension on the obliterated hypogastric artery. Start the dissection and respect the landmarks:
   - *Lateral:* iliac vessels
   - *Medial:* obliterated hypogastric artery and bladder

   The dissection continues inferior to the iliac vessels until the obturator nerve is identified. At this point perform the lymphadenectomy.
7. **Pelvic lymphadenectomy:**
   The extent of dissection reaches from the mid-common iliac vessels and external iliac vessels down to the level of the deep circumflex veins. Use harmonic scalpel.

   Para-aortic lymphadenectomy: incise the peritoneum over the right common iliac artery, extend the incision to the promontory and above the IMA.
   - *Right side:* Identify the right ureter, remove the lymph nodes along the right side of the aorta. Avoid injury to the IVC!
   - *Left side:* more challenging because of the proximity and location of IMA and sigmoid colon. Identify left ureter and remove the nodal package between IMA and the left common iliac vessels.
   - *Aortic bifurcation:* extend the peritoneal incision to the promontory. Grasp the nodal package firmly and dissect it using harmonic scalpel.
8. **Laparoscopic radical hysterectomy – *Pararectal space and uterine artery***
   The uterine artery, coming off the internal iliac artery, can easily be identified by placing the obliterated hypogastric artery on upwards tension. Divide it between clips. The para-rectal space is developed bluntly between the following landmarks:
   - *Medial* – rectum
   - *Lateral* – ureter
   - *Anterior* – uterine artery
   - *Posterior* – sacrum
9. **Laparoscopic radical hysterectomy – *Ureters***
   Unroof the ureters with curved endoshears and make sure you carry the dissection all the way down to the bladder!

10. **Laparoscopic radical hysterectomy – *Colpotomy and specimen removal***
    The uterosacral-cardinal ligament complex and vagina is divided as a whole and the specimen removed through the vagina.
11. **Laparoscopic radical hysterectomy – *Vaginal cuff closure***
    Can be done either vaginally or laparoscopically. Use monofilament sutures in figure-of-eight technique or running fashion.

References

1. Jemal, A., Siegal, R., Ward, E., Hao, Y., Xu, J., Murray, T., Thun, M.J.: Cancer statistics 2008. CA Cancer J. Clin. **58**, 71–96 (2008)
2. Camran Nezhat, F.arr Nezhat., Ceana Nezhat, Nezhat's Operative Gynecologic Laparoscopy and Hysteroscopy. 2008: Cambridge University Press. ISBN 9780521862493
3. Zakashansky, K., Chuang, L., Gretz, H., et al.: A case-controlled study of total laparoscopic radical hysterectomy with pelvic lymphadenectomy versus radical abdominal hysterectomy in a fellowship training program. Int. J. Gynecol. Cancer **17**(5), 1075–1082 (2007)
4. Hertel, H., Kohler, C., Michels, W., et al.: Laparoscopic-assisted radical vaginal hysterectomy (LARVH): prospective evaluation of 200 patients with cervical cancer. Gynecol. Oncol. **90**, 505–511 (2003)
5. Obermair, A., Gebski, V., Frumovitz, M., et al.: A phase III randomized clinical trial comparing laparoscopic or robotic radical hysterectomy with abdominal radical hysterectomy in patients with early stage cervical cancer. J. Minim. Invasive Gynecol. **15**(5), 584–588 (2008)
6. Nezhat, F.R., Datta, M.S., Liu, C., et al.: Robotic radical hysterectomy versus total laparoscopic radical hysterectomy with pelvic lymphadenectomy for treatment of early cervical cancer. JSLS **12**(3), 227–237 (2008)
7. Magrina, J.F., Kho, R.M., Weaver, A.L., et al.: Robotic radical hysterectomy: comparison with laparoscopy and laparotomy. Gynecol. Oncol. **109**(1), 86–91 (2008)
8. Dargent, D., Salvat, J.: L'envahissement Ganglionnaire Pelvien: Place de la Pelviscopie Retroperitoneale. McGraw Hill, Medsi, Paris (1989)
9. Nezhat, C., Burell, O., Nezhat, F.R., Benigno, B.B., Welander, C.: Laparoscopic radical hysterectomy with para-aortic and pelvic lymph node dissection. Am. J. Obstet. Gynecol. **166**(3), 864–865 (1992)
10. Querleu, D., LeBlanc, E., Castelain, B.: Laparoscopic pelvic lymphadenectomy in the staging of early carcinoma of the cervix. Am. J. Obstet. Gynecol. **164**, 579–581 (1991)
11. Tillmanns, T., Lowe, M.P.: Safety, feasibility, and costs of outpatient laparoscopic extraperitoneal aortic nodal dissection for locally advanced cervical carcinoma. Gynecol. Oncol. **106**(2), 370–374 (2007)
12. Plante, M., Renaud, M.C., Tetu, B., et al.: Laparoscopic sentinel node mapping in early-stage cervical cancer. Gynecol. Oncol. **91**, 494–503 (2003)
13. Nezhat, C.R., Nezhat, F.R., Burrell, M.O., Ramirez, C.E., Welander, C., Carrodeguas, J., Nezhat, C.H.: Laparoscopic radical hysterectomy and laparoscopically assisted vaginal radical hysterectomy with pelvic and paraaortic node dissection. J. Gynecol. Surg. **9**(2), 105–120 (1993)
14. Sedlacek, T.V., Campion, M.J., Hutchins, R.A., Reich, H.: Laparoscopic radical hysterectomy: a preliminary report. J. Am. Assoc. Gynecol. Laparosc. **1**(4, Part 2), S32 (1994)
15. Ting, H.C.: Laparoscopic radical hysterectomy: a preliminary experience. J. Am. Assoc. Gynecol. Laparosc. **1**(4, Part 2), S36 (1994)
16. Ostrzenski, A.: A new laparoscopic abdominal radical hysterectomy: a pilot phase trial. Eur. J. Surg. Oncol. **22**(6), 602–606 (1996)
17. Kim, D.H., Moon, J.S.: Laparoscopic radical hysterectomy with pelvic lymphadenectomy for early, invasive cervical carcinoma. J. Am. Assoc. Gynecol. Laparosc. **5**(4), 411–417 (1998)
18. Hsieh, Y.Y., Lin, W.C., Chang, C.C., Yeh, L.S., Hsu, T.Y., Tsai, H.D.: Laparoscopic radical hysterectomy with low paraaortic, subaortic and pelvic lymphadenectomy. Results of short-term follow-up. J. Reprod. Med. **43**(6), 528–534 (1998)
19. Spirtos, N.M., Eisenkop, S.M., Schlaerth, J.B., Ballon, S.C.: Laparoscopic radical hysterectomy (type III) with aortic and pelvic lymphadenectomy in patients with stage I cervical cancer: surgical morbidity and intermediate follow-up. Am. J. Obstet. Gynecol. **187**(2), 340–348 (2002)
20. Lee, C.L., Huang, K.G.: Total laparoscopic radical hysterectomy using Lee-Huang portal and McCartney transvaginal tube. J. Am. Assoc. Gynecol. Laparosc. **9**(4), 536–540 (2002)
21. Lin, Y.S.: Preliminary results of laparoscopic modified radical hysterectomy in early invasive cervical cancer. J. Am. Assoc. Gynecol. Laparosc. **10**(1), 80–84 (2003)
22. Obermair, A., Ginbey, P., McCartney, A.J.: Feasibility and safety of total laparoscopic radical hysterectomy. J. Am. Assoc. Gynecol. Laparosc. **10**(3), 345–349 (2003)
23. Pomel, C., Provencher, D., Dauplat, J., Gauthier, P., Le Bouedec, G., Drouin, P., Audet-Lapointe, P., Dubuc-Lissoir, J.: Laparoscopic staging of early ovarian cancer. Gynecol. Oncol. **58**(3), 301–306 (1995)
24. Abu-Rustum, N.R., Gemignani, M.L., Moore, K., Sonoda, Y., Venkatraman, E., Brown, C., Poynor, E., Chi, D.S., Barakat, R.R.: Total laparoscopic radical hysterectomy with pelvic lymphadenectomy using the argon-beam coagulator: pilot data and comparison to laparotomy. Gynecol. Oncol. **91**(2), 402–409 (2003)
25. Gil-Moreno, A., Puig, O., Pérez-Benavente, M.A., Díaz, B., Vergés, R., De la Torre, J., Martínez-Palones, J.M., Xercavins, J.: Total laparoscopic radical hysterectomy (type II-III) with pelvic lymphadenectomy in early invasive cervical cancer. J. Minim. Invasive Gynecol. **12**(2), 113–120 (2005)
26. Ramirez, P.T., Slomovitz, B.M., Soliman, P.T., Coleman, R.L., Levenback, C.: Total laparoscopic radical hysterectomy and lymphadenectomy: the M. D. Anderson Cancer Center experience. Gynecol. Oncol. **102**(2), 252–255 (2006)

27. Li, G., Yan, X., Shang, H., Wang, G., Chen, L., Han, Y.: A comparison of laparoscopic radical hysterectomy and pelvic lymphadenectomy and laparotomy in the treatment of Ib-IIa cervical cancer. Gynecol. Oncol. **105**(1), 176–180 (2007)
28. Chen, Y., Xu, H., Li, Y., Wang, D., Li, J., Yuan, J., Liang, Z.: The outcome of laparoscopic radical hysterectomy and lymphadenectomy for cervical cancer: a prospective analysis of 295 patients. Ann. Surg. Oncol. **15**(10), 2847–2855 (2008)
29. Pellegrino, A., Villa, A., Fruscio, R., Signorelli, M., Meroni, M.G., Iedà, N., Vitobello, D.: Total laparoscopic radical hysterectomy and pelvic lymphadenectomy in early stage cervical cancer. Surg. Laparosc. Endosc. Percutan. Tech. **18**(5), 474–478 (2008)
30. Malzoni, M., Tinelli, R., Cosentino, F., Fusco, A., Malzoni, C.: Total laparoscopic radical hysterectomy versus abdominal radical hysterectomy with lymphadenectomy in patients with early cervical cancer: our experience. Ann. Surg. Oncol. **16**(5), 1316–1323 (2009)
31. Childers, J.M., Hatch, K.D., Tran, A.N., et al.: Laparoscopic para-aortic lymphadenectomy in gynecologic malignancies. Obstet. Gynecol. **82**(5), 741–747 (1993)
32. Chu, K.K., Chang, S.D., Chen, F.P., Soong, Y.K.: Laparoscopic surgical staging in cervical cancer – preliminary experience among Chinese. Gynecol. Oncol. **64**(1), 49–53 (1997)
33. Dottino, P.R., Tobias, D.H., Beddoe, A., Golden, A.L., Cohen, C.J.: Laparoscopic lymphadenectomy for gynecologic malignancies. Gynecol. Oncol. **73**(3), 383–388 (1999)
34. Vidaurreta, J., Bermúdez, A., di Paola, G., Sardi, J.: Laparoscopic staging in locally advanced cervical carcinoma: a new possible philosophy? Gynecol. Oncol. **75**(3), 366–371 (1999)
35. Altgassen, C., Possover, M., Krause, N., Plaul, K., Michels, W., Schneider, A.: Establishing a new technique of laparoscopic pelvic and para-aortic lymphadenectomy. Obstet. Gynecol. **95**(3), 348–352 (2000)
36. Scribner Jr., D.R., Walker, J.L., Johnson, G.A., McMeekin, S.D., Gold, M.A., Mannel, R.S.: Laparoscopic pelvic and paraaortic lymph node dissection: analysis of the first 100 cases. Gynecol. Oncol. **82**(3), 498–503 (2001)
37. Schlaerth, J.B., Spirtos, N.M., Carson, L.F., Boike, G., Adamec, T., Stonebraker, B.: Laparoscopic retroperitoneal lymphadenectomy followed by immediate laparotomy in women with cervical cancer: a gynecologic oncology group study. Gynecol. Oncol. **85**(1), 81–88 (2002)
38. Holub, Z., Jabor, A., Kliment, L., Lukac, J., Voracek, J.: Laparoscopic lymph node dissection using ultrasonically activated shears: comparison with electrosurgery. J. Laparoendosc. Adv. Surg. Tech. A **12**(3), 175–180 (2002)
39. Abu-Rustum, N.R., Chi, D.S., Sonoda, Y., DiClemente, M.J., Bekker, G., Gemignani, M., Poynor, E., Brown, C., Barakat, R.R.: Transperitoneal laparoscopic pelvic and para-aortic lymph node dissection using the argon-beam coagulator and monopolar instruments: an 8-year study and description of technique. Gynecol. Oncol. **89**(3), 504–513 (2003)
40. Köhler, C., Klemm, P., Schau, A., Possover, M., Krause, N., Tozzi, R., Schneider, A.: Introduction of transperitoneal lymphadenectomy in a gynecologic oncology center: analysis of 650 laparoscopic pelvic and/or paraaortic transperitoneal lymphadenectomies. Gynecol. Oncol. **95**(1), 52–61 (2004)
41. Nezhat, F., Yadav, J., Rahaman, J., Gretz 3rd, H., Gardner, G.J., Cohen, C.J.: Laparoscopic lymphadenectomy for gynecologic malignancies using ultrasonically activated shears: analysis of first 100 cases. Gynecol. Oncol. **97**(3), 813–819 (2005)
42. Nagao, S., Fujiwara, K., Kagawa, R., Kozuka, Y., Oda, T., Maehata, K., Ishikawa, H., Koike, H., Kohno, I.: Feasibility of extraperitoneal laparoscopic para-aortic and common iliac lymphadenectomy. Gynecol. Oncol. **103**(2), 732–735 (2006)
43. Thavaramara, T., Sheanakul, C., Hanidhikul, P., Ratchanon, S., Wiriyasirivaj, B., Leelahakorn, S.: Results of laparoscopic pelvic and/or para-aortic lymphadenectomy in gynecologic oncology patients in Bangkok Metropolitan Administration Medical College and Vajira Hospital. J. Med. Assoc. Thai. **91**(5), 619–624 (2008)
44. Milliken, D.A., Shepherd, J.H.: Fertility preserving surgery for carcinoma of the cervix. Curr. Opin. Oncol. **20**(5), 575–580 (2008)
45. Sonoda, Y., Chi, D.S., Carter, J., Barakat, R.R., Abu-Rustum, N.R.: Initial experience with Dargent's operation: the radical vaginal trachelectomy. Gynecol. Oncol. **108**(1), 214–219 (2008)
46. Chuang, L.T., Lerner, D.L., Liu, C.S., Nezhat, F.R.: Fertility-sparing robotic-assisted radical trachelectomy and bilateral pelvic lymphadenectomy in early-stage cervical cancer. J. Minim. Invasive Gynecol. **15**(6), 767–770 (2008)
47. Magné, N., Chargari, C., Vicenzi, L., Gillion, N., Messai, T., Magné, J., Bonardel, G., Haie-Meder, C.: New trends in the evaluation and treatment of cervix cancer: the role of FDG-PET. Cancer Treat. Rev. **34**(8), 671–681 (2008)
48. Lagasse, L.D., Ballon, S.C., Berman, M.L., Watring, W.G.: Pretreatment lymphangiography and operative evaluation in carcinoma of the cervix. Am. J. Obstet. Gynecol. **134**(2), 219–224 (1979)
49. Holcomb, K., Abulafia, O., Matthews, R.P., Gabbur, N., Lee, Y.C., Buhl, A.: The impact of pretreatment staging laparotomy on survival in locally advanced cervical carcinoma. Eur. J. Gynaecol. Oncol. **20**(2), 90–93 (1999)
50. Odunsi, K.O., Lele, S., Ghamande, S., Seago, P., Driscoll, D.L.: The impact of pre-therapy extraperitoneal surgical staging on the evaluation and treatment of patients with locally advanced cervical cancer. Eur. J. Gynaecol. Oncol. **22**(5), 325–330 (2001)
51. Denschlag, D., Gabriel, B., Mueller-Lantzsch, C., Tempfer, C., Henne, K., Gitsch, G., Hasenburg, A.: Evaluation of patients after extraperitoneal lymph node dissection for cervical cancer. Gynecol. Oncol. **96**(3), 658–664 (2005)
52. Pahisa, J., Martínez-Román, S., Martínez-Zamora, M.A., et al.: Laparoscopic ovarian transposition in patients with early cervical cancer. Int. J. Gynecol. Cancer **18**(3), 584–589 (2008)
53. Iavazzo, C., Vorgias, G., Akrivos, T.: Laparoscopic pelvic exenteration: a new option in the surgical treatment of locally advanced and recurrent cervical carcinoma. Bratisl. Lek. Listy **109**(10), 467–469 (2008)
54. Plante, M., Roy, M.: Operative laparoscopy prior to a pelvic exenteration in patients with recurrent cervical cancer. Gynecol. Oncol. **69**(2), 94–99 (1998)
55. Köhler, C., Tozzi, R., Possover, M., Schneider, A.: Explorative laparoscopy prior to exenterative surgery. Gynecol. Oncol. **86**(3), 311–315 (2002)

56. Ferron, G., Querleu, D., Martel, P., Chopin, N., Soulié, M.: Laparoscopy-assisted vaginal pelvic exenteration. Gynécol. Obstét. Fertil. **34**(12), 1131–1136 (2006)
57. Puntambekar, S., Kudchadkar, R.J., Gurjar, A.M., Sathe, R.M., Chaudhari, Y.C., Agarwal, G.A., Rayate, N.V.: Laparoscopic pelvic exenteration for advanced pelvic cancers: a review of 16 cases. Gynecol. Oncol. **102**(3), 513–516 (2006)
58. Choi, J.C., Ingenito, A.C., Nanda, R.K., Smith, D.H., Wu, C.S., Chin, L.J., Schiff, P.B.: Potential decreased morbidity of interstitial brachytherapy for gynecologic malignancies using laparoscopy: A pilot study. Gynecol. Oncol. **73**(2), 210–215 (1999)
59. Recio, F.O., Piver, M.S., Hempling, R.E., Eltabbakh, G.H., Hahn, S.: Laparoscopic-assisted application of interstitial brachytherapy for locally advanced cervical carcinoma: results of a pilot study. Int. J. Radiat. Oncol. Biol. Phys. **40**(2), 411–414 (1998)
60. Engle, D.B., Bradley, K.A., Chappell, R.J., Conner, J.P., Hartenbach, E.M., Kushner, D.M.: The effect of laparoscopic guidance on gynecologic interstitial brachytherapy. J. Minim. Invasive Gynecol. **15**(5), 541–546 (2008)
61. Mariani, A., Dowdy, S.C., Cliby, W.A., Gostout, B.S., Jones, M.B., Wilson, T.O., Podratz, K.C.: Prospective assessment of lymphatic dissemination in endometrial cancer: a paradigm shift in surgical staging. Gynecol. Oncol. **109**, 11–18 (2008)
62. Nezhat, F., Yadav, J., Rahaman, J., et al.: Analysis of survival after laparoscopic management of endometrial cancer. JMIG **15**(2), 181–187 (2008)
63. Tozzi, R., Köhler, C., Ferrara, A., Schneider, A.: Laparoscopic treatment of early ovarian cancer: surgical and survival outcomes. Gynecol. Oncol. **93**(1), 199–203 (2004)
64. Malur, S., Possover, M., Michaels, W., Schneider, A.: Laparoscopic-assited vaginal versus abdominal surgery in patients with endometrial cancer-a prospective randomized trial. Gynecol. Oncol. **80**, 239–244 (2001)
65. Langebrekke, A., Istre, O., Hallquist, A., Hartgill, t, Onsrud, M.: Comparison of laparoscopy and laparotomy in patients with endometrial cancer. J. Am. Assoc. Gynecol. Laparosc. **9**, 152–157 (2002)
66. Holub, Z., Jabor, A., Bartos, P., Eim, J., Urbanek, S., Pivovarnikova, R.: Laparoscopic surgery for endometrial cancer: long-term results of a multicentric study. Eur. J. Gynaecol. Oncol. **23**, 305–310 (2002)
67. Eltabbakh, G.: Analysis of survival after laparoscopy in women with endometrial carcinoma. Cancer **95**, 1894–1901 (2002)
68. Kuoppala, T., Tomas, E., Heinonen, P.: Clinical outcome and complications of laparoscopic surgery compared with traditional surgery in women with endometrial cancer. Arch. Gynecol. Obstet. **270**, 25–30 (2004)
69. Tozzi, R., Malur, S., Koehler, C., et al.: Laparoscopy versus laparotomy in endometrial cancer: first analysis of survival of a randomized prospective study. JMIG **12**, 130–136 (2005)
70. Zapico, A., Fuentes, P., Grassa, A., Arnanz, F., Otazua, J., Cortes-Prieto, J.: Laparoscopic-assisted vaginal hysterectomy versus abdominal hysterectomy in stages I and II endometrial cancer. Operating data, follow up and survival. Gynecol. Oncol. **98**(2), 222–227 (2005)
71. Gil-Moreno, A., Díaz-Feijoo, B., Morchón, S., Xercavins, J.: Analysis of survival after laparoscopic-assisted vaginal hysterectomy compared with the conventional abdominal approach for early-stage endometrial carcinoma: a review of the literature. JMIG **13**(1), 26–35 (2006)
72. Cho, Y.H., Kim, D.Y., Kim, J.H., Kim, Y.M., Kim, Y.T., Nam, J.H.: Laparoscopic management of early uterine cancer: 10-year experience in Asan Medical Center. Gynecol. Oncol. **106**(3), 585–590 (2007)
73. Kalogiannidis, I., et al., Laparoscopy-assisted vaginal hysterectomy compared with abdominal hysterectomy in clinical stage I endometrial cancer: safety, recurrence, and long-term outcome. Am J Obstet Gynecol, 2007. 196(3): p. 248 e1–8.
74. Malzoni, M., Tinelli, R., Cosentino, F., Perone, C., Rasile, M., Iuzzolino, D., Malzoni, C., Reich, H.: Total laparoscopic hysterectomy versus abdominal hysterectomy with lymphadenectomy for early stage endometrial cancer: A prospective randomized study. Gynecol. Oncol. **112**, 126–133 (2009)
75. Walker, J.L., Piedmonte, M., Spirtos, N., et al. Phase III trial of laparoscopy vs laparotomy for surgical resection and comprehensive surgical staging of uterine cancer: A Gynecologic Oncology Group (GOG) Study founded by NCI. In: Proceedings from the 37th Annual Meeting of the Society of Gynecologic Oncologists, Palm Springs, CA, 22–26 March 2006, Abstract 22
76. Mabrouk, M., Frumovitz, M., Greer, M., et al.: Trends in laparoscopic and robotic surgery among gynecologic oncologists: a survey update. Gynecol. Oncol. **112**(3), 501–505 (2009)
77. Boggess, J.F., Gehrig, P.A., Cantrell, L., et al.: A comparative study of 3 surgical methods for hysterectomy with staging for endometrial cancer: robotic assistance, laparoscopy, laparotomy. Am. J. Obstet. Gynecol. **199**(4), 360 (2008). e1-9
78. Seamon, L.G., Cohn, D.E., Henretta, M.S., et al.: Minimally invasive comprehensive surgical staging for endometrial cancer: robotics or laparoscopy? Gynecol. Oncol. **113**(1), 36–41 (2009)
79. Childers, J.M., Spirtos, N.M., Brainard, P., et al.: Laparoscopic staging of the patient with incompletely staged early adenocarcinoma of the endometrium. Obstet. Gynecol. **83**(4), 597–600 (1994)
80. Spirtos, N.M., Eisekop, S.M., Boike, G., et al.: Laparoscopic staging in patients with incompletely staged cancers of the uterus, ovary, fallopian tube, and primary peritoneum: a Gynecologic Oncology Group (GOG) study. Am. J. Obstet. Gynecol. **193**(5), 1645–1649 (2005)
81. DiSaia, P.J., Creasman, W.T.: Adenocarcinoma of the uterus. In: DiSaia, P.J., Creasman, W.T. (eds.) Clinical Gynecologic Oncology, 6th edn, pp 137–184. Mosby–Year Book, St. Louis (2002)
82. Zullo, F., Palomba, S., Falbo, A., Russo, T., Mocciaro, R., Tartaglia, E., Tagliaferri, P., Mastrantonio, P.: Laparoscopic surgery vs laparotomy for early stage endometrial cancer: long-term data of a randomized controlled trial. Am. J. Obstet. Gynecol. **200**(3), 296 (2009). e1-9
83. Nezhat, F., Prasad Hayes, M., Peiretti, M., Rahaman, J.: Laparoscopic radical parametrectomy and partial vaginectomy for recurrent endometrial cancer. Gynecol. Oncol. **104**(2), 494–496 (2007)

84. http://www.cdc.gov/nchs/products/pubs/pubd/hestats/overweight/overweight_adult.htm
85. von Gruenigen, V.E., Gil, K.M., Frasure, H.E., Grandon, M., Hopkins, M.P., Jenison, E.L.: Complementary medicine use, diet and exercise in endometrial cancer survivors. J. Cancer Integr. Med. **3**, 13–18 (2005)
86. Eisenhauer, E.L., Wypych, K.A., Mehrara, B.J., Lawson, C., Chi, D.S., Barakat, R.R., Abu-Rustum, N.R.: Comparing surgical outcomes in obese women undergoing laparotomy, laparoscopy, or laparotomy with panniculectomy for the staging of uterine malignancy. Ann. Surg. Oncol. **14**(8), 2384–2391 (2007)
87. Gehrig, P.A., Cantrell, L.A., Shafer, A., Abaid, L.N., Mendivil, A., Boggess, J.F.: What is the optimal minimally invasive surgical procedure for endometrial cancer staging in the obese and morbidly obese woman? Gynecol. Oncol. **111**(1), 41–45 (2008)
88. Scribner, D.R., Walker, J.L., Johnson, G.A., McMeekin, D.S., Gold, M.A., Mannel, R.S.: Laparoscopic pelvic and paraaortic lymph node dissection in the obese. Gynecol. Oncol. **84**, 426–430 (2002)
89. Zullo, F., Palomba, S., Russo, T., et al.: A prospective randomized comparison between laparoscopic and laparotomic approaches in women with early stage endometrial cancer: a focus on the quality of life. Am. J. Obstet. Gynecol. **193**(4), 1344–1352 (2005)
90. Kornblith, A., Walker, J., Huang, H., et al.: Quality of life (QOL) of patients in a randomized clinical trial of laparoscopy vs open laparotomy for the surgical resection and staging of uterine cancer: A Gynecologic Oncology Group (GOG) study. In: Proceedings from the 37th Annual Meeting of the Society of Gynecologic Oncologists, Palm Springs, CA, 22–26 March 2006, Abstract 22
91. Childers, J.M., Lang, J., Surwit, E.A., et al.: Laparoscopic surgical staging of ovarian cancer. Gynecol. Oncol. **59**(1), 25–33 (1995)
92. Nezhat, F., Ezzati, M., Rahaman, J., et al.: Laparoscopic management of early ovarian and fallopian tube cancers: surgical and survival outcome. Am. J. Obstet. Gynecol. **200**, 83 (2009). e1-6
93. Park, J.Y., Bae, J., Lim, M.C., Lim, S.Y., Seo, S.S., Kang, S., Park, S.Y.: Laparoscopic and laparotomic staging in stage I epithelial ovarian cancer: a comparison of feasibility and safety. Int. J. Gynecol. Cancer **15**, 2012–2019 (2008)
94. Querleu, D., LeBlanc, E.: Laparoscopic infrarenal paraaortic lymph node dissection for restaging of carcinoma of the ovary or fallopian tube. Cancer **73**(5), 1467–1471 (1994)
95. Nezhat, F., Nezhat, C., Welander, C.E., Benigno, B.: Four ovarian cancers diagnosed during laparoscopic management of 1011 women with adnexal masses. Am. J. Obstet. Gynecol. **167**, 790–796 (1992)
96. Camatte, S., Morice, P., Atallah, D., Thoury, A., Pautier, P., Lhommé, C., Duvillard, P., Castaigne, D.: Clinical outcome after laparoscopic pure management of borderline ovarian tumors: results of a series of 34 patients. Ann. Oncol. **15**(4), 605–609 (2004)
97. Tempfer, C.B., Polterauer, S., Bentz, E.K., et al.: Accuracy of intraoperative frozen section analysis in borderline tumors of the ovary: a retrospective analysis of 96 cases and review of the literature. Gynecol. Oncol. **107**, 248–252 (2007)
98. Amara, D.P., Nezhat, C., Teng, N.N., et al.: Operative laparoscopy in the management of ovarian cancer. Surg. Laparosc. Endosc. **6**(1), 38–45 (1996)
99. Nezhat, F., Nezhat, C., Burrell, M.: Laparoscopically assisted hysterectomy for the management of a borderline ovarian tumor: a case report. J. Laparoendosc. Surg. **2**, 167–169 (1992)
100. Reich, H., McGlynn, F., Wilkie, W.: Laparoscopic management of stage I ovarian cancer. A case report. J. Reprod. Med. **35**, 601–604 (1990)
101. Fauvet, R., Boccara, J., Dufournet, C., et al.: Laparoscopic management of borderline ovarian tumors: results of a French multicenter study. Ann. Oncol. **16**, 403–410 (2005)
102. Brosi, N., Deckardt, R.: Endoscopic surgery in patients with borderline tumor of the ovary: a follow-up study of thirty-five patients. J. Minim. Invasive Gynecol. **14**, 606–609 (2007)
103. Darai, E., Teboul, J., Fauconnier, A., Scoazec, J.Y., Benifla, J.L., Madelenat, P.: Management and outcome of borderline ovarian tumors incidentally discovered at or after laparoscopy. Acta Obstet. Gynecol. Scand. **77**(4), 451–457 (1998)
104. Seracchioli, R., Venturoli, S., Colombo, F.M., Govoni, F., Missiroli, S., Bagnoli, A.: Fertility and tumor recurrence rate after conservative laparoscopic management of young women with early-stage borderline ovarian tumors. Fertil. Steril. **76**(5), 999–1004 (2001)
105. Querleu, D., Papageorgiou, T., Lambaudie, E., Sonoda, Y., Narducci, F., LeBlanc, E.: Laparoscopic restaging of borderline ovarian tumours: results of 30 cases initially presumed as stage IA borderline ovarian tumours. BJOG **110**(2), 201–204 (2003)
106. Desfeux, P., Camatte, S., Chatellier, G., Blanc, B., Querleu, D., Lécuru, F.: Impact of surgical approach on the management of macroscopic early ovarian borderline tumors. Gynecol. Oncol. **98**(3), 390–395 (2005)
107. Romagnolo, C., Gadducci, A., Sartori, E., Zola, P., Maggino, T.: Management of borderline ovarian tumors: results of an Italian multicenter study. Gynecol. Oncol. **101**(2), 255–260 (2006)
108. Chi, D.S., Abu-Rustum, N.R., Sonoda, Y., et al.: The safety and efficacy of laparoscopic surgical staging of apparent stage I ovarian and fallopian tube cancers. Am. J. Obstet. Gynecol. **192**(5), 1614–1619 (2005)
109. Leblanc, E., Querleu, D., Narducci, F., Occelli, B., Papageorgiou, T., Sonoda, Y.: Laparoscopic restaging of early stage invasive adnexal tumors: a 10-year experience. Gynecol. Oncol. **94**(3), 624–629 (2004)
110. Ghezzi, F., Cromi, A., Uccella, S., Bergamini, V., Tomera, S., Franchi, M., Bolis, P.: Laparoscopy versus laparotomy for the surgical management of apparent early stage ovarian cancer. Gynecol. Oncol. **105**(2), 409–413 (2007)
111. Bristow, R.E., Tomacruz, R.S., Armstrong, D.K., et al.: Survival effect of maximal cytoreductive surgery for advanced ovarian carcinoma during the platinum era: a meta-analysis. J Clin. Oncol. **20**, 1248–1259 (2002)
112. Vergote, I., van Gorp, T., Amant, F., Leunen, K., Neven, P., Berteloot, P.: Timing of debulking surgery in advanced ovarian cancer. Int. J. Gynecol. Cancer **18**(Suppl 1), 11–19 (2008)
113. Vergote, I., De Wever, I., Tjalma, W., et al.: Neoadjuvant chemotherapy or primary debulking surgery in advanced ovarian carcinoma: a retrospective analysis of 285 patients. Gynecol. Oncol. **71**, 431–436 (1998)

114. Fagotti, A., Fanfani, F., Ludovisi, M., et al.: Role of laparoscopy to assess the chance of optimal cytoreductive surgery in advanced ovarian cancer: a pilot study. Gynecol. Oncol. **96**, 729–735 (2005)
115. Fagotti, A., Ferrandina, G., Fanfani, F., et al.: A laparoscopy-based score to predict surgical outcome in patients with advanced ovarian carcinoma: a pilot study. Ann. Surg. Oncol. **13**, 1156–1161 (2006)
116. Littell, R.D., Hallonquist, H., Matulonis, U., et al.: Negative laparoscopy is highly predictive of negative second-look laparotomy following chemotherapy for ovarian, tubal and primary peritoneal carcinoma. Gynecol. Oncol. **103**, 570–574 (2006)
117. Nezhat, F.R., Datta, M.S., Lal, N., et al.: Laparoscopic cytoreduction for primary advanced or recurrent ovarian, fallopian tube, and peritoneal malignancies. Gynecol. Oncol. **108**(3), S60 (2008)
118. Krivak, T.C., Elkas, J.C., Rose, G.S., et al.: The utility of hand-assisted laparoscopy in ovarian cancer. Gynecol. Oncol. **96**, 72–76 (2005)
119. Vergote, I., De Brabanter, J., Fyles, A., et al.: Prognostic importance of degree of differentiation and cyst rupture in stage I invasive epithelial ovarian carcinoma. Lancet **357**(9251), 176–182 (2001)
120. Sjövall, K., Nilsson, B., Einhorn, N.: Different types of rupture of the tumor capsule and the impact on survival in early ovarian carcinoma. Int. J. Gynecol. Cancer **4**, 333 (1994)
121. Morice, P., Camatte, S., Larregain-Fournier, D., et al.: Port-site implantation after laparoscopic treatment of borderline ovarian tumors. Obstet. Gynecol. **104**, 1167–1170 (2004)
122. Ramirez, P.T., Wolf, J.K., Leveback, C.: Laparoscopic port-site metastases: etiology and prevention. Gynecol. Oncol. **91**, 179–189 (2003)

Part X

Special Topics: Urology

Cancer of the Kidney

Daniel J. Canter and Robert G. Uzzo

31.1 Introduction

In 2009, there will be approximately 58,000 new cases of kidney cancer and nearly 13,000 deaths [1]. While a small proportion of these renal tumors represent an upper tract transitional cell carcinoma, the vast majority are renal cell carcinomas (RCC) that arise from the tubular epithelium of the kidney. Approximately one-half to two-thirds of renal cell tumors are discovered incidentally on cross-sectional imaging performed for other reasons [2]. In fact, over the past 20 years, there has been an increase in the overall incidence of renal parenchymal lesions. Specifically, small renal masses (SRMs), defined as <4 cm, are now being diagnosed with much higher frequency. Despite this trend, early intervention has yet to translate into proven clinical benefits, as mortality from RCC remains unchanged [3, 4]. Nevertheless, in practice, potential overtreatment must be considered in the context of clinical realities. Approximately 25% of SRMs are clinically aggressive, but prediction of tumor behavior prior to resection remains elusive [5]. Furthermore, prospective identification of benign pathology, which accounts for 15–20% of renal masses and can appear identical to RCC on imaging, is still not possible [5, 6].

31.2 Chemotherapeutic Strategies

In 1969, Robson et al. established a standard for treatment of RCC – radical nephrectomy (RN) [7]. To this day, surgical resection is still the cornerstone of therapy for patients with both localized and metastatic renal cell carcinoma, given the ineffectiveness of chemotherapeutic and radio therapeutic strategies against these tumors. Indeed, two prospective randomized trials have demonstrated a survival benefit of RN in the metastatic setting when surgery was combined with the immunotherapeutic agent Interferon-α [8–10]. Today, immunotherapy is being largely replaced by novel targeted agents that include multikinase inhibitors, antivascular endothelial growth factor agents, and mammalian target of Rapamycin (mTOR) inhibitors [11]. Not only are these agents less toxic than their immunotherapeutic predecessors, but they also have shown a survival advantage when compared to older approaches. For instance, Sunitinib – a multitargeted tyrosine kinase inhibitor – improved survival in patients who underwent cytoreductive nephrectomy, when compared to postsurgical patients who received Interferon. The Sunitinib group demonstrated a progression-free survival of 11 months vs. 5 months when compared to the Interferon group [12]. Similarly, in another prospective randomized trial of patients with a poor prognosis, the mTOR inhibitor Temsirolimus demonstrated a survival advantage over interferon (10.9 vs. 7.3 months) when the drugs were administered in the setting of metastatic disease following nephrectomy [13].

31.3 Evolution of Surgery for Renal Cancer

Traditionally, the surgical approach to the kidney has been through a flank, subcostal, or midline incision. As described by Robson, the classic RN includes removal of the entire kidney, perirenal fat, surrounding Gerota's fascia, and the adrenal gland [7]. With the advent of minimally invasive surgery, laparoscopic techniques have been applied to the kidney. There was initial reluctance to widely adopt laparoscopic renal surgery, because of concerns for tumor seeding of the peritoneum. Also, morcellation of specimens raised concerns for inadequate staging. Today, nephrectomy specimens are removed intact and concerns over tumor seeding have not materialized. Indeed, although, prospective randomized trials of open versus laparoscopic radical nephrectomy (LRN) were never completed, long-term retrospective data suggest oncological equivalence between the two approaches [14–18] (Table 31.1). Today, given significantly lower intra-operative blood loss and shorter convalescence, LRN is the standard of care for renal surgery that requires total removal of the kidney [14].

31.4 The Role of Partial Nephrectomy (PN)

For almost 30 years, RN was used to treat almost all renal tumors regardless of size, location, and depth of penetration. During this era, some patients were treated with an "essential" partial nephrectomy (PN) if a RN would have left them anephric. These patients usually had either an anatomically or functionally solitary kidney or had bilateral renal masses. As the oncologic data from these patients matured, the oncological soundness of PN in the appropriately selected patient became apparent. Indeed, over the past 15 years, open PN, nephron-sparing surgery (NSS), has become the standard of care, not only for essential but also for elective indications [19, 20]. As instrumentation and surgeon comfort with laparoscopy has improved, LPNs have become a more routine treatment for amenable renal masses. There are a few comparative series available looking at oncological outcomes between open and laparoscopic PNs [20–24] (Table 31.2).

31.5 Initial Experience with Laparoscopy for Renal Cancer

The era of laparoscopy in urologic surgery began in the early 1990s with pelvic lymph node dissections for the staging of prostate cancer. In 1990, the first LRN was performed by Clayman et al. for a 3-cm oncocytoma [25]. In that case report, each segmental artery was dissected and individually ligated, because the clips available at that time were not large enough to secure the main renal artery. Furthermore, a preoperative angio-infarction of the kidney was performed, and intra-operatively, a ureteral cather was placed. Since that initial report, laparoscopic renal surgery rapidly gained traction. Presently, at centers of excellence, the vast majority of nephrectomies are performed via a laparoscopic approach. Furthermore, surgery for large

Table 31.1 Oncologic and peri-operative outcome: Open and laparoscopic radical nephrectomy

	Year	n	5-Year cancer-specific survival TNM stage (%)				Complications (%)	EBL (mL)	Hospital stay (day)
			T1	T2	T3	T4			
Tsui et al. [15][a]	2003	643	83%	57%	42%	28%	–	–	–
Permpongkosol et al. [16][b]	2005	121	98% vs. 90%	95% vs. 84%	N/A	N/A	15 vs. 15	289 vs. 309	3.8 vs. 7.2
Hemal et al. [17][b]	2007	112	n/a	95.1% vs. 94.4%	N/A	N/A	12.2 vs. 15.5	246 vs. 537	3.6 vs. 6.6
Colombo et al. [18][b]	2008	116	96 vs. 96[c]	61 vs. 85[c, d]	–	–	7 vs. NR	179 vs. 500	1.4 vs. 5.1
Berger et al. [14]	2009	73	95%	90%	N/A	N/A	14	152	NR

[a]Represents open data for comparative purposes; reported series are laparoscopic only, not direct comparisons
[b]Direct comparison between open and laparoscopic groups at single institution (laparoscopic data listed first)
[c]Reported as 7-year survival data
[d]Not statistically significant
Values are reported as mean

Table 31.2 Oncologic and peri-operative outcome: Open and laparoscopic partial nephrectomy

	Year	n	5-Year disease-free survival TNM stage (%)			Positive margins (%)	Complications (%)	EBL (mL)	Hospital stay (day)
			T1a	T1b	T2				
Fergany et al. [20][a]	2000	107	97.6	95	100	–	–	–	–
Gill et al. [21][b]	2003	200	91 vs. 73[c]	9 vs. 27[c]	N/A	3.0 vs. 1.0	19 vs. 13	125 vs. 250	2.0 vs. 5.0
Permpongkosol et al. [22][b]	2006	143	91.4 vs. 97.2	75 vs. 75	N/A	2.4 vs. 1.7	7.0 vs. 25.9	436.9 vs. 427	3.3 vs. 5.4
Lane and Gill [23]	2007	56	100	–	N/A	4.0	19	–	–
Gill et al. [24][b]	2007	1800	99.3 vs. 99.2[d]	N/A		2.9 vs. 1.3	24.9 vs. 19.3	300 vs. 376	3.3 vs. 5.8

[a]Represents open data for comparative purposes [b]Direct comparison between open and laparoscopic groups at single institution (laparoscopic data listed first)
[c]Represents percent of tumors in each stage – not survival data
[d]3-year survival for pT1 tumors, stage not subdivided
Values are reported as mean

renal tumors and tumors with thrombi extending into the renal vein and, even, the vena cava are now being performed laparoscopically [26–28]. Coincident with the growth of laparoscopy, has been the increased detection of incidental SRMs during the last 2 decades, as cross-sectional imaging has become a routine diagnostic tool [3]. Thanks to the widespread acceptance of NSS and refinement of laparoscopic instrumentation, a patient can be offered a PN via laparoscopic approaches (with and without robot assistance) utilizing only three or four small incisions, none measuring greater than 1.2 cm. Cancer control for appropriately selected patients appears to be preserved [29].

31.5.1 Quantifying Renal Cell Tumor Characteristics

The growth of surgical options for renal masses has been accompanied by a greater understanding of the biology of renal masses. Although beyond the scope of this chapter, the treatment alternatives available for SRMs are numerous [30]. In brief, the goal of treatment must strive first for

- Oncological safety
- Nephron preservation

These choices are largely made based on subjective assessments of various variables. Decision to advise the patient to undergo a PN versus a RN, for instance, currently is largely institution- and surgeon-specific. Variables such as comorbidities, body habitus, perceived tolerance of risk, and surgeon comfort with particular techniques drive decision-making. Furthermore, attributes of the tumor itself play a particularly important role. Until recently tumor characteristics were nonquantifiable and the literature largely communicated tumor attributes with descriptive, nonstandardized terms such as central, hilar, and exophytic.

31.5.1.1 R.E.N.A.L. Nephrometry Scoring System

In order to rectify this reality, the R.E.N.A.L. nephrometry scoring system was recently introduced [31]. This tool allows the surgeon to assign standardized, numerical values to critical tumor characteristics, which include

- **R**adius
- **E**xophycity
- **N**earness to renal sinus/collecting system
- **A**nterior/posterior location
- **L**ocation in relation to the renal poles

Adoption of this system should afford improved communication and meaningful comparisons between treatment options that are available to patients with SRM.

This chapter will provide an overview of the indications and technical considerations for the various forms of minimally invasive surgical options that are currently available to patients with renal mass.

31.6 Surgical Options-laparoscopic Transperitoneal Radical Nephrectomy

31.6.1 Historical Overview

The application of laparoscopy to renal surgery was catalyzed by the experience with laparoscopic cholecystectomy in general surgery. In 1990, Clayman and associates performed the first transperitoneal LRN in an 85-year old female for a 3 cm enhancing right renal mass [25, 32]. In that initial case, the patient underwent preoperative angiography with embolization of the main right renal artery, as well as placement of a ureteral catheter to aid in identification of the right ureter. Each of the five segmental renal arteries were individually clipped and divided. The specimen was extracted by morcellation. Total operative time was 6 h 45 min and the patient remained in the hospital for 6 days. Today, this case would be performed without angiography or placement of a ureteral catheter, and the specimen would be extracted intact. Furthermore, the patient would likely spend 2–3 h in the operating room and leave the hospital in 2–3 days.

31.6.2 Operating Room Set up and Patient Positioning

Although techniques somewhat vary from one institution to the other, the major technical themes of LRN are consistent throughout the world. The usual operating room arrangement is depicted in Fig. 31.1a. The patient's midline is marked with a surgical pen in the supine position in order to maintain orientation following positioning and insufflation. The patient is then placed in the lateral decubitus position with the diseased kidney up. We prefer the patient to be at a 45–60° angle rather than in full flank.

31.6.3 Trocar Placement

31.6.3.1 General Considerations for Placing the Camera Port

Pneumoperitoneum is established using a Veress needle or the Hasson technique. We use cross-sectional imaging to measure the distance from the umbilicus to the hilum.

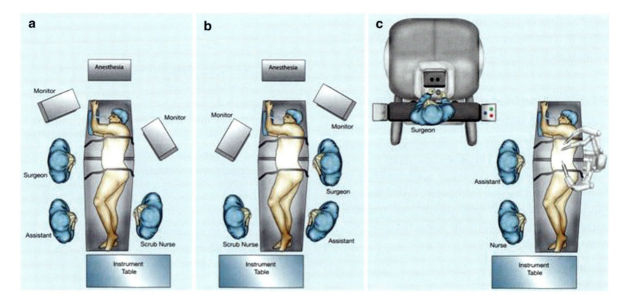

Fig. 31.1 Operating room set-up. (**a**) Left transperitoneal, laparoscopic radical nephrectomy, (**b**) left retroperitoneal, laparoscopic radical nephrectomy, (**c**) transperitoenal robot-assisted laparoscopic partial nephrectomy

This distance helps to guide our placement of the camera port. Some surgeons prefer this 5-mm camera port placed at the level of the renal hilum, whereas others favor its placement slightly inferior to the renal vessels. The renal artery usually sits posterior and a bit superior to the renal vein, thus placement of the camera port inferior to the hilum often affords the surgeon a good view of the artery when a 30° laparascope is used to peer behind the vein.

31.6.3.2 Classical Port Placement

Initially, in addition to the camera port, two working ports are placed. A 5-mm assistant's port will be placed later during the procedure to aid in medial retraction of the colon. In general, a 12-mm working port is placed above the anterior superior iliac spine (ASIS) midway between the umbilicus and the ASIS. Placement of the 12-mm port at this location affords ideal geometry for securing the hilum with an endovascular stapler. At the end of the nephrectomy, this port incision is extended along Langer's lines to aid in removal of the intact specimen. A 5-mm working port is placed medially and inferiorly to the camera port. Additional assistant ports can be placed as needed and according to the surgeon's preference; however, care must be taken when placing these ports such that the instruments and ports are not colliding with each other. In thin patients, the medial ports (i.e., the camera and the medial working port) are often placed in the midline. In obese patients, however, lateral displacement of these ports is often necessary. In these instances the ports are placed "above the hump" of the abdominal curvature following insufflations (Fig. 31.2).

31.6.3.3 Alternative Port Placement

Some surgeons prefer to place the 12-mm port below the camera port instead of above the ASIS as described. In this arrangement, the port above the ASIS is 5 mm in size. This strategy avoids a transverse extraction site and results in an up-and-down final incision. Hernia rates between midline and transverse lower-quadrant incisions appear to be similar; however, some retrospective low-level evidence suggests that paramedian extraction sites result in higher hernia rates [33]. If the

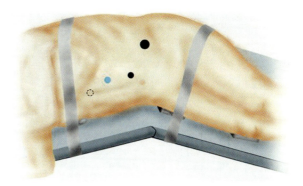

Fig. 31.2 Trocar placement: left transperitoneal laparoscopic radical nephrectomy, *Blue circle* camera port, *dashed circle* assistant port. *Large circle* 12-mm port, while the *small circle* 5-mm port

12-mm port is placed in the medial position, the surgeon must be aware that the angle of attack for the hilum with an endovascular stapler through this port is at times suboptimal. The surgeon must be prepared to use laparoscopic clips for both the artery and the vein when embarking on this approach.

31.6.4 Surgical Technique

31.6.4.1 Mobilization of the Colon

Once the ports have been placed, dissection is initiated by mobilizing the right or left colon incising the line of Toldt superiorly and inferiorly. It is important, during this mobilization, to extend the incision far enough superiorly and inferiorly such that the colon falls far enough medially, exposing the retro-peritoneum. A key technical point during this mobilization is not to incise the kidney's lateral attachments. If these attachments are divided too early in the procedure, the kidney will be too mobile, preventing sufficient traction for dissection of the hilar vessels.

31.6.4.2 Retro-peritoneum and Dissection of the Gonadal Vein

During renal mobilization, it is important to understand the fascial layers of the retro-peritoneum. The intermediate stratum of the retro-peritoneum surrounds the

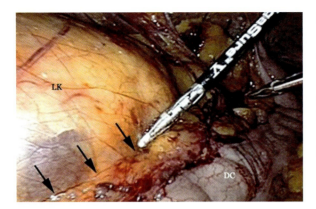

Fig. 31.3 Laparoscopic left radical nephrectomy: *DC* descending colon, *LK* left kidney. The camera is looking in the direction of the patient's pelvis. *Black arrows* indicate the avascular tissue plane along the intermediate stratum of the retroperitoneum along which the dissection advances

kidney. Some surgeons prefer to enter this intermediate stratum while others do not. Regardless of the individual's preference, it is critical to understand the anatomical topography of the retro-peritoneum and to pursue the dissection in a systematic fashion, staying within the same fascial layer (Fig. 31.3). During retroperitoneal dissection, one of the first landmarks that is encountered within the retro-peritoneal fat is the gonadal vein. By pursuing the dissection along the gonadal vessel caudally, safe access to the renal hilum can be established. The ureter travels lateral to the gonadal vein. Establishing a plane lateral to the gonadal vein but medial to the ureter is often most helpful. With the ureter identified, a tissue window onto the surface of the psoas muscle can be developed and the ureter can be lifted superiorly and laterally. Any remaining tissue tethering the gonadal vessels laterally should be divided with thermal energy, dropping the vein medially. Once this dissection is completed, the vein can be transected. This is usually most helpful in the vicinity of the renal vein on the left and the vena cava on the right. The 5-mm LigaSure™ is an excellent tool for transecting this vessel; however, some surgeons prefer to secure the gonadal vein with laparoscopic surgical clips.

31.6.4.3 Exposure of the Lower Pole of the Kidney

With the ureter on upward traction, the lower pole of the kidney can be lifted. This maneuver rotates the kidney in an upward and medial fashion, creating a space between the lower pole of the kidney, the ureter, and the hilar vessels. It is during this part of the operation that active retraction achieved by the surgeon's nondominant hand is most critical. A small bowel clamp or Maryland forceps are used to place lateral traction on the kidney. This traction needs to be assertive and constant during dissection of the renal vasculature.

31.6.4.4 Dissection of the Hilum and Renal Vessels

Careful blunt dissection of the renal vessels can then be undertaken with a combination of the blunt tip of the suction-irrigator device, laparoscopic right angle, laparoscopic peanut, and/or the tip of the LigaSure™ device (Covidien PLC, Dublin, Ireland). During this part of the operation, it is important for the camera operator to maintain appropriate orientation for the laparoscopic surgeon. Depending on laterality of the tumor, the IVC or the aorta should be kept in a left-to-right orientation – often termed "on the horizon."

The main renal vein and artery should be individually identified. The artery lies posterior and superior to the renal vein. Each vessel should be dissected free of its fibro-fatty and lymphatic attachments, so that clips or a stapling device can be placed on the vessel. The vessels can be taken individually or en bloc. Classic teaching has been that the vessels should be transected individually for fear that an arterio-venous fistula can develop, leading to high output congestive heart failure. Recent data suggest that the main vessels can be stapled in tandem without sequelae [34, 35]. If, however, the vessels are to be taken individually, the renal artery must be ligated prior to the renal vein. The surgeon must be certain that all renal arteries have been identified and secured. Ligation of the renal vein before all renal arteries are secured can lead to venous blow-out on the renal side of the ligated vessel, as blood continues to enter but fails to leave the kidney. Even in the absence of this potentially catastrophic event, primary renal vein ligation can lead to significant blood trapping, resulting in postoperative anemia. Ligation of renal vessels is most often accomplished using a laparoscopic

EndoGIA stapler, vascular load, although some surgeons prefer securing both the artery and vein with laparoscopic clips.

31.6.4.5 Addressing Renal Vein Tumor Thrombi

As urologists have become more comfortable with laparoscopic techniques and laparoscopic instrumentation has improved, LRNs are now being safely performed in patients with large renal masses with or without renal vein thrombi [26–28] (Table 31.3). Although the survival data in these series are not mature enough for direct comparisons, it appears that the laparoscopic removal of large renal tumors with venous thrombi is technically feasible with minimal blood loss.

The operative procedure for a LRN with a venous thrombus is essentially the same except when approaching the hilar vessels. After the renal vessels have been identified and the artery has been secured, a flexible laparoscopic ultrasound probe is inserted into the abdominal cavity to image the proximal extent of the thrombus in the renal vein. The renal vein is then ligated proximal to the thrombus. If there is not adequate length on the vein due to the presence of the thrombus, a laparoscopic DeBakey grasper or vessel loop can be placed around the vein to "milk" back the thrombus to allow for an adequate length of exposed vein in order to apply the stapling device. If necessary, a hand port can be placed to assist in this portion of the case.

31.6.4.6 Mobilization of the Kidney and the Adrenal Gland

Once the renal vasculature is controlled, the remainder of the case focuses on freeing the kidney from its surrounding attachments. This can be achieved with a combination of blunt dissection combined with the use of thermal energy as necessary. In general, the adrenal gland should be preserved if preoperative imaging does not suggest invasion of the gland by the tumor. Based on data from heterogeneous cohorts, some authors recommend that the gland be sacrificed in the setting of an upper pole renal tumor that measures 7 cm or greater [36]. Data from our institution show that adrenal preservation is safe, regardless of tumor size and location, provided that the adrenal gland is clearly visualized and uninvolved on imaging [37]. During adrenal preservation, a plane between the adrenal gland and the upper pole of the kidney can be developed in combination of blunt dissection and use of a thermal device, such as the Harmonic scalpel or LigaSure™.

31.6.4.7 Division of the Ureter

The ureter is divided with clips or the LigaSure™ device (Covidien Plc, Dublin, Ireland). The timing of ureteral division is determined by the need for traction on the lower pole of the kidney during the case. Division of the ureter early in the case can facilitate aggressive retraction on the lower pole, in order to better access

Table 31.3 Laparoscopic radical nephrectomy for pT3 tumors: comparative studies

	Year	n	5-Year survival TNM stage (%)		Follow-up (m)	Tumor Size (cm)	EBL (mL)	OR time (min)	Positive margins (n)	Complications (n)
			pT3a	pT3b						
Fergany et al. [20][a]	2000	107	85	59	104	–	–	–	–	–
Desai et al. [26][b]	2003	16	–	–	19.5 vs. 9.4	7.8 vs. 12.4	381.9 vs. 353.6	188.8 vs. 195.7	2/0	1/0
Steinnerd et al. [28]	2007	5	–	–	11.5	5.5	150	119.6	0	0
Guzzo et al. [27]	2009	37	–	–	14	6	200	190	NS	7

[a]Represents open data for comparative purposes
[b]Series divided into known and unknown thrombus (unknown presented first)
Values are reported as mean.

the renal vessels. The potential and unlikely drawback of dividing the ureter early is that the kidney can become hydronephrotic, hindering hilar dissection.

Ureter and Upper Tract Transitional Cell Carcinoma

When performing a laparoscopic nephro-ureterectomy for an upper tract transitional cell carcinoma, we perform the renal dissection and excision as described above. The only difference is that we do not transect the ureter. Depending on the location of the tumor, we will either extend the extraction port as if we were removing an intact kidney and remove the distal ureter from this incision. Or we will reposition the patient and remove the distal ureter with a bladder cuff through a lower midline incision.

31.6.4.8 Extraction of the Specimen and Wound Closure

Once the kidney is circumferentially freed from its attachments, the pneumoperitoneum is reduced under direct vision to demonstrate hemostasis at atmospheric pressure. The inferior 12-mm port is removed and the incision is enlarged slightly to allow passage of the ENDO CATCH™ bag (Covidien PLC) up to the renal fossa. The kidney is then placed within the bag and the purse-strings of the bag are tightened. Once accomplished, all other ports are removed and the incision at the extraction site is extended to facilitate removal of the intact, entrapped specimen. After removal of the kidney, the fascia at the extraction site is reapproximated in two layers. The remaining port sites are closed as per the surgeon's preference.

31.7 Retro-peritoneoscopic Radical Nephrectomy

31.7.1 Indications and Limitations

Due to its location, the kidney can be accessed via a purely retro-peritoneal approach. Retro-peritoneoscopic renal surgery offers the advantage of avoiding the peritoneal cavity, which is especially helpful in patients with prior abdominal surgery who are likely to have extensive abdominal adhesions [38]. Also, a retro-peritoneal approach is preferable in patients in whom the transperitoneal approach is unattractive because of

- Hepatomegaly
- Need for continuing peritoneal dialysis
- Presence of ostomies
- Percutaneous feeding tubes

On the other hand, the retro-peritoneal approach is unfamiliar territory for many urologists. Furthermore, the small working space can make the operation difficult and tedious, especially in patients with copious retro-peritoneal fat, which can impede visualization. Finally, the retro-peritoneum, especially in the presence of copious fat, lacks reliable landmarks that a transperitoneal approach offers. This absence of predictable anatomical cues contributes to a steep learning curve and may lead to catastrophic complications in inexperienced hands. In one multi-institutional report, the IVC was transected in two patients with a stapling device, because it was mistaken for the main right renal vein [39].

Initially, retro-peritoneoscopy was not routinely advocated as an approach to the kidney, because the working space was prohibitively limited. In 1992, Gaur described the technique of dilating the retro-peritoneum with an atraumatic balloon [40]. This strategy allows the retro-peritoneum to be dilated to 800 ml, creating enough working space to afford placement of a camera and instruments to surgically approach the kidney. Even with this advance, the retro-peritoneal approach is challenging and is most often employed by more experienced laparoscopic surgeons [38] [41, 42].

31.7.2 Operating Room Setup and Patient Positioning

The patient is placed in the lateral decubitus position with the kidney of interest facing up. In contrast to the transperitoneal approach, the patient is "flanked" at 90°. The table is then flexed and the kidney bar is elevated to allow for the retro-peritoneal space to expand (Figs. 31.1b and 31.4).

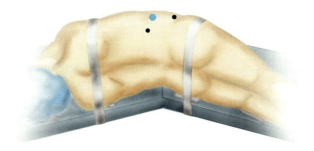

Fig. 31.4 Trocar placement: right retro-peritoneal laparoscopic radical nephrectomy. *Blue circle* camera port, *large circle* 12-mm port, *small circle* 5-mm port

31.7.3 Creation of the Retro-Peritoneal Working Space

Access to the retro-peritoneum for insufflation and placement of trocars is gained by making a small incision just below or off the 11th or 12th rib. Under direct visualization, the retro-peritoneum is entered by incising the three fascial layers and bluntly retracting the muscular fibers with 'S' retractors. The anterior thoraco-lumbar fascia is then entered bluntly. Using manual dissection and palpation, the balloon dilator is placed into the retro-peritoneum. The balloon is directed medially, anterior to the psoas, and the retro-peritoneum is dilated. The balloon is then deflated and directed posterior to the kidney. A second dilation is then performed. This maneuver displaces the kidney antero-medial. During dilation of the retro-peritoneum, care must be taken not to place the balloon into Gerota's fascia.

31.7.4 Trocar Placement

A 12-mm port with a fascial retention balloon is then inserted through the incision and the external adjustment foam cuff is used to create an airtight seal. This port is used for the laparoscopic camera. Two additional ports are then placed under direct visualization in standard fashion. At our institution, we place a 12-mm port just above the ASIS and a second 5-mm working port at the junction of the 12th rib and the paraspinal muscles. It is important to place these ports as far away as possible from each other to prevent intra-operative "sword fighting" of the instruments and camera, which can impede surgical progression. Of note, we favor a 12-mm port just above the ASIS so that we can extend this incision for specimen extraction. We also favor a 12-mm port at this location if exposure to the distal ureter during a nephro-ureterectomy for upper tract urothelial carcinoma is required.

31.7.5 Dissection and Accessing the Hilar Vessels

Once the retro-peritoneum is accessed and the ports have been placed, dissection is commenced. In performing retro-peritoneoscopic renal surgery, one of the most important aspects is maintaining orientation. The primary anatomic landmark used during this approach to the kidney is the psoas muscle. It is critical during this operation for the psoas muscle to be kept in the left to right orientation on the screen by the assistant controlling the camera. With adequate balloon dilation of the retro-peritoneum, the kidney should be freed posteriorly. The kidney is then retracted antero-medial with a small bowel clamp or the suction-irrigator. With the psoas muscle in view and properly oriented, the intermediate stratum of the transversalis fascia is incised from cephalad to caudad. In doing so, the renal hilar vessels should be accessible. The renal vasculature must be individually identified and dissected free of all attachments, so that it can be controlled either individually or en bloc. As in the case of a transperitoneal nephrectomy, either an endovascular stapler or surgical clips can be used. One of the advantages of the retro-peritoneal approach is that the main renal artery is visualized very early in the dissection. The artery can be secured without having to retract the renal vein. Prior to dividing the renal vein on the right side, the suprarenal vena cava must be appropriately dissected in order to avoid injury to this vital structure during stapling. Once the hilar vessels are controlled, the kidney can then be freed of its lateral and superior attachments as well as the attachments to the overlying peritoneum. The ureter is divided and the kidney is bagged and removed intact through an extended incision in the 12-mm working port site.

31.8 Laparoscopic Transperitoneal Partial Nephrectomy

31.8.1 Rational for Nephron Sparing Surgery

For over 30 years, the oncological standard of care for renal tumors was RN which included the removal of

- Kidney
- Perirenal fat
- Gerota's fascia
- Ipsilateral adrenal
- Overlying peritoneum

It was only with the maturation of oncological data in patients who had a PN for "essential" indications that it became evident that oncological principles would not be sacrificed by performing NSS [19, 20]. More recent data has suggested that not only is NSS an oncologic equivalent to radical surgery, but that preservation of renal parenchyma contributes to longer overall survival [43, 44].

Two recent studies have provided further impetus for renal preservation whenever possible. The Mayo clinic showed that patients >65 of age had a statistically significant worse overall survival compared to an age-matched control group who underwent a PN for a similar tumor [43]. Furthermore, Huang et al. showed that patients who underwent a RN suffered more cardio-vascular adverse events when compared to patients who underwent a PN [44]. With this emerging data, the current standard of care is to perform a PN in patients whenever possible, especially if their tumor is less than 4 cm [45]. Unfortunately, research continues to show that PN is underutilized [46, 47].

31.8.2 Transition from Open to Laparoscopic Partial Nephrectomy

The transition from an open to a laparoscopic technique in the case of PN has taken longer to gain traction than the shift from open to LRN. The initial reports of a laparoscopic PN involved only benign disease [48, 49]. There was an early reluctance to perform laparoscopic PNs due to concern for intra-peritoneal tumor spillage. Furthermore, development of appropriate laparoscopic vascular control instrumentation was also a barrier to early adoption of the technique. With the development of the laparoscopic bulldog clamp and laparoscopic Satinsky clamp, however, laparoscopic surgeons are now able to excise small renal tumors in a bloodless field, duplicating open PN techniques [29].

31.8.3 Surgical Technique

31.8.3.1 Patient Positioning and Port Placement

A transperitonal PN is begun in the same manner as a transperitoneal LRN. The patient is placed in 45–60° lateral position and a pneumoperitoneum is achieved. In general, four laparoscopic ports are utilized. The additional port that is needed for a LPN is used as an assistant port for placement of a laparoscopic Satinsky clamp. Alternatively, the instrument can be placed through a stab incision in the skin.

31.8.3.2 Dissection and Accessing the Hilar Vessels

The kidney is mobilized by reflecting the colon medially. The ureter and the gonadal vein is identified and used as a landmark to the hilum. Unlike in the case of the radical procedure, ureteral manipulation must be fastidious in order to avoid injury. The renal hilum is identified and the artery and vein are dissected individually or en bloc. The key to the hilar dissection is creating appropriate tissue windows so that a laparoscopic bulldog or Satinsky clamp can be placed. This dissection is facilitated by the use of the blunt tip suction cannula. Depending on the tumor size, depth, and location, some surgeons will only clamp the renal artery and leave the renal vein untouched. Indeed, under appropriate pneumoperitoneum, venous bleeding is usually minimal. This decision is left to each individual surgeon's discretion.

31.8.3.3 Exposure of the Tumor and Intraoperative Ultrasound

Once the hilum is dissected and exposed adequately to facilitate placement of vascular clamps for hilar control, the kidney is defatted to expose the tumor. Fat overlying the tumor should either be kept on the specimen or sent separately for careful pathologic review. Even with SRMs, fat invasion is possible, necessitating complete resection [50, 51]. Once the tumor is visible, a laparoscopic ultrasound probe is placed through one of the ports and real-time ultrasonographic information is obtained about

- Tumor size
- Depth of invasion
- Distance from the adjacent calyx and renal sinus
- Location of intra-renal vessels close to the tumor or its margins
- Presence of satellite tumors
- Presence of a synchronous tumor

With the ultrasound probe as a guide, the tumor periphery is scored with J-hook electrocautery to mark out the edges of the tumor resection. Heavy sutures and bolsters are placed into the abdominal cavity, so that they are readily available to reconstruct the renal parenchyma once the tumor has been excised. 12.5 g of Mannitol are given to minimize damage to nephrons during ischemia when the hilar vessels are clamped.

31.8.3.4 Excision of the Tumor

After occluding the renal vessels, tumor excision is the next step accomplished by incising deeply into the pre-marked renal parenchyma. The suction cannula is used for tissue counter-traction and also serves to aspirate any bleeding from the tumor bed during excision. Circumferential incision is carried out using either eletrocautery or sharp dissection with laparoscopic scissors. Care is taken to notice any major transected vessels or any violations of the collecting system. The tumor is excised with a small margin of normal parenchyma using a combination of sharp and blunt dissection in a circumferential manner [19]. Once the tumor is completely removed, a deep biopsy is taken for a frozen section margin.

31.8.3.5 Repair of the Renal Parenchyma

Figure-of-eight sutures are used to oversew vessels that were damaged during tumor removal. The collecting system is also reconstructed with 3-zero dissolvable sutures. The edges of the resection bed are then treated with the laparoscopic Argon beam electrocautery. The renal parenchyma is repaired using heavy absorbable suture. An oxidized cellulose bolster is placed in the tumor bed and the suture is then secured over the bolster. The sutures are tightened and secured with Lapra-Ty™ clips. Hemostatic agents can then be applied according to surgeon practice.

31.8.3.6 Removal of the Specimen and Wound Closure

After renal reconstruction is complete, the vascular clamps are released and the kidney is observed to ensure hemostasis and appropriate reperfusion. At this point, the pneumoperitoneum can be lowered to check for significant venous bleeding. Once the frozen sections are confirmed to be free of tumor, a Jackson-Pratt drain is placed posterior to the kidney through one of the 5-mm ports to monitor for a potential urinary leak. The tumor is entrapped in an Endo-catch impermeable bag and removed from the abdomen. The remaining ports are removed; the fascia is closed in standard fashion and the overlying skin is reapproximated.

31.9 Retro-peritoneoscopic Partial Nephrectomy

31.9.1 Indications

The techniques for laparoscopic PN and retro-peritoneoscopic exposure of the kidney have already been described in depth. A retro-peritoneal approach for a laparoscopic PN is ideal for postero-lateral tumors. The retro-peritoneoscopic approach is similar to the approach used for a retroperitoneoscopic RN. There are a few distinctions between a transperitoneal and a retro-peritoneoscopic partial nephrectomy that are worthy of mention.

31.9.2 Technical Differences to a Transperitoneal Approach

Because of the limited working space in the retroperitoneum, the artery and vein should be individually dissected in preparation for placement of laparoscopic

Table 31.4 Robotically-assisted laparoscopic partial nephrectomy: comparative studies

	Year	Tumors (n)	Follow-up	Tumor size (cm)	Mean WIT (min)	Positive margins (n)	Complications (n/%)
Ho et al. [53][a]	2008	20	≥1 year	3.5	21.7	0	0
Wang and Bhayani [52]	2009	40	NR	2.5	19.0	1	6/15
Benway et al. [54][b]	2009	129	1 year	NS	19.7	5	11/8.5
Scoll et al [55].	2010	107	NR	2.8	25.5	5	11/11

[a]Authors do not perform robotic procedure for posterior upper pole tumors
[b]This series contains patients from Wang and Bhayani (2009)
WIT warm ischemia time

bulldog clamps. Unlike a transperitoneal approach where the artery and vein can be occluded individually or en bloc with a Satinsky clamp, the renal artery and vein should be clamped sequentially with one laparoscopic bulldog clamp each during a retro-peritoneal approach. A Satinsky clamp would take up too much working room in an already limited retro-peritoneal space. Nevertheless, it is worth mentioning that some surgeons prefer only to clamp the renal artery regardless of the approach. The renal vein can be left unclamped because the pressure of the pneumoperitoneum is greater than venous pressure, and thus back-bleeding during tumor excision should be minimal. The tumor is then excised and the kidney is reconstructed in a manner similar to a transperitoneal approach.

steep learning curve. Sitting at the console, the robotic user can rotate one's wrists 180° and pass suture from virtually any angle. Renal reconstruction can be performed in 3-D and the passing of suture through the kidney is easier than with pure laparoscopic technique due to the wrist motions of the robot.

With the advent and growth of robotic surgery, robot-assisted laparoscopic PNs (RALPN) have started to gain popularity. Many small series have been published showing that a RALPN is technically feasible without increasing patient morbidity [52–55] (Table 31.4). These series do not have long enough follow-up to show equivalent oncological outcome as do the open or laparoscopic approaches; however, currently there is no suspicion that the technique might be inferior [52–54].

31.10 Robotic-Assisted Laparoscopic Partial Nephrectomy

31.10.1 Advantages of a Robotic Approach

With the introduction and improvement of the DaVinci™ (Intuitive Surgical) robotic systems, robotic surgery has pervaded all surgical specialties. Initially, urologists became familiar with the robot when performing prostatectomies. Since its introduction, the DaVinci™ system has changed the field of prostatic surgery. The advantages of the DaVinci™ system are the improved visualization afforded by its three-dimensional (3-D) vision and the ability to perform intricate reconstructions intra-corporeally with a less

31.10.2 Patient Positioning and Trocar Placement

The procedure for a RALPN has many similarities to a purely laparoscopic PN. Once the midline is marked, the patient is placed in 45–60° flank position with the affected kidney upright. The patient is then secured to the operating table. The kidney bar is elevated and the patient is flexed (Fig. 31.1c). At our institution, prior to placing the camera port, we measure the distances from the umbilicus to the renal hilum and to the renal mass based on the cross-sectional imaging. By measuring the predetermined distance from the patient's umbilicus, we place the camera port at the level of the renal hilum. The pneumoperitoneum is then established. We use two different port arrangements, depending on the location of the tumor (Fig. 31.5).

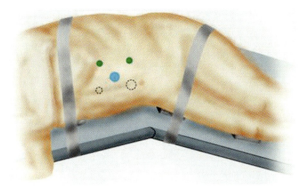 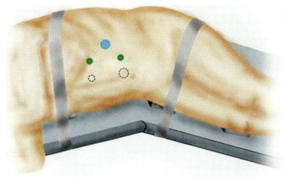

Fig. 31.5 Trocar placement: left transperitoneal robot-assisted partial nephrectomy: two commonly used configurations. *Blue circle* camera port, *dashed circle* assistant port, *large circle* 12 mm port, *small circle* 5 mm port, *green circle* 8 mm robotic ports

31.10.2.1 Trocar Placement – Posterior Tumors

For posterior tumors, we place the camera more laterally so that tumor visualization is facilitated. The two robot arm ports are then inserted more medially and offset by a hand's width from the camera port. We then place two assistant ports at the midline, spaced from the robotic ports so that the assistant is not colliding with the robotic instruments. This port arrangement outlines a pentagon.

31.10.2.2 Trocar Placement – Anterior Tumors

For an anterior or lateral tumor, we place our ports in a more traditional pattern. The camera port is placed at the level of the renal hilum in a more medial position, just lateral to the midline. The robotic ports are then placed superior-lateral and inferio-lateral to the camera port, offset by a hand's width. The two assistant ports are placed medial to the camera port with one port superior and the other port inferior. This arrangement is identical to the pattern of the number five on a face of a die, with the camera port being the dot in the center.

31.10.3 Docking of the DaVinci™ Robot

Once the ports are inserted, the robot is docked at the patient's back. The robotic arms extend around the patient's flank and the robotic instruments are then inserted from the flanked patient's ventrum. We prefer using the monopolar scissors in the right robotic arm and the bipolar Maryland grasper in the left robotic arm. A zero-degree camera is employed, and the assistant sits at the patient's side to help the surgeon at the console throughout the procedure.

31.10.4 Robotic Dissection

Once the robot is docked, the procedure begins in a similar manner to any laparoscopic kidney surgery. The overlying colon is mobilized medially, the ureter is identified inferiorly, the lower pole of the kidney is freed, and the kidney is elevated to place the hilar vessels on traction. The renal artery and vein are dissected free of surrounding adventitia so that a laparoscopic bulldog clamp can be placed across the renal artery and/or vein. Once accomplished, the peri-nephric fat is removed and the kidney is mobilized, so that the tumor excision can be performed. As already mentioned, care must be taken to ensure that the fat overlying the tumor is undisturbed, so that a complete pathological evaluation can be performed. After the kidney has been defatted and the tumor exposed, a laparoscopic ultrasound probe is introduced through the 12-mm assistant port. An ultrasonographic examination of the kidney is performed to confirm the tumor, exclude synchronous tumors, and mark the boundary of the resection. The tumor periphery is marked circumferentially by scoring the renal capsule with the monopolar scissors.

The monopolar scissors are then exchanged for the round tip scissors and vascular occlusion of the main renal artery is then achieved. In general, we prefer the

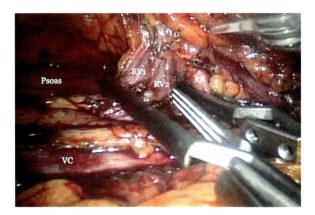

Fig. 31.6 Laparoscopic bulldog clamp being placed on a duplicated renal vein (*RV1/RV2*). The renal artery (*RA*) is already clamped. The vena cava (*VC*) is oriented on the screen in a left to right direction, often referred to as "on the horizon." The lower pole of the kidney is aggressively lifted off of the psoas muscle in order to facilitate access to the renal hilum

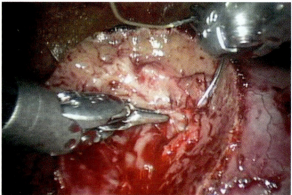

Fig. 31.7 Closure of a violation in the collecting system following tumor resection during a robot-assisted laparoscopic partial nephrectomy. The right robotic arm is preparing to place a suture, while the left robotic arm is facilitating the closure by lifting tissue and thereby displaying the collecting system defect

bedside assistant to place a laparoscopic bulldog clamp through the assistant's 12-mm port (Fig. 31.6). The tumor is then excised and biopsies from the margin are taken for pathologic review.

31.10.5 Reconstruction of the Parenchyma

The reconstruction is performed after robotic needle drivers are substituted for the existing robotic instruments. The assistant passes sutures as needed to the console surgeon for reconstruction. First, the tumor bed is inspected for bleeding and any collecting system entry. We prefer a 3-0 Vicryl with a small needle (CV-23 or GS-22) to close the collecting system or to oversew any tumor-bed bleeding. The Argon beam electrocautery is used to ablate the parenchymal edges, similar to a laparoscopic PN.

2-0 Vicryl sutures with a GS-22 or V-20 needle are passed into the abdominal cavity to close the defect in the renal parenchyma (Fig. 31.7). At the end of each suture, a laparoscopic clip has been placed by the scrub technician. Each suture is passed through both ends of the defect making sure to incorporate the renal capsule. Bolsters of SURGICEL® (Ethicon Inc.) are placed in the middle of the defect before sutures are tightened. It is important to ensure that the suture passes over the bolsters so that maximal tension is assured.

Once the suture is tightened, a Lapra-Ty™ is placed on the Vicryl material to ensure appropriate parenchymal reapproximation. Usually three or four sutures secured in this manner are required to close the tumor bed. Once complete, the vascular clamps are released and the tumor bed is observed to ensure adequate hemostasis.

31.10.6 Removal of the Specimen and Wound Closure

The kidney is then placed into its anatomical position and a closed suction drain is placed next to the renal unit. The tumor is entrapped in an ENDO CATCH™ bag (Covidien PLC) and removed. The specimen is brought out through the camera port. The robot is undocked and all the ports are removed. The fascia is managed in standard fashion, and the overlying skin is reapproximated.

31.11 Conclusions

Laparoscopy and robot-assisted surgery has pervaded all aspects of renal surgery. The growing trend is to perform fewer and fewer open surgeries on the kidney for renal masses. The literature supports the use of minimally invasive techniques to treat renal tumors from an oncologic as well as a renal functional standpoint. Furthermore, these minimally invasive techniques are better tolerated by patients, with a shorter hospital stay, and earlier return to normal activity. Nevertheless, the impetus to use minimally invasive techniques should never compromise utilization of NSS. For instance, open PN must be employed to treat tumors that cannot be resected laparoscopically or robotically. Use of LRN in these situations is not acceptable [45].

Quick Reference Guide

1. **Patient positioning**:
   - Lateral decubitus position
   - Kidney with the mass should be in upright position

   Retro-peritoneal approach:
   - Patient should be at 90°

   Trans-peritoneal approach:
   - Patient can be at 45 to 60°

2. Once the pneumoperitoneum is established and the ports are placed in their appropriate positions, reflect the overlying colon medially by incising the white line of Toldt. Do not dissect the lateral attachments of the kidney at this point or the kidney will be too mobile during the entire procedure and make it harder to dissect the hilar vessels!

3. Incise the intermediate stratum of the retroperitoneum and dissect inferiorly in this layer to identify the gonadal vein and ipsilateral ureter.

4. **Left-sided lesions:**
   The gonadal vein can be dissected superiorly to its junction with the main left renal vein.

   Right sided lesion:
   The gonadal vein inserts into the inferior vena cava (IVC); dissect in a superior direction on the anterior adventitia of the IVC and this will identify the main right renal vein.

5. Isolation of the main renal artery is facilitated by upward traction on the ureter. This traction places the renal hilum on stretch and allows the surgeon to visualize the artery posterior. Remember the main renal artery is usually posterior and superior to the main renal vein.

6. If needed, especially on the left side, the gonadal vein can be ligated to facilitate isolation of the main renal artery.

7. Once dissected, the hilar vessels can be taken individually or en bloc with a stapling device if performing a radical nephrectomy. For a partial nephrectomy, the vessels can be clamped individually or en bloc to achieve a bloodless resection field.

8. **Partial nephrectomy:**
   Intra-operative ultrasound should be used for
   - Visualization of the tumor
   - Determination of its depth
   - Determination of its circumference
   - Determination of the proximity to the intraparenchymal vessels and collecting system

9. **Remember**: Ligate or clamp the renal artery prior to ligating or clamping the renal vein.

10. **Partial nephrectomies:**
    Reconstruct the kidney over oxidized cellulose bolsters with 2-0 vicryl sutures.

References

1. Jemal, A., Siegel, R., Ward, E., Hao, Y., Xu, J., Thun, M.J.: CA: a cancer journal for clinicians. Cancer Stat. **59**, 225–249 (2009)
2. Jayson, M., Sanders, H.: Increased incidence of serendipitously discovered renal cell carcinoma. Urology **51**, 203–205 (1998)
3. Hollingsworth, J.M., Miller, D.C., Daignault, S., Hollenbeck, B.K.: Rising incidence of small renal masses: a need to reassess treatment effect. J. Natl. Cancer Inst. **98**, 1331–1334 (2006). 20 Sep 2006
4. Hock, L.M., Lynch, J., Balaji, K.C.: Increasing incidence of all stages of kidney cancer in the last 2 decades in the United States: an analysis of surveillance, epidemiology and end results program data. J. Urol. **167**, 57–60 (2002)
5. Lane, B.R., Babineau, D., Kattan, M.W., et al.: A preoperative prognostic nomogram for solid enhancing renal tumors 7 cm or less amenable to partial nephrectomy. J. Urol. **178**, 429–434 (2007)
6. Kutikov, A., Fossett, L.K., Ramchandani, P., et al.: Incidence of benign pathologic findings at partial nephrectomy for solitary renal mass presumed to be renal cell carcinoma on preoperative imaging. Urology **68**, 737–740 (2006)
7. Robson, C.J., Churchill, B.M., Anderson, W.: The results of radical nephrectomy for renal cell carcinoma. J. Urol. **101**, 297–301 (1969)
8. Flanigan, R.C., Mickisch, G., Sylvester, R., Tangen, C., Poppel, H.V., Crawford, E.D.: Cytoreductive nephrectomy in patients with metastatic renal cancer: a combined analysis. J. Urol. **171**, 1071–1076 (2004)

9. Flanigan, R.C., Salmon, S.E., Blumenstein, B.A., et al.: Nephrectomy followed by interferon alfa-2b compared with interferon alfa-2b alone for metastatic renal-cell cancer. N. Engl. J. Med. **345**, 1655–1659 (2001)
10. Mickisch, G.H.J., Garin, A., van Poppel, H., de Prijck, L., Sylvester, R.: Radical nephrectomy plus interferon-alfa-based immunotherapy compared with interferon alfa alone in metastatic renal-cell carcinoma: a randomised trial. Lancet **358**, 966–970 (2001)
11. Haas, N.B., Uzzo, R.G.: Tyrosine kinase inhibitors and anti-angiogenic therapies in kidney cancer. Curr. Treat. Options Oncol. **8**, 211–226 (2007)
12. Motzer, R.J., Hutson, T.E., Tomczak, P., et al.: Sunitinib versus interferon alfa in metastatic renal-cell carcinoma. N Engl J Med. **356**, 115–124 (2007). 11 Jan 2007
13. Hudes, G., Carducci, M., Tomczak, P., et al.: Temsirolimus, interferon alfa, or both for advanced renal-cell carcinoma. N. Engl. J. Med. **356**, 2271–2281 (2007)
14. Berger, A., Brandina, R., Atalla, M.A., et al.: Laparoscopic radical nephrectomy for renal cell carcinoma: oncological outcomes at 10 years or more. J. Urol. **182**, 2172–2176 (2009)
15. Tsui, K.H., Shvarts, O., Smith, R.B., Figlin, R.A., De Kernion, J.B., Belldegrun, A.: Prognostic indicators for renal cell carcinoma: a multivariate analysis of 643 patients using the revised 1997 TNM staging criteria. J. Urol. **163**, 1090–1095 (2000). quiz 295
16. Permpongkosol, S., Chan, D.Y., Link, R.E., et al.: Long-term survival analysis after laparoscopic radical nephrectomy. J. Urol. **174**, 1222–1225 (2005)
17. Hemal, A.K., Kumar, A., Kumar, R., Wadhwa, P., Seth, A., Gupta, N.P.: Laparoscopic versus open radical nephrectomy for large renal tumors: a long-term prospective comparison. J. Urol. **177**, 862–866 (2007)
18. Colombo Jr., J.R., Haber, G.P., Jelovsek, J.E., Lane, B., Novick, A.C., Gill, I.S.: Seven years after laparoscopic radical nephrectomy: oncologic and renal functional outcomes. Urology **71**, 1149–1154 (2008)
19. Uzzo, R.G., Novick, A.C.: Nephron sparing surgery for renal tumors: indications, techniques and outcomes. J. Urol. **166**, 6–18 (2001)
20. Fergany, A.F., Hafez, K.S., Novick, A.C.: Long-term results of nephron sparing surgery for localized renal cell carcinoma: 10-year followup. J. Urol. **163**, 442–445 (2000)
21. Gill, I.S., Matin, S.F., Desai, M.M., et al.: Comparative analysis of laparoscopic versus open partial nephrectomy for renal tumors in 200 patients. J. Urol. **170**, 64–68 (2003)
22. Permpongkosol, S., Bagga, H.S., Romero, F.R., Sroka, M., Jarrett, T.W., Kavoussi, L.R.: Laparoscopic versus open partial nephrectomy for the treatment of pathological T1N0M0 renal cell carcinoma: a 5-year survival rate. J. Urol. **176**, 1984–1988 (2006). discussion 8–9
23. Lane, B.R., Gill, I.S.: 5-Year outcomes of laparoscopic partial nephrectomy. J. Urol. **177**, 70–74 (2007). discussion 4
24. Gill, I.S., Kavoussi, L.R., Lane, B.R., et al.: Comparison of 1,800 laparoscopic and open partial nephrectomies for single renal tumors. J. Urol. **178**, 41–46 (2007)
25. Clayman, R.V., Kavoussi, L.R., Soper, N.J., et al.: Laparoscopic nephrectomy: initial case report. J. Urol. **146**, 278–282 (1991)
26. Desai, M.M., Gill, I.S., Ramani, A.P., Matin, S.F., Kaouk, J.H., Campero, J.M.: Laparoscopic radical nephrectomy for cancer with level I renal vein involvement. J. Urol. **169**, 487–491 (2003)
27. Guzzo, T.J., Schaeffer, E.M., McNeil, B.K., Pollock, R.A., Pavlovich, C.P., Allaf, M.E.: Laparoscopic radical nephrectomy for patients with pathologic T3b renal-cell carcinoma: the Johns Hopkins experience. J. Endourol./Endourol. Soc. **23**, 63–67 (2009)
28. Steinnerd, L.E., Vardi, I.Y., Bhayani, S.B.: Laparoscopic radical nephrectomy for renal carcinoma with known level I renal vein tumor thrombus. Urology **69**, 662–665 (2007)
29. Gill, I.S., Desai, M.M., Kaouk, J.H., et al.: Laparoscopic partial nephrectomy for renal tumor: duplicating open surgical techniques. J. Urol. **167**, 469–467 (2002). discussion 75–6
30. Kunkle, D.A., Egleston, B.L., Uzzo, R.G.: Excise, ablate or observe: the small renal mass dilemma – a meta-analysis and review. J. Urol. **179**, 1227–1233 (2008). discussion 33–4
31. Kutikov, A., Uzzo, R.G.: The R.E.N.A.L. nephrometry score: a comprehensive standardized system for quantitating renal tumor size, location and depth. J. Urol. **182**, 844–853 (2009)
32. Clayman, R.V., Kavoussi, L.R., Soper, N.J., et al.: Laparoscopic nephrectomy. N. Engl. J. Med. **324**, 1370–1371 (1991). 9 May 1991
33. Bird, V.G., Au, J.K., Sandman, Y., De Los Santos, R., Ayyathurai, R., Shields, J.M.: Comparison of different extraction sites used during laparoscopic radical nephrectomy. J. Urol. **181**, 1565–1570 (2009)
34. Kouba, E., Smith, A.M., Derksen, J.E., Gunn, K., Wallen, E., Pruthi, R.S.: Efficacy and safety of en bloc ligation of renal hilum during laparoscopic nephrectomy. Urology **69**, 226–229 (2007)
35. Buse, S., Gilfrich, C., Pfitzenmaier, J., Bedke, J., Haferkamp, A., Hohenfellner, M.: En bloc stapler ligation of the renal vascular pedicle during laparoscopic nephrectomy. BJU Int. **101**, 878–882 (2008)
36. O'Malley, R.L., Godoy, G., Kanofsky, J.A., Taneja, S.S.: The necessity of adrenalectomy at the time of radical nephrectomy: a systematic review. J. Urol. **181**, 2009–2017 (2009)
37. Kutikov, A., et al., Routine adrenalectomy is unnecessary during surgery for large and/or upper pole renal tumors when the adrenal gland is radiographically normal. J Urol. Feb 18 (2011)
38. Viterbo, R., Greenberg, R.E., Al-Saleem, T., Uzzo, R.G.: Prior abdominal surgery and radiation do not complicate the retroperitoneoscopic approach to the kidney or adrenal gland. J. Urol. **174**, 446–450 (2005)
39. McAllister, M., Bhayani, S.B., Ong, A., et al.: Vena caval transection during retroperitoneoscopic nephrectomy: report of the complication and review of the literature. J. Urol. **172**, 183–185 (2004)
40. Gaur, D.D.: Laparoscopic operative retroperitoneoscopy: use of a new device. J. Urol. **148**, 1137–1139 (1992)
41. Gill, I.S., Clayman, R.V., Albala, D.M., et al.: Retroperitoneal and pelvic extraperitoneal laparoscopy: an international perspective. Urology **52**, 566–571 (1998)
42. Gill, I.S., Rassweiler, J.J.: Retroperitoneoscopic renal surgery: our approach. Urology **54**, 734–738 (1999)

43. Thompson, R.H., Boorjian, S.A., Lohse, C.M., et al.: Radical nephrectomy for pT1a renal masses may be associated with decreased overall survival compared with partial nephrectomy. J. Urol. **179**, 468–471 (2008). discussion 72–3
44. Huang, W.C., Elkin, E.B., Levey, A.S., Jang, T.L., Russo, P.: Partial nephrectomy versus radical nephrectomy in patients with small renal tumors – is there a difference in mortality and cardiovascular outcomes? J. Urol. **181**, 55–61 (2009). discussion -2
45. Campbell, S.C., Novick, A.C., Belldegrun, A., et al.: Guideline for management of the clinical T1 renal mass. J. Urol. **182**, 1271–1279 (2009)
46. Hollenbeck, B.K., Taub, D.A., Miller, D.C., Dunn, R.L., Wei, J.T.: National utilization trends of partial nephrectomy for renal cell carcinoma: a case of underutilization? Urology **67**, 254–259 (2006)
47. Thompson, R.H., Kaag, M., Vickers, A., et al.: Contemporary use of partial nephrectomy at a tertiary care center in the United States. J. Urol. **181**, 993–997 (2009)
48. Winfield, H.N., Donovan, J.F., Godet, A.S., Clayman, R.V.: Laparoscopic partial nephrectomy: initial case report for benign disease. J. Endourol./Endourol. Soc. **7**, 521–526 (1993)
49. McDougall, E.M., Clayman, R.V., Anderson, K.: Laparoscopic wedge resection of a renal tumor: initial experience. J. Laparoendosc. Surg. **3**, 577–581 (1993)
50. Ukimura, O., Haber, G.P., Remer, E.M., Gill, I.S.: Laparoscopic partial nephrectomy for incidental stage pT2 or worse tumors. Urology **68**, 976–982 (2006)
51. Turna, B., Kaouk, J.H., Frota, R., et al.: Minimally invasive nephron sparing management for renal tumors in solitary kidneys. J. Urol. **182**, 2150–2157 (2009)
52. Wang, A.J., Bhayani, S.B.: Robotic partial nephrectomy versus laparoscopic partial nephrectomy for renal cell carcinoma: single-surgeon analysis of >100 consecutive procedures. Urology **73**, 306–310 (2009)
53. Ho, H., Schwentner, C., Neururer, R., Steiner, H., Bartsch, G., Peschel, R.: Robotic-assisted laparoscopic partial nephrectomy: surgical technique and clinical outcomes at 1 year. BJU Int. **103**, 663–668 (2009)
54. Benway, B.M., Bhayani, S.B., Rogers, C.G., et al.: Robot assisted partial nephrectomy versus laparoscopic partial nephrectomy for renal tumors: a multi-institutional analysis of perioperative outcomes. J. Urol. **182**, 866–872 (2009)
55. Scoll, B.J., Uzzo, R.G., Chen, D.Y., Boorjian, S.A., Kutikov, A., Manley, B.J., Viterbo, R.: Robot-assisted partial nephrectomy: a large single-institutional experience. Urology **75**(6), 1328–1334 (2010)

Cancer of the Prostate

Gino J. Vricella and Lee E. Ponsky

32.1 Introduction

Prostate cancer is the most frequently diagnosed and the second leading cause of death from cancer among men in the USA [1]. An estimated 186,320 cases of newly diagnosed prostate cancer will have occurred in 2008 in the USA, with > 28,000 of these men succumbing to the disease [2]. Over the past 25 years, the 5-year survival rate for all stages combined has increased from 69% to over 98%. According to the most recent data, the relative 10- and 15-year survival is 91% and 76%, respectively [2]. The dramatic improvements in survival, particularly at 5 years, are attributable to both earlier diagnosis and improvements in therapy. Widespread screening with serum prostate-specific antigen (PSA) and digital rectal examination (DRE) has allowed for earlier detection, with the overwhelming majority of cases being detected in a clinically localized stage [3, 4]. Because of this, along with the improved efficacy in treatment modalities, only about 15% of men diagnosed with prostate cancer will ultimately die from it. Both the good and bad news about prostate cancer is one in the same: there are a variety of different treatment options for patients to choose from. These choices can often create anxiety for the patient while they try to learn about the different treatment options and decide which one is best for them. It is in this setting that the physician needs to be an advocate for their patients and help them navigate the different treatment options by presenting an unbiased perspective on the risks and benefits of each therapeutic modality. Subsequently, we review the different treatment options that exist for localized prostate cancer, with particular attention to laparoscopic radical prostatectomy.

32.2 Nonsurgical Management

32.2.1 Active Surveillance and Watchful Waiting

32.2.1.1 Explanation and Reasoning

In patients with localized prostate cancer, the small, well-differentiated prostate cancers are often associated with slow growth rates. These findings have influenced a number of researchers to recommend *active surveillance* or *watchful waiting* for highly selected patients with prostate cancer. Watchful waiting refers to monitoring of the patient until the development of metastatic disease that would require palliative therapy. Active surveillance allows for delayed primary treatment when there is evidence of cancer progression, such as a rising PSA level or biopsy findings consistent with an increase in volume or histological grade. The rationale for this approach stems from the fact that increasing numbers of older men are being diagnosed with prostate cancer as the result of PSA screening. Given the fact that the treatment of older men, who have low-grade disease is unlikely to affect their lifespan, these patients are managed expectantly until the first sign of disease progression, at which point active therapy is instituted [5].

G.J. Vricella and L.E. Ponsky (✉)
Department of Urology, University Hospitals Case Medical Center, 11100 Euclid Avenue, Cleveland, OH 44106, USA
e-mail: gvricella@gmail.com; lee.ponsky@uhhospitals.org

32.2.1.2 Indications

Traditionally, this deferred treatment has been reserved for men with a life expectancy of < 10 years [6]. Early data demonstrate that this approach may be a reasonable alternative to definitive treatment in older men who have low-volume, low-grade prostate cancer [7, 8]. In one case series that involved almost 300 men who were followed with an active surveillance protocol, one-third had evidence of disease progression, but overall, at 8-year follow-up, < 1% had died from cancer [9]. It has also been shown that surveillance offers 10-year survival rates and quality-adjusted life-years similar to those achieved with radical prostatectomy or radiotherapy [10]. This may not be the case, however, for patients with high-risk disease and Gleason scores >7. According to a population-based study by Lu-Yao and Yao, these patients have a better 5-year overall and disease-specific survival with active intervention than with observation [11]. These findings were echoed by a prospective, randomized clinical trial of almost 700 men with localized prostate cancer who were assigned to a watchful waiting protocol versus radical prostatectomy. In this study, Bill-Axelson et al. found that radical prostatectomy reduced disease-specific mortality, overall mortality, and the risks of metastasis and local progression [12].

32.2.1.3 Downfalls

The potential downfalls of active surveillance for men with clinically localized disease would include multiple biopsies, which could complicate subsequent attempts at nerve-sparing surgery, or worse, delay definitive treatment for which the window of opportunity for cure has been missed. A more recent study by Warlick et al., however, found that delayed prostate cancer surgery for patients with small, lower grade prostate cancers did not appear to compromise curability, although longer follow-up will be necessary to confirm these findings [13]. Conservative management is not ideal for patients younger than 65 years of age, because they have the most to lose if the tumor burden is underestimated at the time of diagnosis (this occurs in almost 25% of men with the use of current criteria) [14]. A universal regimen for active surveillance has not been defined, but most reports describe a clinical strategy that includes regular PSA level measurement and DRE with a periodic repeat prostate biopsy along with an option of more active therapy if biochemical (increasing PSA) or histopathologic (increased tumor grade or volume) progression occurs [7].

Radiation Therapy

32.3 External Beam Radiotherapy (EBRT)

32.3.1 Mechanism of Cytotoxicity

The management of urologic oncology has been tied to the use of radiation for over a century. Pasteau and Degrais were the first to describe the use of radiation for the treatment of prostate cancer in 1914 [15]. Since that time, a number of technological advances in planning and delivery systems have been made to offer radiotherapy as one of the main treatment modalities in the armamentarium against prostate cancer.

32.3.2 Planning Strategies

External beam radiotherapy (EBRT) uses beams of gamma radiation (high-energy photons or x-rays) aimed at the prostate through multiple fields. The mechanism of cytotoxicity is thought to be mediated primarily through the induction of unrepaired double-strand breaks in DNA. The expression of radiation damage is not seen until the target cells enter mitosis. In addition, radiation has also been shown to induce programmed cell death, or apoptosis [16].

32.3.3 Definition of Success and Failure

Over the past 20 years, there has been an evolution of radiation technologies, from conventional radiation therapy to three-dimensional conformal radiotherapy (3-D CRT) to intensity-modulated radiation therapy (IMRT). All of these techniques actually use the same high-energy x-rays delivered to the target, and the main difference involves the method of planning the radiation delivery. Conventional radiotherapy planning relies on 2-D fluoroscopic images to design the radiation fields, and these techniques are now considered antiquated for prostate radiation therapy. The incorporation of computed tomography (CT) into radiotherapy was a major advancement, which allows pelvic anatomy to be outlined and reformatted into a 3-D volumetric image. These 3-D images can then be used to design multiple customized fields that conform to the target while minimizing the dose to the surrounding tissues (i.e., bladder and rectum). One of the most influential technological advancements to date in radiation therapy for prostate cancer has been IMRT. Similar to 3-D CRT, IMRT uses a 3-D image set by CT; IMRT, however provides localization of the radiation dose to geometrically complex fields.

32.3.4 Complications

There are no data from well-controlled, randomized trials comparing the treatment outcomes of radiation therapy and surgery. Despite that, observational data suggest that the long-term disease-control achieved with contemporary radiotherapy is roughly similar to radical prostatectomy [17]. This is somewhat misleading, however, because the endpoints for determining treatment success or failure are different for radiation therapy and surgery [18]. Evaluation of the outcomes of radiation therapy is complicated because cancer cells are not killed immediately, but rather sustain lethal DNA damage, and do not die until they attempt to enter into the next cell cycle. Therefore, the PSA level gradually decreases for up to 3 years after the completion of radiotherapy. The most accepted definitions of the biochemical endpoint used to determine treatment outcome after EBRT is the American Society of Therapeutic Radiology and Oncology (ASTRO) definition and now the more recent Phoenix definition of biochemical failure [19, 20]. Using the ASTRO definition, failure requires three consecutive PSA increases measured 6 months apart and backdates to the time of cancer progression to halfway between the PSA nadir and the first rising PSA level. Thus, it often takes a number of years to determine whether or not progression has occurred after radiotherapy. Another limitation of the ASTRO definition is that it incorporates backdating, resulting in an artificial flattening of the Kaplan–Meier curves and overly favorable estimates when follow-up is short [19]. The Phoenix definition of biochemical failure is PSA nadir + 2 ng/mL and is said to improve upon the ASTRO definition by circumventing the limitations listed earlier.

32.3.5 Contraindications

The main adverse side effects of radiation therapy are related to injury to the microvasculature of the bladder, rectum, striated sphincter muscle, and urethra. Approximately one out of three patients will experience dose-related acute symptoms of proctitis or cystitis during a course of radiation treatment; however, these symptoms are transient and resolve in up to 90% of patients or more. Perhaps, the most worrisome, most common, and most permanent sequel of radiotherapy is erectile dysfunction. This is caused by injury to the vasculature of the cavernous nerves and corpora cavernosa of the penis. Impotence is reported in 35–40% of men who were potent before treatment.

A prior transurethral resection of the prostate (TUR-P) is a relative contraindication to EBRT as it is associated with an increased risk for urethral stricture. Other relative contraindications include severe bladder outlet obstructive symptoms (due to risk of acute urinary retention in up to 50%) and inflammatory bowel disease.

With conventional external beam radiotherapy, the 10-year cancer cure rates for patients with clinically localized prostate cancer are nearly 50% [21]. The primary reasons to consider 3-D CRT or IMRT are to escalate the total radiation dose that will improve clinical outcomes without substantially increasing the toxicity. No randomized studies have shown a convincing superiority of 3-D CRT versus conventional EBRT in terms of disease control; however, for a given dose, 3-D CRT has been shown to result in less toxicity [22, 23]. Despite the improvement in post-treatment toxicity, 3-D CRT did not show a significant improvement in disease-specific outcomes when similar doses were used. However, the decreased toxicity of this technique has allowed an escalation of the total dose, which has translated into improved clinical outcomes. A number of prospective studies have shown that higher doses of radiation can be delivered safely with conformal techniques and that such doses are associated with an increase in survival [17, 24, 25]. Pollack et al. randomized just over 300 patients with T1-3N0 prostate cancer between 1993 and 1998 into treatment arms comparing the efficacy of 70 Gy versus 78 Gy of radiation. With a median follow-up of 60 months, freedom from failure in the 78 Gy arm was 70% compared to 64% in the 70 Gy arm, representing a significant difference ($p = 0.03$). The higher dose was associated with a significantly greater risk of grade 2 or higher late rectal toxicity, however (26% for 78 Gy vs 12% for 70 Gy; $p = 0.001$) [24]. A multicenter randomized controlled trial from Loma Linda and Massachusetts General Hospitals reported results for 392 patients with clinical stage T1-2 prostate cancer randomized to 70.2 Gy or 79.2

Gy, using a combination of photon and proton beams. At 5 years, there was no difference in overall survival, but the higher dose therapy conferred a 49% reduction in the risk of biochemical failure ($p < 0.001$). Again, both acute and late grade 2 GI toxicity was significantly more common in the high-dose arm [25].

32.4 Brachytherapy

32.4.1 Historical Approach

Permanent interstitial prostate brachytherapy as a treatment has been performed since the 1960s. Initially, patients were taken to the operating room for an open lymphadenectomy at which time they underwent placement of radioactive seeds inserted directly into the prostate gland via a retro-pubic approach with "finger-guidance" [26]. Given the relatively dismal results, the procedure was largely abandoned until the late 1980s, when ultrasound image guidance was developed with a transperineal approach as a definitive treatment for localized prostate cancer [27].

32.4.2 Treatment Planning

Modern prostate brachytherapy uses a transrectal ultrasound probe with a template that overlies the perineum. Prior to initiating therapy, a transrectal ultrasound-based volume study is performed to assess prostate volume and to determine the number of needles and corresponding radioactive seeds, the isotope, and the isotope strength necessary for the procedure.

32.4.3 Insertion of the Seeds

With the patient under general or local anesthesia, needles are inserted through the perineum via a perineal template and radioactive seeds are deposited into the prostate to achieve a conformal dose distribution. The most common permanent implants are iodine-125 or palladium-103. After the implant has been completed, a post-treatment CT scan or plain film is routinely obtained to check the post-implant dosimetry.

32.4.4 Outcomes

The outcomes for patients treated with interstitial implant have been favorable compared with surgery or EBRT [28]. Long-term (10-year) biochemical progression-free survival for patients at low- and intermediate-risk are up to 90% and 80%, respectively, regardless of the brachytherapy modality or use of adjuvant therapies, such as hormones and EBRT [29, 30]. Urinary symptoms, such as frequency and urgency, tend to be more common during the first 3 months after brachytherapy than after EBRT, but these usually resolve. In a recent study by Crook et al., 484 men with favorable-risk prostate cancer received iodine-125 prostate brachytherapy with a median follow-up of 41 months [31]. Beyond 1 year, 73.3% of men had no significant urinary sequel. Symptoms of retention requiring catheterization or surgical intervention were seen in 3.4% (1.7% stricture, 0.4% transurethral resection of the prostate, 2.7% catheter). Of the 13 men requiring catheterization at any time after 1 year, 1% remain dependent on clean intermittent catheterization. Moderate to severe urinary urgency occurred in 6.4% of patients, but it was unresponsive to anticholinergics in only 0.8% [31]. Proctitis and rectal injury are less common with brachytherapy than with EBRT [32]. The reported rates of significant radiation proctitis were < 5%, rectal bleeding < 10%, and rectal ulcer or fistula < 2% [33]. Erectile dysfunction, which occurs in up to 60% of men post-implant, does so more commonly with brachytherapy than with EBRT [34]. Sildenafil is an effective treatment in the majority of men who suffer from post-implant erectile dysfunction [35].

32.5 Stereotactic Hypo-fractionated Radiosurgery

As discussed earlier, eradication of tumor by radiation is believed to be dose-dependent; however, the dose beyond which no additional benefit is likely largely remains unknown. Newer radiation technologies, such as 3-D CRT, IMRT, and now hypofractionated radiosurgery, have a number of interrelated goals. The ultimate goal in radiation therapy is to provide for precise tumor targeting and safe delivery of higher doses of radiation, while reducing the amount of normal tissue toxicity associated with these higher doses of radiation.

32.5.1 Definition

Hypofractionation refers to the use of larger than conventional dose-per-fraction sizes of radiation. Several investigators have recently argued that the α/β ratio for prostate cancer is much lower than previously thought, which implies a high sensitivity to dose-per-fraction size [36, 37]. If this is in fact true, a hypofractionated regimen would yield high tumor control rates while maintaining an equivalent dose to normal tissues (i.e., bladder and rectum) for late toxicity, and reduce the acute toxicity seen with modern 3-D CRT. In addition, a shortened course of radiotherapy would be a much more appealing option than conventional radiotherapy in terms of logistics (1-week vs a 6- to 9-week course of daily treatment) and cost differential.

32.5.2 Technical Aspects

The demands for high precision of delivery of large dose fractions require a system that is capable of overcoming daily target position variations and potential organ motion to a high degree of precision while delivering conformal radiotherapy. The CyberKnife is a 6MV linear accelerator mounted on a computer-controlled robotic arm. Real-time correction due to target organ daily position changes or motion during radiation delivery is accomplished via an orthogonal pair of digital x-ray imaging devices monitoring the position of fiducial markers placed within the target organ. These fiducial markers consist of three gold "seeds" placed within apex, base, and mid-gland of the prostate (this is done by transrectal ultrasound guidance). Since the planning CT scan is obtained with these seeds in place, it is the relative position of the seeds with respect to the contoured organ that serves as reference points. This allows radiation delivery with a precision of <0.5 mm and a tracking error of <1 mm [38].

32.5.3 Outcomes

Results are limited as few centers in the USA have adapted this technology (originally described for use on intracranial tumors) to treat carcinoma of the prostate. In a recent Phase I/II trial, 40 patients were prospectively enrolled to evaluate the feasibility and toxicity of stereotactic hypofractionated radiotherapy to the prostate for localized, low-risk prostate cancer [39]. The median time to follow-up was 41 months, with five patients dying of non-prostate-related illnesses. Acute and late genitourinary (GU) and gastrointestinal (GI) toxicities were evaluated and PSA values and self-reported sexual function questions were recorded at specific intervals. Acute Grade 2 or less GU and GI toxicities were 48.5% and 39%, respectively; only one patient had an acute Grade 3 GU toxicity, which required catheterization, but resolved with ibuprofen and tamsulosin. Late Grade 2 or less GU and GI toxicities were 45% and 37%, respectively; with no late Grade 3 toxicities reported. The incidence of erectile dysfunction post therapy was 23%. The actuarial 48-month biochemical freedom from relapse was 70% using the ASTRO definition of failure. This study is promising, in that it demonstrates the feasibility of delivering hypofractionated radiotherapy to the prostate with acceptable GU and GI toxicity rates and appropriate biochemical response. The small cohort size and limited follow-up, however, does warrant further clinical validation of hypofractionation before this is widely adopted as an option for the treatment of localized prostate cancer.

32.6 Cryoablation

32.6.1 Historical Approach and Development

Gonder and Soanes were the first to describe the use of cryoablation in the treatment of prostatic disease [40]. A single cryoprobe was inserted transurethrally into the prostate and the freezing process was monitored both rectally by digital exam and by a temperature gauge placed in Denonvillier's fascia. This method, unfortunately, was fraught with a number of complications, among them, urethral sloughing, urinary incontinence, and urethra-rectal fistula. These complications were attributed to a lack of accurate monitoring of the freezing process. Starting in the 1980s with the advent of transrectal ultrasound (TRUS), improvements were made with prostate cryosurgery in terms of enabling real-time imaging of the prostate and using sonography to guide more precise placement of multiple cryoprobes. The introduction of urethral warming catheter also helped to prevent urethral sloughing and resultant strictures [41]. Although these adjustments improved cryoablative surgery immensely, the continued incidence of recto-urethral fistula combined with substandard oncologic outcome pushed cryotherapy again to the wayside. It was not until the late 1990s that again cryoablation was revisited as a formidable technique for prostate cancer treatment. The new gas-driven probes were smaller and a brachytherapy template was used to facilitate more accurate placement of probes transperineally. Multiple temperature sensors are used for better control of the freeze zone and a urethral warming catheter is always placed to protect the urethra [42]. Patient selection has also improved with the optimal prostate size < 50 g.

32.6.2 Method of Action

Cryoablation destroys prostate tissue using extreme cold temperatures. The technique of cryotherapy was first described in the early 1960s by Cooper and Lee using a small-caliber vacuum-insulated liquid nitrogen cryoprobe, which enabled precise organ targeting [43]. Although there are a number of theories to explain the mechanism of tissue injury using cryoablation, the most accepted hypothesis is that freezing tissue directly causes cellular death [44–46]. This is accomplished through two main mechanisms: direct cellular toxicity from disruption of the cellular membrane by iceball crystals, and vascular compromise from thrombosis and ischemia [45].

32.6.3 Complications

With the advent of third-generation cryotherapy technology, there has been a dramatic decrease in morbidity compared to those reported with first-generation cryosurgery. In fact, rectal and bladder complications are now rare (<0.5%) in patients undergoing primary treatment [47–49]. Third-generation cryosurgery is associated with an incontinence rate of up to 5.5%, urethral sloughing rates up to 6.7%, and up to 5.5% of patients have required transurethral resection of the prostate (TURP) for bladder outlet obstruction following cryotherapy [47, 49]. In terms of complications, impotence remains a significant problem after cryosurgery. In most series, even with third-generation techniques, nearly all patients develop impotence [50, 51]. Although in a study by Robinson et al., 13% of patients regained potency and an additional 34% remained sexually active with the assistance of erectile aids, 3 years after cryoablation [52].

32.6.4 Outcomes

Following cryotherapy, PSA levels reach a nadir within 3 months of treatment. Although there are a number of studies that follow biochemical progression-free survival after cryotherapy, recurrence-free outcomes are difficult to interpret because no clear definition of recurrence after cryotherapy has been established [51, 53]. In addition, a number of patients in these studies received neoadjuvant hormone ablation, which further clouds the definition of freedom from biochemical progression. In a pooled analysis by Long et al., with a median follow-up of 24 months, the actuarial 5-year biochemical disease-free survival (bDFS) rates were 60%, 45%, and 36% for low-, intermediate-, and high-risk patients, respectively, using a PSA threshold of 0.5 ng/mL to define failure (as is done in many surgical series), and 76%, 71%, and 45% using a threshold of 1.0 ng/mL to define failure [54], respectively. In an often-cited multi-institutional study by Bahn et al., 590 patients were followed for a mean of 5.4 years [47]. They reported 7-year bDFS rates stratified by the same risk definitions as used by Long et al., using several different definitions for treatment failure [54]. Using an absolute PSA threshold of 0.5 ng/mL to define failure, the bDFS rates were 61%, 68%, and 61% for low-, intermediate-, and high-risk patients, respectively [47]. In another review by Katz and Rewcastle, a comparison of 5-year biochemical progression-free survival rates was measured between different forms of primary therapy for prostate cancer [53]. Patients were stratified into low-, intermediate-, and high-risk groups, and biochemical progression was defined using the ASTRO criteria. According to this review, radical prostatectomy was superior in the low-risk group; however, in both the intermediate- and high-risk groups, there was a decline in the efficacy for all treatment modalities with the exception of cryotherapy, which had the highest PSA progression-free survival within the 5 years of follow-up currently available in the literature.

32.7 High-intensity Focused Ultrasound (HIFU)

32.7.1 Method of Action

High-intensity focused ultrasound (HIFU) is a minimally invasive approach that uses ultrasound beams to treat prostatic disease. With this technique, a probe is inserted transrectally and a high-energy ultrasound beam is focused into the prostate. Acoustic energy absorbed by the prostate tissue is converted into thermal energy with intra-prostatic temperatures reaching upwards of 100°C [55]. This interaction produces coagulating heat, high pressure, cavitation bubbles, and chemically active free radicals; the result is a focal area of tissue destruction by way of coagulative necrosis [56].

32.7.2 Technical Aspects

HIFU of the prostate can be performed under either spinal or general anesthesia with the patient lying on his side or in the dorsal lithotomy position. With both the imaging and treatment probes placed transrectally, the prostate is imaged and a therapeutic plan is created. A series of adjacent target zones are mapped to each cross-sectional level of the prostate gland, and once activated, the machine automatically cycles through the outlined treatment plan. A monitoring device automatically deactivates the machine if the patient moves, and cooling fluid is circulated around the treatment probe to protect the rectal wall. Up to 3 months are required for necrosis to occur and because the energy used is non-ionizing, treatment can be repeated.

32.7.3 Outcomes

HIFU is widely available in Europe (where most of the studies regarding its use in prostate cancer have been done), but outside of clinical trials, is not as accessible in the USA. A large open-label multicenter study in Europe containing just over 400 patients underwent HIFU for prostate cancer between 1995 and 1999. Of the 288 patients who were re-biopsied after treatment, 87% were negative for carcinoma. Complications included urinary incontinence in 13.1% and recto-urethral fistulas in 1.3%. Follow-up was relatively short at just over 13 months and the treatment protocol evolved during the trial, making the interpretation of these results somewhat difficult [57]. In another early study by Beerlage et al., the first 49 of 111 patients were treated by selectively focusing the ultrasound beams to the prostate region believed to harbor the tumor. Of this selectively treated cohort, 72% had residual cancer on repeat biopsy (most likely reflecting the multifocal nature of prostate cancer) demonstrating the limitation of prostate-sparing HIFU. The remaining 62 patients received therapy to the entire prostate, yet the repeat biopsy rate was still relatively high at 32%. Significant side effects included urinary incontinence in 8.1%, rectourethral fistulas in 2.7%, and urethral stenosis in one patient [58]. Initial results by Blana et al. reported a 70% progression-free survival rate with a mean follow-up of 23 months, but the durability of responses has not been documented [59]. In a more recent study, Uchida et al. treated 503 patients between 1999 and 2006 with HIFU for T1-3N0M0 prostate cancer. The bDFR at 5 years for all patients was 63.5%, with actual bDFR in low-, intermediate-, and high-risk groups being 86.3%, 64.8%, and 31.3%, respectively. Negative prostate biopsy findings were found in 80.2%. Complications included urethral stricture, impotence, epididymitis, and urinary incontinence in 16%, 14%, 4%, and 0.8%, respectively [60].

In an effort to decrease complications, groups have continued to modify their techniques to spare tissue at the apex and near the neurovascular bundles. Gelet et al. treated 102 patients, sparing tissue at the apex in an effort to improve continence rates (they also recommended sparing tissue near the neurovascular bundles to preserve potency in selected patients). At 19-month follow-up, 22.5% of patients continued to have some form of urinary incontinence while demonstrating 66%

progression-free survival [61]. Vallancien et al. went as far as performing TURP prior to HIFU in an effort to minimize postoperative retention. Of the 30 patients treated, 73% had negative biopsies at 1 year, the urinary retention rate was lower than other studies (which on average occurs in 20% of patients) at 6.6%, and one patient developed urinary incontinence [62]. The effect that these modifications will have on cure rates is unclear, and long-term biochemical, disease-specific, and overall survival data are not yet available.

Surgery for Prostatic Cancer

There are three main surgical options when treating prostatic cancer
- Traditional open radical prostatectomy
- Laparoscopic prostatectomy
- Robotic prostatectomy, which is becoming more and more popular.

32.8 Open Radical Prostatectomy

32.8.1 Historical Overview

The first radical prostatectomy for prostate cancer was described by Hugh Hampton Young in 1905 through a perineal approach [63]. Millin was the first to describe the radical retro-pubic approach in 1945; however, the procedure remained unpopular because of the frequent complications of incontinence and impotence [64]. The rebirth of the radical prostatectomy as the "gold standard" in terms of treatment modality for clinically localized prostate cancer stems from a better understanding of the surgical anatomy of the pelvis. Description of the anatomy of the dorsal vein complex resulted in modifications in surgical technique leading to reduced operative blood loss. In addition, Walsh's development of the anatomic radical retro-pubic prostatectomy has allowed for the dissection to be performed with better visualization and preservation of the cavernous nerves and external sphincter muscle [65, 66]. This, in turn, has led to a significant reduction in the two most common surgical complications: clinically significant incontinence and impotence, with rates of 3% and 30%, respectively [67].

32.8.2 Extent of Surgery and Choice of Approach

Radical prostatectomy involves removal of the entire prostate and seminal vesicles along with a sufficient amount of surrounding tissue to obtain a negative surgical margin. This procedure is often accompanied by a bilateral pelvic lymph node dissection. Historically, the two main surgical approaches to radical prostatectomy are retro-pubic and perineal. The open retro-pubic approach was preferred by most urologists because of their familiarity with the surgical anatomy. One of the main criticisms of radical perineal prostatectomy (RPP) is its inability to provide access for a pelvic lymph node dissection. With the advent of laparoscopic lymph node dissection, however, this approach has been used and even advocated with RPP at some centers over radical retro-pubic prostatectomy (RRP) [68]. In addition, in the PSA era, the incidence of positive lymph nodes at prostatectomy has decreased significantly and pelvic lymph node dissection is less-often indicated.

32.8.3 Outcomes

Meng and Carroll argued that by using a statistical decision analysis model looking at outcome probabilities of positive lymph node incidence, morbidity from lymph node dissection, sensitivity of frozen section, and RRP morbidity pelvic lymph node dissection can be omitted when the estimated incidence of positive nodes is <18% [69]. When comparing RPP and RRP in terms of oncologic control and urinary incontinence, the results are similar. In comparison to RRP, patients undergoing RPP have less postoperative discomfort, more rapid return of bowel function, more rapid return to work, and a decreased transfusion rate. The advantages of RRP include a lower rate of rectal injury and postoperative fecal incontinence, and a higher rate of maintaining potency [70].

32.9 Laparoscopic Radical Prostatectomy

32.9.1 Evolution of Technique

Laparoscopic radical prostatectomy through a transperitoneal approach was first described by Schuessler et al. in 1992, with the first series of only nine cases reported 5 years later by the same group [71, 72]. The authors concluded, "laparoscopic radical prostatectomy is not an efficacious alternative to open radical prostatectomy as a curative treatment of clinically localized prostate cancer," citing excessive operative times and multiple technical difficulties [72]. Interest in laparoscopic prostatectomy was renewed in 1998 and 1999, when two separate groups from France (Montsouris and Creteil) reported successful adaptations in technique with competitive operative times of < 4 h [73, 74]. With the "Heilbronn technique," Rassweiler described an ascending laparoscopic approach similar to the classic anatomic radical prostatectomy on a series of 100 patients [75]. This evolution of a standardized technique with initial outcomes similar to open procedures led to newfound widespread interest in the laparoscopic approach to radical prostatectomy. It was not until 2001 that Bollens et al. shifted from their initial experience with the transperitoneal approach and published a standardized technique for extra-peritoneal laparoscopic radical prostatectomy [76]. These authors maintained that the extra-peritoneal approach was more comparable with the classic open retro-pubic approach and kept the peritoneal contents out of the operative field, lessening the chance for bowel injury while helping to confine postoperative urine leaks or hematomas. While the extra-peritoneal technique does offer these theoretic advantages, this approach can be much more challenging because of a tighter working space [77].

32.9.2 Indications

Laparoscopic radical prostatectomy, like open radical prostatectomy, is indicated in men with clinically localized carcinoma of the prostate who have a life expectancy of at least 10 years. No standard upper age limit exists for radical prostatectomy and decisions on therapy should be based not only on chronological age, but physiological age as well. The comorbid conditions of the patient should also be taken into account in determining the benefits of treatment.

32.9.3 Contraindications

The only absolute contraindications would be related to medical problems that would preclude an elective laparoscopic procedure, such as bleeding diathesis, severe chronic obstructive pulmonary disease, or end-stage heart failure. Also, because of the prolonged, steep Trendelenburg position used, a history of stroke or cerebral aneurysm is a contraindication.

32.9.4 Preoperative Considerations

The choice of a nerve-sparing versus non-nerve-sparing operation should be extensively discussed with the patient. No role exists for the nerve-sparing operation in patients with locally advanced disease, as this will ultimately compromise the adequacy of cancer control, which is the primary goal of the procedure [78]. Some authors have described challenges with prostate surgery and possible increased morbidity with a prior laparoscopic hernia repair with mesh, as this can obliterate the space of Retzius and complicate the prostate dissection [79]. Others have demonstrated that the challenges of previous mesh placement can be overcome, however. [80].

32.9.5 Getting the Patient Ready for Surgery

Same-day admission is routine and patients are told to report to the preoperative holding area 2 h prior to scheduled surgery time. In addition to the normal preoperative laboratory and radiographic studies, blood is drawn for a type and screen. As discussed later, the need for blood transfusion is significantly reduced with the minimally invasive approach and the routine option for auto-donation of blood is not usually necessary. The patient receives an antibiotic for gram-positive coverage within 30 min of incision. Sequential compression devices (SCD) are placed and activated prior to skin incision and used throughout the procedure.

32.9.6 Technical Steps

32.9.6.1 Patient Positioning

The patient is placed in the dorsal lithotomy position with the arms tucked at the sides and his body secured to the table. All bony prominences and pressure points are supported by foam pads. The abdomen is shaved from the nipples to the pubic bone. The patient is prepped and draped in the usual sterile fashion. A Foley catheter is inserted using sterile technique and kept accessible to the surgeons throughout the procedure.

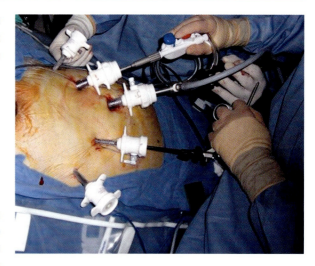

Fig. 32.1 Trocar placement for transperitoneal laparoscopic prostatectomy

32.9.6.2 Establishment of Pneumoperitoneum and Trocar Placement

At this point, a Veress needle or Hassan cutdown technique is used to obtain access to the peritoneum. Once access is achieved, insufflation of the abdominal cavity to 20 cm of pressure is initiated. After the establishment of adequate pneumoperitoneum, five trocars (2 × 12 mm^2 and 3 × 5 mm^2) are placed in an inverted U-shaped configuration (Fig. 32.1).

It should be noted that several trocar placement variations exist and is dependent on surgeon preference. The following description is our preferred method using a standard transperitoneal laparoscopic approach. The first 12-mm trocar is placed infra-umbilically and is used initially for the laparoscope and at the end of the procedure for retrieval of the specimen. A zero-degree lens is used throughout the procedure and the intra-abdominal cavity is inspected. Under direct endoscopic vision, the next two 5-mm trocars are placed two fingerbreadths medially and one fingerbreadth superior to the anterior superior iliac spines (ASIS). The next two trocars are placed midway between the infra-umbilical and ASIS trocars and just lateral to the rectus muscles. These right and left trocars are 12- and 5-mm, respectively. The patient is now placed into the extreme Trendelenburg position to aid in moving the bowel cephalad by gravity.

At this point, a pelvic lymph node dissection may be performed, if warranted.

32.9.6.3 Dissection of Vasa Deferentia and Seminal Vesicles

Once the retrovesical cul-de-sac is clearly identified and any sigmoidal attachments are incised, the first landmarks to be identified are the vas deferens behind the peritoneum and transverse semicircular peritoneal folds on the right and left sides at the level of the internal ring. The more superior of these folds covers the approximate location of the ureters and should be avoided. The more inferior fold is created by the meeting of the vas deferens in the midline, with the seminal vesicles lying just laterally. Using electrocautery, a transverse peritoneotomy along the inferior peritoneal fold is created to reach the vas deferens and seminal vesicles. The vasa deferentia are skeletonized on both sides and dissected down to the level of the seminal vesicles. The vas and its deferential artery, which runs posterior and parallel to it, are clipped and divided (Fig. 32.2). Cephalad traction of the vas allows access to the ipsilateral seminal vesicles, which are completely mobilized circumferentially to their tips, using both sharp and blunt dissection. Of note, the tip of the seminal vesicle (supplied by the vesicular artery) is located in close proximity to the neurovascular bundle, and therefore, excessive electrocautery should be avoided if the nerve-sparing technique is to be utilized. At this point, the bilateral completely mobilized seminal vesicles

32 Cancer of the Prostate

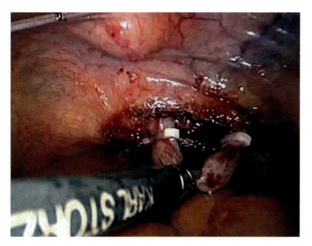

Fig. 32.2 Hemostatic clips around the vas deferens bilaterally

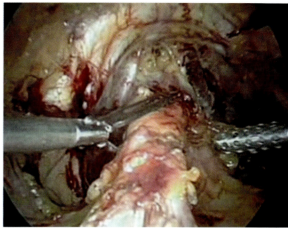

Fig. 32.3 Bladder is dissected from the anterior abdominal wall and the space of Retzius is developed

are retracted anteriorly and Denonvillier's fascia is incised superficially to create a plane between the posterior surface of the prostate and rectum. The visualization of yellow, perirectal fat confirms entry into the correct plane.

32.9.6.4 Mobilization of Bladder and Development of Space of Retzius

Attention is now focused at the level of the bladder. The bladder is filled with 200 cc of sterile normal saline, and using the bipolar cautery, the urachus and both umbilical ligaments are divided. The lateral aspect of the bladder is dissected off the anterior abdominal wall by incising the peritoneum and connecting the points between the incised median umbilical ligaments and the lateral peritoneal reflection. An avascular plane is developed on either side of the bladder and dissection is continued anterior and caudal to the pubic bone (Fig. 32.3). The bladder is emptied and now has been mobilized.

32.9.6.5 Dissection of Deep Dorsal Venous Complex and Exposure of Anterior Prostate

The fatty tissue overlying the endopelvic fascia is swept away laterally and the prostate is held medially, exposing the endopelvic fascia. The point of incision is where the fascia is transparent, revealing the underlying levator ani musculature, lateral to the arcus tendineus fascia pelvis, because the lateral branches of the dorsal venous complex are directly beneath it. This incision is then carried antero-medially to the pubo-prostatic ligaments, bilaterally. In the midline, near the pubo-prostatic ligaments, a small fat pad remains overlying the prostate, which contains the superficial dorsal vein. This is cauterized thoroughly and divided using bipolar forceps. Thus, the anterior surface of the prostate is exposed and the pubo-prostatic ligaments are sharply divided bilaterally with laparoscopic scissors. The deep dorsal venous complex of Santorini runs parallel to the urethra at the level of the prostatic apex and is ligated with a figure-of-eight 0 Vicryl suture ligature on a CT-1 needle. The suture is tied intra-corporeally and the dorsal vein complex is secured, but not divided (Fig. 32.4).

The bladder is retracted cephalad, placing the anterior bladder neck on traction. After incising the fibrous fascia, dissection is continued by following the detrusor muscle fibers and the prostatic base is developed anteriorly. Care is taken to preserve the bladder neck if possible. The anterior bladder wall is incised and the Foley catheter is identified. The catheter balloon is deflated; the catheter is removed and replaced with a male sound. The sound is then manipulated superiorly, exposing the lateral and posterior urethral walls, which are incised (Fig. 32.5). The anterior layer of Denonvillier's fascia is incised to enter the previously dissected retro-vesical plane. The vas deferens and seminal vesicles are then delivered through this opening and brought anteriorly. The remainder of the attachments between bladder and prostate are divided with electrocautery.

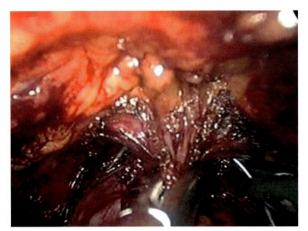

Fig. 32.4 Ligation of deep dorsal venous complex

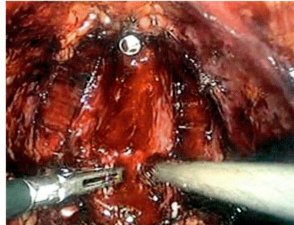

Fig. 32.6 Dissection of the neurovascular bundles completed bilaterally

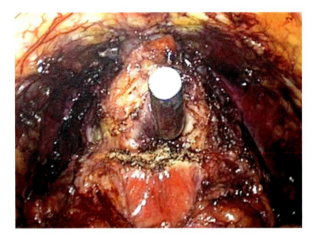

Fig. 32.5 Division of anterior bladder neck

32.9.6.6 Dissection of the Neurovascular Bundles Bilaterally

The next sequence of maneuvers is determined by the decision of whether to perform a nerve-sparing versus non-nerve-sparing approach.

Non-nerve-Sparing Approach

If a non-nerve-sparing approach is performed, the vas deferens and seminal vesicles are lifted anteriorly, placing the lateral pedicles on traction. The surgeon then divides the entire vascular pedicle and neurovascular bundle working towards the apex of the prostate. After division, the lateral border of the prostate and neurovascular bundle is detached from the peri-rectal fat, thereby achieving a wide margin of excision.

Nerve-sparing Approach

If a nerve-sparing approach is attempted, the vas deferens and seminal vesicles are again lifted anteriorly, to place the lateral pedicles on traction. The lateral pedicles are then slowly and meticulously divided close to the lateral border of the prostate using sharp dissection. Apically, the neurovascular bundle can be sharply dissected from the apex of the prostate. At the base, the neurovascular bundle can be dissected free with a combination of right-angle dissection and laparoscopic scissors. Sharp dissection can be used to free the remaining reflection of the endopelvic fascia off the lateral surface of the prostate. Bleeding can result from mobilizing the neurovascular bundles and should be controlled with hemostatic clips, while minimizing the injury to the surrounding neurovascular bundle (Fig. 32.6).

32.9.6.7 Completion of Dissection and Excision of Prostate

The dorsal vein complex is sharply incised following additional bipolar coagulation and the apical notch of the prostate is developed. The anterior urethra is sharply incised, exposing the previously introduced male sound. The tip of the sound is then delivered through the anterior urethrotomy to open the urethral lumen and expose the posterior urethral wall, which is incised in a similar fashion to the anterior urethra. The assistant provides gentle cephalad retraction by grasping the base of the prostate to allow maximum exposure of the urethra. The rectourethralis muscle is sharply incised close to the prostate which completely frees the specimen. The excised prostate (with associated vas deferens and seminal vesicles) is now placed in a non-permeable extraction bag and positioned in the upper abdomen. The pelvis is copiously irrigated and any bleeding addressed with clips or electrocautery (only if necessary). If there is concern for a rectal injury, a 20F Foley catheter is placed into the rectum and the pelvis is filled with saline. Air is then injected through the Foley catheter, while the pool of saline is examined for bubbles. If there is no evidence of leak, it can be assumed that there is no immediate rectal injury.

32.9.6.8 Urethrovesical Anastomosis

The bladder neck is identified and the ureteral orifices are observed for efflux of urine. The urethrovesical anastamosis is performed with two running 2–0 absorbable sutures on an UR-6 needle. The sutures are tied intra-corporeally with the knots on the outside of the bladder. The metal sound with a depressed tip can help guide the needle into the urethra and can also help by allowing the needle to slide along the sound (Fig. 32.7).

32.9.6.9 Reconstruction of Bladder Neck

If necessary, bladder neck reconstruction can be performed anteriorly using another 2–0 absorbable suture on a UR-6 needle. The bladder neck is reconstructed by placing two or three interrupted sutures through the anterior portion of the bladder neck, or a classic running tennis racquet bladder neck reconstruction can be performed.

32.9.6.10 Leak Test

A new Foley catheter is placed under direct visualization after removal of the metal sound prior to completion of the anterior portion of the urethrovesical anastamosis. After completion of the anastamosis, the bladder is tested by instillation of approximately 120 cc of saline, and if a leak is detected, another suture can be placed (Fig. 32.8).

32.9.6.11 Extraction of Specimen and Wound Closure

At this point, the umbilical port is extended for removal of the specimen in the extraction bag. After the specimen is removed and sent to pathology, the abdomen is re-insufflated to check for any obvious areas of hemorrhage. Once adequate hemostasis has been achieved, a

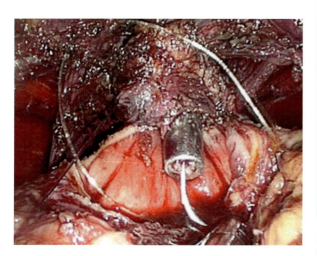

Fig. 32.7 Urethrovesical anastomosis

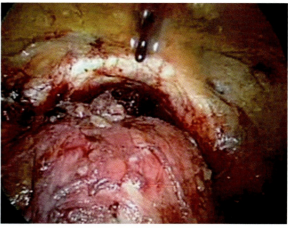

Fig. 32.8 After completion of the urethrovesical anastomosis, the bladder is instilled with normal saline to check for anastomotic leak

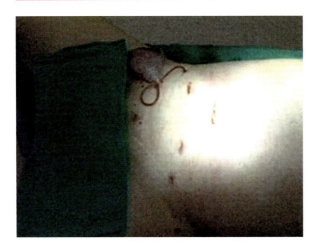

Fig. 32.9 Completion of prostatectomy with Jackson–Pratt drain through right-most port site

Jackson–Pratt drain is placed through the right 5-mm port site into the pelvis and secured in place with a non-absorbable suture. The fascia for port sites of >5 mm are closed with absorbable suture. This can be done with the assistance of a closure tool, such as the Carter-Thomason device, under direct endoscopic vision. All wounds are copiously irrigated and injected with local anesthetic. The skin is closed with a running subcuticular closure. The Foley catheter is left to gravity drainage and the Jackson–Pratt drain is left to bulb suction or gravity drainage (Fig. 32.9).

32.9.7 Postoperative Management

Patients are started on a clear liquid diet on postoperative day 1 and advanced as tolerated. Pain control is achieved with Ketorolac and Morphine initially, and then converted to oral analgesia when tolerating PO. The catheter is typically left in for 7–10 days postoperatively and the patient may undergo a cystogram to check for a leak at the vesicourethral anastamosis. If no leak is identified, the Foley catheter is removed and the patient is given a trial-of-void.

32.10 Robotic Radical Prostatectomy

In 2001, there was another major modification to the laparoscopic radical prostatectomy technique, which incorporated robotic technology using the da Vinci® surgical system (Intuitive Surgical, Sunnyvale, CA). There are many who credit surgical robotics for helping to increase the application of minimally invasive techniques to radical prostatectomy [81]. Some of the main advantages cited by proponents of the robotic system include: three-dimensional stereoscopic visualization, enormous flexibility in performing complex movements, minimal fatigue due to ergonomic design, and perhaps the largest advantage, the ease of intra-corporeal suturing. Robotic prostatectomy may also have a shorter learning curve than standard laparoscopy, potentially allowing novice laparoscopists to complete these procedures [81, 82]. Some criticisms, however, include the loss of tissue resistance or tactile feedback and cost [83]. The surgical robot system requires a tremendous capital investment, the laparoscopic instruments have a finite number of procedures before they must be replaced, and the annual maintenance and per-case disposable instrument costs make this technology prohibitive to many centers, limiting the widespread implementation of such a device.

32.11 Outcomes

32.11.1 Comparison Between Laparoscopic, Robotic, and Open Procedures

The initial reports of laparoscopic and robotic radical prostatectomy mainly focused on its feasibility in terms of operative time, complications, and peri-operative outcomes. As these minimally invasive techniques became more well established, surgeons reported on functional outcomes, namely, urinary continence, potency rates, and oncologic control (where margin status was used as a surrogate for progression-free survival). Undoubtedly, these questions can only be answered by a large-scale prospective randomized study. A recent meta-analysis of 30 comparative studies (none of which were randomized controlled trials) comparing laparoscopic and robotic radical prostatectomies versus open radical retropubic or radical perineal prostatectomies for localized prostate cancer found that there did not appear to be any important differences in complication rates between laparoscopic and open approaches [84] (Tables 32.1 and 32.2).

The initial experiences of the groups from Montsouris and Creteil demonstrated that the laparoscopic approach to radical prostatectomy was safe and that complications

Table 32.1 Transperitoneal laparoscopic radical prostatectomy and open radical retro-pubic prostatectomy: comparison of complications and peri-operative outcomes

	N	Rectal injury (%)	Mean OR time (min)	EBL (m)	Transfusion rate (%)	Mean hospital (d)	Mean catheter (d)	Overall complication rate(%)
Laparoscopic								
Hoznek et al. [85]	134	1.5	240	NA	3	6.1	4.8	9
Turk et al. [86]	125	2.4	265	185	2	8	12	14
Eden et al. [87]	100	1	245	313	3	4.2	NA	8
Guillonneau et al. [88]	567	1.45	200	380	5.3	NA	4.2	3.6
Rassweiler et al. [89]	438	0–1.4	218–288	800–1,100	9.6–30.1	11–12	7	10
Tooher et al. [84][a]	1,351	NA	288	800	2	5	7	17
OPEN								
Dillioglugil et al. [90]	427	0.6	182	NA	26.6	6.2	14–21	27.8
Lepor et al. [91]	1,000	0.5	NA	818	9.7	2.3	NA	6.6
Augustin et al. [92]	1,243	0.2	NA	NA	29.1	NA	15.5	19.9
Rassweiler et al. [89]	219	1.3	219	NA	26.9	16	12	15.9
Tooher et al. [84][a]	1,185	NA	168	1,400	26	7	15	19

[a]This review included 13 comparative studies of transperitoneal laparoscopic prostatectomy versus radical retro-pubic prostatectomy. There is a patient crossover in this study and the Rassweiler data

NA data not available; *EBL* estimated blood loss

and surgeon experience were inversely related [73, 74]. As with other laparoscopic procedures, the reported operative times decreased with increasing surgeon experience [74]. Therefore, one would anticipate that a further reduction in operating times will continue to occur. There are several recent studies that have focused on the complication rates, functional outcomes, and oncologic control of radical prostatectomy in a large series of surgeries performed by surgeons experienced in open and laparoscopic radical prostatectomy. Unfortunately, the conclusions that can be drawn about these comparisons are limited by the nature of the data that is available. The conclusions are drawn mainly from non-randomized, comparative studies, most of which used historical controls. Although, more recently, smaller scale, prospective studies are emerging, which seem to substantiate the conclusions of these older studies.

32.11.2 Complication Rates and Procedure-associated Morbidity

In terms of complication rates and procedure-associated morbidity parameters (e.g. estimated blood loss or transfusion rates), there are a number of studies that compare transperitoneal laparoscopic radical prostatectomy (TLRP) to radical RRP [89, 98–102, 103]. There was little difference in the total percentage of complications reported regarding TLRP versus RRP, which had a median of 17% (0–25) versus 19% (8–25), respectively. The total estimated blood loss (EBL) in mL was less for TLRP than for RRP, with a median EBL of 800 and 1,400, respectively. This higher blood loss translated into a significantly higher transfusion rate requirement among patients undergoing RRP versus TLRP, with a median of 26% and 2%, respectively. The number of days of postoperative catheterization also were less in the TLRP group (median of means = 7) than the RRP group (median of means = 15). Serious intra-operative complications, such as rectal or ureteral injury, were rare in both the techniques, but more common with TLRP than RRP [84]. Perhaps, one of the more intriguing findings came from a prospective study out of Japan comparing open RRP and LRP in terms of QOL differences before and 6 months post surgery. Although the investigators found no significant differences between RRP and LRP, patients who had undergone LRP had a more

Table 32.2 Transperitoneal laparoscopic radical prostatectomy and open radical retro-pubic prostatectomy: comparison of oncologic and functional outcomes

	N	Overall positive margin (%)	% PSA nonrecurrence (interval)	% Urinary continence (follow-up)	% Potency (follow-up)
Laparoscopic					
Hoznek et al. [85]	134	25	89.6 (11 months)	86.2 (12 months)	46 (12 months) BNS
Turk et al. [86]	125	26.4	100 (6 months)	92 (9 months) ≤1 pad	59 (12 months) UNS or BNS
Eden et al. [87]	100	16	100 (3 months)	90 (12 months) No pad	62 (12 months) BNS
Guillonneau et al. [93]	550	16.7	pT2a 92.3 (36 months) pT2b 86.3 (31 months)	82.3 (12 months) No pad	85 (12 months) BNS
Rassweiler et al. [89]	438	22.4	86.8 (30 months)	95.8 (18 months)	NA
Tooher et al. [84]	1,351	23	84–99 (NA)	80 (12 months) No pad	41 (12 months)
Open					
Walsh et al. [94]	64	NA	NA	93 (18 months) No pads	86 (18 months) UNS or BNS
Han et al. (Walsh data) [95]	2,404	11	84 (5 years), 74 (10 years), 66 (15 years)	NA	NA
Kundu et al. (Catalona data) [67]	3,477	NA	NA	93 (18 months) No pad	76 (18 months) BNS
Roehl et al. (Catalona data) [96]	3,478	19	80 (5 years) 68 (10 years)	NA	NA
Bianco et al. (Scardino data) [97]	1,746	12	82 (5 years), 77 (10 years), 75 (15 years)	95 (24 months) No pad	70 (24 months) UNS or BNS
Tooher et al. [84][a]	1,185	29	75–97 (NA)	89 (12 months) No pad	30 (12 months)

[a]This review included 13 comparative studies of transperitoneal laparoscopic prostatectomy versus radical retro-pubic prostatectomy. There is patient crossover in this study and the Rassweiler data

BNS bilateral nerve sparing; *UNS* unilateral nerve sparing; *NA* data not available

favorable attitude towards surgery and significantly more would have chosen that therapy again compared to those who underwent RRP [104].

32.11.3 Biochemical Progression

As stated previously, the primary goal of radical prostatectomy is the cure of the localized prostate cancer. Since the inception of Walsh's anatomical RRP, the reported 5- and 10-year PSA non-progression rates status post open RRP are reported to be 77–80% and 54–75%, respectively [105]. Due to its relatively recent utilization in the treatment of localized prostate cancer, long-term data on biochemical progression after laparoscopic radical prostatectomy are currently unavailable. Short-term data on oncologic control are encouraging, however. A recent prospective analysis done by Pavlovich et al. found that a 3-year actuarial biochemical recurrence-free survival after laparoscopic radical prostatectomy was 98.2% for pT2N0/Nx and 78.7% for pT3N0/Nx/N1 disease ($p < 0.0001$), and it was 94.5% overall. Multivariate analysis controlling for age, preoperative prostate specific antigen, postoperative Gleason score and stage, and margin status showed that only Gleason score and stage (pT3 or any N1 vs pT2) predicted biochemical progression [106]. There also does not appear to be any significant differences in the positive margin rates between laparoscopic and open prostatectomy when tumor stage is taken into account: median percentage of positive margins in T2 and T3 disease using laparoscopic versus open approaches were 10 versus 18 and 40 versus 43, respectively [84]. In another retrospective study from Germany, three consecutive cohorts who underwent radical prostatectomy from 1999 to 2002 were analyzed. The cohorts consisted of 219 patients undergoing open RRP before routine LRP was performed, the initial 219 who underwent LRP during the learning curve (early), and the next 219 who underwent LRP (late). Prostate-specific antigen relapse, defined as an increase in serum levels of > 0.2 ng/mL, was observed in 31 of 178 patients (17.4%) after open and 29 of 219 patients (13.2%) after early laparoscopic radical prostatectomy [89]. These data would seem to indicate that oncologic outcome after laparoscopic radical prostatectomy will not differ from open surgery, but only time will tell as we await long-term oncologic data from laparoscopy.

32.11.4 Urinary Incontinence

Continence is difficult to assess after radical prostatectomy, mainly due to authors' inconsistent definitions of continence and different modalities of acquiring the data. Most authors are now defining patients who do not need to wear a pad at 12 months of follow-up as continent. In a meta-analysis of comparative studies, continence rates after variable follow-ups were 60–90% (median 80%) after TLRP and 67–90% (median 89%) after RRP in three studies [84]. A recent prospective study by Jacobsen et al. found that urinary incontinence rates were comparable 12 months postoperatively between patients undergoing open versus laparoscopic prostatectomy for clinically localized prostate cancer (13% vs 17%, respectively, $p = 0.26$) [107]. In another prospective comparison of 70 patients with RRP and 230 with LRP, there was no significant difference in continence at 1 year, but patients undergoing LRP actually had an earlier return to continence [108].

32.11.5 Sexual Function

Sexual function is another important functional outcome after prostate cancer surgery. Much like continence, the objective evaluation of postoperative erectile dysfunction is somewhat convoluted by the absence of a consensual definition of sexual potency, heterogeneous methods of evaluation, and variable follow-up. There is a consensus that the assessment of recovery of sexual function requires a follow-up of at least 18 months [109]. Other factors that will ultimately influence the operative results are the erection quality prior to surgery, the patient's age, and whether the surgeon is able to preserve both neurovascular bundles. With these caveats in mind, several large series of LRP with bilateral nerve-sparing report potency rates between 58% and 83% [77]. These results are similar to those reported for RRP, which range from 68% to 76% [19, 67, 97].

In summary, early outcomes demonstrate that once the learning curve has been met, TLRP is, at the very least, equivalent to open radical prostatectomy in terms of early oncologic control, continence, and potency rates.

32.12 Future Trends

Laparoscopic and robotic prostatectomies are currently standard treatment options available for the patients with prostate cancer. There are multiple techniques that will likely become more developed in the coming years. Salvage laparoscopic or robotic prostatectomy may provide an advantage over the traditional open approach due to improved visualization, magnification, and decreased blood loss. The incorporation of adjunct imaging (transrectal ultrasound and endorectal MRI) may also serve a role in assisting the surgeon to identify the neurovascular bundles and precise margins of the prostate dissection. There will certainly be more incorporation of ablative therapies in the treatment of prostate cancer, such as cryotherapy and HIFU. The utilization of these techniques for patients who have failed standard radiation therapy will likely provide a potentially curative option for patients with a possible decreased morbidity compared to a salvage prostatectomy. Yet another area on the horizon is the concept of focal therapy. This concept goes against all of the conventional teachings of prostate cancer and its respective therapies, as carcinoma of the prostate is traditionally thought of as a multi-focal disease process. However, with the advancements of ablative therapies and with the appropriately designed and executed studies, treating only part of the prostate (only where the cancer exists) may have a role. It is imperative that as these techniques and technologies are being evaluated, they are studied under institutional review board protocols to ensure patient protection. There is only so much smaller that we can make our incisions and only so much better that we can improve our instruments; however, computers and technology will continue to evolve and progress at astronomical rates. It is with these developments and the appropriate incorporation into the clinical practice of treating patients with prostate cancer that true advancements will be made in the future.

> Two sutures tied together starting on the outside of the bladder at the 6 o'clock position on the bladder neck, and running each stitch up the 12 o'clock position. Care should be taken to avoid the ureteral orifices. A Foley catheter is placed across the anastamosis and the anastamosis is completed and the two sutures are tied together.

Quick Reference Guide

1. Posterior dissection of the seminal vesicles and vas deferens can be done at the beginning of the procedure. It is important to clearly identify the vas to ensure that it is not mistaken for the ureter.
2. When dropping the bladder from the anterior abdominal wall, be sure to dissect in the correct plane as entry into the wrong plane can result in bleeding from the abdominal muscles or fat hanging in the operative field throughout the case.
3. After incising the end-pelvic fascia, continue the incision to divide the lateral pelvic fascia over the prostate to help drop the neurovascular bundles.
4. Develop the neurovascular bundles if indicated.
5. The use of an urethral sound to replace the catheter can assist with the identification of the bladder neck when dividing the anterior bladder neck from the prostate.
6. Care should be taken when dividing the posterior bladder neck, so as not to thin the posterior bladder, while taking care not to cut into the prostate.
7. The posterior dissection of Denonvillier's fascia between the prostate and rectum should be completed as far as possible, with care to avoid injury to the rectum.
8. When ligating the dorsal venous complex, the urethral sound helps to identify the urethra to ensure ligation of the dorsal venous complex and avoid injury to the urethra.
9. When dissecting the apical attachments, care should be taken to avoid injury to the neurovascular bundles.
10. When completing the urethrovesical anastomosis, a running absorbable suture can be utilized.

References

1. Jemal, A., Siegel, R., Ward, E., et al.: Cancer statistics, 2007. CA Cancer J. Clin. **57**(1), 43–66 (2007)
2. American Cancer Society: Cancer Facts and Figures 2008. American Cancer Society, Atlanta (2008)
3. Catalona, W.J., Smith, D.S., Ratliff, T.L., et al.: Measurement of prostate-specific antigen in serum as a screening test for prostate cancer. N. Engl. J. Med. **324**, 1156–1161 (1991)
4. Catalona, W.J., Smith, D.S., Ratliff, T.L., et al.: Detection of organ-confined prostate cancer is increased through prostate-specific antigen-based screening. JAMA **270**, 948–954 (1993)
5. Allaf, M.E., Carter, H.B.: The results of watchful waiting for prostate cancer. AUA Update Ser. **24**, 1–7 (2005)
6. Fowler, F.J., Collins, M.M., Albertsen, P.C., et al.: Comparison of recommendations by urologists and radiation oncologists for treatment of clinically localized prostate cancer. JAMA **283**, 3217–3222 (2000)
7. Carter, H.B., Walsh, P.C., Landis, P., et al.: Expectant management of nonpalpable prostate cancer with curative intent: preliminary results. Urology **167**, 1231–1234 (2002)
8. Johansson, J.E.: Expectant management of early stage prostatic cancer: Swedish experience. J. Urol. **152**, 1753–1756 (1994)
9. Klotz, L.: Active surveillance for prostate cancer: for whom? J. Clin. Oncol. **23**, 8165–8169 (2005)
10. Choo, R., Klotz, L., Danjoux, C., et al.: Feasibility study: watchful waiting for localized low to intermediate grade prostate carcinoma with selective delayed intervention based on prostate specific antigen, histological and/or clinical progression. J. Urol. **167**, 1664–1669 (2002)
11. Lu-Yao, G.L., Yao, S.L.: Population-based study of long-term survival in patients with clinically localised prostate cancer. Lancet **349**, 906–910 (1997)
12. Bill-Axelson, A., Holmberg, L., Ruutu, M., et al.: Radical prostatectomy versus watchful waiting in early prostate cancer. N. Engl. J. Med. **352**, 1977–1984 (2005)
13. Warlick, C., Trock, B.J., Landis, P., et al.: Delayed versus immediate surgical intervention and prostate cancer outcome. J. Natl. Cancer Inst. **98**, 355–357 (2006)
14. Epstein, J.I., Chan, D.W., Sokoll, L.J., et al.: Nonpalpabe stage T1c prostate cancer: prediction of insignificant disease using free/total prostate specific antigen levels and needle biopsy findings. J. Urol. **160**, 2407–2411 (1998)

15. Pasteau, O., Degrais, P.: The radium treatment of cancer of the prostate. Arch. Roentgen Ray **18**, 396 (1914)
16. Sklar, G.: Combined antitumor effect of suramin plus irradiation in human prostate cancer cells: The role of apoptosis. J. Urol. **150**, 1526 (1993)
17. Zelefsky, M.J., Chan, H., Hunt, M., et al.: Long-term outcome of high dose intensity modulated radiation therapy for patients with clinically localized prostate cancer. J. Urol. **176**, 1415–1419 (2006)
18. Gretzer, M.B., Trock, B.J., Han, M., et al.: A critical analysis of the interpretation of biochemical failure in surgically treated patients using the American Society for Therapeutic Radiation and Oncology criteria. J. Urol. **168**(pt 1), 1419–1422 (2002)
19. Abramowitz, M.C., Li, T., Buyyounouski, M.K., et al.: The phoenix definition of biochemical failure predicts for overall survival in patients with prostate cancer. Cancer **112**, 55–60 (2007)
20. Cox, J.D.: The American Society for Therapeutic Radiation and Oncology Consensus Panel Consensus Statement Guidelines for PSA Failure Following Radiation Therapy. Int. J. Radiat. Oncol. Biol. Phys. **37**, 1035–1041 (1997)
21. Zietman, A.L., Chung, C.S., Coen, J.J., et al.: 10-year outcome for men with localized prostate cancer treated with external radiation therapy: results of a cohort study. J. Urol. **171**, 210–214 (2004)
22. Dearnaley, D.P., Khoo, V.S., Norman, A.R., et al.: Comparison of radiation side effects of conformal and conventional radiotherapy in prostate cancer: a randomised trial. Lancet **353**, 267–272 (1999)
23. Morris, D.E., Emami, B., Mauch, P.M., et al.: Evidence-based review of three dimensional conformal radiotherapy for localized prostate cancer: an ASTRO outcomes initiative. Int. J. Radiat. Oncol. Biol. Phys. **62**, 3–19 (2005)
24. Pollack, A., Zagars, G.K., Starkschall, G., et al.: Prostate cancer radiation dose response: results of the M.D. Anderson phase III randomized trial. Int. J. Radiat. Oncol. Biol. Phys. **53**, 1097–1105 (2002)
25. Zietman, A.L., DeSilvio, M.L., Slater, J.D., et al.: Comparison of conventional-dose vs. high-dose conformal radiation therapy in clinically localized adenocarcinoma of the prostate: a randomized controlled trial. JAMA **294**, 1233 (2005)
26. Sogani, P.C., Whitmore Jr., W.F., Hilaris, B.S., et al.: Experience with interstitial implantation of iodine 125 in the treatment of prostatic carcinoma. Scand. J. Urol. Nephrol. Suppl. **55**, 205 (1980)
27. Blasko, J.C., Ragde, H., Grimm, P.D.: Transperineal ultrasound-guided implantation of the prostate: morbidity and complications. Scand. J. Urol. Nephrol. Suppl. **137**, 113 (1991)
28. Quaranta, B.P., Marks, L.B., Anscher, M.S.: Comparing radical prostatectomy and brachytherapy for localized prostate cancer. Oncology **18**, 1289–1302 (2004)
29. Ciezki, J.P.: Prostate brachytherapy for localized prostate cancer. Curr. Treat. Options Oncol. **6**, 389–393 (2005)
30. Potters, L., Morgenstern Calugaru, E., et al.: 12-year outcomes following permanent prostate brachytherapy in patients with clinically localized prostate cancer. J. Urol. **173**, 1562–1566 (2005)
31. Crook, J., Fleshner, N., Roberts, C., et al.: Long-term urinary sequelae following ^{125}Iodine prostate brachytherapy. J. Urol. **179**, 141–146 (2008)
32. Litwin, M.S., Sadetsky, N., Pasta, D.J., et al.: Bowel function and bother after treatment for early stage prostate cancer: a longitudinal quality of life analysis from CaPSURE. J. Urol. **172**, 515–519 (2004)
33. Vicini, F.A., Kini, V.R., Edmundson, G., et al.: A comprehensive review of prostate cancer brachytherapy: defining an optimal technique. Int. J. Radiat. Oncol. Biol. Phys. **44**, 483–489 (1999)
34. Merrick, G.S., Butler, W.M., Wallner, K.E., et al.: Erectile function after prostate brachytherapy. Int. J. Radiat. Oncol. Biol. Phys. **62**, 437–447 (2005)
35. Raina, R., Agarwal, A., Goyal, K.K., et al.: Long-term potency after iodine-125 radiotherapy for prostate cancer and role of sildenafil citrate. Urology **62**, 1103–1108 (2003)
36. Bentzen, S.M., Ritter, M.A.: The α/β ratio for prostate cancer: what is it, really? Radiother. Oncol. **76**, 1–3 (2005)
37. King, C.R., Fowler, J.F.: A simple analytic derivation suggests that prostate cancer α/β ratio is low. Int. J. Radiat. Oncol. Biol. Phys. **51**, 213–214 (2001)
38. King, C.R., Lehmann, J., Adler, J.R., et al.: CyberKnife radiotherapy for localized prostate cancer: rationale and technical feasibility. Tech. Cancer Res. Treat **2**, 25–29 (2003)
39. Madsen, B.L., His, R.A., Pham, H.T., et al.: Stereotactic Hypofractionated Accurate Radiotherapy of the Prostate (SHARP), 33.5 Gy in five fractions for localized disease: first clinical trial results. Int. J. Radiat. Oncol. Biol. Phys. **67**, 1099–1105 (2007)
40. Gonder, M.J., Soanes, W.A., Shulman, S.: Cryosurgical treatment of the prostate. Invest. Urol. **3**, 372–378 (1966)
41. Onik, G.M., Cohen, J.K., Reyes, G.D., et al.: Transrectal ultrasound-guided percutaneous radical cryosurgical ablation of the prostate. Cancer **72**, 1291–1299 (1993)
42. Saliken, J.C., Donnelly, B.J., Rewcastle, J.C.: The evolution and state of modern technology for prostate cryosurgery. Urology **60**, 26–33 (2002)
43. Cooper, I.S., Lee, A.S.: Cryostatic congelation: a system for producing a limited, controlled region of cooling or freezing of biological tissue. J. Nerv. Ment. Dis. **133**, 259–263 (1961)
44. Baust, J.G., Gage, A.A.: The molecular basis of cryosurgery. BJU Int. **95**, 1187–1191 (2005)
45. Gage, A.A., Baust, J.: Mechanisms of tissue injury in cryosurgery. Cryobiology **37**, 171–186 (1998)
46. Hoffmann, N.E., Bischof, J.C.: The cryobiology of cryosurgical injury. Urology **60**, 40–49 (2002)
47. Bahn, D.K., Lee, F., Badalament, R., et al.: Targeted cryoablation of the prostate: 7-year outcomes in the primary treatment of prostate cancer. Urology **60**, 3–11 (2002)
48. Donnelly, B.J., Saliken, J.C., Ernst, D.S., et al.: Prospective trial of cryosurgical ablation of the prostate: five year results. Urology **60**, 645–649 (2002)
49. Ellis, D.S.: Cryosurgery as a primary treatment for localized prostate cancer: a community hospital experience. Urology **60**, 34–39 (2002)
50. Han, K.-R., Cohen, J.K., Miller, R.J., et al.: Treatment of organ-confined prostate cancer with third generation cryosurgery: preliminary multi-center experience. J. Urol. **170**, 1126–1130 (2003)

51. Shinohara, K.: Prostate cancer cryotherapy. Urol. Clin. North Am. **30**, 725–736 (2003)
52. Robinson, J.W., Donnelly, B.J., Saliken, J.C., et al.: Quality of life and sexuality of men with prostate cancer 3 years after cryosurgery. Urology **60**(2 suppl 1), 12–18 (2002)
53. Katz, A.E., Rewcastle, J.C.: The current and potential role of cryoablation as a primary therapy for localized prostate cancer. Curr. Oncol. Rep. **5**, 231–238 (2003)
54. Long, J.P., Bahn, D., Lee, F., et al.: Five-year retrospective, multi-institutional pooled analysis of cancer-related outcomes after cryosurgical ablation of the prostate. Urology **57**(3), 518–523 (2001)
55. Madersbacher, S., Padevilla, M., Vingers, L., et al.: Effect of high-intensity focused ultrasound on human prostate cancer in vivo. Cancer Res. **55**, 3346–3351 (1995)
56. Chapelon, J.Y., Ribault, M., Vernier, F., et al.: Treatment of localized prostate cancer with transrectal high intensity focused ultrasound. Eur. J. Ultrasound **9**, 31–38 (1999)
57. Thuroff, S., Chaussy, C., Vallancien, G., et al.: High-intensity focused ultrasound and localized prostate cancer: efficacy results from the European multicentric study. J. Endourol. **17**, 673–677 (2003)
58. Beerlage, H.P., Thuroff, S., Debruyne, F.M., et al.: Transrectal high-intensity focused ultrasound using the Ablatherm device in the treatment of localized prostate carcinoma. Urology **54**, 273–277 (1999)
59. Blana, A., Walter, B., Rogenhofer, S., et al.: High-intensity focused ultrasound for the treatment of localized prostate cancer: 5-year experience. Urology **63**, 297–300 (2004)
60. Uchida, T., Nitta, M., Hongo, S., et al.: High-intensity focused ultrasound for the treatment in 503 patients with localized prostate cancer. Urology **70**(3 Supp 1), 2 (2007)
61. Gelet, A., Chapelon, J.Y., Bouvier, R., et al.: Transrectal high intensity focused ultrasound for the treatment of localized prostate cancer: factors influencing the outcome. Eur. Urol. **40**, 124–129 (2001)
62. Vallancien, G., Prapotnich, D., Cathelineau, X., et al.: Transrectal focused ultrasound combined with transurethral resection of the prostate for the treatment of localized prostate cancer: feasibility study. Urology **171**, 2265–2267 (2004)
63. Young, H.H.: The early diagnosis and radical cure of carcinoma of the prostate. Johns Hopkins Hosp. Bull. **16**, 315–321 (1905)
64. Millin, T.: Retropubic prostatectomy: a new extra vesical technique. Lancet **2**, 693–696 (1945)
65. Walsh, P.C., Donker, P.J.: Impotence following radical prostatectomy: insight into etiology and prevention. J. Urol. **128**, 492–497 (1982)
66. Walsh, P.C.: The discovery of the cavernous nerves and development of nerve-sparing radical prostatectomy. J. Urol. **177**, 1632–1635 (2007)
67. Kundu, S.D., Roehl, K.A., Eggener, S.E., et al.: Potency, continence and complications in 3, 477 consecutive radical retropubic prostatectomies. J. Urol. **172**, 2227–2231 (2004)
68. Teichman, J.M., Reddy, P.K., Hulbert, J.C.: Laparoscopic pelvic lymph node dissection, laparoscopically assisted seminal vesicle mobilization, and total perineal prostatectomy versus radical retropubic prostatectomy for prostate cancer. Urology **45**, 823 (1995)
69. Meng, M.V., Carroll, P.R.: When is pelvic lymph node dissection necessary before radical prostatectomy? A decision analysis. J. Urol. **164**, 1235 (2000)
70. Janoff, D.M., Parra, R.O.: Contemporary appraisal of radical perineal prostatectomy. J. Urol. **173**, 1863–1870 (2005)
71. Schuessler, W.W., Kavoussi, L.R., Clayman, R.V.: Laparoscopic radical prostatectomy: initial case report [abstr 130]. J. Urol. Suppl. **147**, 246A (1992)
72. Schuessler, W.W., Schulam, P.G., Clayman, R.V., et al.: Laparoscopic radical prostatectomy: initial short-term experience. Urology **50**, 854–857 (1997)
73. Abbou, C.C., Salomon, L., Hoznek, A., et al.: Laparoscopic radical prostatectomy: preliminary results. Urology **55**, 630–634 (2000)
74. Guillonneau, B., Cathelineau, X., Baret, E., et al.: Laparoscopic radical prostatectomy: technical and early oncological assessment of 40 operations. Eur. Urol. **36**, 14 (1999)
75. Rassweiler, J., Sentker, L., Seeman, O., et al.: Heilbronn laparoscopic radical prostatectomy: technique and results after 100 cases. Eur. Urol. **40**, 54 (2001)
76. Bollens, R., Vanden, B.M., Rhoumeguere, T.H., et al.: Extraperitoneal laparoscopic radical prostatectomy: results after 50 cases. Eur. Urol. **40**, 65 (2001)
77. Trabulsi, E.J., Guillonneau, B.: Laparoscopic radical prostatectomy. J. Urol. **173**, 1072–1079 (2005)
78. Shah, O., Robbins, D.A., Melamed, J., et al.: The New York University nerve sparing algorithm decreases the rate of positive surgical margins following radical retropubic prostatectomy. J. Urol. **169**, 2147–2152 (2003)
79. Hsia, M., Ponsky, L., Rosenblatt, S., et al.: Laparoscopic inguinal hernia repair complicates future pelvic oncologic surgery. Ann. Surg. **240**, 922 (2004)
80. Stolzenburg, J.U., Anderson, C., Rabenalt, R., et al.: Endoscopic extraperitoneal radical prostatectomy in patients with prostate cancer and previous laparoscopic inguinal mesh placement for hernia repair. World J. Urol. **23**, 295–299 (2005)
81. Menon, M., Shrivastava, A., Tewari, A., et al.: Laparoscopic and robot assisted radical prostatectomy: establishment of a structured program and preliminary analysis of outcomes. J. Urol. **168**, 945–949 (2002)
82. Aherling, T.E., Skarecky, D., Lee, D., et al.: Successful transfer of open surgical skills to a laparoscopic environment using a robotic interface: initial experience with laparoscopic radical prostatectomy. J. Urol. **170**, 1738 (2003)
83. Guillonneau, B.: What robotics in urology? A current point of view. Eur. Urol. **43**, 103 (2003)
84. Tooher, R., Swindle, P., Woo, H., et al.: Laparoscopic radical prostatectomy for localized prostate cancer: a systematic review of comparative studies. J. Urol. **175**, 2011–2017 (2006)
85. Hoznek, A., Salomon, L., Olsson, L.E., et al.: Laparoscopic radical prostatectomy The Creteil experience. Eur. Urol. **40**, 38 (2001)
86. Turk, I., Deger, S., Winkelmann, B., et al.: Laparoscopic radical prostatectomy. Technical aspects and experience with 125 cases. Eur. Urol. **40**, 46 (2001)
87. Eden, C.G., Cahill, D., Vass, J.A., et al.: Laparoscopic radical prostatectomy: the initial UK series. BJU Int. **90**, 876 (2002)

88. Guillonneau, B., Rozet, F., Cathelineau, X., et al.: Perioperative complications of laparoscopic radical prostatectomy: the Montsouris 3-year experience. J. Urol. **167**, 51–56 (2002)
89. Rassweiler, J., Seemann, O., Schulze, M., et al.: Laparoscopic versus open radical prostatectomy a comparative study at a single institution. J. Urol. **169**, 1689 (2003)
90. Dillioglugil, O., Leibman, N.S., Kattan, M.W., et al.: Risk factors for complications and morbidity after radical retropubic prostatectomy. J. Urol. **157**(5), 1760–1767 (1997)
91. Lepor, H., Neder, A.M., Ferrandino, M.N.: Intraoperative and postoperative complications of radical retropubic prostatectomy in a consecutive series of 1, 000 cases. J. Urol. **166**(5), 1729–1733 (2001)
92. Augustin, H., Pummer, K., Daghofer, F., et al.: Patient self-reporting questionnaire on urological morbidity and bother after radical prostatectomy. Eur. Urol. **42**, 112–117 (2002)
93. Guillonneau, B., Cathelineau, X., Doublet, J.D., et al.: Laparoscopic radical prostatectomy: assessment after 550 procedures. Crit. Rev. Oncol. Hematol. **43**, 123 (2002)
94. Walsh, P.C., Marschke, P., Ricker, D., et al.: Patient-reported urinary continence and sexual function after anatomic radical prostatectomy. Urology **55**, 58–61 (2000)
95. Han, M., Partin, A.W., Pound, C.R., et al.: Long-term biochemical disease-free and cancer-specific survival following anatomic radical retropubic prostatectomy. The 15-year Johns Hopkins experience. Urol. Clin. North Am. **28**, 555–565 (2001)
96. Roehl, K.A., Han, M., Ramos, C.G., et al.: Cancer progression and survival rates following anatomical radical retropubic prostatectomy in 3, 478 consecutive patients: long-term results. J. Urol. **172**, 910–914 (2004)
97. Bianco Jr., F.J., Scardino, P.T., Eastham, J.A.: Radical prostatectomy: long-term cancer control and recovery of sexual and urinary function ("trifecta"). Urology **66**, 83–94 (2005)
98. Bhayani, S.B., Pavlovich, C.P., Hsu, T.S., et al.: Prospective comparison of short-term convalescence laparoscopic radical prostatectomy versus open radical retropubic prostatectomy. Urology **61**, 612 (2003)
99. Bickert, D., Frickel, D.: Laparoscopic radical prostatectomy. AORN J. **75**, 762 (2002)
100. Brown, J.A., Garlitz, C., Gomella, L.G., et al.: Perioperative morbidity of laparoscopic radical prostatectomy compared with open radical retropubic prostatectomy. Urol. Oncol. **22**, 102 (2004)
101. Egawa, S., Kuruma, H., Suyama, K., et al.: Delayed recovery of urinary continence after laparoscopic radical prostatectomy. Int. J. Urol. **10**, 207 (2003)
102. Martorana, G., Manferrari, F., Bertaccini, A., et al.: Laparoscopic radical prostatectomy oncological evaluation in the early phase of the learning curve comparing to retropubic approach. Arch. Ital. Urol. Androl. **76**, 1 (2004)
103. Salomon, L., Anastasiadis, A.G., Levrel, O., et al.: Location of positive surgical margins after retropubic, perineal, and laparoscopic radical prostatectomy for organ-confined prostate cancer. Urology **61**, 386 (2003)
104. Hara, I., Kawabata, G., Miyake, H., et al.: Comparison of quality of life following laparoscopic and open prostatectomy for prostate cancer. J. Urol. **169**, 2045 (2003)
105. Pound, C.R., Partin, A.W., Epstein, J.I., et al.: Prostate-specific antigen after anatomic radical retropubic prostatectomy Patterns of recurrence and cancer control. Urol. Clin. North Am. **24**, 395 (1997)
106. Pavlovich, C.P., Trock, B.J., Sulman, A., et al.: 3-year actuarial biochemical recurrence-free survival following laparoscopic radical prostatectomy: experience from a tertiary referral center in the united states. J. Urol. **179**, 917–922 (2008)
107. Jacobsen, N.-E.B., Moore, K.N., Estey, E., et al.: Open versus laparoscopic radical prostatectomy: a prospective comparison of postoperative urinary incontinence rates. J. Urol. **177**, 615–619 (2007)
108. Anastasiadis, A.G., Salomon, L., Katz, R., et al.: Radical retropubic versus laparoscopic prostatectomy: a prospective comparison of functional outcome. Urology **62**, 292 (2003)
109. Litwin, M.S., Melmed, G.Y., Nakazon, T.: Life after radical prostatectomy: a longitudinal study. J. Urol. **166**, 587 (2001)

Cancer of the Urinary Bladder

Kevin P. Asher and David S. Wang

33.1 Introduction

Invasive bladder cancer remains a clinical challenge for the urologist. In the last 20 years, significant progress has been made unraveling the molecular and genetic pathology of transitional cells cancers. We now have a preliminary understanding of the role of tumor suppressor genes such as p53 and oncogenes such as RAS in the development of this potentially lethal disease. Important breakthroughs have been made in treating superficial tumors with intravesical therapies. Despite these advances, the standard treatment for invasive transitional cell carcinoma (TCC) of the bladder in the absence of metastatic disease remains radical cystectomy and pelvic lymphadenectomy with urinary diversion. Recent experience with laparoscopic urologic surgery has demonstrated that a minimally invasive approach to urologic cancers is associated with a significant decrease in morbidity. While radical cystectomy is effective at providing local control for bladder cancer, there is significant associated operative morbidity and mortality. In recent years the laparoscopic and robotic approaches to radical cystectomy have been explored with encouraging initial results. This chapter describes the laparoscopic and robotic approaches to radical cystectomy and summarizes current worldwide experience with these techniques.

K.P. Asher and D.S. Wang (✉)
Department of Urology, Boston University School of Medicine,
720 Harrison Avenue, Suite 606, Boston, MA 02118, USA
e-mail: davids.wang@bmc.org

33.2 Alternatives to Radical Cystectomy

There are a number of alternative treatments to radical cystectomy for patients with invasive bladder cancer. These treatments are most often offered to patients with significant medical comorbidities or those unwilling to undergo urinary diversion.

33.2.1 Radiation Therapy

Radiation therapy has been used as far back as 1917 for the treatment of bladder cancer, both as a means of primary therapy and as an adjunct to surgical treatment [1]. As many as 50% of patients will achieve a complete response with external beam radiation therapy. The response rate is dependent on several prognostic factors related to tumor staging [2]. Interstitial radiation therapy has recently been described with good results in a select group of patients [3].

33.2.2 Transurethral Resection of the Bladder (TUR-B)

Extensive transurethral resection and partial cystectomy are surgical alternatives to radical cystectomy for invasive bladder cancer, where the aim is to achieve local control while keeping the bladder intact. A number of investigators have described the role of "radical" TUR-B in the treatment of highly selected patients with good results [4–7]. In this procedure, the entire thickness of the bladder wall, including the perivesical fat, is resected endoscopically in an effort to render the patient tumor-free. Similarly, partial cystectomy is an option for the highly selected patient with a solitary tumor at the dome of the bladder, with no prior history of TCC, no associated carcinoma in situ, and with a normally functioning bladder of good capacity. Both of these treatment options offer local control; however, recurrence rates are high, and 30–50% of patients will eventually require radical cystectomy.

33.2.3 Multimodality Treatment

A number of multimodality bladder sparing approaches have been developed to approach muscle-invasive disease. TUR-B combined with systemic chemotherapy has been shown to provide reasonable long-term control for T2 lesions [8]. A variety of protocols combining TUR-B, neoadjuvant or adjuvant chemotherapy, and external beam radiation in various regimens have been reported. Survival rates at 3–5 years range from 37% to 81% [9].

33.3 Radical Cystectomy

33.3.1 General Considerations

For patients who have minimal comorbidities and an otherwise reasonable life expectancy, radical cystectomy with pelvic lymph node dissection provides optimal local disease control. Radical cystectomy is indicated in patients with transitional cell tumors invading into or beyond the muscularis propria without evidence of distant metastasis. Selected patients with tumors deeply invasive into the lamina propria with associated carcinoma in situ (CIS) may also be candidates for radical surgery. Patients who have superficial lesions (Ta, T1) that are unable to be controlled with endoscopic techniques and intravesical therapies, or are technically unresectable using an endoscopic approach, should be considered for radical cystectomy. A subset of patients, those with normal body mass index (BMI), no prior abdominal surgery, normal pulmonary function tests (PFT), no evidence of tumor invasion of adjacent structures, and negative nodes on staging radiologic exams, can be considered for a laparoscopic or robotic approach to cystectomy.

In general, the surgical approach to bladder cancer constitutes of two major parts:

- Resection – The radical cystectomy
- Reconstruction – Creation of a continent or non-continent urinary stoma

33.4 Laparoscopic Radical Cystectomy

33.4.1 Indications

In general, the laparoscopic approach to cystectomy and urinary diversion is best suited to nonobese patients without any previous abdominal surgery, radiation treatment, or chemotherapy. Patients with bulky bladder tumors or large-volume lymphadenopathy are not good candidates for the laparoscopic approach.

Table 33.1 lists the indications and contraindications to laparoscopic radical cystectomy.

Table 33.1 Indications and contraindications to laparoscopic radical cystectomy

Indications		• Muscle-invasive transitional cell carcinoma of the bladder in patients with acceptable operative risk
		• Aggressive, superficial bladder cancer with lamina propria invasion and associated carcinoma-in-situ
		• Recurrent, intractable superficial bladder cancer
Contraindications	Absolute	• Known distant visceral or bony metastasis with limited short-term survival
	Relative	• Morbid obesity
		• Bulky, large volume bladder tumor
		• Radiographic evidence of bulky pelvic lymphadenopathy
		• Prior radiotherapy of pelvis
		• Extensive prior abdominal or pelvic surgery
		• Neoadjuvant chemotherapy

33.4.2 Preoperative Patient Preparation

Preoperatively, each patient is seen by an enterostomal nurse and marked for a urostomy. Patients are given a mechanical bowel prep using a polyethylene glycol solution in combination with antibiotics on a neomycin base. A second-generation cephalosporin is administered in the preoperative area. Sequential compression devices (SCD) are used throughout surgery and hospital stay until the patient is ambulatory. Subcutaneous heparin may be administered throughout the perioperative course as an additional measure to prevent venous thromboembolism.

33.4.3 Patient Positioning

After general anesthesia is administered, the patient is positioned in a low lithotomy position. The arms are carefully padded and tucked at the patient's side. Special attention is given to padding all pressure points from intravenous lines and monitoring devices. The patient is then secured to the table with surgical tape.

33.4.4 Operating Room Setup

The operating surgeon stands at the patient's left side and the assistant surgeon at the right. Monitors are placed at the foot and to the left of the operating room table at the surgeon's eye level.

33.4.5 Port Placement

The patient is placed in a steep Trendelenburg position and a Veress needle is used to achieve a pneumoperitoneum to a pressure of 15 mmHg. We use a set of five trocars with a 12-mm camera port placed supraumbilically. After insertion of the first trocar we inspect the contents of the abdominal cavity for vascular or bowel injury and for evidence of gross metastatic disease. Under direct vision, four additional ports are placed in a semicircular configuration in the lower abdomen (Fig. 33.1).

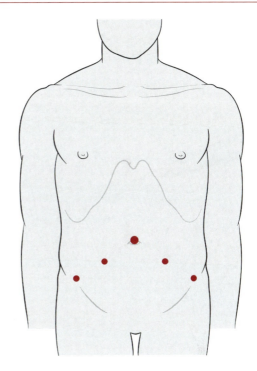

Fig. 33.1 Port placement for laparoscopic radical cystectomy: A set of five trocars is used with a 12-mm camera port placed supraumbilically. Four additional ports are placed in a semicircular configuration in the lower abdomen. (Drawing by Hippmann GbR, Schwarzenbruck, Germany)

33.5 Laparoscopic Radical Cystectomy – Operative Steps

33.5.1 Posterior Peritoneal Incision

Attachments of the sigmoid colon to the abdominal wall are taken down and the colon is retracted cephalad. The initial peritoneal incision is made deep in the rectovesical pouch in the midline, 2 cm above the recess of the Pouch of Douglas (Fig. 33.2). This incision is then continued laterally. The vasa and seminal vesicles are exposed. Denovillier's fascia is then incised in a horizontal fashion and the space between the anterior rectum and posterior prostate is developed (Fig. 33.3). Great care is taken to avoid any rectal injury.

33.5.2 Identification and Transection of the Ureters

The right ureter is identified as it courses over the right common iliac artery. It is dissected down to the level of

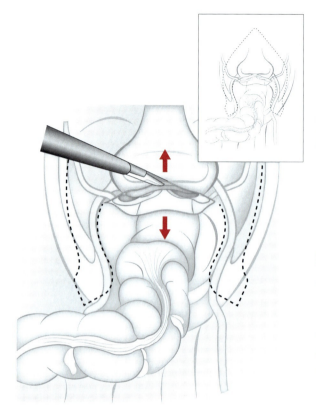

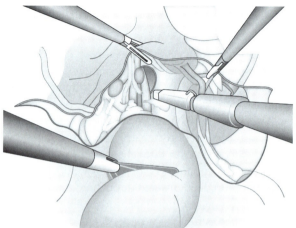

Fig. 33.3 Incision of Denovillier's fascia in a horizontal and development of the space between the anterior rectum and posterior prostate. (Drawing by Hippmann GbR, Schwarzenbruck, Germany)

Fig. 33.2 Initial peritoneal incisions deep in the recto-vesical pouch in the midline, 2 cm above the recess of the Pouch of Douglas. (Drawing by Hippmann GbR, Schwarzenbruck, Germany)

the bladder and clipped. Significant peri-ureteral tissue is preserved. Frozen section of the distal margin of the ureter is performed to ensure that there is no tumor tissue left behind. The ureter is then freed as proximally as possible and a silk stitch at its distal end is placed for later identification. The same procedure is then completed on the left side, and a stitch of different color can be placed and used for later identification of the left ureter.

33.5.3 Anterior Peritoneal Incision

An incision is made on the anterior abdominal wall, opening the peritoneum from the left to the right obliterated umbilical ligament and superiorly to include the urachus. The anterior surface of the bladder is then dissected free from the abdominal wall and the space of Retzius is developed. The pubo-prostatic ligaments are then divided. The endopelvic fascia is opened and the muscle fibers of the levator ani are pushed laterally. A stent is then placed per urethra and the dorsal venous complex is ligated with a 0-Vicryl suture on a CT-1 needle.

33.5.4 Securing the Vascular Pedicles

The assistant retracts the bladder specimen to the left, exposing the right lateral vascular pedicle. This pedicle is then secured with an endoscopic articulating stapler, white load. Alternatively, clips or an ultrasonic ligation device is used. The left vascular pedicle is secured in a similar fashion.

33.5.5 Apical Dissection

At this point the last remaining attachment is at the prostatic apex. The dorsal venous complex is now transected, and a plane between this venous complex and the urethra is established. The proximal aspect of the urethra is then closed with a suture or with a stapler to limit any spillage of urine. The urethra is divided, which completely frees the specimen. Frozen section biopsies are performed at the urethral stump. The specimen is then placed into a laparoscopic specimen bag for later removal.

33.5.6 Extended Pelvic Lymph Node Dissection

There is considerable evidence that a thorough pelvic lymph node dissection not only improves staging but also improves long-term survival in invasive bladder tumors [10, 11]. After the cystectomy is complete, the patient is positioned with the right side 30° up in combination with 30° Trendelenburg.

The boundaries of the pelvic lymph node dissection are:

- Internal inguinal ring distal
- Genitofemoral nerve lateral
- Obturator nerve posterior
- Bladder medial
- Aortic bifurcation superior

Placement of the camera port in a supra-umbilical position allows for further superior dissection, 2–3 cm above the aortic bifurcation.

The lymph node packet is carefully mobilized from the surrounding tissues. It is important to avoid any incision directly into the lymphatic tissue during the dissection to minimize the risk of tumor seeding. Once the lymph node packet is freed, it is placed into a laparoscopic specimen bag for retrieval at the end of the procedure to minimize the contact with other tissue.

33.6 Laparoscopic Urinary Diversion

33.6.1 Introduction

Since the first description of a laparoscopic ileal conduit urinary diversion was reported in 1992 by Kozminski and Partamanian, there has been steady progress in the development of new and innovative techniques to accomplish urinary diversion via the laparoscopic approach [12]. In the initial stages of investigation, this reconstructive element of radical surgery for bladder cancer was considered to be the most difficult element to accomplish using minimally invasive techniques. The development of new techniques, such as the lap-assisted or mini-laparotomy technique, has made laparoscopic urinary diversion more feasible in recent years. Additionally, new developments in laparoscopic instrumentation have aided surgeons to perform more complex reconstructions intracorporeally.

33.6.2 Different Types of Urinary Diversion

Just as in open surgery, there are two general approaches to laparoscopic urinary diversion:

- Noncontinent diversion
  - Ileal conduit
  - Cutaneous ureterostomy
  - Ileo-vesicostomy [13–16]
- Continent diversion
  - Ileal neo-bladder
  - Mainz II recto-sigmoid pouch
  - Various configurations of continent catheterizable stomatas

The simplest and most commonly performed diversion, via the open or laparoscopic approach, is the noncontinent ileal conduit. Continent stomatas utilize the appendix as a catheterizable channel. The indications for each type of diversion are identical to open surgery. The decision to perform a noncontinent versus a continent diversion involves many factors for the patient and the surgeon. The best overall long-term outcome should be the driving force behind the decision for each patient, and difficulties with the laparoscopic techniques should not preclude an appropriate candidate from having a continent diversion.

33.6.3 General Considerations

Another decision point for the surgeon performing laparoscopic radical cystectomy and urinary diversion is whether to perform the diversion via a total laparoscopic technique or using lap-assisted technique. In the total laparoscopic approach, all dissection, incisions, and suturing are performed in-situ using intracorporeal suturing techniques. The lap-assisted technique consists of making a mini-laparotomy incision and exteriorizing the targeted bowel segment and ureters. The uretero-intestinal anastamoses and restoration of bowel continuity are performed extra-corporeally using standard techniques. The first laparoscopic urinary diversion by Kosminski and Partamanian in 1992 was performed via the lap-assisted approach, where an extended port site was utilized to perform the ileal loop diversion [12]. Gill et al. described the first completely intracorporeal laparoscopic radical cystectomy with ileal loop diversion [17].

We describe the basic steps in performing lap-assisted ileal conduit, which is the most commonly performed technique.

33.7 Lap-assisted Ileal Conduit Urinary Diversion

The radical cystectomy and extended pelvic lymphadenectomy is performed as described above. In essence, the reconstruction is performed through a mini-laparotomy. The left ureter is identified via the holding suture placed previously and tunneled beneath the sigmoid mesentery. There must be sufficient ureteral dissection to assure enough length of the ureter to reach the proximal end of the loop without undue tension.

33.7.1 Operative Steps

33.7.1.1 Defining the Small Bowel Loop to Create the Conduit

Next, a port site on the right side of the abdomen is used to exteriorize the small bowel. Alternatively, if the port site is not in an appropriate location, we make a 5-cm incision. The ileum is exteriorized and the vascular arcade examined for sufficient blood flow. A 15–20 cm segment of ileum is then selected, 15–20 cm proximal to the ileo-cecal junction. This segment is isolated with a GIA stapler using blue loads. The isolated segment is then passed posterior to the remaining ileum.

33.7.1.2 Restoration of Bowel Continuity

Bowel continuity is restored via a stapled anastomosis using a standard 55-mm GIA stapler blue load along the antimesenteric border. A 55-mm TA™ stapler is used to close the resulting enterotomy and to complete the anastomosis. We do not routinely oversew the staple line. The mesenteric window is closed with a running silk suture.

33.7.1.3 Preparation and Implantation of the Ureters

The holding sutures on the ureters are then used to deliver the ureters through the previously chosen port site and brought in close proximity to the isolated bowel segment. We spatulate the ureters for a distance of 1 cm. Single J ureteral stents are employed into each ureter and passed into the renal pelvis. 4–0 Vicryl sutures are used in running fashion to implant the spatulated ureters into the proximal aspect of the loop. The distal aspect of the stents is passed through the end of the loop.

33.7.1.4 Creation of the Urinary Stoma

The urinary stoma will usually be created in the right lower quadrant. The ileal segment is anchored to the fascia of the rectus muscle with 2–0 Vicryl sutures. As a last step we evert the mucosa mature a rosebud stoma.

33.7.1.5 Drainage and Wound Closure

We routinely place a #10 flat Jackson-Pratt drain in the pelvis. The mini-laparotomy incision is closed like a regular laparotomy. All port sites greater than 10 mm are closed under direct vision using standard techniques or closure-assist instruments such as the Carter-Thompson device. For wound closure we use 4/0 absorbable suture in a subcuticular technique.

33.8 Results of Laparoscopic Cystectomy

Laparoscopic radical cystectomy and urinary diversion reflects the culmination of the development of significant expertise in ablative and reconstructive urology as well as the introduction of sophisticated laparoscopic instrumentation. Not surprisingly, laparoscopic cystectomy is a technically demanding procedure and

Table 33.2 Laparoscopic radical cystectomy: Worldwide results

	Year	n	Technique	OR time (h)	Blood loss (mL)	Length of stay (min)	Return of bowel function (day)	Complications (n)
Abdel-Hakim [18]	2002	14	Extra-corporeal neobladder	8.3	N/R	N/R	3	None
Gill [17]	2002	3	Intra-coporeal neobladder [2] Extracorporeal Indiana Pouch [1]	9.5	300	8.5	2–4	Bleeding duodenal ulcer [1]
Turk [18]	2001	5	Intra-corporeal Mainz pouch	7.4	250	10	2	None
Denewer [19]	1999	10	Modified ureterosigmoidostomy	3.6	2.2 Units	10–13	N/R	Several serious complications including 1 death from hemorrhage
Gupta [20]	2002	5	Intra-corporeal ileal conduit	7.5	360	7	3	Small bowel obstruction [1]
Puppo [21]	1995	5	Intra-corporeal Ileal conduit	7.2	N/R	10.6	2–4	None

h hour; *N/R* not reported

requires advanced laparoscopic skills. In recent years, a number of small series from around the world have shown that this technique is feasible (Table 33.2). Recently, the first intermediate term oncologic data have become available.

Simnoto et al. reported oncologic results at 30 months in ten male patients undergoing laparoscopic radical cystectomy for recurrent T1 high-grade tumors or T2 tumors [22]. There were no positive margins, no local recurrences, and no port site metastasis. Four of ten patients died of metastatic bladder cancer within 31 months. Six patients underwent urinary diversion with orthotopic ileal neobladder, two had cutaneous ureterostomy, and two a uretero-sigmoidostomy. There were no reported perioperative complications. There was some concern among urologic oncologists regarding the results of this small series, as the rate of metastatic disease was higher than expected in this group of lower risk patients when compared to the open approach.

Haber and Gill reported on their 5 years experience and oncologic outcomes after laparoscopic cystectomy [23]. In a series of 37 patients the mean follow-up was 31 months. Two patients had positive margins, and seven patients had node-positive disease. The average number of lymph nodes harvested was 14. Two patients died from metastatic disease. Five year overall and cancer-specific survival was 63% and 92%, respectively. In this study there were 6 major complications requiring reinterventions, underscoring the technical difficulties of this procedure. As expected, most of these complications, like urine leak and small bowel obstruction, were related to the urinary diversion. At the beginning of this series, all urinary diversions were performed intracorporeally and most of the complications could be attributed to the difficulty with intracorporeal free-hand suturing. As the authors gained experience with the procedure, diversion was performed through an extracorporeal approach. This study represents the longest follow up currently available for laparoscopic cystectomy and urinary diversion, and demonstrates oncologic outcomes similar to that of reported open series.

There has been one case report of port-site recurrence of TCC after a robotic-assisted laparoscopic radical cystectomy and extracorporeal ileal neobladder [24]. This occurred in a 52-year-old man with a pT3 high-grade TCC of the bladder, who presented at 10 months after surgery with a palpable nodule at one

Table 33.3 Robotic Radical Cystectomy: Worldwide results

	Year	n	Technique	OR time (h)	Blood loss (mL)	Length of Stay (day)	Return of bowel function (day)	Complications
Beecken [28]	2003	1	Intra-corporeal Neobladder	8.5	200	N/R	N/R	None
Balaji [29]	2004	3	Intra-corporeal Ileal conduit	11.5	250	7.3	N/R	[1] Ileus, resolved with conservative management
Sala [30]	2006	1	Intra-corporeal Neobladder	12	100	5	N/R	None
Rhee and Theodorescu [31]	2006	30	Extra-corporeal Ileal conduit	10.6	479	11	N/R	N/R
Guru and Mohler [32]	2007	20	Extra-corporeal Ileal conduit [17] Neobladder [2] Not listed [1]	7.3	555	7	4	2 major (1 death due to small bowel obstruction)
Menon [33]	2003	14	Extra-corporeal ileal neobladder	Cystectomy 2.3 Neobladder 2.7	<150	N/R	N/R	N/R
Pruthi [26]	2007	20	Robotic Extra-corporeal diversion Ileal loop [10] Neobladder [10]	6.1	313	4–5	2.1	6 (2 required operative intervention)

N/R not reported

of the laparoscopic trocar sites. The procedure was uncomplicated and the specimen was removed with a specimen retrieval bag. The significance of this complication in laparoscopic cystectomy remains unclear.

33.9 Robot-assisted Laparoscopic Cystectomy

In recent years there has been considerable positive experience with robot-assisted laparoscopic radical prostatectomy [25]. The development of robot-assisted techniques has allowed surgeons to master the steep learning curve associated with laparoscopic abdominal and pelvic procedures, particularly those involving extensive intracorporeal suturing. As the experience with robotic prostatectomy has progressed, innovators in laparoscopic urologic oncology have extended these robotic techniques to develop an approach for robotic-assisted laparoscopic radical cystectomy [26–31]. The fundamental surgical steps are similar in the robotic and the standard laparoscopic approach.

There are several advantages to robotic-assisted radical cystectomy. Improved three-dimensional vision, great magnification, extended degrees of freedom, and especially, a shorter learning curve makes this approach attractive to urologists performing minimally invasive surgery for bladder cancer. A big advantage in applying robotics to prostate or urinary bladder cancer is the fixed nature of these two anatomical structures. As robotic equipment becomes accessible for urologists across the country, the robotic-assisted laparoscopic approach to cystectomy will likely become more popular.

Pruthi and Wallen have recently reported the largest published series of robot-assisted laparoscopic radical cystectomy [26]. In this series, ten men had urinary diversion with an ileal conduit, and ten received an orthotopic neobladder. All diversions were performed extracorporeally. Mean operative time was 6.2 h, and mean blood loss was 313 mL. Nineteen out of 20 patients were discharged home within 5 days. There were six reported complications, two of which resulted in reoperation: postoperative bleeding in one case, peristomal omental herniation in the other. This series shows that robotic-assisted laparoscopic radical cystectomy is feasible and is associated with excellent perioperative outcomes with regard to blood loss and length of hospital stay.

Currently, no long-term oncologic or functional data are available. As such, this innovative procedure is still in the early phases of development, and patients should be informed of the lack of long-term data during the counseling process (Table 33.3).

33.10 Conclusion

Radical cystectomy with lymph node dissection remains the standard approach for most patients with invasive bladder cancer. There are encouraging results with the laparoscopic and robotic approach to this surgical procedure. Although the long-term oncologic data continue to mature, a number of investigators have now demonstrated that this technique offers a feasible and safe approach with short-term results equivalent to standard open surgery. It is likely that in the next 10 years laparoscopic and robotic cystectomy will see widespread application in the management of bladder cancer.

Quick Reference Guide

1. Choose your patient wisely and mark the urostomy site preoperatively
2. Position the patient in lithotomy
3. Use a set of five trocars in a semicircular configuration in the lower abdomen with a 12-mm camera port
4. **The Resection**

    The following operative sequence is strictly followed in each case:

    - *Posterior peritoneal incision*
        - Spare the vasa and seminal vesicles and develop the plane between anterior rectum and posterior prostate.
        - Avoid any rectal injury!
    - *Identification and transection of the ureters*
        - Dissect the ureters down to the level of the bladder and clip them
        - place holding sutures on each ureter
        - Preserve peri-ureteral tissue
        - Obtain a frozen section of the distal margin
    - *Anterior peritoneal incision*
        - Stay between the right and left obliterated umbilical ligament and superiorly to include the urachus
        - Dissect the anterior surface of the bladder of the abdominal wall
        - Develop the space of Retzius
        - Push the levator ani muscle laterally and strictly preserve it
        - Securely ligate the posterior venous complex
    - *Securing the vascular pedicles*
        - Retract the bladder specimen to either side to expose the contralateral vascular pedicle
        - Secure the pedicles with a stapling device, white load
    - *Apical dissection*
        - Transect the dorsal venous complex
        - Develop the plane between this venous complex and the urethra
        - Close off the proximal urethra to avoid spillage of urine
        - Divide the urethra
        - Obtain a frozen section of the urethral stump
    - *Extended pelvic lymph node dissection*
        - Respect all important anatomical landmarks:
            ° Internal inguinal ring distal

- Genitofemoral nerve lateral
- Obturator nerve posterior
- Bladder medial
- Aortic bifurcation superior

5. Place the bladder specimen and lymph nodes in an impermeable retrieval bag
6. **The Reconstruction**
   - Perform the reconstruction through a mini laparotomy
   - Tunnel the left ureter beneath the sigmoid mesentery
   - Ensure that you have sufficient ureteral dissection to avoid any tension on the uretero-ileal anastomosis
   - Exteriorize the terminal ileum through a right-sided port site
   - Choose a bowel segment of 15 to 20-cm length, assess the blood flow, and isolate it with staplers
   - Restore the bowel continuity using standard technique and close the mesenteric window
   - Deliver the ureters through the previously chosen port site
   - Spatulate the ureters on a length of 1 cm and insert stents
   - Implant the ureters into the proximal aspect of the separated bowel loop using a 4/0 running Vicryl and pass the stents through the distal end of the bowel loop
   - Create a rosebud stoma in the right lower quadrant and fixate the ileum conduit to the abdominal wall
7. Remove the specimen
8. Place a #10 flat Jackson-Pratt drain in the pelvis
9. Close the mini laparotomy and all 10-mm ports in standard technique
10. Wound closure is performed with a running, absorbable suture

References

1. Young, H.H., Frontz, W.A.: Some new methods in the treatment of carcinoma of the lower genitourinary tract with radium. J. Urol. **1**, 505–541 (1917)
2. Shipley, W.U., Rose, M.A.: Bladder cancer. The selection of patient for treatment by full –dose irradiation. Cancer **55**, 2278–2284 (1985)
3. Wijnmaalen, A., Koper, P.C., Jansen, P.P., et al.: Muscle invasive bladder cancer treated by transurethral resection, followed by external beam radiation and interstitial iridium-192. Int. J. Radiat. Oncol. Biol. Phys. **39**, 1043–1052 (1997)
4. Barnes, R.W., Dick, A.L., Hadley, H.L., et al.: Survival following transurethral resection of bladder carcinoma. Cancer Res. **37**, 2895–2898 (1977)
5. Herr, H.W.: Conservative management of muscle-infiltrating bladder cancer: prospective experience. J. Urol. **138**, 1162–1163 (1987)
6. Henry, K., Miller, J., Mori, M., et al.: Comparison of transurethral resection to radical therapies for stage B bladder tumors. J. Urol. **140**, 964–967 (1988)
7. Solsona, E., Iborra, I., Ricos, J.V., et al.: Feasibility of transurethral resection for muscle-infiltrating carcinoma of the bladder: prospective study. J. Urol. **147**, 1513–1555 (1992)
8. Hall, R.R., Newling, D.W.W., Ramsden, P.D., Richards, B., Robinson, M.R.G., Smith, P.H.: Treatment of invasive bladder cancer by local resection and high-dose methotrexate. Br. J. Urol. **56**, 558–672 (1984)
9. Wein, A., Kavoussi, L., Novick, A., Partin, A., Peters, C. (eds.): Campbell-Walsh Urology, p 2475. Elsevier, Philapelphia (2006)
10. Herr, H.W., Bochner, B.H., Dalbagni, G., Donat, S.M., Reuter, V.E., Bajorin, D.F.: Impact of the number of lymph nodes reteived on outcome in patients with muscle invasive bladder cancer. J. Urol. **167**(3), 1295–1298 (2002)
11. Konety, B.R., Joslyn, S.A., O'donnell, M.A.: Extent of pelvic lymphadenectomy and its impact on outcome in patients diagnosed with bladder cancer: analysis of data from the Surveillance, Epidemiology and End Results Program data base. J. Urol. **169**(3), 946–950 (2003)
12. Kozminski, M., Partamian, K.O.: Case report of laparoscopic ileal loop conduit. J. Endourol. **6**, 147–150 (1992)
13. Abraham, H.M., Rahman, N.U., Meng, M.V., Stoller, M.L.: Pure laparoscopic ileovesicostomy. J. Urol. **170**(2 Pt 1), 517–518 (2003)
14. Hsu, T.H., et al.: Laparoscopic ileovesicostomy. J. Urol. **168**(1), 180–181 (2002)
15. Loisides, P., Grasso, M., Lui, P.: Laproscopic cutaneous ureterostomy: technique for palliative upper urinary tract drainage. J. Endourol. **9**(4), 315–317 (1995)
16. Puppo, P., et al.: Videoendoscopic cutaneous ureterostomy for palliative urinary diversion in advanced pelvic cancer. Eur. Urol. **28**(4), 328–333 (1995)
17. Gill, I.S., Fergany, A., Klein, E.A., et al.: Laparoscopic radical cystoprostatectomy with ileal conduit performed completely intracorporeally: the initial 2 cases. Urology **56**(1), 26–29 (2000). 29-30

18. Abdel-Hakim, A.M., Bassiouny, F., Abdel Azim, M.S., et al.: Laparoscopic radical cystectomy with orthotopic neobladder. J. Endourol. **16**, 377–381 (2002)
19. Turk, I., Deger, S., Winkelmann, B., Sconberger, B., Loening, S.A.: Laparoscopic radical cystectomy with continent urinary diversion (rectal sigmoid pouch) performed completely intracorporeally: the initial 5 cases. J. Urol. **165**, 1863–1866 (2001)
20. Gupta, N.P., Gill, I.S., Fergancy, A., Nabi, G.: Laparoscopic radical cystectomy with intracorporeal ileal conduit diversion: 5 cases with 2 year follow-up. BJU Int. **90**, 391–396 (2002)
21. Puppo, P., Perachino, M., et al.: Laparoscopically assisted transvaginal radical cystectomy. Eur. Urol. **27**, 80–84 (1995)
22. Simonato, A., Gregori, A., et al.: Laparoscopic radical cystoprostatectomy: our experience in a consecutive series of 10 patients with a 3 year follow up. Eur. Urol. **47**, 785–792 (2005)
23. Haber, G.P., Gill, I.S.: Laparoscopic radical cystectomy for cancer: oncological outcomes at up to 5 years. BJU Int. **100**, 137–142 (2007)
24. El-tabey, N.A., Shoma, A.M.: Port-site metastases after robot-assisted laparoscopic radical cystectomy. Urology **66**, 1110 (2005)
25. Ficarra, V., Cavalleri, S., Novara, G., Aragona, M., Artibani, W.: Evidence from robot-assisted laparoscopic radical prostatectomy: a systematic review. Eur. Urol. **51**, 45 (2007)
26. Pruthi, R., Wallen, E.: Robotic assisted laparoscopic radical cystoprostatectomy: operative and pathological outcomes. J. Urol. **178**, 814–818 (2007)
27. Hemal, A.K., Abol-Enein, H., Tewari, A., Shrivastava, A., Shoma, A.M., Ghonheim, M.A., et al.: Robotic radical cystectomy and urinary diversion in the management of bladder cancer. Urol. Clin. North Am. **31**, 719 (2004)
28. Beecken, W.D., et al.: Robotic-assisted laparoscopic radical cystectomy and intra-abdominal formation of an orthotopic ileal neobladder. Eur. Urol. **44**, 337 (2003)
29. Balaji, K.C., Yohanss, P., McBride, C.L., Oleynikov, D., Hemstreet, G.P.: Feasibility of robot-assisted totally intracorporeal laparoscopic ileal conduit urinary diversion: initial results of a single institutional pilot study. Urology **63**, 51 (2004)
30. Sala, L.G., Matsunaga, G.S., Corica, F.A., Ornstein, D.K.: Robotic-asssted laparoscopic radical cystoprostatectomy and totally intracorporeal ileal neobladder. J. Endourol. **20**, 233 (2006)
31. Rhee, J.J., Lebeau, S., Smolkin, M., Theodorescu, D.: Radical cystectomy with ileal conduit diversion: early prospective evaluation of the impact of robotic assistance. BJU Int. **98**, 1059 (2006)
32. Guru, K., Kim, H., Piacente, P., Mohler, J.: Robot-assisted radical cystectomy and pelvic lymph hode dissection: initial experience at Roswell Park Cancer Institute. Urology **69**(3), 469–474 (2007)
33. Menon, M., et al.: Nerve-sparing robot-assisted radical cystoprostatectomy and urinary diversion. BJU Int. **92**, 232–236 (2003)

Part XI
Special Topics: Pediatrics

34 Minimally Invasive Management of Pediatric Malignancies

Arjun Khosla, Todd A. Ponsky, and Steven S. Rothenberg

34.1 Introduction

Minimally invasive surgery (MIS) is becoming an increasingly important component of the work-up and treatment of pediatric solid tumors. Stephen Gans and George Berci studied the use of laparoscopy in pediatric patients and helped design the first set of pediatric laparoscopic instruments. They stated that laparoscopy is indicated when simpler studies are not definitive and the advantage of this procedure is that it either avoids a laparotomy or establishes the definitive need and plan for an operation [1–3]. During the 1970s and 1980s, Bradley Rodgers and Frederick Ryckman described the use of thoracoscopy in children for the evaluation and biopsy of intrathoracic conditions [4, 5]. Other than these studies, there were very few reports evaluating MIS in children until the late 1980s.

Today, MIS is important in the exploration, diagnosis, staging, palliation, resection, and surveillance of oncologic disease. The development of laparoscopic technology designed specifically for children in the 1990s led to an increased use of MIS in pediatric surgery. Its use in the evaluation and diagnosis of pediatric solid malignancies has been confirmed by numerous studies [6–11]. As experience grows and technology advances, criteria are developed to carefully select patients. Minimally invasive techniques are being used increasingly to treat solid pediatric malignancies [12–17].

Over the past decade, experience in MIS has increased to the point where laparoscopy and thoracoscopy have become acceptable treatment modalities for the work-up and treatment of pediatric solid tumors. MIS has been shown to be a useful method to obtain tissue for both the initial diagnosis of suspicious masses in the peritoneal and thoracic cavities and the diagnosis of recurrent or metastatic disease in patients who have completed initial therapy for malignant disease. Laparoscopy and thoracoscopy are also used in the resection of malignant disease with curative intention in a variety of sites [9]:

- Lungs – thoracoscopic resection of pulmonary and mediastinal metastases
- Adrenal gland – laparoscopic adrenalectomy for neuroblastoma
- Kidney – laparoscopic nephrectomy for Wilms' tumor
- Gonadal tissue – laparoscopic resection of germ cell tumors

In 1996, the National Cancer Institute (NCI) funded a number of studies evaluating MIS in the treatment of various malignancies in adults and children and the effects on patients' quality of life. The NCI also funded the surgical sections of the Children's Cancer Group

A. Khosla
Division of Pediatric Surgery, Rainbow Babies and Children's Hospital, University Hospitals, School of Medicine, Case Western Reserve University, 11100 Euclid Avenue, Cleveland, OH 44106, USA

T.A. Ponsky (✉)
Division of Pediatric Surgery, Rainbow Babies and Children's Hospital, University Hospitals, School of Medicine, Case Western Reserve University, 11100 Euclid Avenue, Cleveland, OH 44106, USA
e-mail: todd.ponsky@uhhospitals.org

S.S. Rothenberg
Department of Pediatrics, Rocky Mountain Hospital for Children, Rocky Mountain Pediatric Surgery, 1601 East 19th Avenue, Suite 5500, Denver, CO 80218, USA
e-mail: steverberg@aol.com

(CCG) and Pediatric Oncology Group (POG) to conduct randomized controlled, surgeon-directed studies to evaluate the role of MIS in children with cancer. These studies, however, closed in 1998 due to a lack of patient accrual. A review examined why these studies failed and found that patient preference of an open technique was not the cause, but rather surgeons themselves favoring an open operation, most likely secondary to lack of experience with MIS. In 2003, a prospective study of 74 pediatric patients with tumors showed that MIS is useful in approximately 25% of oncological patients undergoing surgery [10].

34.2 Benefits of MIS in Pediatric Oncology

The benefits of MIS, including shorter hospitalization with possibly earlier initiation of adjuvant chemotherapy, better pain control, improved cosmesis, and an earlier return to routine activities, have been attributed to a number of factors. MIS has been shown to maintain delayed-type hypersensitivity of T cells and proliferation rates of B and T lymphocytes, while decreasing the rates of tumor cell turnover, increasing monocyte toxicity and tumor cell apoptosis. The cumulative result of these effects is [6]

- More rapid return of normal immune function
- Decreased stress reaction
- Improved ability to fight cancer cell spread

Many studies have shown that because these techniques cause less tissue trauma and because of metabolic properties of the gas used to establish pneumoperitoneum, there is less interference with monocytes, macrophages, polymorphonuclear leukocytes (PMNs), and lymphocytes involved in the host's defense [5]. Many controlled clinical trials have shown that pneumoperitoneum-based surgery results in reduced levels of circulatory cytokines and a better-preserved cell-mediated immune response in patients. In addition, the effects of CO_2 used to establish a pneumoperitoneum have been studied in the peritoneal cavity and distant organs. There was a reduction in pulmonary macrophage reactive oxygen species, a lack of increase in the number of leukocytes, and a reduction in their phagocytic activity. It has been proposed that acidification secondary to the CO_2 insufflation causes these observed phenomena. Currently, there is controversy over the effects of CO_2 in patients with malignancy. Some have proposed that the interference with host defenses affects the clearing of tumor cells as well as the tumor itself, but studies have been inconclusive. Little is known about the effects of CO_2 specifically on pediatric tumor cells. Schmidt studied several pediatric tumor cell lines in vitro and found that it was potentially beneficial. The proliferation rate of neuroblastoma, hepatoblastoma, hepatocellular carcinoma, and lymphoma cells was reduced for 4 days following exposure to CO_2 versus air or helium. It is unclear whether the CO_2 interferes with activation of oncogenes or with inactivation of tumor suppressor genes in pediatric tumors. Iwanaka studied the in vivo effects of CO_2 pneumoperitoneum on neuroblastoma cells and showed no significant difference in survival, tumor growth, or distant metastases when compared to laparotomy [5]. These authors also showed that port-site recurrences were similar between CO_2 and gasless pneumoperitoneum. At present, no clinical studies have confirmed an alteration in tumor cell behavior using MIS in children. Further studies are required to investigate whether long-term survival and recurrence are not compromised by the beneficial immunological effects of MIS.

34.3 Abdominal and Pelvic Tumors

34.3.1 Indications for MIS and General Considerations

Laparoscopy has been used for childhood malignancies

- To establish a diagnosis
- For disease staging
- To obtain a biopsy
- For evaluation of recurrence or metastasis
- For tumor resection

Laparoscopic biopsy has been described in many abdominal and retroperitoneal tumors, including neuroblastoma, nephroblastoma, hepatoblastoma, rhabdomyosarcoma, teratoma, lymphoma, and numerous others (Fig. 34.1). The diagnostic accuracy of laparoscopic biopsies for various malignant diseases has been reported to be as high as 100% and the conversion rate is often low [5]. Many surgeons have expressed concern about port-site metastases, but the reported incidence has been low. Spurbeck and Iwanaka reported

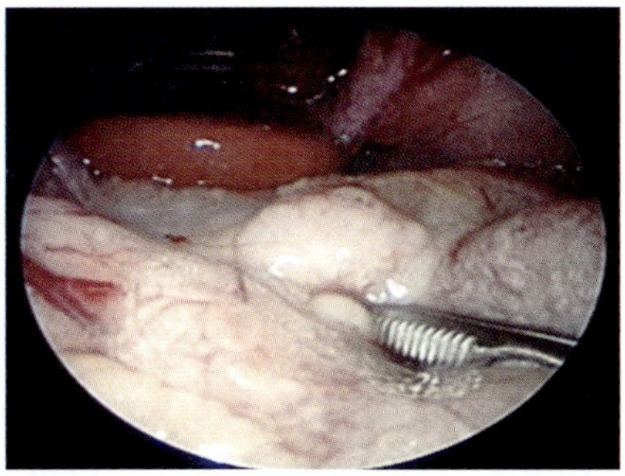

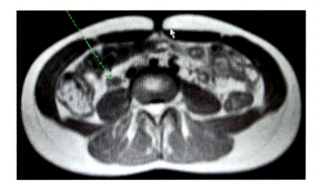

Fig. 34.1 Laparoscopic distal pancreatectomy: adenoma of the pancreatic tail

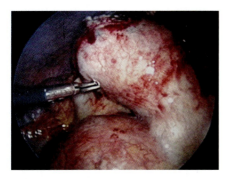

Fig. 34.2 Burkits abdominal lymphoma following chemotherapy, CT scan

Fig. 34.3 Complete resection of Burkits lymphoma following chemotherapy

studied in the evaluation of metastatic spread of hepatoblastoma [21]. Studies from Japan have even proposed laparoscopy for the resection of malignant disease. However, the feasibility of laparoscopic tumor resection is limited in most reported series. In general, large and dense fibrotic tumors are not good candidates for laparoscopic resection. Tumor resection using laparoscopy has most often been presented for neuroblastoma, but has also been reported for pancreatic tumors, nephroblastoma, and numerous other rare conditions. Iwanaka has recommended laparoscopic resection of malignancies such as neuroblastoma and ovarian tumors [13]. Because these tumors were found early, they were ideal candidates for resection using MIS due to their limited extent, small size (less than 5 cm), and being well encapsulated. Patients who underwent minimally invasive resection had a shorter hospital stay as well as a decreased time to postoperative feeding and time to postoperative chemotherapy. The immediate resection of these tumors, however, has also been debated and the authors of the study concluded that, although effective, better indicators were needed for the implementation of such techniques as well as a thorough preoperative work-up in order to avoid complications and subsequent conversion to open procedures. Komuro suggested resection of tumors that do not regress in size or grow larger than 5 cm, while other authors recommended resection of neuroblastomas smaller than 2 cm [22]. Minimally invasive techniques involving laparoscopic resection of extra-osseous Ewing's sarcoma have also been reported in the literature [23]. Solomon et al. demonstrated the use of vaginoscopy for both evaluation and resection of vaginal rhabdomyosarcoma (RMS), which allowed for a less morbid surgical procedure [24]. Stankovic et al. described using minimally invasive therapy for a girl with cervical RMS [25]. Some of the most common tumors treated with minimally invasive approaches are discussed below.

no port-site recurrences in their studies; however, the follow-up may not be long enough to draw final conclusions [6, 13]. Adherence to basic surgical principals and always removing possible tumor specimens through the trocar or using an endoscopic specimen retrieval bag should prevent this (Figs. 34.2 and 34.3).

Laparoscopic resection of liver tumors and the development of animal models have been reported in the literature [18–20]. Laparoscopic fluorescence has been

34.4 Specific Intra-abdominal Malignancies in Pediatric Patients

34.4.1 Wilms' Tumor

MIS is now increasingly being applied to pediatric solid tumors, including Wilms' tumor, in the diagnostic work-up and treatment of these malignancies.

34.4.1.1 Nephrectomy – General Remarks

Generally, radical nephrectomy is performed with sampling of regional lymph nodes, but formal lymph node dissection is not required. Laparoscopic nephrectomy in children has been well described in the literature [26] and urologic tumors of the ureter and kidney are being increasingly treated applying minimally invasive techniques [27]. In fact, laparoscopic nephrectomy with intact specimen extraction has become a routine, effective, and efficacious treatment option for adult patients with T1–T3aN0M0 tumors ≤10–12 cm in size [28]. This study demonstrated that laparoscopic radical nephrectomy allows for a technically adequate dissection with negative margins as well as similar surgical time compared to an open procedure. Significantly decreased blood loss and a quicker hospital discharge are further advantages. Duarte et al. studied laparoscopic nephrectomy for unilateral Wilms' tumor in children following chemotherapy, showing it to be feasible and safe [29].

34.4.1.2 Surgical Technique

Patients are placed in a 30° contralateral supine position. Trocars are placed in the infraumbilical region, near the xyphoid process, at the iliacal fossa and subcostally in the anterior axillary line. Once access to the abdomen has been achieved, it should be explored for evidence of hepatic metastasis, intravascular extension, or intraperitoneal spread. There is no consensus about the limits of tumor size that can be treated with laparoscopic nephrectomy. Retrospective analysis of pediatric patients treated with MIS showed that the tumor's dimension on computed tomography (CT) after chemotherapy did not exceed 10% of the patient's height, which may serve as a possible index [29]. Another important issue is the surgeon's inability to palpate the contralateral kidney when using MIS; however, the International Society for Pediatric Oncology (SIOP) protocol recommends exploration of the other kidney only if preoperative imaging shows bilateral tumor growth.

34.4.2 Neuroblastoma

The treatment for neuroblastoma, like many other solid pediatric tumors, employs multiple modalities, using surgery, chemotherapy, radiation, and bone marrow or stem cell transplantation. Prior to the start of therapy, patients should have their baseline urinary catecholamine metabolites measured because these values can serve as a marker for treatment success, disease persistence, or tumor recurrence. Surgery is the mainstay of treatment of neuroblastoma, used in its evaluation, diagnosis, and treatment. The goals of surgical intervention are resection, if possible, as well as staging by inspection and biopsy. In addition, patients may need second-look operations for evaluation and excision of residual disease. Children with neuroblastoma who experience symptoms of spinal cord compression like paralysis, paresthesias, or incontinence should undergo immediate treatment. Treatment in this situation could consist of laminotomy, radiation, or chemotherapy.

34.4.2.1 Biopsy of Neuroblastoma

Biopsy of a suspected neuroblastoma, which can often be performed laparoscopically, should be done before the initiation of chemotherapy. Fine needle aspiration (FNA) under radiographic guidance has also been demonstrated as an effective technique that decreases the need for open biopsy [30]. One of the main criticisms of this technique is that, although it may provide a tissue diagnosis, it does not provide adequate tissue for multiple histological and cytogenic analyses, which are important to determine prognosis. Laparoscopic wedge biopsy can be employed in such a situation because it provides enough tissue for analysis and is less invasive than a laparotomy. There is debate regarding the best technique for a laparoscopic wedge biopsy. While some perform wedge biopsies using thermic devices such as electrocautery, harmonic scalpel (Ethicon, Cincinnati, OH), or Ligasure™ (Covidien, Connecticut), there is sufficient evidence that heated biopsies may alter the histological analyses [31].

34.4.2.2 Resection of Neuroblastoma

A cooperative trial conducted by the CCG and POG is currently under way to investigate the effect of MIS on neuroblastoma resection. After initial induction chemotherapy, which improves the resectability of the tumor, resection of the primary tumor is undertaken. Because neuroblastomas are infiltrative by nature, they are often not suitable for laparoscopic resection. However, laparoscopic adrenalectomy has been studied for the treatment of small, localized, well-encapsulated adrenal tumors and has been shown to be safe and effective [32–39]. In addition, adrenalectomy for other indications is particularly well suited for a laparoscopic approach because of the relatively small size of the adrenal gland and the associated morbidity of an open approach. Therefore, when considering minimally invasive resection, the patient must undergo a thorough preoperative work-up to properly evaluate the tumor's extent and its size relative to the patient. The surgeon's experience with MIS is also an important factor. Although both transperitoneal and retroperitoneal approaches have been described, the lateral transperitoneal approach offers a more efficient working space and excellent exposure, and therefore has been advocated by many as the preferred approach.

34.4.2.3 Surgical Technique

The transperitoneal approach to laparoscopic adrenalectomy involves placing the patient in 45° lateral decubitus position. Children with bilateral lesions are placed supine. An infraumbilical 5- or 10-mm port is inserted for the 30° or 45° laparoscope and two 3.5- or 5-mm working ports are used, one in the iliac fossa above and medial to the iliac crest and the other placed midway between the umbilicus and the xyphoid process, just off the midline. For bilateral lesions an additional port is added in the ipsilateral iliac fossa. In addition, 5-mm sealing devices such as ultrasonic shears or Ligasure™ are helpful to mobilize tissue and dissect the retroperitoneum. Large blood vessels, such as the inferior vena cava and renal vessels, are mobilized by blunt dissection. For left-sided lesions, the colon, spleen, and tail of the pancreas are mobilized. For right-sided lesions, the liver is elevated and the posterior peritoneum is incised over the gland itself. The adrenal vessels are divided between clips. The specimen is then placed in an endoscopic specimen bag and removed through one of the ports. Additional lymphadenectomy or sampling of the lymph nodes, especially for para-aortic and para-renal lymphadenopathy, may be performed simultaneously. This is a minimum requirement of the International Neuroblastoma Staging System (INSS) for precise staging of abdominal neuroblastoma [40]. MIS has been shown to reduce the time to begin postoperative feeding, the time to begin postoperative chemotherapy, the length of hospital stay, and the estimated blood lost during surgery [39].

Another area where MIS is being applied to the treatment of neuroblastoma is a combination of endoscopy and stereotactic radiosurgery for the treatment of olfactory neuroblastoma, which has offered significant benefits [41]. In addition to less invasive surgical procedures to evaluate and treat neuroblastoma, experimental techniques have been developed, attempting to improve survival in high-risk patients and improve the treatment of all patients with fewer side effects. For example, radioactive metha-ido-benzo-guanidine (MIBG) is being used to deliver treatments specifically targeting neuroblastoma cells, avoiding toxicity to surrounding tissues.

34.4.3 Hepatoblastoma

34.4.3.1 Biopsy of Hepatoblastoma

Work-up for a liver mass in a pediatric patient starts with early tissue diagnosis. In these patients, a needle or laparoscopic biopsy is an acceptable method to obtain tissue. In the laparoscopic approach, a core needle is used to obtain tissue. Hemostasis can usually be obtained by cauterizing the entry site of the needle into the tumor. Typically two or three biopsies should be performed. Some suggest a wedge biopsy of the liver edge but the outer capsule may not be representative of the entire tumor so this should be done in conjunction with a core biopsy. The technique of wedge biopsy has been debated. Most recommend against a heated biopsy using cautery as it may distort the architecture and denature tumor RNA [31].

34.4.3.2 Biopsy – Technique

Usually a tumor biopsy can be performed with one 5-mm port at the umbilicus for a 5-mm 30° laparoscope and another port used for cautery. The second port is usually on the opposite side of the tumor. The core needle can be placed through a third tiny stab incision or can be exchanged with the laparoscopic cautery if no trocar is used.

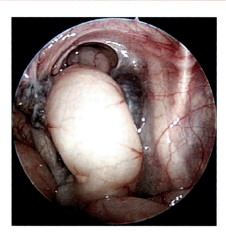

Fig. 34.4 Intra-abdominal sacro-coccygeal teratoma

34.4.4 Sacro-coccygeal Teratoma

Sacro-coccygeal teratoma (SCT) is the most common solid tumor in neonates. Most of these tumors can be removed completely from a posterior-sagittal approach without entering the peritoneal cavity. However, many have discovered the utility of laparoscopy for certain SCTs (Fig. 34.4). Lukish et al. reported laparoscopic division of the median sacral artery prior to posterior-sagittal excision to minimize the chance of bleeding in highly vascular tumors [42].

Minimally invasive approaches to sacro-coccygeal tumors, necessitating ligation of this artery as well as improved access to the presacral area, have been studied in the literature and have demonstrated improved functional results [42, 43]. In highly vascularized lesions, distal control of the aorta allows for temporary vascular occlusion if bleeding occurs. Another role of laparoscopy is to aid in pelvic dissection for those SCTs with a large pre-sacral or pelvic component. This has been shown to be a safe and effective approach as it provides excellent visualization of the tumor and surrounding structures [43, 44].

34.4.5 Ovarian Mass

34.4.5.1 Indications for Management of Ovarian Tumors

Laparoscopy has been widely used in the management of ovarian lesions in children, adolescents, and adults [45–47]. The current recommendations from the Children's Oncology Group (COG) for surgical staging and management of ovarian tumors are [45]

- Intact removal of tumor without violation of the tumor in situ
- Sparing of the fallopian tube if not adherent
- Obtaining ascites for cytology
- Examination and palpation of the omentum with removal of any abnormal areas
- Examination and palpation of the iliac and aorto-caval nodes with biopsy of abnormal areas

Controversy exists in performing a surgical oncology procedure with MIS techniques when the tumor's histology (benign vs malignant) is unknown. In addition, the preoperative work-up does not reliably reveal whether the lesion is benign or malignant and, thus, it is recommended that all ovarian tumors be treated as if malignancy were present. If the lesion is primarily solid or if the serum markers are elevated, an open procedure is indicated. If, however, the serum markers are normal and the lesion is primarily cystic, MIS techniques can be employed in combination with principles of oncologic surgery, taking care to avoid tumor spill. Up to 57% of malignant ovarian tumors have a cystic component.

34.4.5.2 Laparoscopic Access to an Ovarian Cyst

One such minimally invasive technique is laparoscopically excising the tumor from its attachments, placing it in a retrieval bag, and delivering the bag through the umbilical opening. This avoids tumor spill. The cyst is then punctured, the fluid is removed, and the lesion (within the bag) is sent for pathologic examination. In a second technique, used more for large cysts, the cyst is exposed through a 5-cm Pfannenstiel incision, followed by peritoneal washings. The mass is identified and brought up to the incision. A segment of the mass is dried with a lap tape. Dermabond™ (Ethicon, Johnson & Johnson, New Jersey) is applied to an area of the capsule (measuring 3 × 3 cm) and to a sterile ultrasound bag. The bag is then applied directly to the exposed capsule. BioGlue™ (Cryolife Inc., Kennesaw, GA) is then injected into and around the bag/mass interface and allowed to solidify. A Veress needle decompresses the cyst, avoiding tumor spill, and the ovary is delivered out of the peritoneal cavity for either cystectomy or an oophorectomy. Routine surveillance of the omentum, ascites/peritoneal fluid, lymph nodes, contralateral ovary, and peritoneal surface is then performed laparoscopically [45]. This approach markedly reduces the length of the surgical incision while ensuring prevention of peritoneal contamination with cystic fluid. One limitation of the use of MIS is that palpation of the retroperitoneal lymph nodes becomes challenging. However, depending on the child's size and body habitus, a small incision may allow this to be accomplished as well and the 5-cm Pfannenstiel incision allows ample room for examination and palpation of the omentum, iliac nodes, and aorto-caval nodes with biopsy of abnormal areas.

34.5 Specific Thoracic Malignancies in Pediatric Patients

34.5.1 Video-assisted Thoracoscopy – General Remarks

With advances in endoscopic technology, thoracoscopy has become the main alternative to thoracotomy for diagnostic and therapeutic procedures in children and adults. Video-assisted thoracoscopic surgery (VATS), involving both staging and resection, has been used for tumors of the spine, within the lung parenchyma, pleural lesions, mediastinal masses, and evaluation of lymph nodes [48]. VATS has been shown to have a role in pediatric oncology as a diagnostic, staging, and therapeutic tool [49]. Since the 1990s, authors have stressed the benefits of using less invasive muscle-sparing thoracotomies and VATS which include reduced postoperative pain, shorter recovery time, decreased postoperative infection, more immediate postoperative chemo-radiotherapy, and prevention of atrophy and fibrosis secondary to muscle splitting [50, 51]. These techniques also offer a shorter duration of chest tube drainage and postoperative hospital stay, a low morbidity and mortality, and a low conversion rate to open thoracotomy. Even in cases when a tumor is deemed too extensive for thoracoscopic resection and conversion to an open procedure is required, the initial survey can allow for tissue biopsy of the mass and help determine the best open surgical approach to utilize. Rothenberg et al. have reported the safety and efficacy of thoracoscopic resection of mediastinal masses and VATS lobectomy even in infants and children [52, 53]. Koizumi et al. demonstrated the effectiveness of VATS in children less than 6 years of age [54].

34.5.2 Lung Tumors

34.5.2.1 Indications for Biopsy and Metastasectomy

Although primary lung tumors can develop in children, the most common indication for lung resection or biopsy is for metastatic lesions. Excisional biopsy of these tumors can be both diagnostic and therapeutic (Fig. 34.5). A study by Kayton examined the historical development of pediatric pulmonary metastasectomy and described three distinct groups of pulmonary metastasis [55]:

1. Surgical metastasectomy *mandated* for patient survival
   - Adreno-cortical carcinoma
   - Osteosarcoma

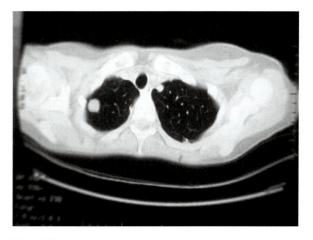

Fig. 34.5 CT scan of patient with pulmonary metastatic osteosarcoma

2. Metastasectomy is *controversial* because tumor is radiation-sensitive
   - Wilms' tumor
   - Ewing's sarcoma
3. Metastasectomy is *rarely performed* except in highly unusual situations
   - Neuroblastoma
   - Differentiated thyroid cancer
   - Rhabdomyosarcoma

One benefit of thoracoscopy is the ability to perform small incisions in immune-compromised children with new lung lesions. Children being treated with chemotherapy will often develop fungal lesions in the lung. Unfortunately, it is difficult to distinguish whether these lesions are infectious, metastases, or new primary lung tumors. Thoracoscopy provides a minimally invasive way to make this diagnosis and to clear these doubts.

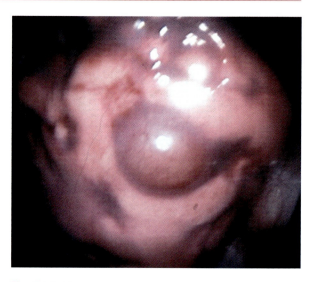

Fig. 34.6 Thoracoscopic resection of lung metastases: osteosarcoma

34.5.2.2 Sub-centimeter Pulmonary Lesion

Unfortunately, for lesions smaller than 1 cm and not peripheral, it may be difficult to identify the lesion thoracoscopically. Several techniques have been developed for these patients. Some utilize intraoperative ultrasound to help identify the lesion, but this is operator-dependent [56]. Others describe labeling the lesion preoperatively with radiographic assistance. For example, the lesion can be identified on CT and a wire can be placed into the tumor, similar to the technique used for breast biopsies. Alternatively, the visceral pleura overlying the lesion can be injected with either methylene blue or a blood patch using CT guidance prior to the operation. [57, 58] Finally, for certain tumors, a core needle biopsy may be sufficient and a CT-guided biopsy may be a better approach.

34.5.2.3 Pulmonary Metastasectomy for Osteosarcoma

A recent topic of debate is the role of thoracoscopy for pulmonary metastasectomy for osteosarcoma. The debate rises from the studies that demonstrate clinical benefit from complete bilateral metastasectomy in patients with osteosarcoma [59]. However, these studies were predicated on a thoracotomy in which the lesions could be identified by both visual and tactile inspection. Some have recently described the use of thoracoscopy to remove these lesions. However, this technique is limited in that only those lesions which can be seen can be removed. Advocates of the MIS approach note that the benefit of removal of small palpable lesions has not been shown [50]. These surgeons recommend that regular surveillance CTs will pick up new lesions which can be treated with repeat VATS and suggest that repeat VATS is a better option than bilateral thoracotomy (Fig. 34.6).

34.5.2.4 Surgical Technique – Thoracoscopic Biopsy

Thoracoscopic biopsy of lung infiltrates can safely be performed in intubated, critically ill children [23]. The standard technique in an adult or big child is placement of one 5-mm port for the scope, one 5-mm port for the grasper, and one 12-mm port for the endostapler. However, in small children, there is little room to deploy the stapler so an alternative approach can be used in which a small segment of lung to be biopsied is encircled by a loop ligature, an adequate specimen is obtained by cutting away the tissue distal to the loop ligature, and the tissue is removed through one of the trocar sites. This technique has been shown to be safe and effective [60]. Recently, this author performed this technique using a single-site approach with an operative laparoscope. Some advocate the use of sealing energy sources, which coagulates and seals the lung tissue [61]. Pulmonary resections are performed similarly. The lungs are freed using sealing energy sources, the bronchus and major vessels are stapled, and the resected lobe is removed through an enlarged trocar site. Numerous studies have confirmed the viability of using thoracoscopy in the evaluation and diagnosis as well as the resection of pediatric malignancy [48, 51, 62–64].

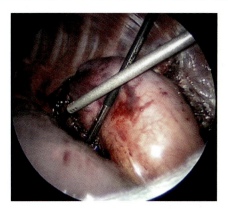

Fig. 34.8 Thoracoscopic excision of a thoracic ganglioneuroma

34.5.3 Mediastinal Tumors

Thoracoscopy is often utilized for diagnosis and treatment of mediastinal masses. Anterior mediastinal masses, such as a lymphoma, can be biopsied thoracoscopically (Fig. 34.7). However, caution should be taken to avoid general anesthesia in any patient with a compressive anterior mediastinal mass.

34.5.3.1 Neuroblastoma

Thoracic neuroblastoma typically presents as a posterior mediastinal mass. Thoracoscopy has been utilized for these tumors for both biopsy and resection. In patients with apparent unresectability, VATS biopsy has been shown to be safe and effective in the evaluation and resection of mediastinal masses [65] (Fig. 34.8). Thoracoscopic resection of neurogenic tumors has demonstrated equivalent local control and disease-free survival, accompanied by shorter hospital stays, when compared with an open resection [66]. Although thoracoscopic resection of neurogenic tumors has become the preferred approach in adults, some have been hesitant to apply it in children due to concerns of higher incidence of malignancy and the larger size of these tumors in children. Studies have demonstrated, however, that malignancy is not a contraindication to thoracoscopic resection [66, 67]. Thoracic neuroblastomas are generally less aggressive than those arising below the diaphragm and are associated with a better prognosis. The rate of tumor recurrence is similar to the open approach and tumor size does not preclude the use of thoracoscopy. Although port-site incisions may need to be extended to remove the tumor, they can be extended to the smallest degree necessary to accommodate the specimen and this does not require a long period of rib retraction. In fact, a survey of pediatric surgical oncology and minimally invasive experts showed thoracoscopic resection of neurogenic tumors to be the best suited application of MIS in pediatric malignancies [68]. Several studies have found no survival difference in patients treated with thoracoscopy compared to thoracotomy and attribute the success of the MIS approach to superior visualization. Petty et al. noted that the VATS group had faster recovery and earlier return to school [17, 67, 68].

One attribute of thoracic neuroblastoma that makes it amenable to thoracoscopy is that complete resection with negative margins may not be necessary to improve survival. This particular tumor's prognosis is based more upon the tumor histology and n-myc oncogene expression.

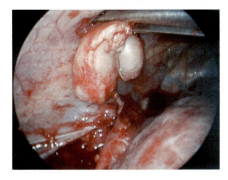

Fig. 34.7 Anterior mediastinal lymph node: Hodgkin's disease

34.5.3.2 Biopsy and Resection Technique

As mentioned above, the ipsilateral lung is collapsed using single-lung ventilation, bronchial blockade, or positive pressure insufflation. The patient is positioned in the lateral decubitus position and rotated partially prone to improve exposure to the mediastinum. Three or four 5-mm ports are used. The tumor is mobilized using a combination of blunt dissection and electrocautery, and once the tumor is free, it is placed in an endoscopic specimen bag and removed through an enlarged port site.

34.6 Future Trends

While most pediatric surgeons resist the idea of utilizing thoracoscopy and laparoscopy in the management of childhood tumors, it is difficult to imagine wide acceptance of future trends. However, many are discussing new, less invasive options for certain patients. The use of Cyberknife has been gaining popularity for certain adult tumors [69]. The fact that Cyberknife may be showing promise for certain adult renal masses makes this technology intriguing for Wilms' tumor as well. Other applications may be for hepatoblastoma, neuroblastoma, or even anterior mediastinal masses such as lymphoma.

Another exciting trend is toward single-site surgery. With new trocars, instruments, and scopes, surgeons are beginning to perform complex operations through a single laparoscopic incision. It is certainly feasible that tumor biopsies can be performed utilizing this technique. In fact, the authors have recently performed a single-site lung biopsy in a child with suspected lung metastases without complication.

34.7 Conclusion

Pediatric surgery as its own specialty is still in its infancy. Techniques and principles are still in evolution. MIS evolved in the adult population decades before it was utilized in children. This is mostly due to the lack of adequate instrumentation. As technology has been adapted for smaller patients, MIS in children has advanced. Appropriately so, any new technique is met with speculation and caution, especially when dealing with cancer in children. However, as more studies emerge, demonstrating the safety and efficacy of MIS for pediatric tumors, this technology will hopefully become accepted as the standard of care.

Quick Reference Guide

1. **Identify goals of procedure:**
   - Is it diagnostic?
   - Is it therapeutic?
2. **Thoracic procedures:**
   - Position the patient to maximize the exposure of the pathology.
     - Prone position: for posterior mediastinal tumors.
     - Supine position: for anterior masses.
   - Obtain single-lung ventilation if possible to aid in exposure.
   - For parenchymal lesions (metastases) less than 1 cm in diameter and not near the pleura consider a CT localization procedure.
3. **Indications for resections of lung metastasis:**
   - Surgical metastasectomy *mandated* for patient survival.
     - Adreno-cortical carcinoma.
     - Osteosarcoma.
   - Metastasectomy is *controversial* because tumor is radiation-sensitive.
     - Wilms' tumor.
     - Ewing's sarcoma.
   - Metastasectomy is *rarely performed* except in highly unusual situations.
     - Neuroblastoma.
     - Differentiated thyroid cancer.
     - Rhabdomyosarcoma.
4. **Abdominal procedures:**
   - Position the patient appropriately to aid with exposure.
   - For renal or adrenal masses consider placing the patient in a modified lateral decubitus position.
5. Ovarian tumor: if preoperative work-up can't distinguish between benign and malignant, then treat the mass as though you were dealing with cancer.

6. Follow basic oncological surgical principles at all times.
7. Place all specimens in an endoscopic retrieval bag if there is any suspicion that they are malignant. Dragging a specimen through a trocar site causes port-site recurrences.
8. While doing a resective procedure place clips to mark the operative field if postoperative radiation therapy is a consideration.
9. Don't compromise technique or patient outcomes. If you are not sure, then convert to an open procedure.
10. Management of a pediatric cancer patient follows the same multidisciplinary rules applied to the adult population.

References

1. Gans, S.L.: A new look at pediatric endoscopy. Postgrad. Med. **61**(4), 91–100 (1977)
2. Gans, S.L., Berci, G.: Advances in endoscopy of infants and children. J. Pediatr. Surg. **6**(2), 199–233 (1971)
3. Gans, S.L., Berci, G.: Peritoneoscopy in infants and children. J. Pediatr. Surg. **8**(3), 399–405 (1973)
4. Ryckman, F.C., Rodgers, B.M.: Thoracoscopy for intrathoracic neoplasia in children. J. Pediatr. Surg. **17**(5), 521–524 (1982)
5. Rodgers, B.M., et al.: Thoracoscopy for intrathoracic tumors. Ann. Thorac. Surg. **31**(5), 414–420 (1981)
6. Spurbeck, W.W., et al.: Minimally invasive surgery in pediatric cancer patients. Ann. Surg. Oncol. **11**(3), 340–343 (2004)
7. Guye, E., et al.: Thoracoscopy and solid tumors in children: a multicenter study. J. Laparoendosc. Adv. Surg. Tech. A **17**(6), 825–829 (2007)
8. Sartorelli, K.H., Partrick, D., Meagher Jr., D.P.: Port-site recurrence after thoracoscopic resection of pulmonary metastasis owing to osteogenic sarcoma. J. Pediatr. Surg. **31**(10), 1443–1444 (1996)
9. Cribbs, R.K., et al.: Minimally invasive surgery and childhood cancer. Surg. Oncol. **16**(3), 221–228 (2007)
10. Metzelder, M.L., et al.: Role of diagnostic and ablative minimally invasive surgery for pediatric malignancies. Cancer **109**(11), 2343–2348 (2007)
11. Holcomb 3rd, G.W., et al.: Minimally invasive surgery in children with cancer. Cancer **76**(1), 121–128 (1995)
12. Esposito, C., et al.: Thoracoscopic surgery in the management of pediatric malignancies: a multicentric survey of the Italian society of videosurgery in infancy. Surg. Endosc. **21**(10), 1772–1775 (2007)
13. Iwanaka, T., et al.: Endosurgical procedures for pediatric solid tumors. Pediatr. Surg. Int. **20**(1), 39–42 (2004)
14. Sailhamer, E., et al.: Minimally invasive surgery for pediatric solid neoplasms. Am. Surg. **69**(7), 566–568 (2003)
15. Leclair, M.D., et al.: Minimally-invasive surgery in cancer children. Bull. Cancer **94**(12), 1087–1090 (2007)
16. Leclair, M.D., et al.: Laparoscopic resection of abdominal neuroblastoma. Ann. Surg. Oncol. **15**(1), 117–124 (2008)
17. Lacreuse, I., et al.: Thoracoscopic resection of neurogenic tumors in children. J. Pediatr. Surg. **42**(10), 1725–1728 (2007)
18. Dutta, S., et al.: Laparoscopic resection of a benign liver tumor in a child. J. Pediatr. Surg. **42**(6), 1141–1145 (2007)
19. Till, H., et al.: Tumor model for laparoscopy in pediatric oncology: subperitoneal inoculation of human hepatoblastoma cells in nude rats. Eur. J. Pediatr. Surg. **16**(4), 231–234 (2006)
20. Yeung, C.K., et al.: Atypical laparoscopic resection of a liver tumor in a 4-year-old girl. J. Laparoendosc. Adv. Surg. Tech. A **16**(3), 325–327 (2006)
21. Till, H., et al.: Laparoscopic fluorescence diagnosis of peritoneal metastases from human hepatoblastoma in nude rats. J. Pediatr. Surg. **41**(8), 1357–1360 (2006)
22. Komuro, H., Makino, S., Tahara, K.: Laparoscopic resection of an adrenal neuroblastoma detected by mass screening that grew in size during the observation period. Surg. Endosc. **14**(3), 297 (2000)
23. Perer, E., et al.: Laparoscopic removal of extraosseous Ewing's sarcoma of the kidney in a pediatric patient. J. Laparoendosc. Adv. Surg. Tech. A **16**(1), 74–76 (2006)
24. Solomon, L.A., Zurawin, R.K., Edwards, C.L.: Vaginoscopic resection for rhabdomyosarcoma of the vagina: a case report and review of the literature. J. Pediatr. Adolesc. Gynecol. **16**(3), 139–142 (2003)
25. Stankovic, Z.B., et al.: Minimal invasive treatment of cervical rhabdomyosarcoma in an adolescent girl. J. BUON **12**(1), 121–123 (2007)
26. Harrell, W.B., Snow, B.W.: Minimally invasive pediatric nephrectomy. Curr. Opin. Urol. **15**(4), 277–281 (2005)
27. Tolley, D.A., Esposito, M.P.: Laparoscopic and renal sparing approaches to tumours of the ureter and kidney. Surg. Oncol. **11**(1–2), 47–54 (2002)
28. Gill, I.S., et al.: Laparoscopic radical nephrectomy in 100 patients: a single center experience from the United States. Cancer **92**(7), 1843–1855 (2001)
29. Duarte, R.J., et al.: Further experience with laparoscopic nephrectomy for Wilms' tumour after chemotherapy. BJU Int. **98**(1), 155–159 (2006)
30. Ganick, D.J., et al.: Clinical utility of fine needle aspiration in the diagnosis and management of neuroblastoma. Med. Pediatr. Oncol. **16**(2), 101–106 (1988)
31. Ridaura-Sanz, C., Asz-Sigall, J.: Histopathological changes in liver biopsy specimens obtained with ultrasonic scalpel. Histopathology **54**(2), 266–268 (2009)
32. Romano, P., et al.: Adrenal masses in children: the role of minimally invasive surgery. Surg. Laparosc. Endosc. Percutan. Tech. **17**(6), 504–507 (2007)
33. Kadamba, P., Habib, Z., Rossi, L.: Experience with laparoscopic adrenalectomy in children. J. Pediatr. Surg. **39**(5), 764–767 (2004)
34. Nassrallah, R.A., et al.: Retroperitoneal minimally invasive endoscopic adrenalectomy in children. Saudi Med. J. **24**(Suppl), S11–S14 (2003)
35. Bentas, W., et al.: Laparoscopic transperitoneal adrenalectomy using a remote-controlled robotic surgical system. J. Endourol. **16**(6), 373–376 (2002)

36. Saad, D.F., et al.: Laparoscopic adrenalectomy for neuroblastoma in children: a report of 6 cases. J. Pediatr. Surg. **40**(12), 1948–1950 (2005)
37. Castilho, L.N., et al.: Laparoscopic adrenal surgery in children. J. Urol. **168**(1), 221–224 (2002)
38. Iwanaka, T., et al.: Surgical treatment for abdominal neuroblastoma in the laparoscopic era. Surg. Endosc. **15**(7), 751–754 (2001)
39. Miller, K.A., et al.: Experience with laparoscopic adrenalectomy in pediatric patients. J. Pediatr. Surg. **37**(7), 979–982 (2002). discussion 979–982
40. Iwanaka, T., et al.: Challenges of laparoscopic resection of abdominal neuroblastoma with lymphadenectomy. A preliminary report. Surg. Endosc. **15**(5), 489–492 (2001)
41. Walch, C., et al.: The minimally invasive approach to olfactory neuroblastoma: combined endoscopic and stereotactic treatment. Laryngoscope **110**(4), 635–640 (2000)
42. Lukish, J.R., Powell, D.M.: Laparoscopic ligation of the median sacral artery before resection of a sacrococcygeal teratoma. J. Pediatr. Surg. **39**(8), 1288–1290 (2004)
43. Bax, N.M., van der Zee, D.C.: The laparoscopic approach to sacrococcygeal teratomas. Surg. Endosc. **18**(1), 128–130 (2004)
44. Chan, K.W., et al.: Minimal invasive surgery in pediatric solid tumors. J. Laparoendosc. Adv. Surg. Tech. A **17**(6), 817–820 (2007)
45. Ehrlich, P.F., et al.: Excision of large cystic ovarian tumors: combining minimal invasive surgery techniques and cancer surgery–the best of both worlds. J. Pediatr. Surg. **42**(5), 890–893 (2007)
46. Cowles, R.A., Gewanter, R.M., Kandel, J.J.: Ovarian repositioning in pediatric cancer patients: flexible techniques accommodate pelvic radiation fields. Pediatr. Blood Cancer **49**(3), 339–341 (2007)
47. Davidoff, A.M., et al.: Laparoscopic oophorectomy in children. J. Laparoendosc. Surg. **6**(Suppl 1), S115–S119 (1996)
48. Al-Sayyad, M.J., Crawford, A.H., Wolf, R.K.: Video-assisted thoracoscopic surgery: the Cincinnati experience. Clin. Orthop. Relat. Res. **434**, 61–70 (2005)
49. Gilbert, J.C., et al.: Video-assisted thoracic surgery (VATS) for children with pulmonary metastases from osteosarcoma. Ann. Surg. Oncol. **3**(6), 539–542 (1996)
50. Smith, T.J., et al.: Thoracoscopic surgery in childhood cancer. J. Pediatr. Hematol. Oncol. **24**(6), 429–435 (2002)
51. Mattioli, G., et al.: Lung resection in pediatric patients. Pediatr. Surg. Int. **13**(1), 10–13 (1998)
52. Ponsky, T.A., Rothenberg, S.S.: Minimally invasive surgery in infants less than 5 kg: experience of 649 cases. Surg. Endosc. **22**(10), 2214–2219 (2008)
53. Rothenberg, S.S., Chang, J.H., Bealer, J.F.: Experience with minimally invasive surgery in infants. Am. J. Surg. **176**(6), 654–658 (1998)
54. Koizumi, K., et al.: Thoracoscopic surgery in children. J. Nippon Med. Sch. **72**(1), 34–42 (2005)
55. Kayton, M.L.: Pulmonary metastasectomy in pediatric patients. Thorac. Surg. Clin. **16**(2), 167–183 (2006). vi
56. Santambrogio, R., et al.: Intraoperative ultrasound during thoracoscopic procedures for solitary pulmonary nodules. Ann. Thorac. Surg. **68**(1), 218–222 (1999)
57. Waldhausen, J.H., Tapper, D., Sawin, R.S.: Minimally invasive surgery and clinical decision-making for pediatric malignancy. Surg. Endosc. **14**(3), 250–253 (2000)
58. Partrick, D.A., et al.: Successful thoracoscopic lung biopsy in children utilizing preoperative CT-guided localization. J. Pediatr. Surg. **37**(7), 970–973 (2002). discussion 970–973
59. Saenz, N.C., et al.: The application of minimal access procedures in infants, children, and young adults with pediatric malignancies. J. Laparoendosc. Adv. Surg. Tech. A **7**(5), 289–294 (1997)
60. Ponsky, T.A., Rothenberg, S.S.: Thoracoscopic lung biopsy in infants and children with endoloops allows smaller trocar sites and discreet biopsies. J. Laparoendosc. Adv. Surg. Tech. A **18**(1), 120–122 (2008)
61. Georgeson, K.: Minimally invasive surgery in neonates. Semin. Neonatol. **8**(3), 243–248 (2003)
62. Lima, M., et al.: Thoracoscopic management of suspected thoraco-pulmonary malignant diseases in pediatric age. Pediatr. Med. Chir. **26**(2), 132–135 (2004)
63. Cury, E.K., et al.: Thoracoscopic esophagectomy in children. J. Pediatr. Surg. **36**(9), E17 (2001)
64. Rodgers, B.M.: Thoracoscopic procedures in children. Semin. Pediatr. Surg. **2**(3), 182–189 (1993)
65. Partrick, D.A., Rothenberg, S.S.: Thoracoscopic resection of mediastinal masses in infants and children: an evaluation of technique and results. J. Pediatr. Surg. **36**(8), 1165–1167 (2001)
66. Iwanaka, T., Kawashima, H., Uchida, H.: The laparoscopic approach of neuroblastoma. Semin. Pediatr. Surg. **16**(4), 259–265 (2007)
67. Petty, J.K., et al.: Resection of neurogenic tumors in children: is thoracoscopy superior to thoracotomy? J. Am. Coll. Surg. **203**(5), 699–703 (2006)
68. DeCou, J.M., et al.: Primary thoracoscopic gross total resection of neuroblastoma. J. Laparoendosc. Adv. Surg. Tech. A **15**(5), 470–473 (2005)
69. Ponsky, L.E., et al.: Initial evaluation of Cyberknife technology for extracorporeal renal tissue ablation. Urology **61**(3), 498–501 (2003)

Part XII

Special Topics: Lung and Mediastinum

Minimally Invasive Management of Intra-Thoracic Malignancies

Philip A. Linden

35.1 Historic Review

Since Evarts Graham first described the first successful single-stage pneumonectomy for lung cancer in 1933 there have been continual reductions in the degree of invasiveness in the field of thoracic surgery [1]. In the 1940s, lobectomy, popularized by Churchill, became an accepted treatment for lung cancer, and eventually replaced pneumonectomy as the standard treatment for resectable lung cancer. The lung cancer study group trial randomizing earliest stage lung cancers to treatment by lobectomy vs. lesser resection (segmentectomy and wedge resection), clearly showed an increase in loco regional recurrence with lesser resection, and established lobectomy as the definitive unit of resection [2]. Recent work on diminishing the "invasiveness" of lung surgery has focused not so much on the amount of parenchyma resected, but on the physiologic insult of the incision. A postero-lateral thoracotomy can decrease FVC by as much as 35% in the immediate postoperative period. Recently, propensity matched analyses have suggested that VATS lobectomy results in fewer complications than thoracotomy and lobectomy (Table 35.1). A propensity matched analysis of lobectomy patients in the national Society of Thoracic Surgery database by the same group has yielded similar results and is currently in press. The VATS approach was developed initially for simple wedge resections and pleural procedures, as a means of minimizing postoperative discomfort and speeding recovery. Although the term VATS stands for video assisted thoracic surgery, strict usage of the term VATS lobectomy dictates no rib spreading or division, no large muscle division, and a working incision about 6 cm in length. Some have adopted the term thoracoscopic lobectomy to describe a strict VATS lobectomy, reserving VATS lobectomy for any lobectomy using video as assistance, often with rib spreading. In this chapter, the term VATS lobectomy implies no rib spreading, no rib division and no large muscle division. Atraumatic instruments have been developed which minimize pressure against the ribs and sub costal nerves (Fig. 35.1).

35.2 The Lung

35.2.1 Anatomic VATS Lobectomy – The Right Lung

35.2.1.1 Right Upper Lobectomy (RUL)

The patient is placed in the left lateral decubitus position, and the operating table is flexed to maximize the working space between the ribs. A 10-mm incision is made just anterior to the anterior axillary line in approximately the seventh interspace. Although a 5-mm incision can be made if a 5-mm camera is being used, a 10-mm incision allows for the introduction of additional instruments alongside the camera, if needed. After inspection of the hemi-thorax for the absence of metastatic disease, the main access incision is made 4–6 cm in length in the anterior axillary line in approximately the fourth interspace. The subcutaneous tissues are spread using self-retaining

P.A. Linden
Department of Thoracic Surgery, Case Medical Center,
University Hospitals, Cleveland, OH 44106, USA
e-mail: philip.linden@uhhospitals.org

Table 35.1 Propensity matched comparison of complications in patients: Lobectomy via thoracotomy (THOR) vs. VATS

Complications	THOR n=284	VATS n=284	P value
Atrial fibrillation, n (%)	61 (21)	37 (13)	0.01
Atelectasis, n (%)	34 (12)	15 (5)	0.006
Prolonged air leak, n (%)	55 (19)	37 (13)	0.05
Bleeding, n (%)	3 (1)	3 (3)	
Transfusion, n (%)	36 (13)	11 (4)	0.002
Wound infection, n (%)	3 (1)	1 (0.4)	0.62
Pneumonia, n (%)	27 (10)	14 (5)	0.05
Empyema, n (%)	2 (0.8)	2 (0.8)	
Bronchopleural fistula, n (%)	3 (1)	1 (0.4)	0.62
Sepsis, n (%)	6 (2)	1 (0.4)	0.12
Renal failure, n (%)	15 (5)	4 (1.4)	0.02
CVA, n (%)	3 (1)	2 (1)	1.0
MI, n (%)	0 (0)	1 (0.4)	0.5
Ventricular arrhythmia, n (%)	2 (0.8)	2 (0.8)	
DVT, n (%)	2 (0.8)	0 (0)	0.5
PE, n (%)	3 (1)	1 (0.4)	0.62
Chest tube duration, median days (25th, 75th quartile)	4 (3.6)	3 (2.4)	0.0001[a]
Length of hospital stay, median days (25th, 75th quartile)	5 (4.7)	4 (3.6)	0.0001[a]
Death, n (%)	15 (5)	8 (3)	0.2
Patients with no complications, n (%)	144 (51)	196 (69)	0.0001

Source: Villamizar NR et al. Thoracoscopic lobectomy is associated with lower morbidity compared with thoracotomy. J Thoracic and Cardiovasc Surg 2009;138:419–425 (reprint with permission)
THOR conventional thoracotomy, *VATS* video-assisted thoracoscopic surgery, *CVA* cerebrovascular accident, *MI* myocardial infarction, *DVT* deep venous thrombosis, *PE* pulmonary embolism
[a] Wilcoxon signed-rank test

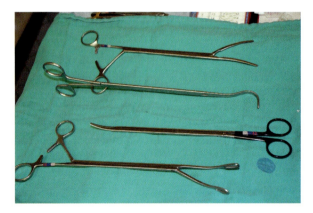

Fig. 35.1 VATS instruments. These instruments are designed with a sliding action mechanism to minimize pressure on the ribs and sub costal nerves from an opening rigid metal instrument. *From top to bottom*: VATS lung compression device, harken instruments, VATS scissors, VATS ring-endograsper

retractor. In order to minimize postoperative discomfort, no rib division, removal, or spreading is employed. An additional 10-mm incision is made in approximately the 8th to 9th interspace just posterior and well inferior to the tip of the scapula (Fig. 35.2). This low incision allows plenty of space in the hemithorax for optimal manipulation of the endoscopic stapler. Some surgeons choose not to make this posterior incision, and instead use a larger camera incision through which staplers may be introduced (2–3 cm in the mid-axillary line).

The upper lobe is pulled forward via the access incision (alternatively a fan retractor may be used), and lymph node dissection of the subcarinal space and right paratracheal space is performed. The posterior and superior aspects of the upper lobe bronchus are

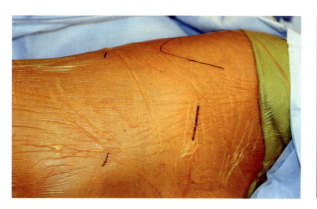

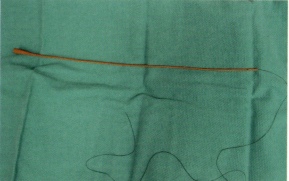

Fig. 35.2 Standard VATS lobectomy incision. The patient's right side is viewed. The patient's head is to the right and anterior is at the bottom of the picture. The tip of the scapula is outlined. Anterior to the tip of the scapula is the working port incision. Inferior to this incision is the camera port. The posterior inferior port is also seen

Fig. 35.3 Endoleader. This device consists of an 8 F red rubber catheter. A 0 silk suture has been passed through the distal side hole out the very center of the tip. Knots in the suture have been made and are then slid into the tip of the red rubber catheter to secure the silk leader

dissected at the same time. Frozen section of the nodes and of the wedge resection of the nodule, if needed, is performed. The lobe is then retracted posterior and dissection of the hilum is performed. The pleura overlying the hilum is incised. The superior pulmonary vein is inspected and dissection begins between the upper lobe vein and middle lobe vein. The loose tissue superficial to the right main pulmonary artery is incised and the superior border of the upper lobe vein is dissected off the main and ongoing pulmonary artery. A large, curved, blunt clamp is used to dissect posterior to the upper lobe vein, taking care not to injure either the ongoing pulmonary artery or any deep venous branches. The endovascular stapler is introduced through the posterior port and may be passed directly around the upper lobe vein if enough dissection has been performed. Alternatively, a red rubber catheter can be passed behind the vein and the narrow tip of the endovascular stapler can be placed in the wide mouth of the red rubber and guided behind the vein (Figs. 35.3 and 35.4). The vein is divided (Fig. 35.5). A sponge on a stick is immediately available to tamponade bleeding if dissection or division of a vascular structure results in bleeding.

Sharp dissection using blunt tipped scissors is then performed on the main pulmonary artery, locating the truncus anterior branch to the right upper lobe. Superiorly and posterior, the truncus anterior is dissected from the bronchus. The stapler is introduced via the posterior port site and guided around the artery in a fashion identical to that used for the upper lobe vein.

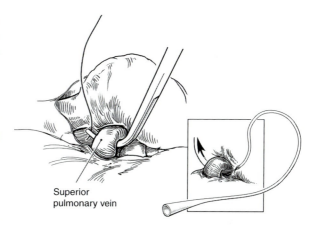

Fig. 35.4 The endoleader mechanism provides an atraumatic means of dilating the tracts behind pulmonary vessels and drawing the stapler around the vessels. In order to reverse the direction of the endoleader, an 0 silk can be passed in the opposite direction and tied to the suture of the endoleader

Further dissection is performed along the ongoing pulmonary artery, identifying and preserving the middle lobe artery, and identifying the smaller ascending branch to the posterior segment of the right upper lobe (also termed the "recurrent" branch) (Fig. 35.6). Occasionally, this branch is absent or arises from the artery to the superior segment of the lower lobe. Division of the minor fissure may allow for better access to this artery. The artery is divided using an endovascular stapler introduced through the posterior port. Further divisions of the minor and major fissures are performed, with care to preserve the ongoing pulmonary artery and the middle lobe

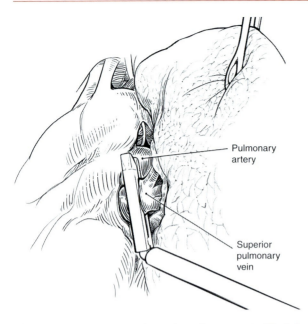

Fig. 35.5 Division of the left superior pulmonary vein. The left superior pulmonary vein has been dissected away from the left main pulmonary artery and is divided with a stapler passed through the inferior, posterior, port

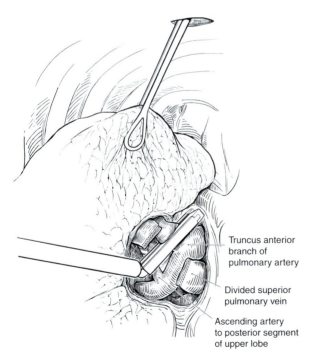

Fig. 35.6 Division of the right truncus anterior artery. The truncus anterior artery to the right upper lobe is divided with an endovascular stapler passed through the inferior, posterior port

arterial branch. After division of the ascending artery to the posterior segment of the right upper lobe, the upper lobe bronchus should be visible. The base of the bronchus is dissected free, sweeping all lymph nodes up on to the specimen. Real-time endo-bronchial visualization with an endoscopic pediatric bronchoscope is useful as the thick tissue stapler is used to close the base of the upper lobe bronchus. If there is any doubt in regard to placement of the stapler, insufflation of the middle and lower lobes is performed to assure patency of these lobar bronchi. The bronchus is divided with the stapler as well the remainder of the major fissure. Any visible bronchial arteries should be clipped. A large endoscopic bag or "lap-sac" is used to collect and remove the specimen. Frozen section margins are checked as indicated, and the inferior pulmonary ligament is lysed with cautery. A single 28 French straight chest tube with an additional hole cut at around the 12–14-cm mark is introduced through the camera port and threaded posterior to the apex of the chest. The lower and middle lobes are fully reinflated under direct vision in order to insure that the middle lobe has not torsed. The remaining two incisions are closed using two deep layers of 2-0 Vicryl and a subcuticular skin layer.

35.2.1.2 Right Middle Lobectomy (RML)

The incision is the same as that used for the upper lobectomy except that the access port is in the fifth interspace and is smaller and slightly more posterior. Dissection begins over the superior pulmonary vein. The middle lobe vein is identified and divided using an endovascular stapler. In 5–10% of patients. the middle lobe vein drains into the inferior pulmonary vein. Dissection in the minor fissure is performed using a combination of cautery and sharp dissection, and the middle lobe artery or arteries (occasionally there are two) are identified. The middle lobe artery is divided using an endovascular stapler introduced through the posterior port. The bronchus to the middle lobe travels deep and medial to the artery. After division of the artery, medial dissection will reveal the bronchus which is stapled. The fissures are completed with a stapler delivered through the posterior and anterior working port. A single chest tube is placed, the lung is inflated, and the ports are closed.

35.2.1.3 Right Lower Lobectomy (RLL)

The 6-cm access incision is made in the fifth interspace overlying the fissure in the mid-to-anterior axillary line. After inspection of the hemi thorax to rule out metastatic disease, a subcarinal and right paratracheal lymph node dissection are performed, if mediastinoscopy has not previously been performed. After ruling out N2 nodal disease, the lower lobe is retracted superiorly, and the inferior pulmonary ligament is lysed with cautery introduced through the posterior port. The inferior pulmonary vein is visualized and is dissected free. The posterior pleural reflection is dissected up to the bronchus intermedius. After ensuring that the middle lobe vein does not drain into the inferior lobe vein, a blunt angled clamp is used to encircle the vein and it is divided with an endovascular stapler (Fig. 35.7). While the lower lobe is retracted superiorly, dissection deep into the vein reveals the posterior surfaces of the bronchus intermedius and lower lobe bronchi. I prefer not to divide the lower lobe bronchi at this point until the pulmonary artery is dissected through the fissure. The lower lobe is allowed to return to its anatomic position, and the fissure is dissected using cautery. As one nears the pulmonary artery, cautery is replaced by sharp dissection. The lower lobe superior segmental artery, basilar trunk artery, and middle lobe artery are dissected free. The superior segmental artery and basilar trunk arteries are generally divided separately using an endovascular stapler delivered through either the posterior or anterior port. Deep to the artery, the lower lobe bronchus is visualized. Medial to the lower lobe bronchus lays the anterior aspect of the major fissure, and this can be divided using an endoscopic stapler. This aids in exposure of the lower lobe bronchi. After sweeping nodes onto the lower lobe specimen, the lower lobe bronchus can be taken as one unit. If so, the middle lobe should be inflated after clamping, but before division. If there is any question about impingement of the middle lobe bronchus, then the superior segmental bronchus and basilar trunk bronchus should be taken separately. After division of the bronchus, the posterior aspect of the fissure is taken using a stapler delivered through the anterior port. The specimen is placed in a bag prior to removal. The right lower lobe is the largest lobe, and occasionally the incision needs to be enlarged in order to facilitate removal. A single chest tube to the apex, with an additional basilar hole may be used.

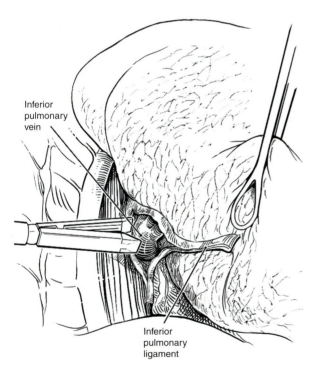

Fig. 35.7 Division of the right inferior pulmonary vein. The inferior pulmonary ligament has been divided with cautery, and the vein has been dissected free. The lower lobe is elevated and the vein is divided with an endovascular stapler passed either through the posterior port (as shown) or through the anterior port

35.2.2 Anatomic VATS Lobectomy – The Left Lung

35.2.2.1 Left Upper Lobectomy (LUL)

The patient is placed in the right lateral decubitus position. The camera is introduced via a 10-mm incision placed in approximately the seventh interspace, anterior axillary line. A working incision, 4–6 cm in length is placed in the fourth interspace overlying the main pulmonary artery and superior pulmonary vein. A 10-mm incision is made just posterior to the scapula, in approximately the 8th–9th interspace at the level where the inferior edge of the lung contacts the diaphragm. The lung is retracted posterior. Virtually all of the dissection is via the access incision. Level 5 (AP window) and level 6 (periaortic) nodes are harvested using sharp and cautery dissection and sent for frozen section. Neoadjuvant chemo-radiation can be considered if either returns positive. Dissection begins at the superior pulmonary vein. At the superior edge of the vein, the vein is dissected free of the main pulmonary artery using a combination of sharp and blunt dissection. Sharp dissection of the main pulmonary artery assists with this portion of the dissection. While dissecting the lower edge of the superior pulmonary vein, the inferior pulmonary vein should be visualized. A blunt angled dissector is alternately introduced from above and below the vein. Dissection from above is safest as the pulmonary artery can be directly visualized. An endoleader is passed from inferior to superior, and an endovascular stapler is introduced and fired (Fig. 35.8). Posterior to the vein, and inferior to the main artery, and anterior to the lingular branches, the bronchus can be seen after dissection of lymph nodes. Sharp dissection of one or two of the first few branches of the pulmonary artery, if accessible, (anterior branches) can be performed prior to dissection of the upper lobe bronchus. Use of the "endoleader" red rubber catheter to guide the endovascular stapler (inserted through the posterior incision) is very helpful with these delicate and large branches. The upper lobe bronchus is then dissected sharply. Posterior to the bronchus lie the lingular branches of the pulmonary artery. The inferior and superior aspect of the bronchus should be dissected first. With anterior traction on the blunt angled dissecting instrument, the bronchus is encircled, taking care not to disturb the lingular arteries. The endoleader guides the tip of the endoscopic stapler around the bronchus, leaving the lingular arterial branches undisturbed. Care must be taken that the left main bronchus has not been encircled, as it is easy to do this with the long left main bronchus. After clamping, but prior to division of the bronchus, the lower lobe should be insufflated (or inspected via pediatric video bronchoscope) to insure patency. After division of the bronchus, the lingular branches and any remaining upper lobe branches are divided with care to preserve the artery to the superior segment of the lower lobe. The fissure may now be divided via a stapler introduced either through the posterior port or anterior camera port. Flipping the upper lobe posterior and then anterior as the stapler is place around the fissure will help avoid injury to the first branch of the lower lobe (superior segmental artery). After completion of the fissure, the lobe is placed in a bag and removed. The inferior ligament is lysed with cautery and a single chest tube is placed.

35.2.2.2 Left Lower Lobectomy (LLL)

Patient positioning and port placement are identical to that described for a left upper lobectomy except the working port is typically in the fifth interspace. The inferior ligament is lysed with cautery and the inferior pulmonary vein is dissected free after lysing the posterior pleural reflection. The superior pulmonary vein is visualized and preserved. The inferior vein is divided with an endovascular stapler introduced via either the working port or posterior port. The lower lobe bronchus is dissected from its inferior aspect as the lower lobe is retracted superiorly. At this point, either the lower lobe bronchus can be completely dissected, with care not to injure adjacent pulmonary arterial branches. Alternatively, the lower lobe arterial branches can be dissected through the fissure. Dissection is begun at the anterior aspect of the fissure with cautery. The most distal lingular branch is typically first encountered. This is followed

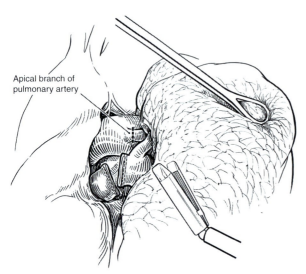

Fig. 35.8 Division of the apical branch of left superior pulmonary artery. The superior pulmonary vein has already been divided. The apical branch of the left upper lobe (the first branch) often can be divided prior to division of the right superior pulmonary vein. It is divided using an endovascular stapler passed through the posterior, inferior port. The stapler is angled superiorly

to the ongoing pulmonary artery and the basilar trunk artery is found and dissected. This artery is divided with an endovascular stapler introduced through the inferior anterior (camera) port. After division of the basilar trunk, the artery to the superior segment of the lower lobe is dissected free and divided with an endovascular stapler. The remaining portion of the fissure is divided with an endoscopic stapler and the specimen is removed in an endoscopic bag.

35.2.3 Nonanatomic Resection – The Wedge

Wedge resection of a tumor and a small rim of normal surrounding lung is the method employed for

- Excisional biopsy
- Definitive treatment of cancer metastatic to the lung
- Compromise resection in the high-risk lung cancer patient

Wedge resection has been shown to carry a three-fold increase in loco-regional recurrence over lobectomy, and possibly result in reduced long-term survival [2]. In general, lesions that are larger than 3 cm, and certainly tumors larger than 5 cm, are usually better managed by lobectomy. The likelihood of local recurrence after wedge resection is not well understood. Based on a small number of patients, Sawabata et al. have recommended that an after stapling margin of at least two centimeters, or a margin greater than that of maximal tumor diameter, be obtained. Of the patients with at least 2 cm margins, 0/7 had microscopic disease detected [3]. As CT scanning has become more prevalent, many cancers are being discovered at very small sizes. Some have proposed that limited resection (either wedge or segmentectomy) may be the preferred operation for such small lesions. CALGB 140503 is currently enrolling patients and randomizes patients with tumors less than 2 cm in diameter to either lobectomy or limited resection.

There is no data to support the use of adjuvant external beam radiation with any negative margin, no matter how small. The use of brachytherapy seeds placed at the time of wedge resection and its effect on loco-regional recurrence is currently being studied by a multi-institutional ACASOG trial.

35.2.3.1 Technique of Wedge Resection

Typically three 10-mm ports are employed. The camera is placed in the 7th interspace between the posterior and anterior axillary line, depending on the position of the tumor. A posterior port is placed inferior to the tip of the scapula, and an anterior port is placed high in the axilla, 3rd interspace for apical or posterior apical lesions, 4th to 6th interspace for lower lesions. The tumor is typically palpated through the anterior port, as the interspaces posterior (especially in a small person) are typically too small to introduce a finger. After palpation of the tumor, an approach is chosen that will, ideally, yield margins equal to the diameter of the tumor.

If the tumor is immediately adjacent to the pleural surface, a crushing clamp can be placed along the anticipated path of the stapler, followed by application of a regular tissue stapler in succession. The specimen is placed in a bag and removed. Care must be taken not to crush a small or soft lesion, as it may be impossible to locate the lesions after it is crushed. If the tumor is not adjacent to the pleural surface, but is near a fissure, then a stapler applied first through the fissure toward the deep margin of the tumor is often the best strategy. A clinical margin equal to the diameter of the tumor is optimal, best obtained by placing the stapler a safe distance away from the tumor. Smaller margins are usually obtained simply by the action of the solid edge of the stapler closing against a firm tumor. As the stapler closes, the tumor is naturally displaced away from the stapled edge. Frozen section of the margins should be obtained whenever the margin is not equal to or greater than the diameter of the tumor.

35.2.3.2 Single Incision Wedge Resection, "UNIVATS"

For small (2 cm), visible, peripheral tumors, a modified technique using a single port incision can be used. I have termed the technique – "UNIVATS." A single 2-cm incision is made anterior to the mid-axillary line and the camera is inserted. The incision should be at least 10 cm away from the target. If the lesion is clearly visible then the incision is enlarged to approximately 3 cm. An angled, long ring forceps is used to grasp the lung via the same incision, and an articulating blue term segmentectomy is applied to anatomic dissection of a segmental bronchus and artery with resection of a segment or a group of segments smaller than an entire lobe. The most commonly performed segmental resections include the superior segments of the lower lobes, the basilar group of segments of the lower lobes, a lingular resection, or a lingular sparing left upper lobectomy.

35.2.4.1 Superior Segmentectomy

Three incisions are made. The camera port and posterior ports are identical to those for VATS lobectomy, while the access port may be smaller and more posteriorly located. The superior segmental vein is identified at the most posterior aspect of the inferior pulmonary vein. Proximal dissection on the inferior vein will reveal this segmental branch. After a combination of sharp and blunt dissection, the segmental vein is isolated and divided with an endovascular stapler. Dissection in the posterior aspect of the fissure will often reveal the segmental artery. In a thick fissure, it may be easiest to identify the large, ongoing artery and follow it to the segmental artery. The segmental artery is divided with an endovascular stapler. The segmental bronchus can be found with additional dissection behind the divided artery. A thick tissue stapler is used to perform the parenchymal divisions.

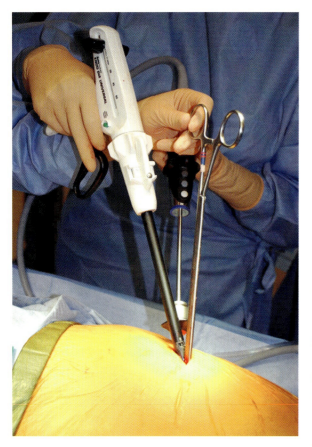

Fig. 35.9 "UNIVATS" technique. All three instruments are passed through a single 3-cm incision in order to perform a single wedge resection

load stapler is passed through the same incision, directed away from the target, and articulated back onto the lung (Fig 35.9). Using successive fires, a wedge resection can be performed. The specimen is placed in a bag prior to removal. This technique is not useful if a lobectomy is being planned, as other incisions are required, but is useful for suspected benign lesions, for metastatic lesions, or for biopsies for interstitial lung disease.

35.2.4 Segmental Resections

In patients with borderline pulmonary reserve and small (less than 3 cm) tumors, segmentectomy may offer a lower chance of recurrence than wedge resection. The

35.2.4.2 Basilar Segmentectomy

The incisions are identical to that used for a VATS lobectomy. The inferior pulmonary ligament is lysed with cautery, the inferior pulmonary vein is dissected free proximally, and the superior segmental vein is identified and preserved. The basilar portion of the vein is divided with an endovascular stapler.

On the right side, the fissure is dissected down to the pulmonary artery. As the artery is identified, the sheath of the artery is incised. Easy access to the sides of the artery will indicate that the correct plane has been entered. The large basilar trunk is easily separated from the superior segmental artery and is divided with an endovascular stapler. It is wise to identify the middle lobe artery and insure that it is more proximal and will not be harmed with division of the basilar trunk. At times the middle lobe artery arises opposite the superior segmental artery. Deeper dissection reveals the bronchus that has a similar branching pattern to that of the artery. The middle lobe bronchus must be preserved. A 3.5-mm thick stapler can be used on the basilar segmental bronchus. The anterior fissure inferior to the middle lobe bronchus is next divided. This is most easily accomplished by passing a blunt angled clamp through the bed of the divided bronchus, inferior to the middle lobe bronchus and toward the hilum. An endoleader can be passed, followed by a 4.8-mm thick stapler. The basilar segment can be retracted posteriorly, and the remaining line between the superior and basal segments can be divided with a thick tissue stapler.

On the left side, the incisions are identical to that for a VATS lower lobectomy. The dissection may begin on the inferior vein, dissecting the superior segmental vein away before the confluence with the inferior pulmonary vein. The basilar vein confluence is divided with an endovascular stapler. I prefer to next begin dissection in the anterior aspect of the fissure, preserving the lingular arteries. The basilar trunk artery is isolated and divided. The bronchus is seen deep into the artery and the superior segemental bronchus is seen and preserved, while the basilar bronchus is divided with and endoscopic stapler. The parenchymal division between the superior and basal segments is completed last.

35.2.5 VATS Lingular Sparing Left Upper Lobectomy

The dissection begins in an identical fashion to that of a VATS left upper lobectomy. The superior pulmonary vein is dissected free, and the lingular division is preserved, while the upper lobe division is divided with an endovascular stapler. The main pulmonary artery is dissected and the first one or two branches are dissected free and divided with an endovascular stapler. Next, the upper lobe bronchus is dissected free deep to the vein and the lingular bronchus and upper lobe division bronchus are cleaned. Simultaneous video bronchoscopy with a pediatric scope through the double lumen tube is useful in insuring that the lingular bronchus remains patent. The posterior aspect of the upper division bronchus is dissected with care, posteriorly, as the lingular branches may be close to the bronchus. The upper lobe division bronchus is divided with a 3.5 -m stapler. Additional upper lobe branches may now be visible and should be divided. Dissection must stop at the superior segmental artery to the lower lobe, which is preserved. The parenchyma between the lingula and upper lobe division is compressed with a clamp and then divided using thick tissue staplers.

35.2.6 VATS Lingular Resection

The VATS lingular resection begins in the anterior fissure. The fissure is dissected with a combination of sharp dissection and cautery until the pulmonary artery is found (often the last lingular artery). After identifying the lingular arteries, I prefer to dissect the superior pulmonary vein and identify and divide the lingular vein. The upper lobe bronchus is usually easily identified after dividing the vein and lingular arteries, and the lingular bronchus is divided (again, simultaneous bronchoscopy with a pediatric video scope helps insure division of the proper bronchus). Care must be taken not to injure the lingular arteries behind the bronchus. One or two lingular arteries are divided with endovascular staplers. The parenchyma is divided with thick tissue staplers (See attached video).

35.3 Lung Cancer: Emerging Therapies

35.3.1 Radiofrequency Ablation (RFA)

Radiofrequency ablation is a means of local tumor destruction that relies on frictional heat generated by alternating currents. Radiofrequency energy created by a generator passes between an active electrode inserted into the tumor and a dispersive electrode usually placed on the patient's lower body. The energy results in heating of tissue adjacent to the active electrode and, at temperatures greater than 60°C, results in local tissue death. The electrodes can be used via a percutaneous, CT guided, or intra operative approach. Currently, three manufacturers produce probes (Boston Scientific, RITA, and Valley Lab), each with a slightly different design.

Initially used in liver tumors, RFA has more recently been applied to primary and secondary tumors of the lung. One initial study examined tumors that were resected after ablation and showed that the majority of tumors had residual viable tumor. Complete necrosis was seen in smaller (<2 cm) tumors [4]. Another early study of lung tumors in 18 inoperable patients showed a 54% incidence of pneumothorax and had one death from severe hemoptysis in a patient with a central lung tumor [5]. Because of the risk of life-threatening hemoptysis associated with central lesions, most centers exclude these patients. A recent study of intra operative RFA from the Brigham and Women's Hospital however shows that some patients with central tumors may be treated safely if the tumor is dissected away from vital structures prior to RFA [6].

One of the largest long-term studies of RFA for pulmonary tumors involved 189 primary or metastatic tumors in 153 inoperable patients [7]. The 30-day mortality rate was 3.9%. The overall pneumothorax rate was 28%; the chest tube insertion rate was only 10%. The 2 and 5 year survival rates for non small cell lung cancer were 57% and 27%. A significant difference was seen in recurrence rates in tumors larger than 3 cm in diameter. The 2- and 5-year recurrence rate for tumors less than 3 cm was 64% and 47%, while it was 25% (2- and 5-year recurrence) for tumors larger than 3 cm. This increase in recurrence rate at 3 cm has been confirmed in several other series. Thus, RFA may allow for control of tumor growth in a proportion of tumors, and may be associated with long term survival in some patients, but is not without risk.

35.3.2 Stereotactic Radiosurgery

External beam radiation has long been the alternative to primary surgical resection for the treatment of localized lung cancers in patients who are not medically fit to undergo surgical resection. The limitations of external beam radiation include significant bystander injury to functioning adjacent lung, and dose limitations to nearby vital structures such as the spinal cord, trachea and mainstem bronchi, heart and esophagus. The effectiveness of external beam radiation is limited, with 5 year survival rates around 20% or less, and local tumor progression in about half of all patients [8]. In an effort to maximize the effective radiation dose and minimize toxicity to adjacent lung, stereotactic radiosurgery has been advocated. Computed tomography-based three-dimensional planning is used in conjunction with multiple individual radiation beams for improved targeting and avoidance of vital structures. In addition, various techniques have been used to minimize toxicity to intrathoracic structures during the respiratory cycle including breath holding, abdominal compression to minimize diaphragmatic excursion, and respiratory tracking and gating. The Cyberknife Stereotactic Radiosurgery Sytem (Accuray, Sunnyvale, CA) is perhaps the most sophisticated stereotactic system. A linear accelerator radiation source is mounted on a robotic arm, and individual beams of radiation are delivered gated to a vest worn by the patient and synchronized to the patient's respiratory cycle. The system requires that fiducial markers be placed in and around the tumor either via percutaneous or endobronchial techniques. Typically three treatment sessions of 20 Gy each are employed. The biologic effective dose (BED) is estimated to be 180 Gy with this regimen, far greater than the 70–80 Gy given in a 1.8 Gy 40 fraction conventional external beam radiation regimen. Tumors within 2 cm of lobar bronchi are generally excluded from receiving these high doses, because there has been a high incidence of lobar bronchomalacia and collapse. In a recent study employing this dosage scheme, local failure was seen in about 21% of patients [9].

In the largest series to date, conducted in Japan, 254 Stage I non small cell lung cancer patients, underwent stereotactic radiosurgery [10]. After a median follow up of 38 months, the local recurrence rate was 43% when a BED of <100 Gy was used and 8.4% when a BED of >100 Gy was used. The loco-regional (parenchymal plus regional nodal areas) recurrence rate was 17.7% with the higher dose, similar to the 5-year loco-regional recurrence rate seen with wedge resections. Perhaps the most intriguing statistic from this study is a 5-year survival rate of 71% in medically operable patients treated with a BED of >100 Gy. A current RTOG protocol, 0618, is enrolling medically operable stage I non-small cell lung cancer patients. If, on follow up CT scans, enlargement is seen and a PET scan or biopsy is positive, then the tumors will be surgically resected. Unfortunately, only 2-year objectives are planned.

35.4 The Pleura

35.4.1 Review of Current Literature

Malignant pleural effusions occur in about half of all patients with cancer, and can cause dyspnea and coughing. Common malignancies associated with pleural effusions are nonsmall cell lung cancer and breast cancer, although any malignancy may cause fluid to accumulate in the potential space between the lung and chest wall. The goals in treatment of malignant pleural effusions are complete drainage of the pleural fluid, and adhesion of the lung to the chest wall to obliterate the pleural space. Initial thoracentesis is useful in diagnosing a pleural effusion which will have a high total protein and LDH level, should show no organisms on gram stain and should have a pH greater than 7.2. Cytology may or may not show malignant cells. Improvement of the patient's symptoms with drainage of a significant amount of fluid is an indication for a procedure to prevent fluid re-accumulation. Re-expansion of the lung after large volume thoracentesis suggests that the patient may be a candidate for pleurodesis. If the mainstem bronchus is obstructed or significant intra parenchymal disease is present that prevents functioning of the lung, then removal of fluid may not improve the patient's breathing. Malignant effusions often recur. A systemic review of the 36 randomized-controlled trials involving 1,499 patients by Shaw and Agarwal demonstrated that the administration of a sclerosant was superior to drainage alone in the prevention of effusion recurrence. Talc pleurodesis was found to be more effective than pleurodesis using bleomycin or tetracycline. Further, thoracoscopic instillation was superior in preventing recurrence as compared to bedside procedures through talc sclerosis through tube thoracostomy [11].

An alternative to pleurodesis is placement of a chronic indwelling drainage catheter. The Pleur-X catheter (Denver Biomedical) is a soft, cuffed catheter with several side holes designed to be inserted into the pleural space and tunneled under the skin, with a cuff that sits just under the skin. The cuff helps prevent migration of bacteria and helps secure the catheter. Patients who are very weak, have lymphangitic spread of cancer through the lung, or have significant disease in the contra lateral lung may have significant respiratory distress after unilateral talc pleurodesis, and these patients are often best served by simple placement of a Pleur-X catheter. Patients whose lung is encased by tumor and is unable to expand are obviously not candidates for fusion of the pleural space and may also benefit from a Pleur-X catheter. The catheter is typically drained several times per week. Often the catheter will induce a gradual pleural inflammatory response allowing for eventual fusion of the pleural space and removal of the catheter in the office.

35.4.2 Pleurodesis – The Technique

Both talc pleurodesis and insertion of a Pleur-X catheter are typically done under general anesthesia with lung isolation. Bronchoscopy should be done prior to incision in order to rule out bronchial obstruction from tumor. The patient is placed in the lateral decubitus position and a 10-mm incision is made in approximately the 6th or 7th interspace in the anterior axillary line. Fluid is drained and the pleural space is inspected. Biopsies of tumor nodules or inflamed pleura can be obtained. The surface of the lung is inspected. If obvious encasement with tumor is seen, then placement of a Pleur-X catheter is chosen. Positive pressure ventilation with direct visual inspection helps the surgeon determine if the lung will expand and if fusion with the parietal pleural space is an option. After documentation of lung expansion the lung is collapsed and up to five grams of talc are insufflated diffusely into the pleural space. The talc inside a Luken's trap is attached to oxygen tubing, and 4 L/min is used to deliver the talc through a curved Yankauer into the pleural space. Afterward a 28 F chest tube is inserted posteriorly and suction applied for 48 h. A decrease in the chest tube output to less than 100 cc over 24 h is a good indicator of long term success. High chest tube output can be managed by repeat administration of talc through the chest tube at the bedside.

If the lung does not expand, then placement of a Pleur-X catheter is considered. Via a separate stab incision, the catheter is tunneled and inserted into the pleural space via the 10-mm incision. The incision is closed over the catheter in three layers: a muscle layer, subdermal layer, and subcuticular layer. Either thoracoscopy with talc or Pleur-X placement can be done under sedation and local anesthesia, with limited visualization.

35.5 The Mediastinum

35.5.1 The Pericardium

35.5.1.1 Review of Current Literature

Malignant pericardial effusions can be managed by observation, catheter drainage, drainage with balloon dilation of the pericardium, or removal of a portion of pericardium (pericardial window). Effusions commonly recur after simple drainage, although there have been some descriptions of success with catheter drainage and balloon dilation of the pericardial tract. Two common surgical approaches to pericardial drainage for recurrent effusions are a subxyphoid incision with creation of a pericardial window and drainage of the fluid into the preperitoneal space, and thoracoscopic pericardial window with drainage into the pleural space. A recent met-analysis reviewed the pros and cons of both procedures, concluding that thoracoscopic pericardial windows, while slightly more invasive, provides longer freedom from re-accumulation of the effusion the thoracoscopic procedure had no difference in time of chest tube drainage, length of stay, or mortality [12]. A thoracoscopic approach also allows for evaluation of the pleural space, with simultaneous treatment of any malignant pleural effusion. The disadvantages of a thoracoscopic approach include the need for single-lung ventilation, and the increased time needed for positioning after induction prior to incising the pericardium.

If tamponade is present upon induction, immediate incision and drainage may be needed. If there are any clinical or echocardiographic signs of tamponade, it is usually best to have the pericardial effusion drained percutaneously in the catherization lab prior to induction of anesthesia.

35.5.1.2 Pericardial Window – The Technique

VATS pericardial window is done via two or three incisions in the lateral decubitus position. The first incision is a 5-mm camera port placed just inferior to the tip of the scapula. The patient is rotated posteriorly. A 5-mm incision in the fifth interspace mid-clavicular line is used to grasp the pericardium. A 5-mm incision 2–3 interspaces below the tip of the scapula is used to retract the lung and incise the pericardium with a long tipped cautery. Drainage of the pericardial fluid prior to operation helps the surgeon grasp the pericardium from the fifth interspace incision, and cautery is used to resect at least a 3 cm in diameter window of pericardium. Large swaths of pericardium should probably not be resected, at least on the right side, so as to avoid herniation of the heart with subsequent torsion and arrest. Loculations in the pericardium can be broken with a blunt tipped curved plastic suction device or a blunt curved ring forceps. It is not necessary to leave a drain in the pericardium; a chest tube should be left in the pleural space and can usually be removed the following day.

35.5.2 The Thymus

35.5.2.1 Review of Current Literature

The goal of any surgical procedure for thymoma is complete removal of all thymic tissue. Non-thymomatous Myasthenia Gravis is the most common indication for thymectomy, and up to 30% of these patients may have a thymoma [13]. Other patients may have thymoma without myasthenia. With either condition, completely removal of all thymic tissue is important.

Many different techniques have been developed to remove thymic tissue and the amount of extra capsular mediastinal and cervical fat that is resected with the thymic tissue varies. The traditional approach to thymectomy has been full sternotomy and removal via blunt and cautery dissection of all inferior aspects of the thymus (extending laterally down the pericardium), the main body of the thymus, and both superior thymic horns, which usually run anterior to the innominate vein into the neck. If tumor invades adjacent tissues, then en-bloc resection of all structures involved by tumor with preservation of at least one phrenic nerve is performed. Three minimally invasive approaches have been developed as an alternative to full sternotomy. A partial sternotomy may be performed extending from the sternal notch down to the fourth interspace. Although such an incision has been shown to decrease risk of operation and bleeding during reoperative aortic valve surgery, its advantages are less clear in surgery for thymectomy; moreover, exposure to the inferior aspects of the thymic gland can be very limited. Two other techniques are a transcervical approach and video-assisted thymectomy. Kaiser and colleagues advocate the extended transcervical thymectomy for myasthenia, reporting 43% and 45% 3 and 6 year rates of complete stable remission [14]. Although there are no prospective randomized trials of open versus minimally invasive techniques, several retrospective publications have examined the different approaches. Sonnet et al. compared six different surgical techniques for nonthymomatous myasthenia and concluded that transcervical thymectomy and video assisted thymectomy operations were superior to other less radical procedures [15]. Maggi, et al., compared video-assisted thymectomy with an additional cervical incision to extended transternal thymectomy in a retrospective review of thymomatous myasthenia gravis patients. There was no difference between video assisted thymectomy and extended trans-sternal thymectomy in disease recurrence or complete stable remission rates [16]. A non-randomized prospective study evaluated VATS resection vs. median sternotomy in the treatment of Masaoka stage II thymomas and showed less blood loss in the VATS group, but no differences in operation time, duration of chest tube drainage, or length of hospital stay. All patients were disease-free at 3 years, though this is not considered long term follow up for this disease [17].

35.5.2.2 VATS Thymectomy – The Technique

Although unilateral VATS approaches have been described, a bilateral approach is detailed here for completeness:

The patient is positioned in the supine position elevated on blanket rolls several inches off the table. Both arms are extended to the sides or folded and elevated over the head and suspended with padding. The table is angled 30°. A 10-mm camera port is placed in the anterior axillary line in approximately the seventh interspace. Two separate 5-mm ports are placed in the sub mammary crease in the female or the equivalent positions in the male. These are approximately in the midaxillary line, fourth interspace and 2 cm anterior to the axillary line in the fifth interspace. Alternatively, a more cosmetic approach can be three small incisions placed in the submammary crease extending from the midclavicular line to the midaxillary line. For patients with non thymomatous conditions, these small ports may allow for removal of the specimen (Fig. 35.10). The phrenic nerve

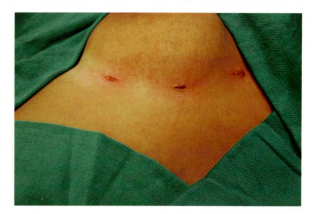

Fig. 35.10 Submammary thymic incisions. These incisions are highly cosmetic, being hidden in the sub mammary crease and in the axilla. 3- to 5-mm ports are used. The two working ports and camera ports may be interchanged during the procedure

is identified along its entire course. On the left side, dissection is performed with an ultrasonic scalpel and begins inferiorly and posteriorly on the pericardium, anterior to the phrenic nerve. The thymus and adjacent mediastinal fatty tissue are grasped and dissected off the pericardium. Care must be taken when using any cautery or ultrasonic dissection near the phrenic nerve. As dissection proceeds toward the thoracic inlet, the innominate vein is identified and dissection of perithymic tissue begins with the innominate vein, with care to clip thymic veins draining into the innominate vein. Dissection of the left superior thymic horn is performed with hand-over-hand dissection anterior to the vein. Dissection is also performed between thymic tissue and the sternum. Some surgeons find carbon dioxide insufflation of the chest cavity helpful to help with anterior dissection. Dissection is usually possibly well past the midline. A small-bore chest drain is inserted, and near identical incisions are made on the on the right side. Along the right side dissection is begun anterior to the phrenic nerve freeing perithymic tissue off the pericardium. Dissection proceeds cranially along the anterior aspect of the superior vena cava. The anterior superior horn of the thymus is pulled down hand over hand. Anteriorly the thymus is dissected away from the sternum. The specimen is placed in a small bag and retrieved through the 10-mm camera port incision. A small Blake drain is left on the right side. The drains can be removed in the recovery room if the postoperative CXR shows no significant pneumothorax and there is no air leak. Typically patients leave the hospital the next day.

35.5.3 The Lymphatic Tissue

35.5.3.1 Mediastinal Node Dissection

Mediastinal nodal dissection is typically performed through the same incisions used for VATS lobectomy, detailed earlier in this chapter. The technique differs on each side. Mediastinal nodes are:
- 2 – High paratracheal nodes generally not accessed via the chest
- 4 – Paratracheal
- 5 – AP window
- 6 – Paraaortic arch
- 7 – Subcarinal
- 8 – Paraesophageal
- 9 – Inferior pulmonary ligament

Right Sided Nodal Dissection

Subcarinal Nodal Dissection

The patient is angled forward, the camera is moved to the posterior inferior port, and the lung is grasped at the junction of the superior segment of the lower lobe and the posterior segment of the upper lobe and retracted anteriorly. Via the anterior working port incision, a blunt curved instrument (pediatric suction tip) can be used to disrupt the pleural reflection. The medial aspect of the right main bronchus is found opposite from the origin of the right upper lobe bronchus. Blunt dissection is used cranially up under the azygous vein and subcarinal nodes are encountered. If dissection is difficult, then both the camera and retraction instrument can be inserted through the anterior inferior port, and an additional instrument can be inserted through the posterior port to aid in dissection.

Right Para-tracheal Nodal Dissection

The patient is kept at 90°. Via the posterior inferior port, a long grasper is used to retract the apex of the lung inferiorly and posteriorly. Via the anterior working port incision the pleura overlying the trachea is incised down to the junction of the azygous vein and superior vena cava. All lymph nodes can be removed from the right paratracheal position, with care to preserve the vagus nerve.

Other mediastinal nodes: level 9 (inferior ligament nodes) are routinely accessible with division of the inferior pulmonary ligament. Level 8 (paraesophageal) nodes are accessible with the lung retracted anteriorly.

Left Sided Nodal Dissection

Levels 5 (AP window) and 6 (aortic arch) nodes are easily dissected via the standard left anterior VATS working incision. These are routinely exposed as one dissects the proximal branches of the left pulmonary artery. Subcarinal nodes (level 7) are more difficult to access on the left as compared to the right, but can be reached with the patient and lung retracted anteriorly. The main bronchus is identified posteriorly adjacent to the aorta and dissection is extended toward the hilum to access subcarinal nodes. Left sided paratracheal nodes are generally not accessible via a left sided approach, although certain centers in Japan have shown approaches to the trachea after division of the ligamentum arteriosum.

Quick Reference Guide

Anatomic Vats Lobectomy

1. Complete preoperative work up includes
   - CT chest w/wo contrast
   - PET-CT
   - Lung function tests
   - Cardiac clearance if necessary
2. Always perform a diagnostic thoracoscopy to rule out metastatic disease before placing the utility incision
3. Avoid any rib division, rib removal or rib spreading
4. All anatomic dissections follow the same sequence
   - Dissection and division of *vein*
   - Dissection and division of *artery*
   - Dissection and division of *bronchus*
5. Right Upper Lobectomy (RUL)
   - Patient positioning:
     – Left lateral decubitus, operating table flexed to open up the intercostals space

- Trocar placement:
  - 10mm trocar in the 7th interspace, anterior to the anterior axillary line
  - Utility incision of 4–6 cm anterior axillary line, 4th interspace
  - 10mm trocar 8th/9th interspace posterior and inferior to the tip of the scapula. (will be used for stapler insertion)
- Operative steps
  - Pull upper lobe forward via the access incision and perform subcarinal and paratracheal LN dissection. This maneuver exposes the bronchus as well.
  - Retract the lobe posterior to dissect the hilum
- *Vein dissection*
  - Start the dissection of the superior pulmonary vein between upper lobe vein and middle lobe vein
  - Do not injure the ongoing pulmonary artery or deep venous branches
  - Divide the vein with a stapler through the posterior incision
- *Artery dissection*
  - Use sharp dissection and avoid cautery
  - Locate the truncus anterior branch to the right upper lobe
  - Identify and preserve the middle lobe artery
  - Divide the artery with a stapler through the posterior incision
- *Bronchus dissection*
  - Dissect the base first and sweep all lymph nodes up on to the specimen
  - Before firing the stapler ventilate the lung to assure that you are only dividing the upper lobe bronchus
  - Any visible bronchial arteries should be clipped
- *Final steps*
  - An impermeable retrieval bag for specimen removal is mandatory
  - Perform frozen section on the bronchial stump
  - Lyse the inferior pulmonary ligament
  - Placement of one 28 Fr chest tube is sufficient and will be brought in through the camera port and placed posterior
  - Before closing inflate the lower and middle lobe under direct vision to assure that the middle lobe is not torsed

6. Right Middle Lobectomy (RML)
   - Access port 5th interspace, smaller and slightly more posterior
   - Operative steps
     - *Vein dissection*
       - In 5–10% the middle lobe vein drains into the inferior pulmonary vein
     - *Artery dissection*
       - Dissect the minor fissure first to gain access to the middle lobe artery
     - *Bronchus dissection*
       - Middle lobe bronchus travels deep and medial to the artery
       - Complete the fissure and insert single chest tube

7. Right Lower Lobectomy (RLL)
   - Access port 5th interspace, 6 cm of length, mid to anterior axillary line, overlying the fissure
   - Operative steps
     - Rule out N2 nodal disease
     - Retract the lower lobe superior and lyse the inferior pulmonary ligament through the posterior port
     - *Vein dissection*
       - Identify the inferior pulmonary vein
       - Be certain that the middle lobe vein does not drain into the inferior lobe vein before you divide it.
     - *Artery dissection*
       - Dissect the pulmonary artery through the fissure
       - Divide the superior segmental artery and basilar trunk artery separately
     - *Bronchus dissection*
       - Divide the lower lobe bronchus only after dissection of the pulmonary artery
       - The lower lobe bronchus can be taken as one unit after assuring that the middle lobe inflates properly

- The right lower lobe is the largest lobe and you might have to enlarge the incision for specimen removal.
8. Left Upper Lobectomy (LUL)
   - Trocar placement mirrors the one for the right lung
   - Access port is placed in 4th interspace
   - All dissection is done via the access incision
   - Operative steps
     - Perform lymph node dissection Level 5/6 and send for frozen. If + on frozen section, consider to abort the procedure and refer the patient for neo-adjuvant therapy.
     - Dissection from above is safest as the pulmonary artery can be directly visualized
     - An 'endoleader' red rubber catheter facilitates dissection of the vascular supply
     - Make sure not to encircle the left main bronchus!
9. Left Lower Lobectomy (LLL)
   - Access port 5th interspace
   - Operative steps
     - *Vein dissection*
       - Visualize superior pulmonary vein and preserve
       - Divide the inferior vein with a stapler through the posterior port
     - *Artery dissection*
       - Follow the most distal lingular branch to the ongoing pulmonary artery to find the basilar trunk artery and divide it

Wedge Resection

1. Use three 10mm ports
2. Lesions larger than 3cm should not be wedged because of a threefold increase in loco regional recurrence
3. Obtain a margin of at least 2cm or equal to the diameter of the lesion
   - Port placement
     - Camera port: 7th interspace between posterior and anterior axillary line
     - Posterior port: Inferior to the tip of the scapula
     - Anterior port: High in axilla
       - 3rd interspace for apical or posterior apical lesions
       - 4th interspace for lower lesions
4. Palpate the tumor through the anterior port
5. If the tumor is close to the fissure, fire a stapler through the fissure first towards the deep margin of the lesion.
6. Always obtain frozen section!

Lymphadenectomy

- Right sided lymphadenectomy
  - *Subcarinal nodal dissection*
    - Angle the patient forward and bring the camera in through the posterior inferior port
    - Grab the lung at the junction of the superior segment of the lower lobe and the posterior segment of the upper lobe and retract it anteriorly
    - Bluntly disrupt the pleural reflection
    - Use blunt dissection only up under the azygos vein where you will encounter the subcarinal nodes.
  - *Paratracheal nodal dissection*
    - Keep the patient at 90 degrees
    - Retract the apex of the lung inferiorly and posteriorly.
    - Incise the pleura overlying the trachea down to the junction of the azygous vein and superior vena cava
    - Remove the nodes
    - Do not injure the vagus nerve
- Left sided lymphadenectomy
  - Level 5/6 are easily exposed when dissecting the proximal branches of the left pulmonary artery.
  - Level 7 can be reached with the patient and lung retracted anteriorly
  - Identify the main bronchus and extend the dissection toward the hilum to access subcarinal nodes.
  - Left sided paratracheal nodes are generally not accessible via a left sided approach.

References

1. Graham, E., Singer, J.: Successful removal of an entire lung for carcinoma of the bronchus. JAMA **101**, 1371 (1933)
2. Ginsberg, R., Rubinstein, L.: Randomized trial of lobectomy versus limited resection for T1N0 non-small cell lung cancer. Ann. Thorac. Surg. **60**, 615–623 (1995)
3. Sawabata, N., Ohta, M., Matsumura, A., et al.: Optimal distance of malignant negative margin in excision of nonsmall cell lung cancer; A mutlicenter prospective study. Ann. Thorac. Surg. **77**, 415–420 (2004)
4. Yang, S., Askin, F., et al.: Radiofrequency ablation of primary and metastatic lung tumors: analysis of an ablate and resect study. Presented at the American Association of Thoracic Surgery 82nd annual meeting, Washington DC, 2002
5. Herrera, L., Ferannddo, H., Perry, Y., et al.: Radiofrequency ablation of pulmonary malignant tumors in nonsurgical candidates. J Thorac. Card. Surg. **125**, 929–937 (2003)
6. Linden, P., Wee, J., Jaklitsch, M., Colson, Y.: Extending indications of radiofrequency ablation of lung tumors through an intraoperative approach. Ann. Thorac. Surg. **85**, 420–423 (2008)
7. Simon, C., Dupuy, D., DiPetrillo, T., et al.: Pulmonary radiofrequency ablation: long-term safety and efficacy in 153 patients. Radiology **243**, 268–275 (2007)
8. Zierhut, D., Betttscheider, C., Schubert, K., et al.: Radiation therapy of stage I and II non-small cell lung cancer. Lung Cancer **34**, S39–S43 (2001)
9. McGarry, R., Papiez, L., Williams, M., et al.: Stereotactic body radiation therapy of early-stage non-smallcell lung carcinoma: phase I study. Int. J. Radiat. Oncol. Biol. Phys. **63**(4), 1010–1015 (2005)
10. Onishi, H., Shirato, H., Nagata, Y.: Hypofractionated stereotactic radiotherapy for stage I non small cell lung cancer: updated results of 257 patients in a Japanese multi-institutional study. J. Thorac. Oncol. **2**, S94–S100 (2007)
11. Shaw P, Agarwal R.: Pleurodesis for malignant pleural effusions. Cochrane Database Syst. Rev. (1), (2004), CD002916. doi:10.1002/14651858.CD002916
12. O'Brien, P., Kucharczuk, J., Marshall, M., et al.: Comparative study of subxyphoid versus video-assisted thoracoscopic pericardial window. Ann. Thorac. Surg. **80**, 2013–2019 (2005)
13. Okumura, M., Shiono, M., Minami, M., et al.: Clinical and pathological aspects of thymic epithelial tumors. Gen. Thorac. Cardiovasc. Surg. **56**, 10–16 (2008)
14. Shrager, J., Nathan, D., Kaiser, L., et al.: Outcomes after 151 extended transcervical thymetomies for myasthenia gravis. Ann. Thorac. Surg. **82**, 1863–1869 (2006)
15. Sonnet, J., Jaretzki, A.: Thymectomy for nonthymomatous myasthenia gravis: a critical analysis. Ann. NY Acad. Sci. **1132**, 315–328 (2008)
16. Maggi, L., Andreeta, F., Antozzi, C., Mantegazza, R., et al.: Thymoma-associated myasthenia gravis: outcome, clinical and pathological correlations in 197 patients on a 20 year experience. J. Neuroimmunol. **15**, 237–244 (2008)
17. Cheng, Y., Kao, E., Chou, S.: Videothoracoscopic resection of stage II thymoma: prospective comparison of the results between thoracoscopy and open methods. Chest **128**, 3010–3012 (2005)

Index

A

Abdominal cavity endoscopic exploration, pioneers of
  Christian Jacobeus, 5
  George Kelling, 6
  Heinz Kalk, 6
  John Ruddock, 6
  Michael J. Mack, Mark J. Krasna, 6
  Swierenga J, 6
Abdominal dissection, esophageal cancer
  antrum and fundus, division of, 130
  conduit, maintaining rotation of, 132
  diagnostic laparoscopy and decision, 129
  dissection
    left gastric artery and vein, 130
    retrogastric dissection, 129
  feeding jejunostomy, placing of, 131–132
  gastric conduit, creation of, 130
  mobilization
    gastric antrum, 129–130
    gastric fundus, 129
    greater curvature, 129
  operating room set-up and trocar placement, 129
  patient positioning and on-table endoscopy, 128
  pyloroplasty–Heinecke-Mikulicz, 131
Abdominal tumors, pediatric, 502–503
Abdominoperineal resection
  anal opening, closure of, 244
  IMA, 245
  IMV, 245
  left colon
    mobilization of, 245
    proximal division, 245–246
  operating field, exposure, 245
  pelvic wound closure, 246
  perineal dissection and specimen exteriorization, 246
  positioning, patient and equipment, 244–245
  rectum, mobilization of, 245
  trocar placement positioning, 244–245
  trocar sites and colostomy creation, 246
ADEPT. *See* Advanced Dundee Endoscopic Psychomotor Tester (ADEPT)
Adjuvant/neo-adjuvant therapy, 102
Adjuvant therapy, 103
Adrenal gland cancer
  adrenal incidentaloma
    catecholamine hypersecretion, 392
    follow-up metabolic testing, 392
    general considerations, 391–392
    hyperaldosteronism, 392
    hypercortisolism, 392
  adrenal surgery, clinical indications
    Cushing's syndrome, 390–391
    functional adrenal mass, 390
    isolated adrenal metastasis, 390, 391
    suspected malignancy, 389–390
  laparoscopic adrenalectomy, 393
  perioperative considerations, 392–393
  radiologic findings, 390
  surgical anatomy, 395
  surgical technique
    advantages and disadvantages, 394
    anterior transabdominal adrenalectomy, 395, 400–401
    lateral transabdominal adrenalectomy, 394, 396–400
    retroperitoneal adrenalectomy, 394–395, 401
Adrenal metastasis, 390, 391
Advanced Dundee Endoscopic Psychomotor Tester (ADEPT), 17
Aging patient, minimally invasive surgery
  adjuvant therapy role, 103
  epidemiology, cancer, 97–98
  minimally invasive management
    colorectal cancer, 101
    esophageal cancer, 100–101
    gastric cancer, 101
    lung cancer, 100
  pathophysiological changes
    cardiovascular, 98
    endocrine, 99
    gastrointestinal, 99
    immunological, 99
    musculoskeletal, 99
    neurological, 99–100
    pulmonary, 98
    renal, 98–99
  surgical approach
    intraoperative management, 102–103
    postoperative management, 103
    preoperative management, 101–102
Anaplastic thyroid cancer, 334, 338

Anatomical liver resections
  hepatectomies
    classification, 284
    surgical technique, 284–294
  intra-operative ultrasound
    objectives, 281
    role, 275–276
    technique and major steps, 281–282
  laparoscopic liver surgery, 276–278
  laparoscopic resections
    indications, 273–274
    liver transplants, role in, 274–275
    vs. open approach, 274
    primary liver tumors and HCC, 274
    vs. radiofrequency ablation, 275
  leak test, 283–284
  minimally invasive liver surgery, 275
  parenchyma dissection
    CUSA® system, 282
    EnSeal®, 283
    Harmonic Scalpel® and Sonosurg®, 282
    Ligasure®, 282
    parameters, 282
    personal technique, 283
    stapling devices, 283
    TissueLink™, 283
  specimen removal, 283
  surgical approach
    anesthesia, special considerations, 280–281
    operating room setup and equipment, 278–280
    patient positioning, 280
    preoperative evaluation, 278
    trocar placement, 280, 281
Anterior transabdominal adrenalectomy (ATA)
  adrenal gland dissection, 400–401
  advantages and disadvantages, 394
  difficulties in, 395
  patient positioning and trocar placement, 400
Appendiceal malignancies
  carcinoid tumors, 203–204
  histological subtypes, 200–201
  laparoscopy role, 202–203
  mucinous neoplasm, 201–202
  non mucinous tumor, 201
  peritoneal carcinomatosis therapy, 202–203
Aromatic fatty acids, 338
Arterial angiography, 357
ATA. *See* Anterior transabdominal adrenalectomy (ATA)

B
BABA. *See* Bilateral axillary-breast approach (BABA)
Benign small bowel tumors, 187–188
Bilateral axillary-breast approach (BABA), 346–347
Brachytherapy, prostate cancer, 468

C
Calcitonin, 333
Catecholamine blockade, 393
Catecholamine hypersecretion, 392
CD markers, 74–75
CD31 surface marker, 75

Cellular immunity
  lymphocytes, 74–76
  natural killer cell activity, 73–74
  systemic monocyte function, 72–73
  T-cell function, 71–72
Central hepatectomy, 288–289
Cervical cancer
  advanced stage
    interstitial radiation implant, 424
    laparoscopic ovarian transposition, 424
    pelvic and para-aortic lymphadenectomy, 423
    pelvic exenteration, 424
  early stage
    laparoscopic lymphadenectomy, 417
    radical vaginal hysterectomy, 415–416
    robotic radical hysterectomy, 416–417
    sentinel lymph node sampling, 417–421
    total laparoscopic radical hysterectomy, 416
    trachelectomy, 422–423
  indications for laparoscopy, 407
  surgical technique
    general considerations and instruments, 408
    laparoscopic radical hysterectomy, 408–412
    lymphadenectomy, 413–415
Chemotherapy
  Burkits abdominal lymphoma, 503
  gallbladder cancer, 300
  parathyroid cancer, 360
Chronic lymphocytic leukemia (CLL), 315
Chronic myeloid leukemia (CML), 313, 316
CLL. *See* Chronic lymphocytic leukemia (CLL)
Clusters of differentiation, 74–75
CML. *See* Chronic myeloid leukemia (CML)
Colorectal cancer
  aging patient, 101
  laparoscopy, 63
Computed tomography (CT)
  esophageal cancer staging, 128
  pancreatic cancer, 363
  parathyroid cancer, 357
Concurrent and construct validity, 14
Conn's syndrome, 392
Content validity, 14
CO_2 pneumoperitoneum, 77–78
Cryoablation
  liver tumors, 29
  prostate cancer
    complications, 470
    history and development, 469–470
    method of action, 470
    outcomes, 470–471
  tumor tissue ablation, 29
CT. *See* Computed tomography (CT)
CUSA® system, 282
Cushing's syndrome, 390–391
Cyberknife, 510, 524
Cyclin D1, 356
Cytokines, humoral immunity
  C-reactive protein (CRP), 70
  inflammatory cascade, 70
  interleukin-1 (IL-1), 71

interleukin-6 (IL-6), 70–71
tumor necrosis factor alpha (TNF-α), 71

D
da Vinci oncological trends, 52
DaVinci™ robot, 459
Differentiated thyroid cancer (DTC)
  anaplastic thyroid cancer, 338
  follicular thyroid cancer
    clinical presentation and prognosis, 337
    FNA, 338
    guidelines, 338
    pathological features, 337
  papillary thyroid cancer
    early thyroidectomy, 336
    features, 335
    guidelines, 336–337
    lobectomy *vs.* total thyroidectomy, 336
    management, 337
    Mount Sinai approach, 336
    patient differentiation, 336
Disseminated peritoneal adenomucinosis (DPAM), 202
Distal pancreatectomy, 117
DPAM. *See* Disseminated peritoneal adenomucinosis (DPAM)
DTC. *See* Differentiated thyroid cancer (DTC)
Duodenojejunostomy, 384

E
Early gastric cancer (EGC)
  complications, 175
  endoscopic resection (*see* Endoscopic resection)
  outcomes, 178
  postprocedure management, 175, 178
  risk factors, 167
EBRT. *See* External beam radiotherapy (EBRT)
EGC. *See* Early gastric cancer (EGC)
Elderly patients. *See* Aging patient, minimally invasive surgery
EMR. *See* Endoscopic mucosal resection (EMR)
Endoluminal procedures, EGC
  complications, 175
  endoscopic resection
    endoscopic submucosal dissection (ESD), 168
    indications, 169–170
    patient selection, 168–169
    techniques, 170–177
  outcomes, 178
  postprocedure management, 176, 178
  risk factors, 167
Endometrial cancer
  conditions, 425
  laparoscopic surgical staging, 426–427
  patient positioning and technique, 425
  quality of life assessment, 430
  recurrence management, 428–429
  robotic-assisted staging of, 427–428
  special considerations
    elderly, 430
    obesity, 429–430
  staging completion, 428–429

Endoscopic mucosal resection (EMR)
  nonsuction technique–"lift-and-cut," 170–171
  suction technique–"suck-and-cut," 171–173
Endoscopic resection
  endoscopic submucosal dissection (ESD), 168
  indications
    extended indications, 169–170
    standard indications, 169
  patient selection
    endoscopic staging, 168
    pathologic staging, 169
  techniques
    endoscopic mucosal resection (EMR), 170–172
    endoscopic submucosal dissection (ESD), 172–177
Endoscopic staging
  chromoendoscopy, 168
  endoscopic ultrasound (EUS), 168
  virtual gastroscopy, 168
Endoscopic submucosal dissection (ESD), 168, 172–177
Endoscopic thyroid surgery
  non-cervical approach
    BABA, 346–347
    transaxillary approach, 347
  oncological outcome, 344
  patient selection, 344
  rationale for, 343
  risks and benefits, 343–344
  transcervical approach
    instrumentation, 345–346
    operative steps, 346
    patient positioning, 345
    trocar configuration, 344
  video-assisted thyroidectomy, 347–348
Endoscopic TV Vidicon tube camera, 9
Endoscopy
  abdominal cavity, 5–6
  definition and evolution, 3
  illumination, 6–7
  image transmission, 7–8
  light source, 3–4
  light source, Bozzini and Desormeaux, 3–4
  open tube, 4
  telescope, 4–5
  television image, 8–10
EnSeal® vessel fusion system, 283
ENT, robotic applications, 53–54
ESD. *See* Endoscopic submucosal dissection (ESD)
Esophageal cancer
  aging patient, 100–101
  laparoscopy role, 126
  nonsurgical management, 127
  staging of, 128
  surgical management
    abdominal dissection, 128–132
    esophagogastric end-to-side anastomosis, 133–134
    thoracic dissection, 132–133
Esophagogastric end-to-side anastomosis
  drain placement and wound closure, 134
  postoperative management, 134
  two-cavity approach, 133–134

Esophagus and gastroesophageal junction
　　transhiatal approach
　　　　Barret's dysplasia, 144
　　　　cervical anastomosis, 142
　　　　endoluminal treatment, 144
　　　　fundoplication, 142, 143
　　　　gastric conduit, 141–142
　　　　history, 138
　　　　minimal invasive esophagectomy, 137
　　　　postoperative management, 142–143
　　　　staging laparoscopy, 143, 144
　　　　suitable approach, 137–138
　　　　surgical management, 139–141
　　　　traditional open surgical approaches, 143
　　two-cavity approach
　　　　anatomy, 125
　　　　laparoscopy role, 126
　　　　minimally invasive techniques, 126–127
　　　　nonsurgical management, 127
　　　　postoperative management, 134
　　　　preoperative considerations, 128
　　　　resections, 125–126
　　　　staging, esophageal cancer, 128
　　　　surgical management, 128–134
External beam radiotherapy (EBRT)
　　gallbladder cancer, 300
　　prostate cancer
　　　　complications, 467
　　　　contraindications, 467–468
　　　　cytotoxicity, 466
　　　　planning strategies, 466
　　　　success and failure, 466–467
Extrahepatic bile duct cancer. See Gallbladder cancer

F
Face validity, 14
FDG-PET. See Fluorodeoxyglucose-positron emission tomography (FDG-PET)
Fine needle aspiration (FNA), 335
Flow cytometry, 357
Fluorodeoxyglucose-positron emission tomography (FDG-PET), 300
FNA. See Fine needle aspiration (FNA)
Follicular thyroid cancer, 337–338

G
Gallbladder cancer
　　controversies, surgical resection, 306
　　FOX CHASE data, 305
　　incidence of, 298
　　management
　　　　FDG-PET, 300
　　　　historical overview, 298
　　　　preoperative workup, 298, 300
　　　　staging and re-resection, 298, 299
　　non-surgical management of, 300
　　porcelain gallbladder, 298
　　risk factors, 297
　　surgical management of, 300–302
　　surgical procedures

　　　　hepatoduodenal lymphadenectomy, 302–304
　　　　laparoscopic common bile duct excision, 304–305
　　　　laparoscopic radical cholecystectomy, 302–304
　　　　laparoscopic Roux-en-Y choledocho-jejunostomy, 304–305
Gartner's hype cycle of innovation, 40–41
Gastric cancer
　　aging patient, 101
　　laparoscopy, 62–63
Gastroesophageal junction. See Esophagus and gastroesophageal junction
Gastrointestinal stromal tumor (GIST), 186
Gastro-jejunal anastomosis
　　creation of, 155
　　techniques, 154–155
Genetic surgery, 42–43
GIST. See Gastrointestinal stromal tumor (GIST)
Global operative assessment of laparoscopic skills (GOALS), 17–18
Gynecological surgery, robotic applications, 53
Gynecologic malignancies
　　cervical carcinomas, laparoscopy and applications
　　　　advanced stage, 423–424
　　　　early stage, 415–423
　　　　indications for, 407
　　　　surgical technique, 408–415
　　endometrial cancer, laparoscopy and applications
　　　　conditions, 425
　　　　laparoscopic surgical staging, 426–427
　　　　patient positioning and technique, 425
　　　　quality of life assessment, 430
　　　　recurrence management, 429
　　　　robotic-assisted endometrial cancer staging, 427–428
　　　　special considerations, 429–430
　　　　staging completion, 428–429
　　fallopian tubal and primary peritoneal carcinomas, 430–438
　　ovarian cancer, laparoscopy and applications
　　　　advanced stage invasive, 434–437
　　　　borderline ovarian tumors, 432
　　　　early stage invasive, 432–434
　　　　laparoscopic management of, 438
　　　　management pitfalls, 437–438
　　　　surgical staging, 431
　　　　surgical technique, 431–432

H
Haemostasis, MIS
　　laser, 26
　　mechanical methods, 26
　　thermal methods, 26
　　tissue sealants, 26
Hand-assisted laparoscopic splenectomy (HALS)
　　indication for, 320
　　intermediate splenomegaly, 320–321
　　massive splenomegaly, 321
　　patient positioning, 320
　　specimen extraction, 322
　　splenectomy and, 325–326
　　splenic hilum, dissection of, 321–322
Hand-assisted laparoscopic surgery, 27–28, 269

Haptics, MIS, 33–34
Harmonic Scalpel®, 282
Hepatectomies
    central hepatectomy, 288–289
    classification, 284
    extended
        hepatectomy left, 289
        hepatectomy right, 289–290
    hemihepatectomies, 284–288
        major hepatectomy left, 286–288
        major hepatectomy right, 284–286
    limited hepatectomies-segmentectomies, 290–294
Hepaticojejunostomy, 384
Hepato-biliary system
    extrahepatic cholangiocarcinoma
        adjuvant therapy, 258
        advantages and disadvantages, 257
        classification, 256
        conventional surgical therapy, 256
        endoscopic diagnosis and unresectable disease palliation, 257
        endoscopic photodynamic therapy, 257–258
        epidemiology, 255
        pathology, 257
        preoperative workup, 256
        risk factors and symptoms, 256
        staging, 256–257
    gallbladder carcinoma
        epidemiology, 253
        preoperative workup, 253
        staging of, 253–254
        surgical therapy, 254
        symptoms, 253
    nonanatomical resection (See Liver, nonanatomical resection)
    operating room
        adjuvant therapy, 255
        intraoperative bile spillage problem, 254
        intraoperative positive frozen section management, 254
        laparoscopy and incidental, 254
        port site metastasis, 255
        staging, 255
Hepatoblastoma, pediatric, 505
Hepatoduodenal lymphadenectomy, 302–304. See also Laparoscopic radical cholecystectomy
High-intensity focused ultrasound (HIFU), 28
    prostate cancer, 471–472
    tissue ablation, 28
Hodgkin's disease (HD), 315
Hodgkin's lymphoma (HL), 311–312
Hopkins flexible fiber image transmission, 7
Hopkins rod lens telescope, 8
Human leukocyte antigen DR (HLA-DR), 72
Humoral immunity, 70–71
Hyperaldosteronism, 392
Hypercortisolism, 392

I
ICSAD. See Imperial College Surgical Assessment Device (ICSAD)
Illumination, Heinrich Lamm, 6–7

IMA. See Inferior mesenteric artery (IMA)
Image transmission, 7–8
Imperial College Surgical Assessment Device (ICSAD), 17
Inferior mesenteric artery (IMA)
    identification of, 224–225
    sigmoid branches, division, 225–226
Intra-operative ultrasound
    anatomical liver resections
        objectives, 281
        role, 275–276
        technique and major steps, 281–282
Intra-thoracic malignancies
    lung
        anatomic VATS lobectomy, left lung, 519–521
        anatomic VATS lobectomy, right lung, 515–519
        cancer, 523–524
        segmental resections, 522–523
        VATS lingular resection, 523
        VATS lingular sparing, 523
        wedge resection, 521–522
    mediastinum
        lymphatic tissue, 528
        pericardium, 526
        thymus, 526–527
    pleura, 525
Iodine, 332
^{131}Iodine, 332
IPMN. See Pancreatic intraductal papillary mucinous neoplasm (IPMN)
Ivor Lewis esophagectomy, 126

J
Japanese Society of Endoscopic Surgery (JSES), 163, 164

K
Kidney cancer
    chemotherapeutic strategies, 447
    laparoscopic transperitoneal partial nephrectomy
        nephron sparing surgery, 456
        open to laparoscopic partial nephrectomy, transition, 456
        surgical technique, 456–457
    laparoscopic transperitoneal radical nephrectomy
        operating room set up and patient positioning, 450
        overview of, 450
        surgical technique, 451–454
        trocar placement, 450–451
    laparoscopy for, 448–450
    partial nephrectomy, 448, 449
    retro-peritoneoscopic partial nephrectomy
        indications, 457
        technical differences, 457–458
    retro-peritoneoscopic radical nephrectomy
        hilar vessels, dissection and accessing, 455
        indications and limitations, 454
        operating room setup and patient positioning, 454–455
        trocar placement, 455
        working space creation, 455
    robotic-assisted laparoscopic partial nephrectomy
        advantages, 458
        DaVinci™ robot, 459

parenchyma reconstruction, 460
patient positioning and trocar placement, 458–459
robotic dissection, 459–460
specimen removal and wound closure, 460
surgery, 447–448

L
LADG. *See* Laparoscopy-assisted distal gastrectomy (LADG)
Laparoscopic adrenalectomy, 393
Laparoscopic-assisted total gastrectomy (LATG)
complications and technical difficulties
esophago-jejunostomy, reconstruction methods, 164–165
intra-and postoperative complications, 163, 165
evaluation, 165
gastro-splenic ligament
greater omentum, 161
indications, 159–160
irrigation, drainage, and wound closure, 163
Japanese Society of Endoscopic Surgery (JSES), 163, 164
surgical technique
Braun's anastomosis, 163
duodenum transection, 162–163
esophago-jejunostomy, 163
esophagus transection, 162
greater omentum, 161
hepatic artery dissection, 162
irrigation, drainage, and wound closure, 163
left gastric vessels division, 162
lesser omentum and right gastric vessels division, 161–162
mini-laparotomy, 163
patient positioning, 160
posterior gastric artery division, 162–163
right gastro-epiploic vessels, 161
Roux-en-Y reconstruction, 163
trocar placement, 160
Laparoscopic cholecystectomy (LC), 11. *See also* Surgical residency training
Laparoscopic common bile duct excision, 304–305
Laparoscopic distal pancreatectomy
fundamental categories, 365–366
multiple endocrine neoplasia (MEN), 367
patient selection, 366
preoperative tumor localization, 366
surgical technique, 367–371
Laparoscopic lymphadenectomy, cervical cancer, 417
Laparoscopic pancreaticoduodenectomy (LPD)
challenges, 380
historic review, 380
patient outcomes, 385–387
patient positioning and trocar placement, 381
patient selection, 380–381
perioperative care, 384–385
reconstruction, 383–384
resection, 381–383
robotic-assisted approach, 386
training, 387

Laparoscopic radical cholecystectomy
patient positioning and operating room setup, 303
postoperative detected gallbladder cancer, dissection for, 304
preoperative evaluation, 302
preoperative suspected gallbladder cancer, dissection for, 303–304
trocar placement, 303
Laparoscopic radical cystectomy
anterior peritoneal incision, 490
apical dissection, 490
extended pelvic lymph node dissection, 491
general considerations, 488
indications, 488
operating room setup, 489
patient positioning, 489
port placement, 489
posterior peritoneal incision, 489
preoperative patient preparation, 489
ureters, identification and transection, 489–490
vascular pedicles, securing, 490
worldwide results, 492–494
Laparoscopic radical hysterectomy, cervical cancer
adnexa, 410, 411
diagnostic laparoscopy, 408, 410
para-rectal space and uterine artery, 411
para-vesicle space, 411
recto-vaginal space, 408, 410
robotic equipment, 408, 409
trocar placement, 408, 410
ureter, dissection of, 412
uterus, transection of, 412
vaginal cuff closure, 412
vesico-vaginal space, 408, 410, 411
Laparoscopic radical prostatectomy
contraindications, 473
evolution of, 473
indications, 473
postoperative management, 478
preoperative considerations, 474
technical steps
bladder mobilization and Retzius space, 475
bladder neck reconstruction, 477
deep dorsal venous complex, dissection of, 475–476
leak test, 477–478
neurovascular bundle, dissection of, 476–477
patient positioning, 474
prostate dissection and excision, 477
specimen extraction and wound closure, 478
trocar placement, 474
urethrovesical anastomosis, 477
vasa deferentia and seminal vesicles, dissection of, 475
Laparoscopic rectal procedures
abdominoperineal resection
anal opening, closure of, 244
IMA, 245
IMV, 245
left colon, mobilization of, 245
left colon, proximal division, 245–246
operating field, exposure, 245

pelvic wound closure, 246
perineal dissection and specimen exteriorization, 246
positioning, patient and equipment, 244–245
rectum, mobilization of, 245
trocar placement positioning, 244–245
trocar sites and colostomy creation, 246
laparoscopic Hartman's procedure, 246
low anterior resection (LAR)
anastomosis, creation of, 243
IMA, 241
IMV, 241, 242
left colon and splenic flexure, mobilization, 242
operating field, exposure of, 241
pneumoperitoneum desufflation and trocar sites closure, 244
positioning, patient and equipment, 239–240
rectum, mobilization and division, 242, 243
surgical specimen, exteriorization of, 243
trocar placement, 240
minimally invasive palliative surgery, 246–247
preoperative staging and workup, 235–236
preoperative treatment, 236
surgical approach
laparoscopic loop ileostomy, 238
laparoscopic rectal resections, 239
laparoscopic surgery, rectal cancer, 238
preoperative planning and strategy, 238
surgical option
LAR vs. APR, 237
locally advanced tumors, surgery, 237
minimally invasive approaches, 237–238
resection margins, 237
transanal excision and transanal endoscopic microsurgery, 236
transanal intersphincteric mobilization, 244
Laparoscopic Roux-en-Y choledocho-jejunostomy, 304–305
Laparoscopic splenectomy (LS)
anterior and lateral approach, 319–320
complications
diaphragm perforation, 323
hemorrhage, 322–323
miscellaneous, 323
pancreatic tail injury, 323
essential equipment, 318
HALS, 320–322, 325–326
indications, 317
patient positioning, 319
preoperative workup and considerations, 318
Laparoscopic trachelectomy, cervical cancer, 422–423
Laparoscopic transperitoneal partial nephrectomy
nephron sparing surgery, 456
open to laparoscopic partial nephrectomy, transition, 456
surgical technique, 456–457
Laparoscopic transperitoneal radical nephrectomy
operating room set up and patient positioning, 450
overview of, 450
surgical technique
colon mobilization, 451
gonadal vein dissection, 451–452
hilum and renal vessels, dissection of, 452–453
kidney and adrenal gland mobilization, 453

renal vein tumor thrombi, 453
specimen extraction and wound closure, 454
ureter division, 453–454
trocar placement, 450–451
Laparoscopic urinary diversion
general considerations, 491–492
types, 491
Laparoscopy
elderly
adjuvant therapy, 103
epidemiology, aging and cancer, 97–98
minimally invasive management, 100–101
pathophysiological changes, 98–100
surgical approach, 101–103
esophageal cancer, 126
and immunology
anesthesia, 77
angiogenesis-related plasma protein changes, 78–79
cellular immunity, 71–76
CO_2 pneumoperitoneum, 77–78
humoral immunity, 70–71
peritoneal immunity, 76–77
surgery and tumor resistance, 78
and malignancy
cancer–carcinomatosis, 60
cancer–curative intent, 59–60
cancer–palliation, 60
colorectal cancer, 63
gastric cancer, 62–63
immune system influence, 60–61
liver tumors, 63
pneumoperitoneum, 60
port-site metastasis, 61–62
staging, 63–64
moral and ethical issues
Gartner's hype cycle of innovation, 40–41
intracellular surgery, 43
micro-robots, 43
OSATS, 40
robotic surgery, 41–42
surgeon and patient, dissociation of, 39
suspended animation, 44
tissue engineering and regeneration, 43–44
small bowel tumors (see Small bowel tumors)
theories, 61
Laparoscopy-assisted distal gastrectomy (LADG)
complications and technical difficulties, 163–165
diagnostic laparoscopy, step I, 151
dissection and division procedure, step II, 151–153
duodenum, division of, 152–153
gastro-jejunal anastomosis, step IV, 154–155
indications, 149
left gastric artery, step III, 154
lymph node dissection and Japanese classification, 149–150
results and complications, 155
sentinel lymph node mapping, 150
surgical technique
instruments, 150–151
patient positioning, 150
trocar placement, 151

LAR. *See* Low anterior resection (LAR)
Lateral transabdominal adrenalectomy (LTA)
    advantages and disadvantages, 394
    left side
        adrenal gland dissection, 397–398
        operating room setup and patient positioning, 396, 397
        trocar placement, 396–397
    right side
        adrenal gland dissection, 399–400
        patient positioning and trocar placement, 398–399
LATG. *See* Laparoscopic-assisted total gastrectomy (LATG)
Left hemicolectomy and sigmoid colon
    complications and pitfalls
        abdominal organs, puncture injuries of, 231
        bleeding from abdominal wall, 230
        port site metastasis, 230–231
        trocar site hernias, 230
        ureteral injuries, 231
    operative technique
        anastomosis, creation of, 229–230
        colon, proximal division of, 228
        instruments and equipment, 221
        operative field, exposure of, 223–224
        patient positioning, 221
        preoperative considerations, 221
        proximal mesorectum, dissection of, 228
        rectum, distal division of, 228
        sigmoid and descending colon, 226–227
        splenic flexure, mobilization, 228–229
        surgical specimen, extraction of, 229
        team positioning, 221, 222
        trocars, placement of, 222, 223
        vascular approach, 224–226
        wound closure, 230
    SAGES and ASCRS, 219–220
    surgical approach, 219, 221
Ligasure®, 282
Light transmission principles, 6
Liver, nonanatomical resection
    complications, 265
    HALS, 269
    laparoscopic hepatectomies, 264
    liver malignancies, 263–264
    minimal invasive approach, 264
    surgical technique
        diagnostic laparoscopy and dissection line, 265, 267
        dissection, operative steps, 267–268
        operating room setup and patient positioning, 265, 266
        specimen, 269
        trocar placement, 265, 266
Liver tumors
    cryoablation, 29
    laparoscopy, 63
Lobectomy *vs.* total thyroidectomy, 336
Low anterior resection (LAR)
    anastomosis, creation of, 243
    IMA, 241
    IMV, 241, 242
    left colon and splenic flexure, mobilization, 242
    operating field, exposure of, 241
    pneumoperitoneum desufflation and trocar sites closure, 244
    positioning, patient and equipment, 239–240
    rectum, mobilization and division, 242, 243
    surgical specimen, exteriorization of, 243
    transanal intersphincteric mobilization, 244
    trocar placement, 240
LPD. *See* Laparoscopic pancreaticoduodenectomy (LPD)
LS. *See* Laparoscopic splenectomy (LS)
Lung cancer
    aging patient, 100
    radiofrequency ablation (RFA), 523–524
    robotic resection of, 54
    stereotactic radiosurgery, 524
Lung tumors, pediatric
    biopsy and metastasectomy, 507–508
    osteosarcoma, pulmonary metastasectomy, 508
    sub-centimeter pulmonary lesion, 508
    thoracoscopic biopsy, 508–509
Lymphadenectomy, cervical cancer
    para-aortic lymph node dissection, 413–414
    pelvic lymphadenectomy, 413
    retroperitoneal, 414–415
    trocar placement, 413
Lymphatic tissue, 528
Lymph node dissection and Japanese classification, 149–150
Lymphocytes, 74

M
Malignancy
    laparoscopy
        cancer–carcinomatosis, 60
        cancer–curative intent, 59–60
        cancer–palliation, 60
        colorectal cancer, 63
        gastric cancer, 62–63
        immune system influence, 60–61
        liver tumors, 63
        pneumoperitoneum, 60
        port-site metastasis, 61–62
        staging, 63–64
    pneumoperitoneum (*see* Pneumoperitoneum)
Malignant cells
    insufflation gas effect, 88–89
    in vitro studies, 86–87
    in vivo studies, 87–88
Malignant small bowel tumors, 184–186
Maryland virtual patient (MVP), 19–20
MCT. *See* Microwave coagulation therapy (MCT)
Mechanical/box trainers
    limitations, 16
    mechanical model, 14
    MISTELS, 15
    reliability and validation, 15
    simulation training, 14–15
    vs. virtual reality, 17
Mediastinal tumors
    pediatric
        biopsy and resection technique, 510
        neuroblastoma, 509

robotic applications, 54
robotic thymectomy and resection, 54
Mediastinum, intra-thoracic malignancies
   lymphatic tissue, 528
   pericardium, 526
   thymus, 526–527
Medullary thyroid cancer (MTC), 333
Metastatic tumors, 187
Micro-robots, laparoscopy, 43
Microwave coagulation therapy (MCT), 264
Minimally invasive open thyroidectomy (MIT)
   definition, 341
   Mount Sinai approach
      instrumentation, 342
      operative steps, 343
      patient positioning, 342
      postoperative management, 343
      regional anesthesia, 342
   patient selection, 342
   risks and benefits, 341
Minimally invasive surgery (MIS)
   Cuschieri's view, 23
   device technology and research
      HALS, 27–28
      tissue ablation, 28–29
   ergonomic and operating theatres technology, 34–35
   haptics, 33–34
   imaging technology and research
      head-mounted display, 32
      image-guided surgery, 30–31
      image transmission, 29–30
      light sources, 29
      magnifying endoscopy, 31–32
   instrument technology and research
      haemostasis, 25–26
      instrument development, 24–25
      NOTES and instrument development, 26–27
      problems, 24
      tissue approximation and anastomosis, 25
   robotics, 32–33
   surgery without external scars, 35
   telemedicine, 34
MISTELS, 15
MIT. See Minimally invasive open thyroidectomy (MIT)
Monocyte function
   clinical research and animal research, 73
   HLA-DR, 72
Morbid obesity, 207
Multiple endocrine neoplasia (MEN), 367
MVP. See Maryland virtual patient (MVP)
Myelofibrosis, 313, 315

N
Natural killer cell activity
   animal research, 73–74
   clinical research, 74
   mechanism of action, 73
Natural Orifice Surgery Consortium for Assessment and Research (NOSCAR), 108–109
Natural orifice transluminal endoscopic surgery (NOTES)
   animal models and human applications, 109–112
   ethical issues, 42
   gastro-jejunostomy, 115–116
   intestinal resection, 118
   lymph node biopsy, 115
   and oncology, 109, 112
   optimal access, 118–119
   peritoneoscopy, 112–114
   routine endoscopic procedures, 109–110
   solid organ resection, 117–118
   surgical procedures, 108
   thoracoscopy and mediastinoscopy, 114–115
Nephrectomy, 117
Neuroblastoma, pediatric
   biopsy, 504
   resection, 504–505
   surgical technique, 505
Non-Hodgkin's lymphoma (NHL), 185–186, 312, 314
NOSCAR. See Natural Orifice Surgery Consortium for Assessment and Research (NOSCAR)
NOTES. See Natural orifice transluminal endoscopic surgery (NOTES)

O
Objective structured assessment of technical skills (OSATS), 15, 40
Oophorectomy, 117
Open radical prostatectomy
   choice of approach, 472–473
   history, 472
   outcomes, 473
Open tube, Kussmaul, 4
OSATS. See Objective structured assessment of technical skills (OSATS)
Ovarian carcinomas
   advanced stage invasive
      clinical risk factors, 435
      cytoreductive surgery, 436–437
      resectability determination, 435
      second-look laparoscopy, 436
   borderline ovarian tumors, 432
   early stage invasive, 432–434
   management algorithm, 438
   management pitfalls
      cyst rupture, 437
      inadequate staging, 437
      port-site metastases, 437–438
   surgical staging, 431
   surgical technique, 431–432
   tumor, pediatric
      laparoscopic access, 506–507
      management of, 506

P
PACE. See Preoperative assessment of cancer in the elderly (PACE)
Pancreatic cancer
   complications and recovery, 374, 376
   interventional laparoscopy
      central pancreatectomy, 368
      enucleation, 369, 372–373

laparoscopic distal pancreatectomy, 365–371
  splenic preservation, 370
laparoscopic resection
  neuroendocrine lesions, 371, 374
  pancreatic cystic lesions, 374
laparoscopic staging of
  accuracy, 364
  context-dependent approach, 363
  criticisms, 365
  disease deemed resectable, 364
  efficacy, 364–365
  historical perspective, 363
  patient selection, 365
  unresectable disease, 364
patient study, 374, 375
whipple procedure
  adjuvant/neoadjuvant therapy, 379
  evolution of, 380
  IPMN, 380
  minimally invasive approach, 380–381
  patient outcomes, 385–387
  robotic whipple, 386
  surgical technique, 381–385
  training, 387
  vascular resection, 379
Pancreatic cystic lesions, 374
Pancreatic intraductal papillary mucinous neoplasm (IPMN), 380
Pancreaticojejunostomy, 383–384
Pancreatic tail injury, 323
Papillary thyroid cancer, 335–337
Para-aortic lymph node dissection, 413–414
Parathyroid adenoma1 (PRAD1), 356
Parathyroid cancer
  clinical features and laboratory findings, 356
  diagnostic modalities, 357
  etiology and risk factors, 355
  histology, 356–357
  hypercalcemia, 360
  incidence of, 355
  molecular pathogenesis, 356
  nonfunctioning carcinoma, 360
  outcome and prognosis, 361
  surgical treatment
    en bloc resection, 359
    intraoperative findings, 358
    operative strategy, 358–359
    postoperative surveillance, 359
    recurrent and metastatic parathyroid cancer, 359
    role of, 358
  systemic therapy, 360
  TNM staging, 357–358
Parenchyma dissection, liver resections
  CUSA® system, 282
  EnSeal®, 283
  Harmonic Scalpel® and Sonosurg®, 282
  Ligasure®, 282
  parameters, 282
  personal technique, 283
  stapling devices, 283
  TissueLink™, 283

Partial hysterectomy, 117
PECAM1, 75
Pediatric malignancies
  Cyberknife, 510
  intra-abdominal malignancies
    hepatoblastoma, 505
    neuroblastoma, 504–505
    ovarian mass, 506–507
    sacro-coccygeal teratoma, 506
    Wilms' tumor, 503–504
  minimally invasive surgery (MIS)
    abdominal and pelvic tumors, 502–503
    benefits, in oncology, 502
    overview, 501–502
  thoracic malignancies
    lung tumors, 507–509
    mediastinal tumors, 509–510
    video-assisted thoracoscopy for, 507
Pelvic lymphadenectomy, 413
Pelvic tumors, pediatric, 502–503
Pericardium, 526
Peritoneal immunity, 76–77
Peritoneal mucinous carcinomatosis (PMCA), 202
Physiologic changes, whole patient
Pleura, 525
Pleurodesis, 525
Pneumoperitoneum, 60
  insufflation gas effect, 88–89
  malignant cells
    in vitro studies, 86–87
    in vivo studies, 87–88
  physiologic changes, whole patient
    cardiac effects, 85–86
    central nervous system, 85
    deep venous thrombosis, 84
    hypercoagulability, 84
    pulmonary effects, 86
    pulmonary embolism, 84
    systemic immunity, 84–85
    visceral effects, 86
  port-site recurrence
    clinical studies, 91–92
    laboratory studies, 90–91
    prevention, 92–93
  tumor cells, 89–90
Porcelain gallbladder, 298
Portal vein thrombosis, 326
PORTLAND approach
  esophagectomy, stage II
    mobilization, curvature, 140–141
    patient positioning and trocar placement, 140
  staging laparoscopy, stage I
    laparoscopic feeding jejunostomy, 140
    left gastric artery, lymphadenectomy and division, 139–140
    patient positioning and trocar placement, 139
Port-site recurrence
  clinical studies, 91–92
  laboratory studies
    abdominal wall trauma, 90
    aerosolization, tumor cells, 90

Index

immunosuppression theory, 91
port composition, 91
port placement, 91
wound closure type, 90–91
prevention, 92–93
Preoperative assessment of cancer in the elderly (PACE), 101–102
Prostate cancer
brachytherapy, 468
cryoablation
complications, 470
history and development, 469–470
method of action, 470
outcomes, 470–471
external beam radiotherapy (EBRT)
complications, 467
contraindications, 467–468
cytotoxicity, 466
planning strategies, 466
success and failure, 466–467
high-intensity focused ultrasound (HIFU), 471–472
laparoscopic radical prostatectomy
contraindications, 473
evolution of, 473
indications, 473
postoperative management, 478
preoperative considerations, 474
technical steps, 474–478
nonsurgical management, 465–466
open radical prostatectomy
choice of approach, 472–473
history, 472
outcomes, 473
patient outcomes
biochemical progression, 481
complication rates, 480
laparoscopic vs. robotic and open procedures, 479–480
procedure-associated morbidity, 480
sexual function, 481
urinary continence, 481
robotic radical prostatectomy, 478
stereotactic hypo-fractionated radiosurgery, 468–469
Proteomics and structural genomics, 49
Pseudomyxoma peritonei (PMP), 202

R
Radiation therapy
gallbladder cancer, 300
parathyroid cancer, 360
urinary bladder cancer, 487
Radical nephrectomy, pediatric, 504
Radical vaginal hysterectomy
Schauta–Amreich, 415–416
Schauta–Stoeckel, 416
Radioactive iodine (RAI), 331
Radiofrequency ablation (RFA), 28, 264
hepatocellular carcinoma, 275
liver malignancies, 264
lung cancer, 523–524
tissue ablation, 28
REA. See Retroperitoneal adrenalectomy (REA)

Retinoid therapy, 338
Retrogastric dissection, esophageal cancer, 129–132
Retroperitoneal adrenalectomy (REA)
advantages and disadvantages, 394–395
surgical technique, 401
Retroperitoneal lymphadenectomy, 414–415
Retro-peritoneoscopic partial nephrectomy, 457–458
Retro-peritoneoscopic radical nephrectomy
hilar vessels, dissection and accessing, 455
indications and limitations, 454
operating room setup and patient positioning, 454–455
trocar placement, 455
working space creation, 455
Reverse transcription polymerase chain reaction (RT-PCR), 335
RFA. See Radiofrequency ablation (RFA)
Right hemicolectomy and appendix
appendiceal malignancies
carcinoid tumors, 203–204
histological subtypes, 200–201
laparoscopy role, 202–203
mucinous neoplasm, 201–202
non mucinous tumor, 201
peritoneal carcinomatosis therapy, 202–203
colorectal cancer, factors associated with
after cholecystectomy, 199–200
hyperplastic polyps, 200
serrated adenoma, 200
complications, 213, 214
eliminating skin incisions/surgery with no scars, 214
laparoscopic right hemicolectomy
patient positioning and operating room setup, 209
pre-operative and intra-operative, tumor localization, 208
preoperative preparation, 208
surgical steps, 208, 210–213
trocar placement, 209–210
mini laparoscopy, 214
postoperative care, 213
right colon cancer treatment
non surgical therapies, 205
surgical treatement, 205–208
single-port endoscopic surgery, 214
Robot-assisted laparoscopic cystectomy, 494–495
Robotic applications
artificial intelligence, 48
cancer cells, automated identification of, 48–49
da Vinci oncological trends, 52
dynamic active constraints and haptics, 50
general surgery, 55
genetic abnormalities, 48
gynecological surgery, 53
MIS, 32–33
oncologic predictive algorithms, 47–48
overlay, arterial targets, 51
proteomics and structural genomics, 49
registration difficulties, 50
robotic brachytherapy, 52
robotic stereotactic radio-surgery, 51–52
robotic surgery, 41–42

skull base surgery and ENT, 53–54
thoracic surgery, 54
tumor localization, 49–50
tumor tracking and motion compensation, 51
urology
    renal cancer, robotic resection of, 53
    robotic prostatectomy, 52–53
Robotic-assisted laparoscopic partial nephrectomy
    advantages, 458
    DaVinci™ robot, 459
    parenchyma reconstruction, 460
    patient positioning and trocar placement, 458–459
    robotic dissection, 459–460
    specimen removal and wound closure, 460
Robotic esophageal resection, 54
Robotic gastric surgery, 54–55
Robotic large bowel procedures, 55
Robotic radical hysterectomy, 416–417
Robotic radical prostatectomy, 478
Robotic resection
    esophageal resection, 54
    lung cancer, 54
    mediastinal tumors, 54
    renal cancer, 53
    solid organ lesions, 55
Robotic thymectomy, 54
Robotic whipple, 386

S
Sacro-coccygeal teratoma (SCT), 506
Salpingectomy, 117
Sentinel lymph node mapping, 150
Sentinel lymph node sampling, 417–421
Single port access (SPA), 42
Skull base surgery, robotic applications, 53–54
Small bowel tumors
    benign small bowel tumors
        hamartoma, 187–188
        hemangioma, 188
        leiomyoma, 187
        lipoma, 188
        small bowel adenoma, 187
    diagnostic work-up, endoscopic evaluation
        balloon-assisted endoscopy, 189
        capsule endoscopy, 188–189
        intraoperative enteroscopy, 189
        push enteroscopy and overtubes, 188
    epidemiology, 183–184
    malignant small bowel tumors
        adenocarcinoma, 184–185
        carcinoid tumor, 185
        GIST, 186
        metastatic tumors, 187
        non-Hodgkin's lymphoma (NHL), 185–186
    postoperative management and outcome, 194
    preoperative management
        anastomosis, creation of, 192–193
        contraindications, 190
        diagnostic laparoscopy, 192
        dissection and transection, 192
        hand-assisted approach, 193
        indications, 189–190
        patient positioning, 191
        preoperative considerations, 190–191
        preoperative localization, 190
        specimen and wound closure, 194
        trocar placement, 191
        tumor size, relevance of, 190
Solid organ lesions, robotic resection of, 55
Sonosurg®, 282
Spleen, hematological disorders
    Barcelona data
        CLL, 315
        CML, 316
        diagnostic laparoscopy, 316–317
        Hodgkin's disease, 315
        myelofibrosis, 315
        NHL, 314
        perioperative outcome after LS, 315
        primary and secondary splenic lymphoma, 314
        secondary tumors, 316, 317
        Waldenstrom's macroglobulinemia, 316
    classification and current nonsurgical therapies
        chronic myeloid leukemia, 313
        Hodgkin's lymphoma, 311–312
        myelofibrosis, 313
        non-Hodgkin's lymphoma, 312
    laparoscopic splenectomy, 311
    laparoscopic splenectomy, complications
        diaphragm perforation, 323
        hemorrhage, 322–323
        pancreatic tail injury, 323
    massive splenomegaly, 324
    MIS, 311
    portal vein thrombosis, 326
    preoperative splenic embolization, role of, 325
    primary tumors, 313
    secondary tumors, 313–314
    splenectomy
        HALS and, 325–326
        malignancy and, 325
    splenic vessels, 325
    splenomegaly, 323–324
    surgical technique
        anterior approach, 319
        essential equipment, 318
        general considerations, 318–319
        hand-assisted laparoscopic splenectomy, 320–322
        laparoscopy staging, 322
        lateral approach, 319–320
        lymph node biopsy, 322
        patient positioning, 319
        preoperative imaging, 318
        preoperative workup and special considerations, 318
        SAE, 318
        specimen extraction, 320
        splenectomy, 317
Splenectomy, 117
Splenic artery embolization (SAE), 318
Splenomegaly
    massive, 324
    spleen weight, 323–324

Stereotactic radiosurgery
    lung cancer, 524
    prostate cancer, 468–469
Surgical residency training
    cognitive skills, 19–20
    cost considerations, 18–19
    fellowship council, 12–13
    laparoscopic training, 12, 20
    objective metrics, 17
    proctoring and preceptoring, 12
    resident education guidelines, 13
    simulation training
        box trainers, limitations of, 16
        broad categories, 13–14
        GOALS, 17–18
        mechanical/box trainers, 14–16
        MISTELS, 15
        reliability and validation, 14
        virtual reality, limitations and challenge, 16–17
    transfer of training, 18
    value and relevance, 19
    work-hour restrictions, 18

T

T-cell function
    animal research, 72
    clinical research, 72
    delayed type hypersensitivity (DTH), 71–72
    significance, 72
Telescope, pioneers of
    Fritz Lange and C.A. Meltzing, 5
    Galileo Galilei, 4
    Johann Mikulicz, 4–5
    Maximilian Frederick Nitze, 4–5
    Theodor Rosenheim and Rudolf Schindler, 5
Telesurgery technology
    MIS, 34
Television bronchoscopy, 9
Television image, 8–10
T-helper 1 and T-helper 2, 75
Thoracic dissection, esophageal cancer
    diaphragm, retraction of, 132
    dissection
        azygos vein, 133
        conduit and completion, 133
    lateral dissection and thoracic duct, 133
    operating room set-up and trocar placement, 132
    subcarinal node package, 132–133
Thoracic surgery, robotic applications, 54
Thymus, 526–527
Thyroglobulin (Tg), 333
Thyroid cancer
    differentiated, management of
        anaplastic thyroid cancer, 338
        follicular thyroid cancer, 337–338
        papillary thyroid cancer, 335–337
    minimally invasive approaches
        adjunctive techniques and equipment, 340–341
        endoscopic thyroid surgery, 343–348
        general considerations, 338–339
        minimally invasive open technique, 341–343

        patient selection, 339–340
        risks and benefits, 339
        video-assisted lateral neck dissection, 348
    palpable thyroid mass
        definition, risk factors and clinical presentation, 334
        fine needle aspiration, 335
        hot and cold nodules, 334
        molecular testing, 335
        ultrasound evaluation, 334
    pathology
        anaplastic thyroid cancer, 334
        differentiated thyroid cancers, 333
        medullary thyroid cancer, 333
    physiology
        calcitonin, 333
        iodine and ^{131}iodine, roles, 332
        para-follicular C cells, 332
        thyroglobulin, 333
        thyroid hormones – T3/T4, 332
        thyroid stimulating hormone, 332
    radioactive iodine, 331
    recurrence rate, 331
Thyroid stimulating hormone (TSH), 332
Thyroxine (T4), 332
Tissue ablation
    cryoablation, 28–29
    HIFU, 28
    microwave ablation, 28–29
    RFA, 28
Tissue engineering and regeneration, 43–44
TissueLink™ device, 283
Total laparoscopic radical hysterectomy, 416
Transhiatal approach
    Barret's dysplasia, 144
    endoluminal treatment, 144
    esophageal cancer, surgical management
        esophagectomy, stage II, 140–141
        staging laparoscopy, stage I, 139–140
    esophageal resection, 137–138
    fundoplication, 142, 143
    gastric conduit
        creation, 141–142
        pull up, 142
    history, 137–138
    minimal invasive esophagectomy, 137
    staging laparoscopy, 143–144
    traditional open surgical approaches, 143
Transhiatal esophagectomy, 125
Transluminal surgery
    minimally invasive techniques, 107
    NOSCAR, 108–109
    NOTES
        animal models and human applications, 109–112
        gastro-jejunostomy, 115–116
        intestinal resection, 118
        lymph node biopsy, 115
        and oncology, 109, 112
        optimal access, 118–119
        peritoneoscopy, 112–114
        solid organ resection, 116–118

surgical procedures, 108
  thoracoscopy and mediastinoscopy, 114–115
Transurethral resection of bladder (TUR-B), 487–488
Triiodothyronine (T3), 332
Tumor resistance, 78–79
Two-cavity approach. *See* Esophagus and gastroesophageal junction

U

Ultrasound
  endoscopic, EGC resection, 168
  esophageal cancer, 128
  in liver surgery, 275–276
  palpable thyroid mass, 334
  parathyroid cancer, 357
  prostate cancer, 471–472
  tissue ablation, 28
Urinary bladder cancer
  laparoscopic radical cystectomy
    anterior peritoneal incision, 490
    apical dissection, 490
    extended pelvic lymph node dissection, 491
    general considerations, 488
    indications, 488
    operating room setup, 489
    patient positioning, 489
    port placement, 489
    posterior peritoneal incision, 489
    preoperative patient preparation, 489
    ureters, identification and transection, 489–490
    vascular pedicles, securing, 490
    worldwide results, 492–494
  laparoscopic urinary diversion
    general considerations, 491–492
    types, 491
  lap-assisted ileal conduit urinary diversion, 492
  multimodality treatment, 488
  radiation therapy, 487
  robot-assisted laparoscopic cystectomy, 494–495
  transurethral resection of bladder (TUR-B), 487–488
Urology, robotic applications
  renal cancer, robotic resection of, 53
  robotic prostatectomy, 52–53

V

Vascular approach, 224–226
Venography, 357
Video-assisted lateral neck dissection, 348
Video-assisted thoracic surgery (VATS) lobectomy
  left lung
    left lower lobectomy (LLL), 520–521
    left upper lobectomy (LUL), 519–520
  lingular resection, 523
  lingular sparing, LUL, 523
  right lung
    right lower lobectomy (RLL), 519
    right middle lobectomy (RML), 518
    right upper lobectomy (RUL), 515–518
Video-assisted thoracic surgery (VATS) thymectomy, 527
Video-assisted thoracoscopy, 507
Video-assisted thyroidectomy, 347–348
Virtual reality (VR)
  vs. box /mechanical trainers, 17
  limitations and challenges, 16–17
  simulators, 13–14, 16

W

Waldenstrom's macroglobulinemia, 316
Wilms' tumor, 503–504